Occupational Therapy Interventions

Function and Occupations

Occupational Therapy Interventions
Function and Occupations

Catherine Meriano, JD, MHS, OTR/L
Quinnipiac University
Hamden, Connecticut

Donna Latella, EdD, OTR/L
Quinnipiac University
Hamden, Connecticut

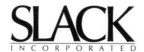

Delivering the best in health care information and education worldwide

ISBN: 978-1-55642-732-9

Occupational Therapy Interventions: Function and Occupations Instructional Material for the Educator is also available from SLACK Incorporated. Don't miss this important companion to *Occupational Therapy Interventions: Function and Occupations*. To obtain the *Instructor's Manual*, please visit: http://www.efacultylounge.com

SLACK Incorporated uses a review process to evaluate submitted material. Prior to publication, educators or clinicians provide important feedback on the content that we publish. We welcome feedback on this work.

Published by: SLACK Incorporated
                 6900 Grove Road
                 Thorofare, NJ 08086 USA
                 Telephone: 856-848-1000
                 Fax: 856-853-5991
                 www.slackbooks.com

Contact SLACK Incorporated for more information about other books in this field or about the availability of our books from distributors outside the United States.

Library of Congress Cataloging-in-Publication Data

Occupational therapy interventions : function and occupations / [edited by] Catherine Meriano, Donna Latella.
      p. ; cm.
   Includes bibliographical references and index.
   ISBN 978-1-55642-732-9 (pbk. : alk. paper) 1. Occupational therapy. I. Meriano, Catherine. II. Latella, Donna.
   [DNLM: 1. Occupational Therapy--methods. 2. Occupational Therapy--psychology. WB 555 O1481 2007]

RM735.O353 2007
615.8'515--dc22
                             2007029137

For permission to reprint material in another publication, contact SLACK Incorporated. Authorization to photocopy items for internal, personal, or academic use is granted by SLACK Incorporated provided that the appropriate fee is paid directly to Copyright Clearance Center. Prior to photocopying items, please contact the Copyright Clearance Center at 222 Rosewood Drive, Danvers, MA 01923 USA; phone: 978-750-8400; website: www.copyright.com; email: info@copyright.com.

Printed in the United States of America.

Last digit is print number: 10 9   8   7   6   5   4   3

DEDICATION

We wish to dedicate this text to our families: John, Kathleen, and Jay Meriano and Domenic, Kristy, and Dylan Latella. Your support and patience through the writing of this text was greatly appreciated. This is also dedicated to the talented faculty and students of the Occupational Therapy Department of Quinnipiac University, as well as all of our former clients and their families, who have assisted in teaching *us* about the intervention process.

CONTENTS

Occupational Therapy Interventions: Function and Occupations Instructional Material for the Educator is also available from SLACK Incorporated. Don't miss this important companion to *Occupational Therapy Interventions: Function and Occupations*. To obtain the *Instructor's Manual*, please visit: http://www.efacultylounge.com

ACKNOWLEDGMENTS

We would like to thank Kimberly Hartmann, PhD, OTR/L, FAOTA, Chair of Occupational Therapy at Quinnipiac University, and Roseanna Tufano, MFT, LFT, OTR/L, Assistant Professor of Occupational Therapy at Quinnipiac University, for their extensive support throughout this project. Their guidance and suggestions provided valuable input.

ABOUT THE AUTHORS

Donna Latella, EdD, OTR/L is a tenured Associated Professor of Occupational Therapy and Director of Academic Integrity at Quinnipiac University, Hamden, Connecticut. Her clinical background is in acute care, outpatient rehabilitation, and nursing home practice. Presently, Donna's clinical practice is at High Hopes Therapeutic Riding, Inc., as a Registered Therapist in Hippotherapy and a Certified Therapeutic Riding Instructor. Her teaching responsibilities include Adult Interventions, Health Conditions, Problem-Based Learning, Fieldwork I, Splinting, Capstone Graduate Project, and Service Learning. Donna volunteers with her certified therapy dog, Griffin, providing animal-assisted therapy in reading programs, hospitals, and day centers. Her publications and presentations have covered topics such as evaluation of the upper extremity, dysphagia, leadership, service learning, animal-assisted therapy, educational malpractice, and learning styles. Donna enjoys jogging, horseback riding, and boating with her husband, two children, and many pets.

Catherine Meriano, JD, MHS, OTR/L is a tenured Professor of Occupational Therapy at Quinnipiac University, Hamden, Connecticut. Her clinical background is in acute care, outpatient rehabilitation, and nursing home practice. Catherine is the President of the Board of Directors for the Center for Academic Integrity, and a recent member of the Roster of Accreditation Evaluators for the American Occupational Therapy Association. Her teaching responsibilities include Evaluation Process, Problem-Based Learning, Development of the Older Adult, Legal Issues in Occupational Therapy, and Neurology Screens. Her publications and presentations have included topics such as evaluation of the upper extremity, dysphagia, academic integrity, and legal issues in health care. Catherine enjoys spending time in the clinic, traveling with her family, and spending time with her husband and two children.

CONTRIBUTING AUTHORS

Amy P. Burns, MOT, OTR/L
Staff Therapist/Manager in Training
Lord Chamberlain Nursing and Rehabilitation
  Center
Stratford, Connecticut

Marilyn B. Cole, MS, OTR/L, FAOTA
Professor Emeritus
Quinnipiac University
Hamden, Connecticut

Jennifer Ruisi Cosgrove, EdD, OTR/L
Independent Consultant
North Kingstown, Rhode Island

Amy Darragh, PhD, OTR/L
Assistant Professor
Department of Occupational Therapy
College of Health Sciences
University of Wisconsin—Milwaukee
Milwaukee, Wisconsin

Robert DeMatteo, OTR/L
Behavioral Health Program
Saint Mary's Hosptial
Waterbury, Connecticut

Margo Ruth Gross, EdD, LMFT, LMT, OTR/L
Assistant Professor
Sacred Heart University
Fairfield, Connecticut

Kimbery Hartmann, PhD, OTR/L, FAOTA
Chairperson, Occupational Therapy
Quinnipiac University
Hamden, Connecticut

Cristina Klippel-Tancreti, MBA, OTR/L
Occupational Therapist
Department of Outpatient Rehabilitation Services
Connecticut Mental Health Center
New Haven, Connecticut
Occupational Therapist
Athena Healthcare Systems
Southington, Connecticut

Kim Mikenis, MPH, OTR/L
Occupational Therapist II
Connecticut Mental Health Center
Department of Mental Health and Addiction
  Services
New Haven, Connecticut

Deanna Proulx-Sepelak, MHA, OTR/L
Assistant Dean, School of Health Sciences (EC-ALD)
Quinnipiac University
Hamden, Connecticut

Martha J. Sanders, MA, MSOSH, OTR/L, CAPS
Assistant Professor of Occupational Therapy
Quinnipiac University
Hamden, Connecticut

David M. Santoro, MBA, OTR/L
Administrator
Southington Care Center
Southington, Connecticut

Mary Ellen Santucci, OTR/L
Level III Occupational Therapist
Hospital of Saint Raphael
New Haven, Connecticut

Rebecca L. Simon, MS, OTR/L
Faculty, Occupational Therapy Assistant Program
New England Institute of Technology
Warwick, Rhode Island

Karen Sladyk, PhD, OTR, FAOTA
Bay Path College
Longmeadow, Massachusetts

Sylvia Valerio Sobocinski, MA, OTR/L
Department of Outpatient Rehabilitation Services
Connecticut Mental Health Center
New Haven, Connecticut

Robert Wright, OTR/L
Wright2Work
Colchester, Connecticut

PREFACE

In 2002, the American Occupational Therapy Association created the *Occupational Therapy Practice Framework (Framework)* that replaced the medical terminology used by many clinicians. This new document re-emphasized the role of occupational therapists working with clients to improve or maintain skills in functional activities, both in institutional settings and community settings. This practice framework was designed to clearly delineate the evaluation and intervention processes, as well describe all of the factors that impact functional activities. While the main focus is these functional tasks, or areas of occupation, the foundational skills required for these tasks have also been addressed. These foundational skills include motor skills and processing skills. In addition, the client's patterns of activity have also been addressed.

This text has been created to blend the *Framework* with the entry-level clinical skills in use today for the intervention of adults with physical disabilities. In addition, this text will assist more experienced clinicians to integrate the *Framework* terminology and its purpose into practice. There are several interventions which are discussed only briefly as these are not typically entry-level skills. These are interventions that require advanced training, such as advanced dysphagia techniques, aquatics, the use of physical agent modalities, driver training, etc. Resources for additional education can be found in the Appendix at the end of the text.

As students emerge from universities well-versed in the *Framework* document, they will need tools which discuss intervention using the most current terminology. As well, experienced clinicians also require these same tools to remain current and grow with the field of occupational therapy.

INTRODUCTION

This text will begin with a thorough review of the *Occupational Therapy Practice Framework: Domain and Process (Framework)* (AOTA, 2002). Following this, Chapter 2 will discuss the foundational skills required for all areas of occupation. While the *Framework* document is a very thorough document, it does not include every aspect of clinical intervention. When an area requires further definition, such as in perceptual skills, other references will be utilized to supplement the *Framework* document. The Foundational Skills chapter is primarily discussing remediation techniques for these skills. Once the foundational skills have been reviewed, each area of occupation—activities of daily living (ADL), instrumental activities of daily living (IADL), work, retirement/volunteer, education, leisure, and social participation—will be discussed. While information regarding evaluation is contained within these chapters, with a sampling of evaluation provided in Appendix B,, the primary focus of the text is intervention. Remediation, adaptation/compensation, and maintenance are addressed in the chapters. Because much remediation focuses on practicing a task, the emphasis in these chapters is on adaptation/compensation. Wellness will be addressed in Chapter 9 regarding education to address both disability prevention and health promotion.

Throughout these chapters, information more specific to the topic will be provided regarding frames of references, pathologies, psychosocial considerations, the role of the OTA, safety, and more. Chapter 1 provides a general overview of these topics, and reference back to this first chapter is often recommended.

The chapters that cover more traditional areas of occupation for adult interventions have similar formats. These chapters are Foundational Skills for Functional Activities, Activities of Daily Living, and Instrumental Activities of Daily Living. The remaining chapters—Education, Work, Retirement/Volunteer and End of Life Issues, Leisure, Social Participation, and Wellness—cover much of the same information as the *Framework* document, but in a more narrative and general format.

At the end of many chapters, a case study is presented. Appendix A, at the end of the text, is a resource guide compiled from all of the chapters. This contains useful web resources, ordering information, and continuing educational opportunities (for more advanced skills training). Appendix B is a grid that provides information pertaining to a sampling of evaluations.

It should be noted the term "occupational therapist," "occupational therapy practitioner," or "therapist" throughout the text does not indicate OTR only. It is important to emphasize the collaborative relationship that exists between the registered occupational therapist (OTR) and the occupational therapy assistant (OTA). According to AOTA, both OTRs and OTAs are responsible for providing quality occupational therapy services including direct intervention with clients (AOTA, 2004). The focus of this text is intervention, and therefore, the majority of the information can apply to both types of practitioners. Some information related to nonstandardized evaluation and specialized topics may pertain to the OTRs; however, standardized evaluations, as well as collaboration, on the part of the OTA are vital in establishing intervention plans.

Bibliography

American Occupational Therapy Association. (2002). *Occupational therapy practice framework: Domain and process.* Bethesda, MD: AOTA.

American Occupational Therapy Association. (2004). *The reference manual of the official documents of the American occupational therapy association* (10th ed.). Bethesda, MD: AOTA.

Introduction

Catherine Meriano, JD, MHS, OTR/L
Donna Latella, EdD, OTR/L

CHAPTER OBJECTIVES

By the end of this chapter, the student will be able to:

- ☑ Comprehend the **domain and process** of the *Occupational Therapy Practice Framework (Framework)* as it relates to occupational therapy's focus on occupation and daily living skills.
- ☑ Comprehend related occupational therapy **models/frames of reference.**
- ☑ Comprehend the impact of **modes of injury** upon occupational performance.
- ☑ Describe and give examples of the specific categories of the *Occupational Therapy Practice Framework*, including p**erformance areas, performance skills, performance patterns, context, activity demands,** and **client factors**.
- ☑ Describe the **evaluation process** and it's components as related to engagement in occupation.
- ☑ Describe the **intervention proces**s and its components as related to engagement in occupation.
- ☑ Comprehend **occupational therapy intervention approaches**, and recognize the differences between them, in order to establish an appropriate intervention plan.
- ☑ Comprehend the types of **occupational therapy interventions.**
- ☑ Describe and understand the **outcome process** as it relates to successful engagement in occupation.
- ☑ Understand and apply specific **documentation** skills to occupational therapy intervention.
- ☑ Understand the role of the **family/caregiver** during the intervention process.
- ☑ Understand the importance of **evidence-based practice** in occupational therapy practice.

OCCUPATIONAL THERAPY FRAMEWORK DOMAIN AND PROCESS: DOMAIN OF OCCUPATIONAL THERAPY

The *Occupational Therapy Practice Framework: Domain and Process* (American Occupational Therapy Association, 2002), guides the core concepts and constructs of occupational therapy practice. The *Framework* was created in order to evolve with the current needs of the profession.

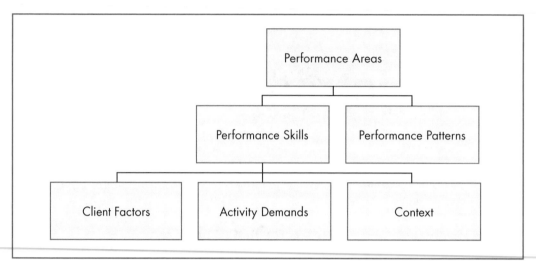

Figure 1-1. Domain of occupational therapy (adapted from American Occupational Therapy Association. (2002). Occupational therapy practice framework. *American Journal of Occupational Therapy*, 56 (6), 609-639).

The purpose of the *Framework* is to describe the domain of human activity as well as the process of occupational therapy evaluation and intervention as they relate to occupation. Specifically, it guides the profession of occupational therapy to focus on the *individual client's* engagement in daily occupations throughout the evaluation and intervention processes (AOTA, 2002).

The **domain** of occupational therapy sets the stage for, and encompasses, the evaluation and intervention processes. It focuses on the client's ability to engage in meaningful and purposeful daily activities, or occupations, in whatever context is appropriate for those occupations. *Each aspect of the domain is seen as equally important in the occupational therapy process. For example, evaluating the motor skills of a client who has sustained a wrist fracture is considered to be as important as evaluating the client's ability to perform daily routines.* **Occupations** are "everything we do in life, including actions, tasks, activities, thinking, and being" (Law, Baum, & Dunn, p. 6, 2005). The multiple occupations of every individual are unique, each with its own context and meaning to a particular client. *Therefore, how will the working mother who enjoys yoga continue her meaningful occupations and roles with an upper extremity injury?*

According to the *Framework* document, the domain of occupational therapy consists of performance areas, which are made up of performance skills and patterns, which are impacted by the context, activity demands, and individual client factors (AOTA, 2002). Figure 1-1 depicts this information visually, and each term is defined below.

Performance Areas

The occupational therapy practitioner must first examine the individual client's **Performance in Areas of Occupation**. These are general categories of areas where individuals typically perform activities or occupations that are meaningful to them. For the adult population, these areas are (AOTA, 2002):

- Activities of Daily Living (ADL).
- Instrumental Activities of Daily Living (IADL).
- Education.
- Work/Volunteer.

- Leisure.
- Social Participation.

Within occupational therapy practice, the therapist considers the many areas of occupation, as above, in which the individual or group may engage. Occupational therapy then addresses the performance issues affecting the individual's or group's abilities to perform these occupations. In order to work on performance issues, the occupational therapist must know which performance skills and patterns are needed for the specific areas addressed, as follows.

Performance Skills	Performance Patterns
Motor skills	Habits
Process skills	Routines
Communication/Interaction skills	Roles

Since skills are small components of performance and have functional purposes, they must be analyzed for their effectiveness (or lack of) during performance. **Motor skills** include posture, mobility, coordination, and strength. *Using the example of the client with the wrist fracture, a motor skill deficit may be decreased ability to perform bilateral fine motor tasks as the client's affected upper extremity may be immobilized in a cast.* **Process skills** include knowledge, temporal organization, and attending to task. *This client may have difficulty with the process skill of attending to work responsibilities while on pain medication.* **Communication/interaction** skills include relations, physicality, and information exchange. *A client who typically uses upper extremity gesturing to communicate may be significantly limited while immobilized in a cast.* Performance skills are impacted by, but not dictated by context, activity demands, and client factors (AOTA, 2002). As another example, a client may have limited body function but may have learned to compensate for this limitation and still be able to complete necessary motor skills in a particular activity. In this example, the unusual method of attaining motor skills may impact performance, but will not necessarily dictate a new method.

Performance patterns include **habits**, which are automatic behaviors; **routines**, which are established sequences of occupations/activities that provide daily structure; and **roles**, which are a set of socially accepted behaviors. The performance patterns are activities that we do on a frequent basis until they become a common behavior in our daily tasks (AOTA, 2002). *Therefore, how will the working mother who does yoga on a daily basis perform her daily routines, roles, and responsibilities after sustaining a wrist fracture?*

These performance patterns are influenced by context (AOTA 2002). **Contexts** are interrelated, internal, or external conditions that are within and surround the individual and influence performance. Context includes the cultural, physical, social, and spiritual environment in which the individual functions on a daily basis. In addition, the individual's personal data (age, socioeconomic status, etc) and temporal information (when activity is performed, stage of life, etc) must be reviewed. Virtual contexts occur when a client is surfing the Internet, taking an online course, or using email. The OT considers specific contexts that may influence the performance of a specific activity or occupation (AOTA, 2002). *Consider the spiritual context of an adult who has attended church as a daily routine for many years. This is a meaningful activity for the client, although the routine may be limited post-CVA, particularly if the client is no longer able to drive. How might this contextual limitation be evaluated and adapted for this client?* The OT must also assess the **activity demands** placed on an individual in order to partake in a particular occupation (AOTA, 2002). Activity demands are unique to each activity completed by the client, whereas context may be similar for a group of activities. *An example of activity demands is as follows: Once the dilemma of transporting the client to church is solved, the space demands and required actions for accessibility*

Table 1-1

CONTEXT, ACTIVITY DEMANDS, AND CLIENT FACTORS

Context	Activity Demands	Client Factors
Cultural	Objects used and their properties	Body functions
Physical	Space demands	Body structures
Social	Social demands	
Personal (age, gender, education, socio-economic status)	Sequencing and timing	
Spiritual	Required actions	
Temporal (day/year, stage of life)	Required body functions	
Virtual	Required body structures	

Adapted from American Occupational Therapy Association. (2002). Occupational therapy practice framework. *American Journal of Occupational Therapy, 56* (6), 609-639.

into and around the church may be additional issues. Lastly, the OT assesses the **client factors** such as physiological function and anatomical structure that may influence performance. Specifically, illness, disease, and disability may affect the ability of an individual to engage in chosen occupations such as the mental, sensory, and movement-related functions involved with attending church. Specifically, post-CVA, a client may not have sufficient memory to participate in church as he/she did in the past. In addition, how might vision and endurance limitations affect ability to participate in this meaningful activity? (AOTA, 2002). Table 1-1 summarizes these areas.

The Process of Occupational Therapy

The process of occupational therapy begins with evaluation of the client's occupational needs, issues, meaningful activities, and desires. The results determine intervention strategies that focus on engagement in occupations. These intervention strategies are then assessed in the outcome process to determine if appropriate outcomes have been achieved (AOTA, 2002).

Evaluation Process

The evaluation process of occupational therapy is aimed at assessing a client's goals and needs, as well as barriers to performance. The evaluation process focuses on the entire domain of practice (as above) and how each area may influence client performance. The OT uses skilled observation and applicable assessment tools in order to determine a problem list. The process has two steps.

- Step One: The *occupational profile* determines the client's needs, problems, and concerns about daily performance of occupations. This process includes the clients' history, background, values, and priorities in terms of his/her occupations.

- Step Two: The evaluation of occupational performance, which focuses on identifying specific issues and evaluating those that may affect performance.

It is important to note that the client's input, priorities, and goals guide the evaluation process

(AOTA, 2002). Specifically, when evaluating occupational performance, the therapist should ask the client questions such as:

"What are your goals in the recovery process?"

"What do you do for fun?"

"What is important to you during the recovery process or upon discharge from therapy?"

STEP ONE: THE OCCUPATIONAL PROFILE

As stated previously, the occupational profile is completed to determine the client's interests and goals. The profile can also assist the therapist when determining what forms of intervention to use. Therefore, if a client is having difficulty completing ADLs because of decreased fine and gross motor coordination, the therapist can certainly practice ADLs with him/her. Typically, however, clients dress only once per day, and in some settings, such as hospitals, clothes may not be available. To allow for additional coordination training, the therapist could pull out the pegs and Thera-Putty, which would probably result in a bored individual. On the other hand, if the therapist knows from the occupational profile that this client enjoys painting, then the therapist has an activity for therapy that will engage the client while improving coordination.

STEP TWO: EVALUATION OF OCCUPATIONAL PERFORMANCE

Each of the chapters in this text will discuss the evaluation of occupational performance specifically for the chapter topic: Foundational skills, ADL, IADL, Education, Work/Retirement, Leisure, Social Participation, and Wellness. In addition, a smapling of evaluations is provided in Appendix B.

Intervention Process

AOTA (2002) separates the intervention process into three sub-steps: Intervention Plan, Intervention Implementation, and Intervention Review.

The **Intervention plan** is based on the results of the evaluation process. It guides the intervention process, and is designed to enhance participation in occupations and activities. The intervention plan is created in collaboration with the client and considers the following (AOTA, 2002):

1. Client goals, beliefs, values, and health as determined by the occupational profile and the medical history.

2. Performance skills and patterns, which are influenced by context, activity demands, and client factors as determined by the evaluation process.

3. The setting or circumstance surrounding the interventions, including any limitations on intervention imposed by the setting or the payment source.

4. Applicable theories or models/frames of reference.

5. The appropriate approach (create, promote, establish, restore, maintain, modify).

6. The interaction with family and caregivers.

7. Evidence-based research.

In addition, the OT uses the knowledge of occupation, human performance/development, and the effects of disease and disability as a guide to the intervention process. Each of the topics listed will be discussed later in this chapter.

Intervention implementation puts the plan into action in order to enhance client performance. It involves a skilled process that includes collaboration with the client in order to enhance occupation and activity participation. Interventions focus on changing the context, activity demands, client factors, performance skills or patterns, as appropriate. Change in one area usually affects another, resulting in a dynamic process. *For example, interventions that involve increasing functional mobility (ADL area) will enhance the client's return to independent performance patterns (roles, routines, and responsibilities).* Outcomes are identified and documented throughout interventions while clients are continuously reassessed through this dynamic inter-relationship (AOTA, 2002). The role of the OT may also change as this dynamic intervention process continues. The process includes the therapeutic use of self, the therapeutic use of occupations or activities, consultation, and/or education (AOTA, 2002).

Therapeutic use of self is not unique to occupational therapy; however, with the holistic approach to intervention, rather than the medical model of intervention, OTs have multiple opportunities to utilize this skill. OTs provide interventions regarding such personal issues as bathing, toileting, and sexual activity, as well as individual interests of leisure, social participation, and work. In these sessions, therapist have the opportunity to "use personality, insights, perceptions, and judgments as part of the therapeutic process" as described in the AOTA *Framework* document (2002, p. 628). In addition, therapists working in the area of adult physical dysfunction include psychosocial issues in the intervention plan, not just physical issues. Lastly, behavioral issues may also require intervention and modeling of proper behaviors by the therapist is required as an essential component of the intervention plan. For example, this form of intervention may be required following a cerebral vascular accident or a traumatic brain injury with *clients who have impaired mental/cognitive functions such as thought, personality, or temperament issues.*

As therapists utilize the skill of therapeutic use of self, they must be aware of their own attitudes, beliefs, and values. Clients may have different ways of completing occupations or have different attitudes regarding an occupation. For example, beliefs and values regarding "appropriate" forms of sexual activity may differ between the therapist and the client; some cultures put a great deal of emphasis on food, and will vehemently resist when told feeding is unsafe; a family's unwillingness to take a parent home may seem inappropriate to a therapist, but the therapist should not judge that family; and what is deemed "appropriate dress" for work or leisure may differ from the client's perspective. In all of these situations, the therapist must acknowledge his/her own beliefs and values, but not impose them on the clients or caregivers. For a more in-depth discussion of therapeutic use of self, please refer to Chapter 8.

According to the *Framework*, **therapeutic use of occupations or activities** can include occupation-based/purposeful activities or preparatory methods (AOTA, 2002). Throughout this text, occupation-based and purposeful activities will be described together as functional activities. Preparatory methods are described as foundational skills. One of the determinations an OT must make is whether to begin intervention with these foundational skills or through the use of functional activities. According to Zoltan (1996, p.3), these forms of intervention are called a top-down or bottom-up approach. With a top-down approach, the OT adjusts the activity or occupational performance with the goal of promoting independence with the use of adaptive and compensatory techniques. *Consider the client with memory function deficits. He/she may need to use a planner as a compensatory technique to complete a daily routine or schedule.* Conversely, the bottom-up approach addresses underlying dysfunction in the foundation skill areas and assumes the client will improve in functional ability as a result. This indicates foundational skills are the building blocks for the functional activities. With some clients, it will be necessary to work on these skills in isolation, prior to beginning or in conjunction with functional activities. With other clients, intervention of functional activities will also improve foundational skills through their incorporation in the functional activities. *For example, the client with a memory deficit may initially work with memory games before or while attempting the above compensatory technique.* While the beginning of this text does review the remediation of foundational skills, the majority of the text will concentrate on the remediation, adaptation/compensation, and maintenance of functional activities.

The top-down approach has been refined by Fisher in the Occupational Therapy Intervention Process Model (Fisher, 2002). In this model, Fisher has further broken down the top-down approach into "simulated occupation" and "restorative occupation" finding the interventions utilizing actual activities were preferred over the simulated situations. While simulations do have some benefit, the client will find greater meaning completing actual activities, thus improving carryover (Fisher, 2002).

While the most common settings for **consultation** are in the areas of work/volunteer and adult education, consultation can occur in any setting. According to the *Framework*, consultation occurs when the therapist collaborates with the client to identify problems and possible solutions. The therapist "is not directly responsible for the outcome of the intervention" (AOTA, 2002). Because the expertise of therapists is so varied, consultation can be requested of therapists in community, educational, vocational, medical, and many other environments. *Consider the therapist who may evaluate the client's home environment and make recommendations for accessibility and safety, but does not implement them.* The therapist is functioning as a consultant in this example.

Education, on the other hand, should occur in all environments. Even though the *Framework* defines education as, "imparting knowledge and information about occupation and activity and which *does not* result in the actual performance of the occupation/activity" (AOTA, 2002, emphasis added), this does not mean education should occur on a limited basis. Education regarding the purpose of occupational therapy, the occupations of individuals, and the importance of purposeful activity is ongoing for most therapists in all settings. *Consider the therapist who provides in-services regarding the role of occupational therapy to new medical interns every year in a hospital setting.* It is also important to note, while AOTA has distinguished education in this manner, most settings and payers do acknowledge, and require documentation for, ongoing education regarding the completion of functional activities with clients.

The second portion of the intervention implementation process is to monitor the client's response and progress through continuous assessment. The **Intervention Review** process continually assesses the effectiveness and progress of the plan by reviewing the actions and/or interventions that were completed, and the outcomes that were achieved, not achieved, or no longer a priority for the client. The intervention plan is adjusted accordingly in collaboration with the client. The intervention review process also includes a determination and recommendations for discharge, additional referrals, or continuation of services as appropriate (AOTA, 2002).

Performance Skills and Patterns

Prior examples illustrated how performance skills can impact an individual's function. Throughout this book, the emphasis of intervention will be on functional activities. As OTs, however, we utilize the task analysis process to break down these functional activities into performance skills and performance patterns, and view how context, activity demands, and client factors impact these functional tasks. This means goals associated with performance skills, such as coordination, for example, are acceptable as long as they lead toward a functional goal, as in ADLs.

The intervention plan may also have goals specifically related to performance patterns, context, activity demands, and client factors as well, provided that these relate back to the occupations of interest for the individual client.

The Setting

If a client's performance skills and performance patterns will be impacted by the context where the functional activity occurs, it would appear the ideal setting for intervention would be in the client's actual context. Unfortunately, this is not always possible, particularly when you consider the vast institutional and community programs where OTs practice. This forces many therapists to simulate the context and activity as much as possible.

Some of these settings further limit the simulation, however, for safety, insurance, or financial reasons. For example, using a cooking task can be limited because of safety concerns or structural issues. *While working at an adult day center on a wellness program, clients may not be allowed to put food into or take food out of the ovens because the director may have concerns about the clients' safety. If one works in a prison system, there are restrictions regarding use of sharp cooking utensils. In a hospital setting, there may be a kitchen, but it is not tailored to simulate each client's home kitchen.*

Financial concerns also play a role in settings, particularly in clinics that receive Medicare funds, private insurance, or workers' compensation. The caseworker often is not an OT, yet can limit the amount of visits allowed to therapy. The recent Medicare caps have resulted in clients receiving less care than recommended by the therapist.

Lastly, the setting itself can limit the context of therapy. Hospital therapists are able to complete home visits, but typically this is to gather information for clinic simulations and to prepare for discharge. The client does not usually attend these visits to practice any skills in his/her home. The school-based therapist is limited to interventions that impact education. While the school-based therapist does have broad areas in which to provide intervention (self-help/adaptation, communication, cognition, motor, and social emotional), the intervention must still relate back to educational goals.

Introduction to Occupational Therapy Models and Occupational Performance

The roots of occupational therapy are founded on the humanistic philosophy, which is a client-centered focus (Crepeau, Cohn, & Schell, 2003). Intervention is focused on the needs, interests, values, desires, goals, and perspectives of the client (Reed, 2001).

Specific concepts of humanism relate directly to well-known individuals such as Carl Rogers and Abraham Maslow. Rogers believed the client should be allowed to set his/her own goals, direct therapy, and find solutions to problems. Maslow believed the client should be viewed as the expert of his/her own life and the therapist should guide the client to self-actualization through the use of genuineness, nonjudgmental acceptance, and understanding (Cole, 1998). Today, components of the humanistic approach are seen in many of the client-centered theories that will be discussed in this section.

The occupational therapy models discussed below are intended to provide the backdrop or framework for the assessment and intervention processes. The first section includes examples of frames of reference or models that are client-centered in nature and have been chosen because they are collaborative in nature, and according to Law (1998), are more likely to engage clients in the occupational therapy process. In turn, this engagement has been shown to increase satisfaction, success in therapy, and positive outcomes. In addition, Christiansen & Baum (1997) discuss the importance of client-centered models involving the activities, tasks, and roles of the individual. The second section includes examples of systems models that are holistic in nature and include the interaction of systems inside, as well as outside of, the client. Systems models focus on occupational function/dysfunction and everyday routines that may be impacted (Bruce & Borg, 2002). Other chapters throughout the text will also discuss frames of reference or models that are appropriate to the specific chapter.

SECTION 1: CLIENT-CENTERED MODELS

Client-Centered Approach

The client-centered approach involves the therapist working with the client in order to decide which areas of occupational performance should be focused on. Depending on their ability to participate, clients will contribute to the decision-making process and make choices. If the client is cognitively unable to participate, then the family-centered therapy approach is attempted with the family representing the client.

The client-centered approach to occupational therapy practice focuses on the respect for, and collaboration with, the individual receiving services. This approach, then, facilitates the client to find meaning in his/her own daily occupations. The ultimate goal of the client-centered approach is to empower the clients by allowing them to direct the course of intervention and contribute to the process. For example, part of their contribution may include looking at their own strengths and areas of limitations, in order to prioritize the intervention plan. Through person-centered communication, the therapist facilitates and enables the client to be responsible for decision making. In order for this approach to be successful, the therapist must have a good understanding of the client. The environment in which this empowerment occurs must be caring, respectful, visionary, and supportive (Law, 2002; Law, 1998).

The Person-Environment Occupational Performance Model

Christiansen & Baum (1997) state that the Person-Environment Occupational Performance Model (PEOP) focuses on elements that describe what individuals do in their daily lives, what motivates them, and how their personal characteristics interact with occupations that are undertaken to influence occupational performance. "A basic belief of the model is that people are naturally motivated to explore their world and demonstrate mastery within it. Their success in doing so is a measure of how successfully they have adapted" (Christiansen & Baum, 1997). Adaptation describes how well individuals are able to meet their daily challenges in everyday life through achieving set goals. This model also discusses the belief that individuals are motivated to face new challenges with increased confidence when they are in a setting that encourages success. In addition, a sense of fulfillment and a development of identity come from feelings of mastery and accomplishment of goals within everyday occupations. As a result of these meaningful experiences, individuals begin to understand who they are and their place in the world. The following will discuss pertinent issues in regard to the elements of the model.

THE PERSON AND MOTIVATION

Motivation can be divided into two categories—the **intrinsic theories** and the **cognitive theories** of motivation. The intrinsic theories of motivation look at internal drives and needs which occur as a result of free choice and without external reward. The intrinsic need for satisfaction can be relevant to the importance of everyday occupation through the following example: an individual has an intrinsic need for self-satisfaction in his/her work environment in order to be motivated to return each and every day. Cognitive theories of motivation show individuals motivate themselves through setting goals, planning actions, and achieving goals. Cognitive influences look at explanations for why things happen, expectations and goals (Christiansen & Baum, 1997).

THE PERSON AND SELF-EFFICACY

Self-efficacy describes an individual who views him- or herself as competent. This element is vital for success in occupational performance tasks because an individual's feelings of competence may influence the outcome.

THE PERSON AND PERSONALITY

Personality involves the interests, values, and attitudes of an individual, which influence his/her behavior, attention, and response to new events. Differences in personality can be seen in choice, satisfaction, and environments that are most comfortable for each individual. According to Christiansen & Baum (1997), "because an individual's preferences for occupation are an expression of his or her personality type, psychologists have shown increasing interest in studying the occupations of daily life as a means for understanding personality."

THE PERSON AND VALUES

Values are beliefs that influence choice, behavior, thinking, feeling, and overall meaning in life that, consequently, are central to understanding occupation (Christiansen & Baum, 1997).

THE PERSON AND MEANING

Meaning reflects how events are interpreted in our lives based on present goals, values and past experiences. Individual perceptions, which contain signs and symbols, convey meaning, influence actions, and enrich engagement in occupation. Christiansen & Baum (1997) state that there are individual, as well as collective or shared meanings, which are influenced socially and culturally. "When a person pays special attention to the way in which an occupation is done and the place in which it is performed, it becomes an opportunity for having special meaning" (Christiansen & Baum, 1997). In addition, Yerxa (1998) emphasizes the importance of engagement in meaningful occupations in order to restore and maintain health and well-being.

THE ENVIRONMENT

The environment is a direct influence upon successful occupational performance. This includes an individual's ability to interact with and explore the environment, as well as his/her level of arousal within the environment. Arousal consists of physical and psychological characteristics that can affect an individual's level of performance. *For example, a client may be underaroused (bored) or overaroused (agitated).* The quality of the environment, based on a person's needs, will affect the inclination as to whether or not he/she will explore or interact with the environment (Christiansen & Baum, 1997). Additional properties of the environment include: physical, cultural, societal, and social support factors that affect performance.

OCCUPATIONAL PERFORMANCE

Christiansen & Baum (1997) describe occupational performance as the "doing of occupation." The authors discuss a hierarchy of occupation-related behaviors and abilities that have increasing levels of complexity as follows:

- *Roles*: Positions in society that have responsibilities and privileges (e.g., grandparent).
- *Occupations*: Meaningful, goal-directed activities (e.g., caring for a child).
- *Tasks*: Actions that have a purpose (e.g., mopping the floor).
- *Actions*: Behaviors that are observed and recognized (e.g., reaching for an item).
- *Abilities*: Characteristics that support occupational performance (e.g., upper extremity strength).

More specifically, occupations are purposeful and have a temporal dimension within the context of work, pleasure, or self-maintenance. Within the PEO Performance Model, the OT will consider these factors and apply them within a client-centered focus. The client and therapist work together to identify issues related to living skills and performance of occupations. The two will collaborate on appropriate goals, intervention, and outcomes of therapy. "The Person-

Environment Occupational Performance Model offers a balanced Model for viewing the client and jointly planning intervention" (Christiansen & Baum, 1997).

The Person-Environment Occupation Model

The Person-Environment Occupation Model (PEO) focuses on occupational performance and its link to people, occupation, roles, the environment, work, and play as a dynamic, interwoven process. The approach to occupational therapy also acknowledges the importance of context, temporal conditions, physical and psychological aspects, and influences of behavior. Because the environment is always in flux, individuals need the behaviors necessary to shift while working toward goals.

Assumptions (Law, Cooper, Strong, Stewart, Rigby, & Letts, 1996):

1. The *person* is a unique being who has many roles that are dynamic and variable across time and context, duration, and importance.

2. Within this model, the *environment* includes cultural, socioeconomic, institutional, physical, and social aspects.

3. *Occupation* is considered to be self-directed, functional tasks, and activities engaged in over a lifetime.

4. *Occupational performance* is the dynamic experience and outcome of the interaction between the person, environment, and occupation. It involves meaningful, purposeful activities, and tasks in which an individual engages over a lifetime.

5. The model assumes that the *person, environment, and occupation* interact continually over time and space. Occupational performance is optimized when these are considered compatible.

When following the PEO model, the focus of the occupational therapy evaluation and intervention should be to elicit change and facilitate improved occupational performance. This occurs by collaborating with the client, involving his/her occupation, and considering the environment specific to the individual.

Occupational Adaptation Model

First introduced by Schultz & Schkade (1992a&b), this model encourages the therapist to assist the client to identify occupations to which he/she is interested in returning. Based equally on the individual, the environment, and the client's interactions, this model emphasizes the use of meaningful occupations to allow the client to experience adaptation. When the client responds to the challenges, adaptation occurs and leads to mastery. Because the client is completing tasks that hold meaning, internal motivation is present. While foundational skills, such as range of motion (ROM) and edema are addressed, they are focused toward the activity that the client desires to complete. Gibson & Schkade (1997) later found that occupational therapy intervention focused on the roles and contexts that were identified as important by the clients resulted in higher levels of independence and less restrictive discharge environments.

SECTION 2: SYSTEMS MODELS

The Model of Human Occupation

Kielhofner and Burke (1980) described the Model of Human Occupation (MOHO) as an open or dynamic system, which influences occupational behavior in individuals. "Being engaged in occupation means doing culturally meaningful work, play, or daily living tasks in the stream of time and in the context of one's physical and social world" (Kielhofner, 1995, p, 3). Occupation, according to Kielhofner and Burke (1980), is the action or doing in which humans occupy their world. Occupational behavior occurs when one makes choices and takes action. Humans are occupational by nature, and thus need to be active.

MOHO describes the human open system as a cycle that influences occupational behavior. This systems theory calls information coming into the human being *input*. This information is internally processed as *throughput*. Based on how an individual processes and forms beliefs about this information, he/she will perform behavior or react emotionally. This response is called *output*. Lastly, information that comes back into the system from the environment is called *feedback* (Kielhofner & Burke, 1980).

This model emphasizes how individuals continuously engage in this feedback loop. Information is processed (step two of the cycle) via three subsystems:

1. The *Volition subsystem* consists of three components: personal causation, valued goals, and interests. These components influence behavior and are differentiated out of an individual's innate urge to explore and master the environment. Individuals also incorporate information from experience to form internal symbolic representation. The enactment of occupational behavior and performance is guided by these components (1980).

2. The *Habituation subsystem* consists of habits and roles. Habits guide human automatic behavior and do not always require conscious attention (1980). According to Bruce & Borg (2002), many people find security in their habits and may feel uncomfortable when changing them. Kielhofner, (1995) explains how roles are images individuals keep regarding the positions held in various social groups and of the obligations with those positions.

3. *Performance* is responsible for influencing occupational behaviors via skills and the constituents of skills. Skills are further defined as perceptual motor skills, process skills, and communication/interaction skills (Kielhofner & Burke, 1980). Bruce & Borg (2002) also state that this subsystem is constantly interchanging information between the constituents and the environment in the processing of information during problem solving and actions.

The environment significantly impacts an individual's behavior by providing feedback about the output, or actions taken. The environment is believed to be comprised of components: objects, tasks, social groups, and culture (Kielhofner, 1995). Objects are used by individuals to perform tasks. Tasks are used for performance in the environment. Social groups are natural collections of individuals such as clubs or families. Culture refers to the values and technology that can affect an individual's performance.

Kielhofner (1995) discussed an individual's functional status as being in order or disorder. *Order* connotes a state of health with positive feedback loops and successful performance of daily living tasks. To explain this concept further, the term *occupational function* has also been used to suggest that the individual is able to choose, organize, or perform occupation without difficulty (Bruce & Borg, 2002). The individual is able to meet social demands with positive feedback from the environment. *Disorder* connotes the inability to perform occupational tasks, decreased or absent role performance, and the inability to meet role responsibilities (Kielhofner, 1995). Bruce and Borg (2002) discussed the concept further using the term *occupational dysfunction* to reflect impaired occupational performance. Dysfunction occurs when an individual has difficulty performing, organizing, or choosing occupations, or when occupational behavior results in a decreased quality of life. Occupational dysfunction can impact the cycle negatively including one's habits, volition, performance, and the ability to negotiate in the environment.

MOHO looked at the development of occupation as a lifelong process, which includes changes in the individual as well as the environment. As developmental changes naturally occur, the human system must learn, relearn, and adapt in order to respond to, and maintain, an appropriate level of function. Occupational development is a process of transformation with periods of stability followed by transition and then, eventually, a new order of behavior.

The Ecology of Human Performance

The Ecology of Human Performance is based on the premise of how human behavior and task performance are affected by the interaction between a person and the context (or the ecology). In turn, the person, the context, and task performance affect each other through the transactional process of human performance. A specific transaction will affect an individual's performance as the person, context, or performance range are changed by the actual experience. Within this model, the occupational therapy intervention process is designed to improve the client's performance by changing variables such as the person, the context, the task, or the transaction between them. The intervention process involves the client, the family, and the OT in collaboration (Crepeau, Cohn, & Schell, 1998).

Within this model, occupational therapy intervention strategies may include (2003):

1. Establishing or restoring an individual's abilities/performance in a specific context.

2. Changing the context or task.

3. Modifying or adapting the contextual characteristics and task demands to reflect performance in context.

4. Preventing barriers to performance in context.

5. Designing interventions to enhance performance.

The Ecology of Human Performance model has four basic assumptions (1998):

1. Persons and contexts are unique and dynamic.

2. Natural contexts are not the same as contrived contexts.

3. Occupational therapy involves improving self-determination and inclusion of individuals with disabilities in any context.

4. Contextual supports are included when achieving independence.

Definitions (2003):

- *Person*: An individual with unique abilities, experiences, and needs, such as cognitive and psychosocial. A person is not predictable because everyone is unique and complex. The meaning attached to a person's tasks and contexts influences performance.

- *Task*: A set of behaviors needed to reach a goal. Tasks are influenced by a person's roles.

- *Performance*: Comprised of the process and results of interactions within the context when engaging in a task.

- *Context*: Includes the temporal and environmental aspects.

- *Temporal Aspects*: Includes an individual's age, developmental stage, place in life phases, and disability status.

- *Environmental Aspects*: Include physical, social, and cultural aspects.

- *Person-Context-Task Transaction*: The major variable that affects performance.

In summary, when the occupational therapy evaluation and intervention process are considered within the Ecology of Human Performance Model, the variables of person, context, and task performance have an affect on, and are affected by, human performance.

THE APPROACH

The *Framework* delineates five intervention approaches: create, restore, maintain, modify, and prevent (AOTA 2002). Law, Baum, & Dunn (2005) discuss how intervention strategies, which reflect the *Framework,* tend to fall in the above five categories. The first two categories (create and restore) involve changing the individual's environment including physical, social, and institutional issues, as well as technological strategies such as devices and aids. The third category (maintain) focuses on the person and on the approaches to recovery/adaptation of neurological, sensory, and motor issues. The last two categories (modify and prevent) involve the delivery of services and the strategies the OT will use to facilitate changing attitudes, policies, and laws that affect the rehabilitation process. For the purposes of this text, the five intervention approaches have been modified slightly. The Chapter 9 will focus on create (health promotion) and prevent (disability prevention), the Chapter 2 will focus on remediation (restore) and the remaining occupational area chapters will discuss remediation (restore), compensation/adaptation (modify), and maintenance of each occupational area.

The occupational profile will tell the therapist which approach the client is interested in. This approach should be a starting point. However, if a client has a progressive disease, such as Parkinson's disease, and the client's desire is to address only remediation of skills, the therapist has an obligation to educate the client/family about the disease process and attempt to combine some remediation along with environmental adaptations and other compensatory strategies.

Within these approaches, there are general principles that require definition and discussion. Grading of activities in these approaches, carryover/generalization by the client, and the purchase of adaptive or durable medical equipment are three such topics.

Grading of activities is more commonly used in the remedial approach, but can also be utilized at times when using the adaptive/compensatory approach. Grading is defined as, "viewing an activity on a continuum from simple to complex, typically grading an activity more challenging as a person gained skill" (Jacobs & Jacobs, 2004, p. 96). As a client gains skill in a particular foundational task or occupational task, the expectations will increase. Grading can include asking the client to complete more of the task, complete the task with higher quality, complete a task with greater complexity, or complete a task with less time allotted. Because a complete task analysis is completed prior to initiation of intervention, the therapist has a clear understanding of what components of a task can be graded as improvement is noted. *A specific example of grading is as follows: Upon discharge from a rehab facility, the client must independently make his own lunch each day. The intervention may begin with the client preparing a "light" meal of a cold cheese, lettuce, tomato, and mayonnaise sandwich. After this goal has been achieved, meal preparation may be upgraded to making a grilled cheese sandwich or a cheese omelet. In the event the initial "light" meal was unsuccessful, the activity may be downgraded to one step (e.g., of just adding one ingredient, such as the cheese).*

One form of grading is referred to as *chaining. Backward chaining* is when a therapist begins a task and then asks the client to complete the task (Trombly & Radomski, 2002). This allows the client a sense of accomplishment when he/she finishes a task. As the client demonstrates improvement, the therapist completes less and less of the task, eventually requiring the client to complete the entire task independently. *Forward chaining* can also be used. This is when the client begins the task and once unable to complete the task the therapist steps in (Trombly & Radomski, 2002). As improvement is noted, the therapist will offer assistance later and later in the process. While both of these methods offer grading, forward chaining can often lead to a feeling of failure for the client because he/she had to be "saved" by the therapist. For this reason, backward chaining is preferred. *A typical example of grading involves tying shoes. This multi-step, cognitive, and fine motor task may be broken down by either forward or backward chaining the activity.*

Cuing can also be used as grading. The amount of cues, either visual or auditory, should be decreased as the client's skills improve. If cues are required postdischarge, they become a maintenance tool.

Whether or not grading of activities is required, the OT is observing for carryover and generalization during ongoing sessions. While these terms are similar, they are not identical. *Carryover,* as defined by the *American Heritage Dictionary* (2000), is "something transferred or extended from an earlier time or another place." Relating this definition to occupational therapy, instructions given or tasks learned will be repeated at later sessions of therapy or by the client in a setting similar to the original setting of instruction. This alone will not allow a client to be independent, because settings often change for the client. Because of this, generalization is required. While most individuals think of *generalization* as making a general statement, as seen in the *American Heritage Dictionary's* (2000) definition of, "a principle, statement or idea having general application," OTs think of generalization as the ability to complete carryover in a variety of settings. According to Jacobs & Jacobs, the occupational therapy definition is, "skills and performance in applying specific concepts to a variety of related solutions" (2004, p.94). Therefore, successful occupational therapy intervention requires not only carryover, but also generalization. Toglia (1991) has taken this concept even further by defining levels of generalization. These levels are near, intermediate, far, or very far depending on the degree of change from the original task to the new task. If the new task is similar to the one already mastered, then the generalization is near. Likewise, if there is a great deal of difference between the two tasks, the generalization is very far. The characteristics of the tasks which are changed are referred to by Toglia (1991) as *surface characteristics,* such as variations in size, directions given or how a task is presented, or *underlying concepts,* such as a change in the planning required by the client in order to complete the task. The further down the continuum of Toglia's generalization, the further away from simple carryover the client moves. It is the responsibility of the OT to move the client from simple carryover to generalization.

The third general topic is *adaptive equipment/durable medial equipment* (DME). An interesting study was completed by Mann, Llanes, Justiss, & Tomita that asked over 1000 elderly people what their most important assistive device was and the top five (when controlled for number of people using the devices) were oxygen tanks, dentures, three-in-one commodes, computers, and wheelchairs (2004). This same study states the participants had an average of 14 pieces of equipment and used 12 (2004). This suggests, while adaptive equipment/DME may not be on the top of all clients' lists of favorites, they are utilizing the equipment for the most part. It also demonstrates the fact that clients have a different definition of "assistive device" than most therapists. This is an important consideration when educating clients regarding equipment.

When suggesting equipment to a client, there are several considerations that must be reviewed with the client. These are:

- Prospective use of the equipment: Required frequently or on rare occasions?

- Desire of the client: Does he/she want this or do you, as the therapist, think he/she needs it?

- Cost of the equipment: Adaptive equipment and bathroom DME generally are not covered. Is there an alternative that is available in the general population?

- Functionality: Is the piece of equipment going to be functional in all appropriate environments for the client?

MODES OF INJURY

While this text is not a pathology manual, prior examples have demonstrated that knowledge of pathology and the anticipated course of illness is important when determining the most appropriate intervention approach. The OT must utilize his/her knowledge of human performance/development, and the effects of disease and disability when determining which approach to utilize with a particular client. Examples of pathologies will be mentioned throughout the book, but a general review is provided here for reference in all chapters. Wellness, by definition, does not focus on injury and will not be reviewed.

Nearly all injuries/illnesses will result in limitations of at least one foundational skill. As discussed later in this chapter, these skills can be addressed individually or during functional activities. Chapter 2 will emphasize the remediation of each skill, while other chapters will address the foundational skills in relationship to the areas of occupation. The modes of injury for foundational skills are addressed throughout Chapter 2 as each skill is addressed. While these skills are addressed individually, it is important to note that many clients have deficits in multiple areas and overlap of deficits will also occur, such as decreased ROM secondary to edema of the hand.

Modes of Injury for Areas of Occupation

While modes of injury for specific skills can be delineated, occupationally based deficits can relate to a large number of injuries. Often, clients do not have just one diagnosis that is impacting the areas of occupation, but a few to several. In addition, an original injury may result in future diagnosis such as chemical dependency, depression, etc. Someone who is diabetic may experience sensory, visual, and cardiac symptoms, while someone with a spinal cord injury may have depression along with all of the other medical complications associated with this diagnosis. Nearly any injury or illness can result in a limitation to the areas of occupation; however, minor injuries, such as a well-healing hand fracture, can be easily overcome without the intervention of occupational therapy. When skilled intervention is required, the injuries or illness are usually more significant. The most common injuries/illnesses fall into two categories: orthopedic and neurological. Common orthopedic injuries are lower extremity fractures, joint replacements, amputations, or spinal surgeries. Upper extremity fractures and joint replacements can also indicate the need for occupational therapy.

Neurological injuries can result from trauma, such as spinal cord injuries or brain injuries, or from nontraumatic events such as cerebral vascular accidents, brain aneurysms, or cancer. Specific neurological diseases can also impact function, such as Parkinson's disease, Guillain-Barré syndrome, amyotrophic lateral sclerosis, multiple sclerosis, etc.

Many of the orthopedic injuries and some of the neurological illnesses will have a typical course that includes improvement in function. For these individuals, a remedial approach or a combination of remediation and adaptation will be appropriate. Some of these illnesses, however, will be progressive in nature and less remediation is typically appropriate while greater emphasis is placed on adaptation and maintenance of skills.

INTERACTION WITH FAMILY AND CAREGIVERS

As mentioned above, the family and caregivers will impact the intervention plan. If working with a child, the parents/caregivers should be involved throughout the process of intervention planning, as they will be completing many tasks at home with the child. When working in adult settings, the anticipated support of the family after discharge can impact the intervention plan significantly. In addition, it is essential to know how much time and interest family members and caregivers have for training by the OT.

EVIDENCE-BASED PRACTICE

The process of evidence-based practice involves the use of research studies in order to select the most clinically and cost-effective approaches to evaluation and intervention. This approach to practice may also enhance clinical reasoning skills, particularly through the evaluation of the evidence and the appropriate application/integration into therapy.

Evidence-based practice also allows the occupational therapy practitioner to educate the client regarding the effectiveness of the evaluation and intervention processes chosen. Specifically, it involves informing the client of the intervention's benefits and risks, as well as positive and negative implications. This further enhances the client-centered environment by allowing the client to make informed decisions about the services provided (Law, Baum, & Dunn, 2005).

Law, Baum, and Dunn (2005) discuss three challenges of evidence-based practice: the responsibility of the therapist to keep up on current literature, to develop good communication skills, and to understand how to evaluate the evidence within the literature.

In addition, Christiansen & Baum (1997) identify the challenges of evidence-based practice as being able to access, evaluate, and interpret the literature; collect data to support intervention recommendations; and communication of possible outcomes to the client.

Law (2002) emphasizes the need for OTs using evidence-based practice to become reflective practitioners. Reflective practice involves the use of clinical reasoning skills for decision making. Law uses the *E Model* as a decision-making tool and means of reflection. It is explained in five categories (Law, 2002):

1. *Expectations* are shaped by the client's needs and the therapist's knowledge of theory in order to formulate assumptions.

2. The *Environment* influences thoughts, beliefs, and actions. Recommendations are only effective to current environmental contexts.

3. *Experience* may be formal or informal. It involves reflection and objectivity.

4. *Ethics* are guided by governing bodies and personal philosophy.

5. *Evidence* gathering has improved with increased access to and emphasis on the process.

Law (2002) emphasizes that in the evidence-based practice process, evidence should not be considered alone. A competent therapist should consider all of these factors before making recommendations.

OUTCOME PROCESS

While the intervention review is completed informally on an ongoing basis, the outcome process measurement is a formal reassessment of the progress toward the anticipated outcomes. The outcome process involves choosing a measurement for each anticipated outcome and then measuring the progress toward achieving the outcomes. The therapist should choose outcomes and measures such as those related to occupational performance, client satisfaction, adaptation, role competence, health/wellness, prevention, and quality of life (AOTA, 2002). It is important to create outcome measures early in the process because this will help to define the focus of intervention. These outcome measures should be valid, reliable, sensitive to client change, match targeted outcomes, and be selected to complement the client goals. It is also important to review the ability of an outcome measure to predict future outcomes (2002).

Once outcome measures have been determined, it is just as important to utilize this information appropriately. Therapists should compare progress to the targeted outcomes throughout the intervention process, and assess the outcomes results in order to adjust the intervention plan. Figure 1-2 summarizes the occupational therapy process in the form of a decision tree for therapists.

DOCUMENTATION IN INTERVENTION

Introduction

Documentation in occupational therapy intervention involves the practitioner's contribution to the client's record. It is a method of communication of services provided for the health care team as well as third-party payers. Whether documentation is collected/presented through a medical record or any other form of record-keeping, it remains a vital component of the intervention process. This important component requires appropriate terminology and professionalism, which, in occupational therapy, is driven by the *Occupational Therapy Practice Framework* (AOTA, 2002), as well as the *Guide to Occupational Therapy Practice* (Moyers, 1999; Crepeau et al, 2003).

Purpose of Documentation

Through the use of written words, documentation is completed as a chronological record of the client's progress, status, and condition (Trombly & Radomski, 2002). It serves as a basis for judgment, evidence of appropriate decision making (Crepeau et al, 2003), effectiveness of intervention, and need for occupational therapy services. Appropriate documentation should reflect sound clinical reasoning (Crepeau et al, 2003), while investigating the unknown. Also, the practitioner should use documentation to ponder probing questions regarding the client's progress or lack of progress during the intervention process (Trombly & Radomski, 2002).

AOTA (1995) describes four general purposes of documentation:

1. Facilitation of effective intervention.
2. Justification of reimbursement.
3. Documentation as a legal document.
4. A communication tool for the health care team, client, and family.

Additional specific purposes of documentation:

- Accountability for actual intervention and time spent with client.
- A method of recording results of evaluation, intervention, and re-evaluation.
- A method for recording and measuring progress, status of client's condition, and response to intervention.
- Documentation is a legal requirement.
- Documentation is required in order to see progress and validate reimbursement by third-party payers.
- Documentation is an ethical responsibility of health care professionals.
- A baseline of function will be documented.
- Continuity of care is provided through proper documentation.

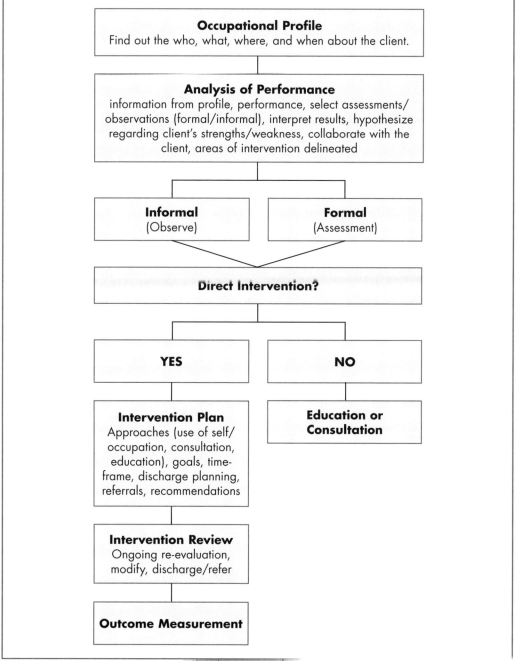

Figure 1-2. Decision tree for occupational process (adapted from American Occupational Therapy Association. [2002]. Occupational therapy practice framework. *American Journal of Occupational Therapy*, 56[6], 609-639).

- Documentation is a communication tool for any potential audience.
- Documentation provides a permanent record of occurrences.
- Documentation allows for emphasis on observable, measurable changes in progress.

- Appropriate documentation may communicate meaningful and functional outcomes.
- Documentation provides a chronological sequence—paints a picture of what occurs from beginning to end of session in a "clinically sound sequence" (Sames, 2005).
- Appropriate documentation will demonstrate clinical reasoning—intervention methods/tools are chosen with a specific strategy and outcome in mind.
- Documentation informs other team members of the specifics of each intervention session and allows a smooth transition into the next session. In addition, in the event that the assigned therapist is unable to work with the same client, documentation should be specific and descriptive enough for the covering therapist to easily conduct the session.
- Documentation demonstrates the effectiveness of occupational therapy intervention.
- Documentation may be used for legal issues such as evidence in court cases.
- Documentation provides data for research and education.

Important Considerations of Documentation

Good documentation skills are developed over time and close supervision/training (Crepeau et al, 2003). It is important to consider **who** will read your documentation. Therefore, *words must be chosen carefully* (Sames, 2005). Remember, it is not only other OTs who will read the documentation. Potential audiences may include (Aquaviva, 1998):

- Other team members.
- Peers.
- Peer reviewers.
- Accrediting agencies such as Joint Commission on Accreditation of Health care Organizations (JCAHO) and Commission on Accreditation of Rehabilitation Facilities (CARF).
- Insurance companies/third-party payers.
- Client/family.
- Administrators.
- Lawyers.
- Researchers.
- Any other chart reviewers.

General Guidelines for Documentation

Documentation should be completed in a timely manner, not only because it is easy to forget the details of every client on a caseload, but also to provide up-to-date information on your client. For example, the client may have demonstrated new safety issues or recent progress in therapy. The next individual working with the client needs to know this information for safe and appropriate interventions and interactions. The therapist must demonstrate good time management skills, allowing for appropriate documentation time for each client. Typically, the last 5 minutes of an intervention session is used for documentation (Sames, 2005). This does not include the time required for documentation of initial evaluations, weekly reassessments, and/or discharge summaries. Typically, documentation is entered into the progress section of the client's chart/medical record.

Additional guidelines include the following:

- Be accurate and collect accurate information.
- Be complete.
- Use proper spelling and grammar.
- Be concise and clear.
- Avoid jargon. Jargon includes words that are typically understood by one discipline or group of professionals such as "compensatory techniques" or "minimal set-up." Unacceptable abbreviations should also be avoided (Sames, 2005).
- Avoid arrows, hyphens, etc.
- Be careful with buzzwords and "red flag" words. Buzzwords are considered to be popular or currently-used words such as "collaborative" or "active" learning. The problem is that these terms may be unfamiliar to some audiences and may become unpopular over time. Red flag are terms that may, for example, put reimbursement of services in jeopardy. These words include "maintain" and "continued" (Sames, 2005).
- "If it is not documented, it did not happen/exist!!!" (Sames, 2005).
- Timely for accuracy of memory and not take away from time with client
- "Paint a verbal picture" (Sames, 2005).
- Focus on function, underlying cause, progress, and safety (Aquaviva, 1998).
- State expectations for progress, slow, or lack of progress (Aquaviva, 1998).
- Summarize needed skilled services (Aquaviva, 1998).

When to document:

- Upon admit.
- Daily.
- Weekly.
- Monthly formal re-evaluation.
- When change occurs, with progress, or lack of progress.
- Medical changes/complications, client placed "on hold" for therapy.
- When physician needs information.
- Discharge summary: show barriers to progress or effectiveness of intervention.

Note basics:

- Think about what you will write before doing it (students should do rough drafts on field-work until cleared by supervisors).
- Sign and date.
- Check for grammatical/spelling errors.
- Use blue/black pen—no erasing.
- Errors are neatly crossed out ed a single line and "error, initials, and date" is written next to the error.
- Limit use of abbreviations—only use accepted ones.
- Write legibly, including signature (or print name underneath/beside).

Documentation Standards

The AOTA (2004) standards for documentation recommend the following components of documentation (Sames, 2005):

- *Client Identification*: This includes the client's name and medical record number on each page of documentation.
- *Date and type of contact*: Each type of documentation should always be dated. Occasionally, it is also required to state the time of day and length of session provided. A heading should be given for the type of contact, such as a screening or evaluation.
- *Type of documentation*: The name of the department (OT/Rehab, etc) should be given as well as clearly delineated type of documentation, such as a SOAP note.
- *Signature/countersignature*: The practitioner must legibly sign his/her name followed by the professional title (e.g., OTR/L). Room must be left for any required countersignatures, such as for students. Signatures should be placed at the end of the documentation.
- *Terminology*: Only facility-accepted, professionally-recognized terminology and abbreviations should be used.
- *Corrections*: Errors should be corrected by drawing a line through the word(s), initialing by the error, and dated. Only blue or black ink should be used. No erasable pens or correction liquid should be accepted.
- *Confidentiality and handling of records*: All official rules and regulations for confidentiality, storage, and disposal of records must be followed.

Documentation Process

1. Screening: Chart review and actual screen.

2. Evaluation: Use of assessment tools such as: interview/profile, observation, standardized/nonstandardized formats, synthesize results.

3. Planning Intervention: Setting of collaborative goals, select approaches, methods, tools, and strategies.

4. Service delivery: How intervention is delivered and implemented.

5. *Monitoring progress*: Re-evaluate and adapt plan.

6. *Discharge therapy*: Maintenance program and follow-up plans (Trombly & Radomski, 2002).

Types and Formats of Documentation

The type and format of documentation used will depend upon the setting in which the services take place. For example, many community-based settings do not have formal client charts or computerized systems of documentation. The facility may only have a folder that is considered the client's record. The documentation approach may also vary, depending upon the team approach. For example, with a transdisciplinary approach to intervention where the health care team's responsibilities are blurred, the contributors to the documentation process may not be the same with each session. This documentation may take a very formal format, such as a daily subjective, objective, assessment, and plan (SOAP) note or a less formal approach, such as a weekly narrative note, depending upon the third-party payer. A second example is Medicare as a third-party payer. The multidisciplinary approach to documentation typically involves standardized forms such as the Minimum Data Set (MDS) and the 701 form. For the most part, the type of documentation used is driven by the third-party payer, the intervention setting, and the client population (Crepeau et al, 2003).

SPECIFIC TYPES OF DOCUMENTATION

Screening Note

A **screening note** is a quick hands-off chart review, interview, and observation of client in order to determine if full evaluation is needed. No referral or billing is required. Brief contact note or specific screening form documented to either state further evaluation not recommended or request for referral and evaluation.

Contact Note

A **contact note** is a brief narrative note containing the time spent with the client, the reason, and the type of screening, such as (Trombly & Radomski, 2002):

- To communicate the referral was received, evaluation/discharge note completed, or reasons why not completed.
- To document screenings.
- Documenting all contacts with client and family.
- Missed sessions/refusals.
- To state the evaluation was completed.
- Equipment given/splint fabricated and instructions issued.
- Any other pertinent issues that may occur between intervention sessions. For example, if a client is observed to have a significant safety issue, such as a fall when a practitioner happens to be walking by the room, the details of the event and how this was handled must be documented.

Formats for Contact Notes

- *Evaluation report*: After the physician referral is received, the therapist may be begin the process of gathering data through documentation review, observation, interview, and full hands-on assessments. Data is interpreted, documented, goals set with timeframe, and intervention plan/recommendations communicated. Precautions and contraindications are highlighted along with the client's goals/expectations. The report is documented on an evaluation sheet (Trombly & Radomski, 2002).

- *Intervention/progress note*: The documentation of the actual intervention session may take many forms as discussed later in this section. The practitioner will also objectively discuss the amount of assistance required to complete tasks, as well as the instructions and cuing needed. The assessment of the session may include documentation of the client's response to intervention and overall participation in therapy. A summary of progress towards goals with updates of goals and plan are documented (Trombly & Radomski, 2002). Typical components of the intervention may include:
  - The date.
  - Type of interventions: The practitioner will list the methods, modalities, group/individual, strategies, activities, adaptive equipment and/or techniques used during the session.
  - Length of session.
  - Progress toward goals with updates and changes, as appropriate.
  - Client's response to intervention.
  - Comparison with previous reports and status.
  - Timeframe changes and recommendations.
  - Equipment recommendations.
  - Home program.
  - Caregiver instruction.
  - Plan/discharge recommendations with revised goals and plan, as appropriate.
- *Re-evaluation report/note*: As evaluation is an ongoing process, it is very much interwoven within each intervention session. As such, the practitioner is informally re-evaluating on a continuous basis. Formal re-evaluations, and the forms used to complete them, will be conducted according to the facility's policy, as well as third-party payer needs. Re-evaluations may include:
  - Data recorded and reported regarding reassessment.
  - Comparative analysis of findings and summary.
  - Modification of goals.
  - Update plan.
  - Need for discharge.
- *Discharge note/discontinuation summary*: Discharge from therapy may be due to the client achieving set goals or maximum benefits of therapy, insurance caps, or the client refusing to participate in therapy. The summary involves a "review of occupational therapy assessment, intervention, and outcome" (Trombly & Radomski, 2002). It may take various formats including a specific discharge form that may be created by the facility/program. The documentation summarizes the client's evaluation/intervention processes from beginning to end. Components of a discharge note should include:
  - The beginning and ending date of services.
  - The therapy process/summary of intervention strategies.
  - Re-evaluation, goal status, attainment, progress in therapy, why goals not achieved.
  - Functional outcome of services.
  - Number of completed sessions (Trombly & Radomski, 2002).
  - Home programs, maintenance programs, and caregiver instructions.
  - Recommendations/equipment needed.
  - Follow-up plans and/or referrals for continued occupational therapy as well as other services in the continuum of care.

➢ The "client's assessment of efficacy of occupational therapy" (AOTA, 2003; Sames, 2005).

- *M.D. report*: Often reports are sent to the physician regarding the client's progress either on a monthly basis or with each scheduled visit. The format of the report depends upon where the client is within the intervention process. For example, if the client is seeing the physician at a time for re-evaluation, this format may be used. If the client is close to discharge time, the particular note may be used. Certain physicians may have a specific format that he/she requires/desires.

FORMATS OF DOCUMENTATION

SOAP Note

The SOAP note is a very well known form of progress note. The acronym represents the four components of the note: the *subjective, objective, assessment, and plan*. This format provides a consistent structure for all disciplines to follow. The format also allows for a quick review of the client's status prior to intervention. The structure allows the therapist to follow trends and patterns that may occur during the intervention process, which makes the SOAP format very interdisciplinary in nature.

Details of a SOAP Note

- *S=Subjective*: This is the client's report/perceptions of the problem, which are often documented as a quotation such as: "Client stated..." or, "client reported...".

- *O=Objective*: The objective section consists of factual or professional information that is confirmed or validated by the therapist. Baseline data and/or progress on goals, observations, and client performance may be included. The information is often presented in a chronological or story format. The data is not interpreted here. Hints for beginning the objective section may be: Client was seen for... or, the intervention consisted of... Then, the chronological listing of the interventions participated in are listed.

- *A=Assessment*: The assessment is directly related to the subjective and objective sections. The therapist's professional opinion and analysis are documented. This analysis includes: clarification of client goals and problems, and therapist's ratings of client progress. In this section, the subjective and objective data may be interpreted and a prioritized list of problems to be addressed developed.

- *P=Plan*: The plan section specifies the type, frequency, and duration of interventions to use in next session and/or in response to progress or lack of. Updated goals may be listed here. This section also includes discharge plans and home programs, as appropriate. Specifically, this section should provide enough information for a substituting therapist to take over the next session, if needed.

Example of a SOAP Note

- S: "My right shoulder hurts only when I sleep on it."

- O: Intervention consisted of: Heat pack to right shoulder for 10 minutes; Bilateral assitive active range of motion (AAROM) exercises including towel and dowel exercises, 15 repetitions/2 sets; Client donned bra and shirt with moderate assist for right upper extremity (RUE). Client replaced clean clothes on low shelves of closet with minimal (a), ice pack placed on right shoulder for 5 minutes at end of session. During activity, client's pain assessed at right shoulder 6/10 (on a scale of 0 to 10).

- A: Despite level of pain, client appeared happy with today's progress with AROM and ADLs. Client seems to have a high tolerance for pain and occasionally requires cues to not push herself too hard.

- P: Educate client on pain management techniques such as visualization. Educate client on alternative positioning when sleeping to decrease shoulder pain. Increase AAROM to 20 repetitions, as tolerated. Attempt above ADL activities with no assistance, as tolerated.

DAP Note

The DAP note format is very similar to the SOAP note. The acronym represents the three components of the note: *description, assessment, and plan*. This format also provides a consistent structure for all disciplines to follow, although it is not used as frequently. Similarly to the SOAP note, the interdisciplinary format also allows for a quick review and the ability to follow trends and patterns.

Details of a DAP Note

- *D=Description*: This is the findings section of the note, which combines the Subjective and Objective components of the SOAP note. This section documents quotes or paraphrases regarding the client's perceptions, description of the session, observations, results/findings, and facts.

- *A=Assessment*: This section documents exactly the same information as in the Assessment section of the SOAP note.

- *P=Plan*: This section documents exactly the same information as in the Plan section of the SOAP note.

Example of DAP Note (Adapted From Above SOAP Note)

- D: "My right shoulder hurts only when I sleep on it." The intervention consisted of: Heat pack to right shoulder for 10 minutes; Bilateral AAROM exercises including towel and dowel exercises, 15 repetitions/2 sets; and client donned bra and shirt with moderate assist for RUE. Client replaced clean clothes on low shelves of closet with minimal (a), ice pack placed on right shoulder for 5 minutes at end of session. During activity, client's pain assessed at right shoulder 6/10 (on a scale of 0 to 10).

- A: Despite level of pain, client appeared happy with today's progress with AROM and ADLs. Client seems to have a high tolerance for pain and occasionally requires cues to not push herself too hard.

- P: Educate client on pain management techniques such as visualization. Educate client on alternative positioning when sleeping to decrease shoulder pain. Increase AAROM to 20 repetitions, as tolerated. Attempt above ADL activities with no assistance, as tolerated.

Narrative Note

The narrative notes do not have a specific structure like SOAP and DAP notes. This format typically begins with objective data, follows with interpretive/assessment information, and ends with a review of objectives met as well as plans for next session. This narrative note also tells a story that allows for more flexibility in communicating information. The writer is responsible for including all information in a smooth, flowing note, with as much detail as needed. The SOAP or DAP note can be easily converted to a narrative format (Sames, 2005).

Example of Narrative Note (Adapted From Above SOAP Note)

Today, the client stated she is experiencing right shoulder pain when sleeping on it. She was seen for: Heat pack to right shoulder for 10 minutes; Bilateral AAROM exercises including towel

Table 1-2

SAMPLE DOCUMENTATION FORM

Client Name	Date	Date	Date	Date
Heat Pack	Time and body part			
Therapeutic Exercise	Body part(s), exercises, repetitions, sets			
Physical Agent Modalities	Modality used, intensity, duration, other settings			
ADL activities	Activity, level of assistance needed, adaptive equipment			
Client Education	Topic and materials issued			
Ice Pack	Time and body part			

Adapted from American Occupational Therapy Association. (2002). Occupational therapy practice framework. *American Journal of Occupational Therapy, 56* (6), 609-639.

and dowel exercises, 15 repetitions/2 sets; and client donned bra and shirt with moderate assist for RUE. The client replaced clean clothes on low shelves of closet with minimal (a), ice pack placed on right shoulder for 5 minutes at end of session. During activity, the client was assessed for right shoulder pain 6/10 (on a scale of 0 to 10). Despite her level of pain, the client appeared happy with today's progress with AROM and ADL. She seems to have a high tolerance for pain and occasionally requires cues to not push herself too hard. The next session should provide client education on pain management techniques such as visualization and on alternative positioning when sleeping to decrease shoulder pain. If tolerated, increase AAROM to 20 repetitions. Also, if tolerated, attempt above ADL activities with no assistance.

Flow Sheet/Checklist

There are several advantages to using flow sheets when documenting. These include a concise format for tracking progress, allowing for a quick look at the documentation, much data is compiled in a small space, and the format allows for easy coverage of the client's care, if needed. Flow sheets may also include formatting data with graphs, tables, and charts.

The disadvantages of a flow sheet/checklist primarily involve the limited space for documenting any psychiatric issues, descriptions, or client reactions that are necessary for holistic client-centered interventions. This format cannot replace progress notes that should also be completed on a weekly, biweekly, or as-needed basis. A basic example of a flow sheet for an outpatient setting (based on the above example) can be found in Table 1-2.

Computerized Forms

Many large facilities are now using computers for documentation of evaluations, interventions, and discharge summaries. Any of the above formats may be used when creating computer programs for documentation.

Documentation Examples

- *Screening*: Contact, SOAP note, DAP note, narrative note, or screening form created. Frequency: Typically one time with possible follow-up as needed.

- *Contact*: Narrative note, checklist/flow sheet (Trombly & Radomski, 2002). Frequency: Depends on purpose of note.

- *Evaluation*: Standardized/nonstandardized forms. Frequency: One formal evaluation.

- *Intervention*: SOAP note, DAP note, narrative note, flow sheet/checklist, or computerized forms. Frequency: Depending upon format(s) used may be daily, weekly, or monthly.

- *Re-evaluation*: Standardized/nonstandardized forms, SOAP note, DAP note, or narrative note.

- *M.D. Report*: SOAP note, DAP note, narrative note, or re-evaluation format. Frequency: Written on-appointment-basis, monthly, or upon discharge.

- *Discharge summary*: Discharge summary form, re-evaluation form, narrative note. Frequency: Upon discharge (Trombly & Radomski, 2002).

WRITING GOALS

Effective goal writing is a vital component of the evaluation and intervention processes. It is a collaborative process that includes the therapist, COTA, client, and family/caregivers. The purpose of goal-setting is to measure the effectiveness of the chosen interventions (Sames, 2005). In addition, goal writing serves to indicate changes in baseline skills that are expected to occur as the result of the intervention plan.

The specific goal writing methods used depend upon the frames of reference chosen, the intervention setting, the types of outcomes anticipated (Moyers, 1999), as well as the intervention approach in the *Framework* (2002). This section will discuss these specifics mentioned above.

Considerations when writing goals:

- Goals should be created in collaboration with client/family.

- Consider the client's present condition or diagnosis.

- Consider the client's limitations and strengths.

- Does the client have any complications secondary to his/her conditions?

- Client's past medical history, precautions, and prognosis.

- What is the facility, environment, or setting in which therapy will occur?

- What is the client's discharge environment?

- What is the timeline for therapy?

- Are there any clinical pathways, standards, protocols when working with this client?

- What frames of reference will be followed?

- Does the client have insurance? What is the client's insurance? Are there any insurance limitations? Is the client paying?
- What are the desired outcomes of therapy?
- What is the predicted length of stay for this client?
- What are the considered continuum of care and discharge plans/options for this client?
- What are the client's/family's needs and goals?

General Types of Goals (Sames, 2005)

REMEDIATIVE/RESTORATIVE/REHABILITATIVE

This type of goal is used when a client no longer can perform task due to an illness or injury. The goals are written to change a functional level or achieve a stated function. *For example, within 2 weeks, the client will toilet herself independently while using the dominant upper extremity.*

HABILITATIVE

This type of goal attempts to teach a client new skills that were never taught previously. Often, this type of goal is used with clients who have developmental delays. *For example, by the end of the school year, the client will be able to participate in physical education for 15 minutes at a time.*

MAINTENANCE

This type of goal is used when the client has not demonstrated further progress in therapy. Maintenance attempts to sustain the client at the present level of function without losing gains. This approach to goal writing is typically used in long-term settings and upon discharge from therapy. *For example, upon discharge from therapy, the client will continue to be independent in her assisted living situation.*

MODIFICATION/COMPENSATION/ADAPTATION

This type of goal adapts the context, environment, or the tools regarding the activity, instead of changing the client's abilities. *For example, within 1 week, the client will independently don socks with the use of a sock aide.*

PREVENTATIVE

This type of goal addresses potential "at risk" issues with occupational performance. *For example, the client will demonstrate three proper body mechanic techniques when caring for her child, within 3 weeks.*

HEALTH PROMOTION

This type of goal may be used more frequently in emerging practice areas. The emphasis of this approach is on enhancing contexts and activities in order to enable maximize occupational participation. Goals may be addressed with clients individually, in a group, a community, or organization. *For example, within 1 month, all students of Anytown Elementary School will be educated by the OT in proper body mechanics when wearing backpacks.*

These types of goals actually parallel the Occupational Therapy Intervention Approaches, as listed in Table 7 of the *Framework* document (AOTA, 2002). Therefore, the goal-writing process will guide the choice and process of the interventions. Before beginning intervention, it is important to consider the goal-writing and intervention approaches.

Formats and Methods of Goal Writing

There are many formats or guides for writing goals. Generally, goals involve the "who, what, where, and when" approach. The *who* is typically the client and/or caregiver involved in the goal/ intervention. The *what* is the occupational performance skill or behavior to be addressed. The *where* may be included to state the environment in which the behavior or skill will occur. The *when* may be included to address the time of day when the skill or behavior will be addressed.

Action words or *verbs* should be used when writing goals to describe the client's behavior or skill to be addressed. Action words include: bathes, dresses, eats, walks, reaches, and zippers.

Goals must be measurable, observable, and functional. They must describe a change in the client's occupational performance skill or behavior, how much (*measurable*) the behavior will change, and how this behavior will be measured. The ultimate intent in goal writing is to measure to show progress.

When considering the functional aspect/functional outcomes of goal writing, it is important to consider relating the goal to meaningful, purposeful aspects of the client's life. This is achieved through a collaborative approach with the client. Functional goals may include those that enhance occupational performance, improve skills, improve role performance, promote health and wellness, prevent dysfunction, and/or improve quality of life.

Five Kinds of Functional Goal Outcomes

1. Occupational performance

2. Prevention

3. General health

4. Satisfaction

5. Quality of life (Moyers, 1999)

More specifically, there are several formal methods that guide goal writing. One will be described in the following.

ABCD METHOD

The ABCD method of writing goals was developed by Ginge Kettenbach (1990). Each letter describes a specific component included in each client-centered goal.

- A: The **audience** is typically the client, although in certain circumstances, the goal may be specific to the caregiver. (This text refers to the audience as the "client." Depending upon the facility/environment, the audience may be referred to as the "patient," the "consumer," or the "student.")

- B: The **behavior** is specifically what is expected of the audience. Sames (2005) describes the behavior as something that is seen, heard, done, or said. The behavior represents an action such as dressing, bathing, eating, speaking, or walking. The choice of words in the goal-writing should represent these actions.

- C: The **conditions** are specific circumstances under which behavior must occur, support the behavior, clarify the goal, or state how much cuing or assistance is needed (Sames, 2005). For example, the client may need minimal assistance to feed himself or maximal verbal cuing for safety in the shower.

- D: The **degree** represents the measurement component of the goal. In order for a goal to be measurable, it must include a realistic, specific timeframe and a duration, frequency, percentage, or degree that quantifies the amount of function the client will attempt to achieve.

Sample Goal Using ABCD Method

Within 2 weeks (**degree**), the client (**audience**) will independently (**degree**) feed herself (**behavior**) using an adapted fork and spoon (**condition**).

Specific Types of Goals

The two specific types of goals are long-term goals (LTG) and short-term goals (STG). LTG tend to be more global in nature and generally address occupational performance. Most often, only one LTG is written in order to set the stage for the STG. The duration of a LTG is typically set to discharge time or the time when therapy will end. Although LTG are measurable, observable, and functional, they again tend to be more general in nature.

Examples:

- Client will achieve full independence in order to be discharged to live alone at home in 4 weeks.
- Client will complete a 4-hour workday, independently, within 4 weeks.

STG are often referred to as objectives. The duration of STG is typically shorter and they are very specific in nature, particularly in terms of being measurable, observable, and functional. STG address occupational performance areas *or* components and are written in order to be up- or downgraded as the client's functional abilities change. Typically, multiple STG are written that directly relate back to the LTG. STG should also have functional outcomes.

Examples:

- Client will attend to a group task for 30 minutes with only one verbal cue for redirection in order to prepare for return to work within 2 weeks.
- Client will complete upper extremity (UE) dressing with min (a) using reacher and sock aide within 2 weeks in order to live alone.
- Client will increase RUE shoulder flexion by 40 degrees within 2 weeks in order to complete ADLs.
- Client will ambulate to bathroom, using rolling walker and contact guard within 2 weeks in order to return home.

PROGRESS LEVELS

- Total assistance (dependence)=Client does 0%.
- Maximum assistance=Client does 25%.
- Moderate assistance=Client does 50%.
- Minimum assistance=Client does 75%.
- Standby assistance=Client does 100% (I) and has supervision.
- Independent status=(I).
- Contact guard.
- Close supervision.
- Distant supervision.
- Different types of cuing (Trombly & Radomski, 2002).

LEGAL CONSIDERATIONS

- Accuracy.
- Completeness.
- Timeliness.
- Gaps in documentation/blanks.
- Objectivity.
- Corrections/erasing.
- Negative statements.
- Sufficient MD orders.
- Possible denials of payment.
- Tamper-free.
- Client can see their records.
- You cannot alter them later.
- Include date and time.
- Legible signature.
- Confidentiality.
- **Health Insurance Portability and Accountability Act** (HIPAA).
- Abbreviations.
- Document correspondence and teaching sessions.
- Grammar/spelling.
- Fraud/plagiarism (Aquaviva, 1998).

CONFIDENTIALITY ISSUES

- Do not take work home with client's name.
- Permission from client to use/share.
- Right to see.
- HIPAA.
- **Family Educational Rights and Privacy Act** (FERPA).
- Storage of documents (Aquaviva, 1998).

COMMON MISTAKES IN DOCUMENTATION

- Failure to state affected body part or side of body.
- Failure to state actual motion.
- Failure to put in measurable terms.

- Failure to attach time frame.
- Failure to use functional outcome.
- Failure to include functional activities.

Summary Questions

1. Describe the *Occupational Therapy Practice Framework* as if to another health care professional.
2. Name and discuss the components of the evaluation and intervention processes.
3. Discuss the general differences between the approaches to intervention.
4. Discuss the components of the documentation process in occupational therapy intervention.
5. Discuss the "bottom-up" approach to intervention.

References

American heritage dictionary of the english language (4th ed.). (2000). Boston: Houghton Mifflin.

American Occupational Therapy Association. (1995). Elements of clinical documentation (revision). *American Journal of Occupational Therapy, 47,* 1087-1099.

American Occupational Therapy Association. (2002). Occupational therapy practice framework. *American Journal of Occupational Therapy, 56*(6), 609-639.

American Occupational Therapy Association. (2004). *The reference manual of the official documents of the American Occupational Therapy Association* (10th ed.). Bethesda, MD: AOTA.

Aquaviva, J. D. (Ed.). (1998). *Effective documentation for occupational therapy* (2nd ed.). Bethesda, MD: AOTA.

Bruce, M. A. G., & Borg, B. A. (2002). *Psychosocial frames of reference* (3rd ed.). Thorofare, NJ: SLACK Incorporated.

Christiansen, C., & Baum, C. (1997). *Occupational therapy: Enabling function and well-being* (2nd ed.). Thorofare, NJ: SLACK Incorporated.

Cole, M. (1998). *Group dynamics in occupational therapy* (2nd ed.). Thorofare, NJ: SLACK Incorporated.

Crepeau, E. B., Cohn, E. S., & Schell, B. A. (2003). *Willard and Spackman's occupational therapy for physical dysfunction* (10th ed.). Philadelphia: Lippincott Williams & Wilkins.

Gibson, J. W., & Schkade, J. K. (1997). Occupational adaptation intervention with patients with cerebrovascular accident: a clinical study. *American Journal of Occupational Therapy, 51*(7), 523-529.

Fisher, A. G. (2002). A model for planning and implementing top-down client-centered, and occupation-based occupational therapy intereventions. Short course presented at University of New Hampshire.

Jacobs, K., & Jacobs, L. (2004). *Quick reference dictionary for occupational therapy* (4th ed.). Thorofare, NJ: SLACK Incorporated.

Kettenbach, G. (1990). *Writing SOAP notes.* Philadelphia: F.A. Davis.

Kielhofner, G., & Burke, J. P. (1980). A model of human occupation, Part I: Conceptual framework and content. *American Journal of Occupational Therapy, 34*(9), 572-581.

Kielhofner, G. (1995). *A model of human occupation: Theory and application.* (2nd ed.) Baltimore: Williams and Wilkins.

Law, M., Cooper, B., Strong, S., Stewart, D., Rigby, P., & Letts, L. (1996). The person-environment-occupation model: A transactive approach to occupational performance. *Canadian Journal of Occupational Therapy, 63,* 9-23.

Law, M. (1998). *Client-centered occupational therapy.* Thorofare, NJ: SLACK Incorporated.

Law, M. (2002). *Evidence-based rehabilitation: A guide to practice.* Thorofare, NJ: SLACK Incorporated.

Law, M., Baum, C., & Dunn, W. (2005). *Measuring occupational performance* (2nd ed.). Thorofare, NJ: SLACK Incorporated.

Mann, W. C., Llanes, C., Justiss, M. D., & Tomita, M. (2004). Frail older adults' self-report of their most important assistive device. *Occupational Therapy Journal of Research, 24*(1), 4-14.

Moyers, P. (1999). The guide to occupational therapy practice. *American Journal of Occupational Therapy, 53,* 247-322.

Reed, K. (2001). *Quick reference to occupational therapy* (2nd ed.). Gaithersburg, MD: Aspen Publishers.

Sames, K. (2005). *Documenting occupational therapy practice.* Upper Saddle River, NJ: Pearson/Prentice Hall.

Schultz, S., & Schkade, J. K. (1992a). Occupational adaptation: Toward a holistic approach for contemporary practice, part 1. *American Journal of Occupational Therapy, 46*(9), 829-837.

Schultz, S., & Schkade, J. K. (1992b). Occupational adaptation: Toward a holistic approach for contemporary practice, part 2. *American Journal of Occupational Therapy, 46*(10), 917-925.

Toglia, J. (1991). Generalization of intervention: A multicontext approach to cognitive perceptual impairment in adults with brain injury. *American Journal of Occupational Therapy, 45*(6), 505-516.

Trombly, C. A., & Radomski, M. V. (Eds.). (2002). *Occupational therapy for physical dysfunction* (5th ed.). Philadelphia, PA: Lippincott, Williams & Wilkins.

Yerxa, E. J. (1998). Health and human spirit of occupation. *American Journal of Occupational Therapy, 52,* 412-418.

Zoltan, B. (1996). *Vision, perception, and cognition* (3rd ed.). Thorofare, NJ: SLACK Incorporated.

2 Foundational Skills for Functional Activities

Deanna Proulx-Sepelak, MHA, OTR/L

CHAPTER OBJECTIVES

By the end of this chapter, the student will be able to:

- ☑ Comprehend the **underlying or foundational skills** an individual requires to successfully engage in functionally meaningful tasks.
- ☑ Describe specific **theories/frames of reference** as related to foundational skills.
- ☑ Comprehend **safety issues** as related to foundational skills.
- ☑ Delineate between the role of the **occupational therapist** (OT) and the **occupational therapy assistant** (OTA) as they pertain to foundational skills.
- ☑ Comprehend and identify related **psychological implications** as related to impairments in foundational skills.
- ☑ Comprehend the impact of **modes of injury** upon foundational skills.
- ☑ Identify **remedial techniques** for impairments in specific foundational skills.
- ☑ Identify general activities of daily living (ADLs) **maintenance** strategies that incorporate foundational skills.
- ☑ Identify general precautions and contraindications for various foundational skill interventions such as Physical Agent Modalities (PAMs) and therapeutic exercise.

CHAPTER OVERVIEW

The goal of this chapter is to outline the underlying skills that an individual requires to successfully engage in functionally meaningful tasks. These foundational skills, in the order that they are presented within this chapter, include pain and edema, sensation, joint range of motion (ROM), strength, endurance, coordination, muscle tone, and skills of cognition and perception. Material within this chapter is presented using a focus on remedial approaches. Subsequent chapters within the text will then analyze the adaptive/compensatory approaches as related to the specific Areas of Occupation outlined by the *Occupational Therapy Practice Framework* document (*Framework*) (American Occupational Therapy Association [AOTA], 2002).

As a precursor to this chapter, it is important to reiterate the collaborative relationship that exists between the registered OT and the certified OTA. As health care becomes increasingly driven by the efficient utilization of resources, many rehabilitative establishments are trending towards the use of registered OTs as evaluative administrators and OTAs as both collaborators in developing the client-centered intervention plan, as well as actual facilitators of that plan given appropriate supervision. This chapter is written using "OT" as a general term and with full reference to both OTs and OTAs as vital components of the rehabilitative team.

How do remedial approaches differ from those of a compensatory focus? Remediation, per the *Framework* document, is "an intervention approach designed to change client variables to establish a skill or ability which has not yet developed or to restore a skill or ability which has been impaired" (AOTA, 2002, p. 627). This definition is further simplified by Thomas in *Tabers' Medical Dictionary* (1997) as those techniques implemented with the "intention of remedy" or to "cure and relieve disease (or illness)." In general, approaches considered remedial are those that OTs implement with the goal of curing an underlying impairment, while those approaches considered compensatory in nature are implemented by OTs with the intent of adapting to an underlying condition or deficit that has been deemed long-standing.

According to Zoltan (1996), intervention takes one of two forms: a *top-down or bottom-up approach*. With a top-down approach (refer to Chapter 1), the OT adjusts the activity or occupational performance with the goal of promoting independence by using adaptive and compensatory techniques. Conversely, the bottom-up approach addresses underlying dysfunction in the foundation skill areas and assumes that the client will improve in functional ability as a result. An example of the concept of remediation is as follows: The OT may conduct an ADL session with a client who demonstrates deficits in the areas of coordination, strength, ROM, and cognition. Here, the OT is fostering improvement in the foundational skills through repetition in a familiar task, not adapting the task as one would in a compensatory or top-down approach. Remediation, therefore, focuses on the execution of foundational performance skills within the context of personally meaningful activity in order to facilitate a return to maximal independence.

OTs emphasize the importance of the client-centered or client-driven approach. OTs formulate intervention with clients, not for clients. In doing so, it is the OT's responsibility to recognize and respect all clients as individuals with their own personal interests, beliefs, values, habits, roles, and, most importantly, prioritization of the occupations they choose to pursue. This principle reflects the OT's unique ability to recognize the personal contexts in which client occupations occur. The contextual emphasis dictates a client-centered approach for the field of occupational therapy and is outlined more specifically in Chapter 1. The concept of context is re-emphasized here as it relates to attention the OT must pay to effectively compile a remedial intervention plan sensitive to each individual client. Specifically, respect is paid to a client's safety, psychosocial adaptation to illness or injury, and the perception of pain. A clear respect for these areas not only fosters overall well-being in clients, but also contributes to the degree of therapeutic rapport that one is able to achieve with clients during the ever-critical, initial stages of intervention and healing.

As mentioned, OTs must also be considerate of the impact that illness and/or injury has on the client in the context of their personal lives. All clients are individuals with their own personal means of coping and adaptation to a life-altering event such as illness or injury. This process occurs at differing levels and time frames for each client. As outlined by Falvo in *Medical and Psychosocial Aspects of Chronic Illness and Disability* (2005), "Some actively confront their condition, learning new skills or actively engaging in intervention to control or manage the condition. Others defend themselves from stress and the realities of the diagnosis by denying its seriousness, ignoring intervention recommendations, or refusing to learn new skills... Still others cope by engaging in self-destructive behavior... Which has detrimental effects on their physical condition" (p. 4). In all, OTs must respect that this process of acceptance is occurring during the intervention process, must be sensitive to it, and whenever possible, provide education and advocacy to support clients and their families or caregivers.

The OT will then develop the intervention plan both in collaboration with the client and with careful attention paid to the specific aspects of any given activity that enables success in the execution of occupation. The *Framework* (AOTA, 2002) identifies this as **Activity Demands**. Of significance to the discussion on foundational skills for functional activity is the manner in which activity demand aspects are categorized. This includes such items as required actions, body functions, and body structures. Required actions are defined by the *Framework* document as "the usual skills that would be required by any performer to carry out the activity" (2002, p. 624). These include physical motor skills, process or cognitive skills, and communication skills. Required body functions are defined as "the physiological functions of body systems ... required to support the actions used to perform the activity" (2002, p. 624). And required body structures are "anatomical parts of the body such as organs, limbs, and their components (which support body function)" (2002, p. 624). In essence, these three aforementioned aspects of activity demands per the *Framework* (2002) identify specifically those underlying, foundational skills necessary for the engagement in all meaningful activity. It is here we will focus the attention of this chapter.

Each foundation skills subsection within this chapter specifically presents any applicable and related definitions, potential modes of injury, or illness that may lead to a deficit in that foundation skill area, and typical occupational therapy remediation techniques for improving that skill. Diagrams, figures, and tables are provided as a means of summarizing data within each subsection. In addition, special considerations and possible maintenance program components have been included.

REMEDIAL TECHNIQUES FOR PAIN AND EDEMA

The consideration of individually-perceived pain for each of our clients is critical to the success an OT will have during the remedial or healing stage of recovery. In most cases, the degree of perceived pain will present one of the greatest enablers or barriers to the degree of success a client will experience during the rehabilitative process. Remedial intervention generally begins just after an injury or onset of illness, and as a result, much of our intervention choices may further aggravate the degree of discomfort our clients experience. Therefore, the OT must prioritize pain management within the development of the intervention plan, making it a foundational skill for functional activity within the context of this textbook.

Pain is notoriously difficult to measure accurately. This is due to the subjective nature in which our clients report it; a symptom experienced internally by our clients may not necessarily be observed externally by the therapist. Although clients may be asked to report their pain using the traditional rating scale method, it is the therapist's ethical duty to establish priority of that identified pain and infuse strategies that address them in the daily, weekly, or even monthly intervention sessions. These strategies should not only allow clients an avenue to openly express perceived pain, but also to include techniques within the realm of occupational therapy that allow for the management and relief of the pain.

Definitional Analysis

Pain is defined by the *Framework* (AOTA, 2002) as a body function specific to sensation. For further analysis, pain is described in *Taber's Cyclopedic Medical Dictionary* (1997) as "an unpleasant sensory and emotional experience arising from actual or potential tissue damage or described in terms of such damage. Pain includes not only the perception of an uncomfortable stimulus but also the response to that perception" (p. 1387). Through these definitions, one is better able to observe the vastness of pain, not only as a basic body function, but also as a foundational skill required for the successful engagement in all meaningful occupation. For example, the perception or fear of exacerbating pain may inhibit a client's ability to sleep sufficiently (**global mental function**), to attend to others (**specific mental function**), or to produce efficient movement (**neuromusculoskeletal and movement-related functions**). A client's pain may then affect their performance skills including motor skills, process skills, and possibly even communication/interaction skills such as gesturing, posturing, engaging, or expressing oneself. It is through analyzing the specifics of this definition that we are able to recognize the true, potentially devastating affects of our clients' experiences with pain.

Modes of Injury or Illness

A review of the typical modes of injury or illness is not, and should not, be emphasized when discussing pain specifically. Again, pain is a subjectively-perceived sensation with potentially large effects on a client's ability to succeed with occupational therapy intervention. What is of importance is not necessarily the mode from which the pain occurs, but rather, the existence of it.

Pain may exist secondary to a very wide array of health conditions. In many cases, pain perceived by a client is not in isolation, but secondary to another cause such as an injury to the body. Therefore, when considering effective remedial techniques to address pain, the OT will also employ methods that address any potential underlying causes for the pain. Most often, this includes attention to the natural reaction of the body to injury or insult—the inflammatory response or edema.

Remedial techniques for addressing pain and edema are appropriately selected given careful attention to the natural healing process of the human body. As described by Cameron (2003), injuries to tissues require the body system to initiate a repair response. This response calls upon both the vascular and immune systems to reduce loss of blood, accumulate leukocytes and lymphocytes as protective measures, and begin the process of tissue regeneration. This repair response occurs over the period of days to months and directly dictates the type of methods that are appropriate and effective for the OT to implement. Per Bracciano (2000), the initial phase, or *inflammatory phase* of healing, begins immediately following the injury and is characterized by erthromatosis (condition of redness) or cyanosis (blueness of skin), warmth, swelling, and pain at the site of injury. "The normal acute inflammatory process lasts for no more than 2 weeks. If it continues for more than 4 weeks, it is known as *subacute inflammation*" (Cameron, 2003, p. 30). This quotation clearly places a timetable on the healing process and, therefore, acts as a guideline for appropriate method selection when addressing pain and edema in conjunction with the biological healing process.

Conditions typically related to the sudden, or acute, onset of pain and localized edema include fractures, sprains, strains, tears, lacerations, arthritides, and musculoskeletal disorders such as exacerbated lateral epicondylitis or carpal tunnel syndrome. In addition, neurological damage resulting in a lack of motor function may also contribute to edema and pain. Refer to Table 2-1 for a summary of remedial techniques in both the acute or subacute phase of healing as they relate to addressing pain and Table 2-2 for those related specifically to edema.

When symptoms of pain and edema last for greater lengths of time following the onset of injury, they are often considered chronic in nature. Pain or edema that has not been properly addressed in the acute phase, and is further exacerbated by such factors as prolonged immobility and general deconditioning, is often associated with the development of chronic conditions. According to Cameron (2003), "pain persisting beyond what is normally expected of a given condition is considered chronic in nature," while "chronic inflammation is inflammation that lasts for months or years" (p. 30). Conditions that may result in chronic pain or edema include cancers, amputations, fibromyalgia, complex regional pain syndrome, and nerve injuries or entrapments to name a few. Longer-term symptoms associated with multiple exacerbations of arthritis and musculoskeletal disorders, such as lateral epicondylitis or carpal tunnel syndrome, may also be considered chronic in certain circumstances. Therefore, a discussion as to techniques used by OT

Table 2-1

REMEDIAL PAIN TECHNIQUES OF THE BIOMECHANICAL THEORY ACCORDING TO PHASE OF HEALING

Health Condition	*Remedial Techniques per Phase of Healing*
Pain, including soft tissue injuries, fractures, lacerations, sprains, strains, tears, arthritides, musculoskeletal disorders	Acute Phase: Cold thermal modalities, nonthermal ultrasound, splinting for protection, passive range of motion (PROM), active assistive range of motion (AAROM), active range of motion (AROM), iontophoresis.
	Subacute Phase: Hot and/or cold thermal modalities, ultrasound, PROM, AAROM, AROM, manual therapies, phonophoresis, aquatic rehabilitation.

Table 2-2

REMEDIAL EDEMA TECHNIQUES OF THE BIOMECHANICAL THEORY ACCORDING TO PHASE OF HEALING

Health Condition	*Remedial Techniques per Phase of Healing*
Edema, including soft tissue injuries, fractures, lacerations, sprains, strains, tears, arthritides, musculoskeletal disorders.	Acute phase: Cold thermal modalities, nonthermal ultrasound, compression garments, compression pumps, compression wrapping, elevation, PROM, AAROM, AROM.
	Subacute phase: Hot and/or cold thermal modalities, thermal ultrasound, compression garments, compression pumps, compression wrapping, retrograde massage, elevation, PROM, AAROM, AROM, aquatic rehabilitation, manual lymph drainage.

for addressing chronic pain and edema (see Table 2-5) can be found below in the "Maintenance" subheading of this section.

Intervention choices for edema are based not only on whether it is acute or chronic in nature, but also on other contributing factors. As described by Burkhardt, these factors include the cause of the edema (single injury or systemic diagnosis) and other contributing factors, such as blood clots and cardiac function (Gillen & Burkhardt, 2004). The cause of the edema itself will dictate if the intervention approach is localized or generalized and is executed with careful attention paid to potential contributing factors. For a complete list of precautions, see Table 2-22.

Remedial Techniques: Biomechanical Approach

Remedial strategies for pain (Table 2-1) and edema (Table 2-2) are widely based within the Biomechanical Theory and recognize the kinetic and kinematic principles of voluntary movement within of the human body (Pedretti & Early, 2001). Frequently methods implemented within this theory include the use of PAMs.

Physical Agent Modalities

It is important to note that the use of physical agent modalities (PAMs) by OTs is often regulated by state-specific legislation and licensure laws. This legislation is enacted as a means of protected clients from the array of potential contraindications that may arise secondary to the implementation of a PAM. Refer to Tables 2-21 through 2-24 for a summary of the potential indications and contraindications of PAMs most readily employed by the OT. These regulations vary from state to state; some requiring continuing education or certification beyond the competency level required for registration, while others require the prescription of the medical doctor. It is the OT's responsibility to be readily aware of their own governing state's legislature regarding the use of modalities as well as the AOTA's position paper on the use of PAMs in general. The AOTA position paper regarding the use of PAMs is available for purchase from the AOTA (refer to Appendix A for additional contact information). PAMs, as discussed in the content of this chapter, will be outlined in general so as to accurately illustrate this point.

Superficial thermal modalities include the use heat and/or cold for their counteractive effects on injury. Cold modalities, including ice packs, ice baths, and contrast baths are implemented for the purpose of desensitizing pain receptors and minimizing edema in the acute stages of healing. In general, ice packs are applied with one layer of toweling between the ice pack and the client's skin and left in place for 10 to 20 minutes. Ice baths are carried out by submerging the affected extremity in an ice-filled bucket of water (preferably placed on the ground or other stabile surface) for "3 to 5 seconds, repeating 2 to 3 times, causing quick vasomotor restriction" (Gillen, 2004, p. 226). Contrast baths are similar in procedure; however, warm water and ice water are used alternately to further elicit the vasomotor response (Cochrane, 2004). Vapocoolant sprays are also utilized for short term relief pain caused by muscle spasms. When utilizing vapocoolant sprays, a client is typically positioned with the identified muscle on passive stretch or lengthened state. The spray bottle is then inverted and applied 2 to 3 times at a 30-degree angle approximately 45 cm from skin surface in a unidirectional, sweeping motion along the muscle length (Michlovitz, 1996). It should be noted that if either the client or therapist is pregnant, this modality is contraindicated.

Heat modalities tend to be strictly contraindicated in the acute phase, but are implemented widely in the subacute and chronic phases of the healing process. The OT may use commercial hot packs, paraffin wax baths that provide circumferential heating to all surfaces (very popular in subacute arthritis), fluidotherapy (Chattanooga Group, 2005) units in which the extremity is placed and warmed air (also has a nonheated setting) circulate grated corn husks within the enclosure, or ultrasound at a continuous setting to produce the desired effects of heat on subacute or chronic pain and edema. Each of these identified PAMs is applied for the duration of approximately 15 to 20 minutes, and with the use of a protective barrier for the skin, to promote tissue healing (Cameron, 2003).

Iontophoresis (Figure 2-1) is indicated to promote healing, decrease pain, and minimize edema. Under the direction of a physician, this PAM uses electric currents to deliver prescription medications such as corticosteroids (anti-inflammatory) or analgesics (Cameron, 2003) transcutaneously to the direct site of injury. This remedial pain and edema technique is found to be very effective for many clients. However, careful attention must be paid by the OT to the precautions and contraindications (see Table 2-21) inherent to the use of this PAM and to the client-specific tolerance of this electrical modality.

Ultrasound, briefly mentioned previously, can also be implemented with the use of medication to produce a similar response to that of iontophoresis. When ultrasound is used in this manner, it is titled phonophoresis (Figure 2-2). This process uses transcutaneous prescription medications, such as corticosteroids, which are permeated through the skin and directly to the site of injury via sound waves. The sound waves provided by the ultrasonic transducer are set to a nonthermal or pulsed level of delivery in this application. "The nonthermal effects are used primarily for alter-

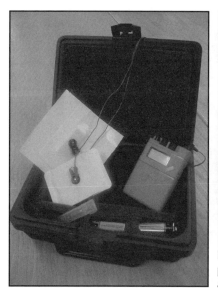

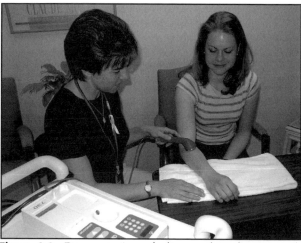

Figure 2-2. Demonstration of ultrasound application with prescribed medication, formally termed phonophoresis, as an intervention for pain and edema associated with subacute lateral epicondylitis.

Figure 2-1. Iontophoresis unit.

ing membrane permeability in order to accelerate tissue healing" (Cameron, 2003, p. 196). This process includes the removal of excess fluids seen in edema and is most commonly implemented in the subacute phases of healing.

Transcutaneous electrical nerve stimulation (TENS) is another type of therapeutic electrical modality, with the goal of interrupting the pain cycle (Cameron, 2003). In contrast to those previously described, the TENS modality is frequently reserved for use in conditions characterized by long term pain or chronic pain, as seen in nerve entrapments and complex regional pain syndromes, for example.

Compression techniques may also be implemented by the OT to promote a mechanical decrease in acute, subacute, or chronic cases of edema. The underlying theory for compression-related techniques is to facilitate the return of edematous fluids to the heart for efficient removal from the system (Cameron, 2003). Techniques as simple as elevating an affected area above the heart allows for gravitational forces to engage in removing excess fluids in the acute and subacute stages. In addition, aquatic rehabilitation techniques recruit the principles of hydrostatic pressure to circumferentially compress affected areas and achieve the same outcome in mostly subacute or chronic situations (Salzman, 1998). Bandage wrappings, garments (such as fitted gloves [Figure 2-3]), or electric pumps that provide timed, intermittent, and circumferential compression via filling a plastic sleeve that encloses the affected area with air are all flexible enough in nature to be implemented in either acute, subacute, or chronic stages of recovery. The intensity and frequency of these types of strategies are generally high and often considered a laborious process secondary to the natural accumulation of fluids from upright posture versus gravity alone. Careful attention must be paid to ensure appropriate circulation is maintained during any mechanical compression techniques.

Splinting is also a remedial technique used as a means to protect from further injury and to foster rest during the acute healing process. Of critical importance in this application is that the OT additionally provides education to the clients and caregivers as to the appropriate wear schedule for the splint. This wear schedule must be designed to balance rest and use in accordance with the recommendations of the physician and based on the type of injury. The importance of this issue is found in the potential ramifications of fostering disuse of affected muscles and joints. Prolonged

Figure 2-3. Demonstration of massage technique for subacute edema within the hand. Massage is performed in a distal to proximal direction using a lanolin-based lotion. Also pictured is a compression glove that provides circumferential compression to the hand during continuous wear outside of the OT session as is tolerated.

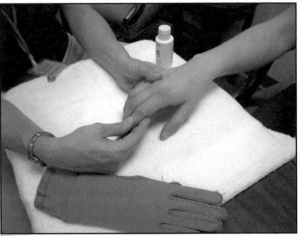

disuse will promote shortening of muscle tissue and potentially cause further disability. Therefore, the use of the splint should be implemented by the OT in conjunction with a program promoting joint ROM within the limits presented by the acute injury.

Retrograde massage techniques facilitated manually by the OT provide temporary compression to the tissues affected by edema. With firm-pressure massage specifically, the therapist provides manual compression (using a lanolin-based lotion to decrease friction) along the affected extremity and in the direction of the heart where excess fluids are then removed. Refer to Table 2-22 for a general outline of this procedure. This technique is provided in conjunction with appropriate positioning the client against gravity, as was discussed previously. This form of massage is specifically reserved for the subacute stage in order to avoid any possibility of further injury to susceptible tissues during acute healing. Another form of massage is titled, *manual lymph drainage*, and is used in cases of chronic edema specifically. Here, the therapist manually performs techniques designed to elicit a release of "trapped" lymph within the circulatory system. Lymph is produced when excess fluids, such as seen with edema, permeate into the interstitial space at the cellular level (Cameron, 2003). The lymphatic system attempts to remove these fluids through circulation to expel them from the system via the kidneys. In lymphedema, there tends to be a blockage in this system, which, in turn, causes an abnormal accumulation of the lymph. "This change in the quality of the connective tissue is also referred to as lymphostatic fibrosis" (Zuther, 2003, p. 40) and may be caused by congenital factors, trauma, pregnancy, and cancers (Cameron, 2003). Lymphedema is a specialty area within occupational therapy and requires additional training for proficiency. Appendix A offers more information and resources on lymphedema training.

RANGE OF MOTION

In accordance with the individualized injury and precautions set by the physician, the occupational therapist may recruit passive range of motion (PROM), active-assisted range of motion (AAROM), and active range of motion (AROM) regimes as additional remedial techniques to address acute pain and edema. As a natural reaction to discomfort, clients tend to avoid use of the affected joints, thereby fostering further accumulation of fluids and impeding the healing process in general. These "healing" fluids are comprised of proteins and cells necessary for preventing infection and, when left in a static state, create a "glue" that adheres to surrounding tissues and prohibits available range of motion (Cameron, 2003). This illustrates the significance of edema as a potential complication in healing and, therefore, the importance of implementing remedial techniques for effective management. Gentle muscle contraction, as seen with ROM, acts as a

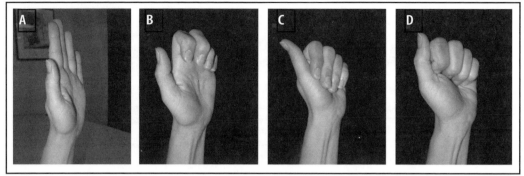

Figure 2-4. Tendon gliding exercises implemented to maintain smooth motion among tendons of the hand in the presence of edema. A) All joints of digits 2-5 are in extension. B) Distal interphalangeal (DIP) and proximal interphalangeal joints (PIP) are flexed while metacarpophalangeal joints (MCP) remain extended. C) MCPs move into flexion while DIPs become extended and PIPs remain flexed. D) All DIPs, PIPs, and MCP joints are flexed.

vasopneumatic pump to encourage return of the excess fluids to the heart, prevent the adhesion of surrounding tissues, and minimizing resulting discomfort in the acute stage of healing. OTs encourage this process by means of teaching range of motion programs, such as tendon gliding exercises for edema accumulating in the hand (Figure 2-4). Tendon gliding exercises specifically are completed at the intensity of five repetitions twice daily at regular intervals, until the edema has diminished (Prosser & Conolly, 2003).

MANUAL TECHNIQUES

Manual therapies is a collective term describing remedial techniques implemented by the OT that require the use of therapeutic touch. Lymphedema techniques, described previously, are also categorized here in addition to craniosacral, myofascial release, and techniques of strain counter-strain. Though each has its own unique approach, collectively these techniques are founded on the belief that dysfunction arises from tensions occurring within the fascia layer of the body and techniques implemented are intended to restore uniformity throughout that system. Each represent purely manual or hands-on techniques; therefore, these are typically contraindicated in the acute healing stages and more commonly used in the subacute and chronic phases. However, due to the potential for hands-on techniques to further aggravate painful tissues, they are often used in conjunction with other pain minimizing PAMs such as superficial heat or vapocoolant sprays. Due to the specialized nature of these techniques, continuing education is required to ensure safe and successful implementation. Refer to Appendix A for additional information and resources on these specialized technique options.

Techniques at a Glance

Refer to Table 2-3 for pain-specific techniques and Table 2-4 for edema-specific techniques, as well as the summary provided in Table 2-21 that outlines general procedures and precautions.

Special Considerations

As stated earlier in this section, when indicating the use of PAMs, it is the responsibility of the OT to be both knowledgeable about the specific modality and well aware of state licensure and legislation that governs their use. This procedure is recommended as a safeguard to clients and therapists alike as a result of the delicate contraindications and precautions their use presents in each individual application. "Although a number of conditions, including pregnancy,

---

Table 2-3

REMEDIAL TECHNIQUES FOR PAIN

- Superficial thermal modalities
- Iontophoresis
- Joint ROM and positioning
- Phonophoresis

- TENS
- Manual therapies
- Aquatic rehabilitation techniques

Table 2-4

REMEDIAL TECHNIQUES FOR EDEMA

- Massage
- Compression garments
- Compression wraps and pumps
- Positioning/splinting

- Elevation
- Joint ROM
- Manual lymph drainage
- Aquatic rehabilitation techniques

---

malignancy, the presence of a pacemaker, impaired sensation, and impaired cognitive status indicate the need for caution with the use of most physical agents, the specific contraindications and precautions for the specific agent being considered and the specific (client) situation must be evaluated before an intervention may be used or should be rejected" (Cameron, 2003, p. 423). For example, fractures or tendon lacerations are situations where, traditionally, the use of heat modalities is contraindicated due to the potential effect they may have on the healing tissues. However, of recent, research shows ultrasound may actually foster healing of bone (Cameron, 2003). Additionally, in arthritis, heat modalities are *strictly* contraindicated when symptoms are of *acute* exacerbation; however, the literature recommends their use in the *subacute* and *chronic* stages. Overall, the OT must carefully consider all of these issues when evaluating the use of PAMs as remedial techniques to address pain and edema on a case-by-case basis.

An additional consideration lies in the effectiveness of a multidisciplinary approach to the remediation of pain specifically. For example, the physician is ideally prescribing pharmaceutical agents designed to diminish the perception of the client's pain, psychology and social work departments are providing support systems to the client as avenues of coping with the pain, and rehabilitative services are implementing remedial approaches to address the underlying causes for the pain. It is only through this collaboration of professionals that pain can be effectively addressed.

Thermal injuries (or burns) were intentionally omitted from this discussion of pain, regardless of the fact that the pain is produced as a primary result of this injury. Pain is a critical issue for any client who has sustained a thermal injury and is directly related to the degree and extent of the burn itself. In many cases, high-dose medications are the primary and most effective means of controlling pain associated with burns over the duration of the healing process and the presence of edema may be minimal due from direct trauma to the tissue itself. OTs may implement techniques described below in the management subsection, yet these are not remedial in nature. Compression garments are traditionally implemented and are considered remedial, although their purpose is not to diminish edema as was described above, but rather to minimize scarring of the healing tissues. It is because of these and other unique situations presented by thermal injuries that it is discussed here generally and not in the context of other remedial strategies for addressing pain and edema reviewed earlier.

Table 2-5
MANAGEMENT TECHNIQUES FOR MANAGING CHRONIC PAIN AND EDEMA

Health Condition	Management Techniques
Pain including cancers, amputations, fibromyalgia, complex regional pain syndrome, arthritides and musculoskeletal disorders, and nerve injuries.	Biofeedback, TENS, Imagery, Reiki, Yoga, Tai Chi, Ai Chi
Edema including cancers, arthritides, and congestive heart failure.	Ai Chi, compression garments, compression pumps

Maintenance Programs

Conditions that cause chronic pain and edema were previously deferred to this portion of the subsection. The reason for this is found in the fact that techniques implemented by the OT in chronic pain and edema are not considered remedial approaches. Rather, these are maintenance strategies that allow clients to effectively cope with chronic symptoms while engaging in meaningful daily activity. These techniques are summarized in Table 2-5.

Occupational therapy intervention for chronic pain heavily emphasizes education regarding a variety of alternate coping methods. Biofeedback provides clients with an auditory cue as to how they can effectively decrease various body rhythms, such a heart rate and blood pressure, as indicators of stress or discomfort (Jamil, 1997). Imagery is often facilitated by the therapist in a controlled environment guiding client's attention away from uncomfortable symptoms. Participation in complimentary therapies may also be encouraged by the OT and includes Reiki, Yoga, and Tai Chi, again as methods of promoting wellness and healthy coping in the presence of chronic symptoms (Jamil, 1997). Ai Chi has also become a more common recommendation as it combines the therapeutic effects of Tai Chi and heat in addressing pain management. Ai Chi is, in essence, Tai Chi performed in a warm water pool (Salzman, 1998).

As for management techniques in cases of chronic edema, the delineation from methods for remediation becomes less obvious. Management tools are the very same those implemented in the subacute stages of recovery or healing, however, in this application, they are intended for long term use. Predominantly, OTs recommend the use of compression garments or intermittent pumps to clients experiencing long-term issues with fluid accumulation. Ai Chi is again mentioned here due to the mechanical principles that directly aid in the return of excess fluids to the heart—chiefly, hydrostatic pressure. The importance of traditional elevation must also be emphasized to clients and carried over whenever possible as an effective method for the management of chronic edema.

As discussed earlier, the efficacy of acute, subacute, or chronic pain and edema techniques require aggressive intensity to yield efficient results. This requires the OT to educate clients on the importance of carrying over strategies throughout the day outside of the occupational therapy session and within the context of everyday life. The effective implementation of PAMs in occupational therapy intervention requires the OT to also create an individualized program for clients to carry out independently in order to achieve the overall treatment goal. Also of consideration is that many of these clients are discharged from occupational therapy services early in the healing process, further emphasizing the importance of a well-developed and understood individualized maintenance program. For example, clients receiving cold modalities for pain and edema while in the occupational therapy session should also be educated and deemed safe to independently follow an individualized home program. Similarly, those receiving massage should be taught self-massaging techniques. In addition, to ensure successful execution of either technique used above as examples, the OT must consider the intensity or frequency expected of the client and the tools available to the client for effective execution. For example, recommending the use of a bag of frozen vegetables rather than the purchase of commercially available (and often costly) cold packs before and after each meal daily. Overall success is better achieved when working within the context of the client rather than placing demands on the client.

REMEDIAL TECHNIQUES FOR SENSATION

Definitional Analysis

Sensation is defined by the *Framework* (AOTA, 2002) as a client factor requiring functions of seeing, hearing, and other sensory interpretations. The category of "Other Sensory Interpretations" recruits contributions from the vestibular, proprioceptive, olfactory, gustatory, and tactile systems. Jacobs & Jacobs (2004) go further in defining sensation as inclusive of both the peripheral and cortical processing centers. This additional consideration then allows the subdivision of sensation into two distinct categories: those sensory functions obtained via the peripheral nervous system (PNS), including pain and temperature, and those functions obtained via the central nervous system (CNS) including discrimination of touch or the integration of righting reactions required by postural control. As OTs, sensation, or lack thereof, holds a vital role in overall intervention planning. As discussed in the previous subsection, continuous sensory signals of pain can impede a client's ability to engage in personally-meaningful occupations. This principle also hold true for a client who has diminished, or complete lack of, sensation. This subsection describes the remedial approaches OTs commonly implement to address both exaggerated and diminished sensory responses.

Modes of Injury or Illness

Sensation is affected primarily by two modes of injury or illness: those affecting the CNS and those affecting the PNS. This delineation assists in discussing the typical modes of injury or illness that yield sensory disturbances.

The CNS receives sensory messages by way of receptors located throughout the body. These receptors convey messages directly to the brain regarding characteristics of touch, temperature, taste, vibration, sound, position, and pain. Sensibility, or the ability to interpret sensory stimuli, is a result of the accurate interpretation of these stimuli within the brain, which, in turn, results in our ability to respond accordingly. Sensation serves many other functions as well. These include protective responses to noxious stimuli and the ability to recognize familiar touch, smells, and tastes. Therefore, sensation is considered a body function per the *Framework*, specific to the sensory receptors that are located throughout the body or as part of the PNS. However, the ability to accurately interpret senses and execute appropriate responses to those senses is a cognitive function occurring within the brain and CNS.

The CNS, including the brain and spinal cord, is responsible for interpreting sensory information. The brain and spinal cord are vulnerable to an array of illnesses or injuries manifested either internally, such as stroke, meningitis, abscesses, and tumors, or externally, such as with traumatic brain injury (TBI) or spinal cord injuries (SCI) to name a few. Each portion or lobe of the brain harbors its own unique contributions to the body as a whole. Specifically, the parietal lobe houses the primary somatosensory cortex where the receptor information from throughout the body is interpreted. Therefore, trauma, either internal or external to the parietal lobe or surrounding area of the brain, may affect sensory interpretation. Likewise, a condition that causes degeneration of this critical area of the brain, such as multiple sclerosis (MS), would produce similar results. Degenerative types of sensory disturbances vary greatly in both extent and intensity from client to client regardless of diagnosis; one may have a complete loss of sensation on the left side of the body, another both lower extremities, while another, only the right arm. Also, degenerative CNS conditions tend not to follow a specific dermatome distribution, as is typically the case with peripheral injuries or illnesses.

Most all sensory information travels to the central nervous system (the brain and spinal cord) for interpretation via the PNS or sensory receptors throughout the body. The exception exists only in reflexive responses to noxious stimulus that harbor the explicit purpose of protection by way of reflexes at the spinal level. Injury or illness affecting sensation may, therefore, occur at the level of the PNS, sparing the CNS, and present with sensory deficit in given dermatomes areas. This can also result secondary to trauma or degenerative diseases of the peripheral nerves themselves. Trauma affecting the PNS is most commonly the result of direct nerve damage, such as can be the case with fractures, edema, burns, lacerations, or impingements which theyby halt the sensory messages sent to the brain. The conduction of sensory information via the PNS can also be impeded by illnesses like diabetes, neuropathies, Guillain-Barré syndrome, post-polio syndrome, systemic sclerosis, and tumors within the PNS to name a few. MS may also cause PNS deficits if the characteristic plaques form along the peripheral nerves specifically.

Disruption of the sympathetic nervous system may also contribute to disturbances of sensation. Complex regional pain syndrome (CRPS) is a health condition characterized by pain, vascular changes, abnormal hair growth and/or nail growth, muscular weakness and atrophy, as well as changes in the overall degree of sensitivity of the affected extremity. Though etiology is unknown, much of the literature indicates that symptoms develop secondary to pre-existing conditions and are linked with sympathetic nervous system dysfunction, or the control center for vasomotor activity and sweat gland functions within the body (Reed, 2001). OTs regularly implement desensitization programs for clients experiencing symptoms of CRPS; however, much emphasis is also placed on the management of chronic pain symptoms. These are briefly outlined in Table 2-5 within this chapter and are further explored in a compensatory frame within the remaining chapters of this text.

Remedial Techniques: Cognitive Perceptual Theory

Remedial techniques for sensation are based primarily within the Cognitive Perceptual Theory and are summarized in Table 2-6 and Table 2-9. Sensation must first be perceived and accurately interpreted so as to respond accordingly through motor output. It is through the sensory perceptions that one is able to interact with their environment efficiently.

Remedial techniques include providing clients with an array of opportunities to provide engagement in familiar sensory experiences of all types. The following example illustrates this in the context of an everyday task: While at a restaurant, a person orders a root beer float that arrives to the table in a frosty mug. They then reach for the mug to take a refreshing sip and the root beer spills down their front and on the tabletop. What has happened? Misinterpretation of a sensory experience: what appeared to be a frosty *glass* mug was actually a *plastic* rendition weighing much less than anticipated based on a subconscious recollection of similar sensory experiences. Therefore, the motor response was miscalculated and too forceful for a plastic mug causing it to spill. The inaccurate perception caused an inaccurate response.

Remedial techniques for impaired sensibility take the form of either re-education of receptors (in cases of a loss or decrease in sensation) or desensitization (in cases of heighten sensory responses). Depending upon the mode of injury or illness, as well as the extent of that injury or

Table 2-6

REMEDIAL SENSIBILITY TECHNIQUES OF THE COGNITIVE PERCEPTUAL THEORY ACCORDING TO ORIGIN OF INJURY OR ILLNESS

Origin of Injury or Illness	Remedial Techniques
CNS impairment such as seen with traumatic brain injury, stroke, spinal cord injuries, or brain tumors with generalized effects.	• Sensory retraining program • Desensitization programs with dowels and/or immersion bins
PNS impairment in sensation such as seen with neuropathies, impingements, burns, and tumors located outside of the CNS with localized effects.	• Pressure garments • Massage techniques • Fluidotherapy at a nonthermal setting

illness, all clients will present individually and with highly variable levels of hypersensitivity or hyposensitivity. With this said, the following discussion of remedial techniques is intended to represent a general overview; much of the specifics are determined by the OT given a particular case with independent indicators of sensory dysfunction.

SENSORY RETRAINING TECHNIQUES FOR HYPOSENSITIVITY

When hyposensitivity or anesthesia (lack of sensation) is present, the OT typically will implement a sensory training or retraining program. This is defined as a "general term for therapy aimed at enabling a person to regain contact with his or her environment: (via sensory input and) ...includes ...body awareness exercises and sensory activities utilizing objects" (Jacobs & Jacobs, 2004, p. 213).

When considering the use of sensory retraining techniques, it is also important to discuss the typical pattern of recovery with regard to sensibility following injury or illness to the CNS or PNS. This process is summarized in Table 2-7 and is very case specific; this table represents only a generalization. Some clients may never experience a complete absence of sensation, while others may never achieve a full recovery of sensation. Some may have maximal degrees of impairment involving all senses, while others may only have select loss of only the thermal or light touch receptors with all others remain intact.

In cases of sensory loss, remedial techniques of retraining are intended to provide the body with experiences that will remind the system of how everyday items and movements feel. Tasks of retraining may include an array of activities such as a fine motor task in identifying coins to those of a gross motor nature such as moving the arm above the head so as to successfully brush one's hair. Emphasis is not so much placed on the type of item or movement, but rather the recruitment of other perceptions, such as vision, in retraining the "sense" of the particular task. Therefore, the OT must use their skills of grading activity, or adjusting the degree of difficulty a given task presents, to provide challenge, though allow success. For example, the OT may encourage the client's use of vision to identify common everyday items by touch, then grade the task over time by occluding vision, therefore, placing the demands of identification solely on the interpretation of touch. This can be achieved by beginning with the identification of large, textured items of different shape, and then grading to those that are small, nontextured, and of similar shape. See Table 2-8 for examples of textures that may be used, however, many occupational therapy clinics create textured items from simple materials purchased at local merchants. The rate of gradation will depend on the client, the degree of sensory loss, and the individual rate of recovery.

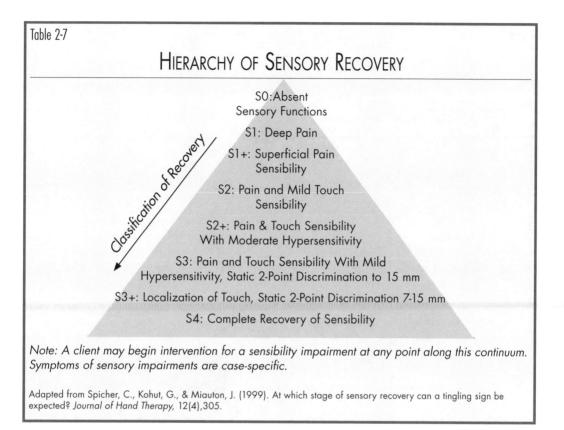

Table 2-7

HIERARCHY OF SENSORY RECOVERY

SO:Absent
Sensory Functions

S1: Deep Pain

S1+: Superficial Pain
Sensibility

S2: Pain and Mild Touch
Sensibility

S2+: Pain & Touch Sensibility
With Moderate Hypersensitivity

S3: Pain and Touch Sensibility With Mild
Hypersensitivity, Static 2-Point Discrimination to 15 mm

S3+: Localization of Touch, Static 2-Point Discrimination 7-15 mm

S4: Complete Recovery of Sensibility

Classification of Recovery

Note: A client may begin intervention for a sensibility impairment at any point along this continuum. Symptoms of sensory impairments are case-specific.

Adapted from Spicher, C., Kohut, G., & Miauton, J. (1999). At which stage of sensory recovery can a tingling sign be expected? *Journal of Hand Therapy*, 12(4),305.

DESENSITIZATION TECHNIQUES FOR HYPERSENSITIVITY

Clients experiencing hyperesthesia (increased sensitivity) or paresthesias (abnormal or misinterpreted sensation) benefit from remedial techniques focusing on the desensitization of sensory receptors. These symptoms can be seen in either PNS or CNS disturbances. The OT will initiate an individually appropriate program of remediation using dowels (or sensory wands) and immersion bins that provide graded exposure to various textures. Figure 2-5 provides illustrations of these techniques. Table 2-8 depicts this concept of techniques as specifically outlined by Barber (1990); however, the textures used may vary depending on manufacturer. Additionally, a third phase may be employed in this process (Waylett-Rendall, 2002), whereby vibration is introduced to provide a more vigorous sensation than that of phases one and two described above. Refer to Appendix A for listing of rehabilitation equipment manufacturer's Web sites and information on obtaining product catalogs. Some occupational therapy clinics, as mentioned previously, will autonomously create their own desensitization programs using textures readily available at local merchant stores. Occupational therapy intervention is initiated by having the client organize the sensory stimulation bins or dowels in a sequence of least to most abrasive, then begin with stimulation via the texture that is most tolerated for 10 minutes, 3 to 4 times per day as a home program, applied directly to the affected area (Waylett-Rendall, 2002). Graded progression to increasing more abrasive textures is then guided by the therapist with particular attention to the client's level of tolerance.

Physical Agent Modalities for Hypersensitivity

OTs may also use sensory experiences, such as continuous pressure by way of pressure garments, massage techniques, or fluidotherapy at a nonthermal setting, in effort to desensitize. These techniques are employed to further amplify the bombardment to sensory receptors, regain

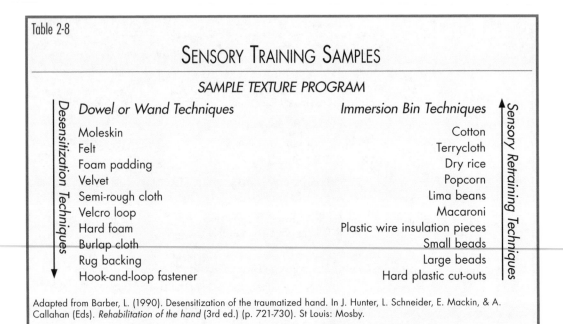

Table 2-8

SENSORY TRAINING SAMPLES

SAMPLE TEXTURE PROGRAM

Desensitization Techniques	*Dowel or Wand Techniques*	*Immersion Bin Techniques*	*Sensory Retraining Techniques*
	Moleskin	Cotton	
	Felt	Terrycloth	
	Foam padding	Dry rice	
	Velvet	Popcorn	
	Semi-rough cloth	Lima beans	
	Velcro loop	Macaroni	
	Hard foam	Plastic wire insulation pieces	
	Burlap cloth	Small beads	
	Rug backing	Large beads	
	Hook-and-loop fastener	Hard plastic cut-outs	

Adapted from Barber, L. (1990). Desensitization of the traumatized hand. In J. Hunter, L. Schneider, E. Mackin, & A. Callahan (Eds). *Rehabilitation of the hand* (3rd ed.) (p. 721-730). St Louis: Mosby.

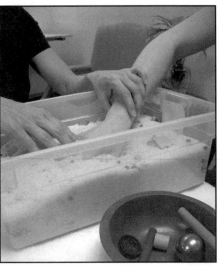

Figure 2-5. Demonstration of the use of immersion for desensitization. In this example, small items are placed in a bin of rice and the client is being asked to retrieve the items. The rice medium provides extra sensory input to the receptors as tolerated by the client. Many therapists also choose to use immersion as a sensory retraining method in situations of decreased sensibility again asking the client to locate items within the immersion bins without using the adaptation of vision.

accurate perception, and are typically used in conjunction with the more traditional, desensitization program. Note, fluidotherapy is also a modality of sensory bombardment at a nonthermal setting only, due to the contraindication of using a heat setting in the presence of abnormal sensation. Without a reliable sensory feedback system, all other PAMs are contraindicated secondary to the potential for injury to tissues. Refer to Table 2-22 for contraindications of PAMs in general.

QUANTIFYING SENSORY REMEDIATION TECHNIQUES

Also illustrated in Table 2-7 is the mention of static, two-point discrimination measures. This is included as a method of objectively measuring sensation. This sense is of particular importance in that two-point discrimination (in contrast to one-point) requires collaboration of multiple senses to interpret accurately. Hence, improvement in a client's performance with two-point discrimination translates to improved sensibility. This is pointed out as a means of illustrating the efficacy

Table 2-9

REMEDIAL TECHNIQUES FOR SENSIBILITY

- Nonthermal or electrical physical agent modalities.
- Sensory retraining emphasizing the graded use of vision.
- Desensitization provided via immersion bins or sensory wands (dowels).

of both desensitization and sensory re-education techniques. However, it is also vital to mention that remediation can be directly influenced by the client's level of motivation as well as by the degree of severity in sensory impairment. This concept will also be further explored as a special consideration with regard to the potential comorbidity of cognitive compromise in CNS injuries and the resulting barriers it poses to addressing sensory disturbance.

Techniques at a Glance

Table 2-9 and Table 2-22 illustrate the most commonly implemented techniques of remediation for sensibility in general.

Special Considerations

The issue of safety is paramount when discussing intervention for a client experiencing compromise in sensibility. Education of the client and caregivers is required to minimize the possibility of injury given the nature of impairment. In the absence of accurate sensory input, the body is subject to an array of injuries including burns, cuts, and decubiti, for example. The OT must emphasize to clients and caregivers alike that sensation is a protective response of the body system and when absent the client must use added caution in all ADLs. For example, reaching blindly into a knife drawer in the kitchen or testing the temperature of the running water prior to entering the bathtub. The client should be educated to rely on the visual sense as a compensatory measure to promote safety until accurate responses of the sensory system can be re-established. This concept is further discussed in Chapters 3 and 4 as techniques of adaptation and compensation.

OTs must also recall each client coming to therapy in need of sensory remediation does so as an individual with his/her own set of previously acceptable and nonacceptable sensory experiences. Some may have strictly avoided certain textures such as woolen garments, tight socks, or even caps that cover the ears. Others may not remotely be bothered by these sensory experiences. In all, it is the duty of the OT to create an individualized program that is sensitive to not only the client's current level of tolerance, but also the prior level of tolerance before the onset of sensory impairment.

Of equal importance to the aforementioned considerations is a client's cognitive status. Many of the underlying modes for compromised sensibility are a result of trauma to the CNS. Therefore, the OT must assess the client's cognitive status and adjust methods accordingly. For example, a client unable to respond accurately to a simple question, such as gender or name, may be experiencing impaired attention or even a barrier in communication, such as aphasia. Given these points, the client cannot be expected to partake in a sensory program without concern for potential safety issues secondary to cognitive disability alone. It is imperative that the OT identify the cognitive status of any client with a sensory impairment in order to ensure the optimal outcome of remediation efforts as well as the general safety of the client.

As a final consideration, the degree to which a sensory program is successful relies heavily on frequency. The OT should enable the carryover of clinic-based techniques into the client's everyday life so as to allow for continuous sensory input both within and outside of the clinic. As in a desensitizing program, clients may be provided with a scrap of denim, a piece of moleskin, or an illustration of massage procedures, for example, and then be educated as to the procedure of providing the stimulus. With sensory retraining, clients should be encouraged to actively engage in daily routines, while recruiting vision as a measure of safety in order to expose the area of impairment to as many traditional sensory experiences as possible. This frequently represents a key factor in the overall success of techniques for sensory impairment.

Maintenance Programs

As mentioned in the previous section, it is important to engage clients in their individualized sensory programs outside of the occupational therapy clinic. The characteristic timeframe wherein nerve regeneration occurs is challenged regularly by clients who regain function weeks, months, and even years following the original onset of sensory impairments. Therefore, those who have not reached full recovery at the time of discharge should continue with techniques of sensory remediation as tolerated. The maintenance program should also specifically outline any potential safety issues the client must continue to observe in the future given their status at time of discharge. Recently, other complementary therapies, such as participation in Reiki, Tai Chi, Ai Chi, and yoga, are also being recommended to foster holistic health while also drawing exaggerated attention to the sense of body position. This provides an excellent opportunity for sensory retraining by means of active engagement in meaningful, leisure tasks inherently motivating for the client (Crepeau, Cohn, & Shell, 2003). Additionally, aquatic techniques are growing in popularity as a measure of remediation due to the compressing forces of hydrostatic pressure. This force, inherent to a water environment, also provides an opportunity for sensory bombardment and an additional intervention option for desensitization (Ruoti, Morris, & Cole, 1997).

REMEDIAL TECHNIQUES FOR RANGE OF MOTION

Definitional Analysis

ROM is defined by the *Framework* (AOTA, 2002) as a subcomponent of client factors in the category of Neuromusculoskeletal and Movement-Related Functions. This subcomponent elaborates upon the definition, adding that ROM is also a function of joints and bones, including the mobility of joints structures, the stability of joint structures, and the mobility of skeletal bones.

Mobility of joints refers to the biomechanical roots of arthrology—the composition of joint structure and functions as they relate to a "junction or pivot point between two or more bones" (Neumann, 2002, p. 25). Neumann (2002) goes on to describe how the nature of normal aging, long term immobilization, trauma, or disease processes all potentially affect the structure, and, therefore, function of our joints. This statement then considers other potential factors such as the integrity of articular bone surfaces, synovial membranes, intraarticular fluids, and the bursa to name a few. Illness or injury may compromise these components as is seen in osteoarthritis, rheumatoid arthritis, and gout.

In considering the stability of joints, one must recall the integral nature of capsular ligaments and muscle integrity. For example, muscles lacking in sufficient tone, such as is commonly seen in neurological conditions, will often impede ROM due to poor joint stability. An illustration can briefly be made by the condition of a subluxation in the shoulder joint. Here, the head of the humerus is displaced downward from the glenohumeral cavity as a result of decreased tension in the proximal shoulder musculature. Without the underlying structural integrity of the shoulder joint itself, range of motion is hindered and can even be harmful due to the increased potential for soft tissue impingement.

The mobility of our bones can be classically portrayed by the scapulohumeral rhythm or interplay between the scapula and humerus during glenohumeral motions above 90 degrees. For example, in analyzing glenohumeral abduction to a maximum of 180 degrees ROM, upward rotation of the scapula is responsible for 60 degrees, while humeral abduction is responsible for the remaining 120 degrees of the total movement. An illness or injury resulting in compromised motion at the scapula would then affect the overall ROM available at the shoulder joint due to immobility of bone alone.

Modes of Injury or Illness

Many modes of injury or illness exist that either primarily or secondarily affect ROM. This section presents an overview of the more commonly recognized injuries and illnesses for which remedial approaches are implemented.

Primary modes of injury or illness are described as "first in time or order" (Thomas, 1997, p. 1560). Therefore, the injury itself is the reason for the limitation observed in ROM. These include such health conditions as bone fractures, spinal cord injuries, muscular or soft tissue injuries such as a rotator cuff tear, simple sprain, or tendon lacerations, and inflammation of the joint cavity as seen with arthritic conditions.

Secondary modes of injury or illness are considered as those "produced by a primary cause" (Thomas, 1997, p. 1732). These health conditions that secondarily affect range of motion can include all types of acquired brain injuries, such as external trauma, cerebrovascular accidents, brain abscesses or tumors, or neurologically based infections (e.g., meningitis). Also included as a potential secondary mode are the degenerative diseases, such as MS, amyotrophic lateral sclerosis (ALS), Guillain-Barré, and myasthenia gravis (MG), where general debility gives rise to prolonged immobility of joints. Prolonged immobility impedes range by means of adhesion or contracture formations and though mentioned here, often cause permanent limitation in available ROM. This is discussed further in the *Special Considerations* segment of this subsection.

Remedial Techniques: Biomechanical Theory

In most cases, issues of ROM are addressed by OTs under the Biomechanical Theory. Refer to Table 2-10 and 2-23 for a summary of the remedial techniques most frequently implemented by occupational therapy to address limits in ROM.

So often, the lingering barrier clients continually face in their recovery from illness or injury is the functional significance found in ROM and strength. Therefore, the facilitation of repetitive range through the available arc of motion is one of the most commonly used remedial strategies across diagnoses or health conditions. The main goal of this technique is to maintain or increase the ROM as well as prevent contractures or adhesions that can potentially form secondary to immobility.

RANGE OF MOTION

As a technique, ROM itself is broken into three main types: PROM, AAROM, and AROM. The type of range elicited as an intervention approach depends heavily on the client's physical status at the given point in time. For example, a client with little or no active range would then require the therapist to passively move the joint through its full arc of motion, termed PROM. Also included here would be the implementation of pendulum exercises; exercises designed to facilitate PROM using gravity as the passive force, rather than that of the therapist. In addition, a client can be taught techniques of using a nonaffected extremity to passively guide the affected limb through its' arc of motion. This technique is referred to as self-ROM, commonly executed in cases of hemiparesis. This may be further encouraged through the use of a dowel, a cane or by an overhead pulley system. Refer to Figure 2-6 for an illustration of commonly implemented self-ROM motion exercise. The OT may

Table 2-10

REMEDIAL RANGE OF MOTION TECHNIQUES OF THE BIOMECHANICAL THEORY ACCORDING TO HEALTH CONDITION

Health Condition	Remedial Techniques
Fractures	Subacute phases of recovery: PROM, AAROM, Self-ROM, AROM
Soft tissue injury including tears, sprains, tendon lacerations, etc	
Spinal cord injuries	PROM, AAROM, Self-ROM, AROM
Acquired brain injury including TBI, CVA, brain cancers, abscesses, meningitis, etc	
Degenerative diseases including MS, ALS, Guillaine-Barré, and MG	

also employ techniques of AAROM where the therapist or assistive device, such as pulleys, work collaboratively with the client sharing effort necessary to achieving full ROM. Figure 2-7 provides an illustration. Finally, AROM is implemented once clients are able to move their joints through the arc of motion independently. Here, the OT will create a client-specific program to be executed independently so as to maintain or increase available AROM. Prefabricated card file systems are used frequently to facilitate this goal. These tools are readily available through manufacturers (listed in Appendix A) and provide a wide array of simply illustrated and narratively described active-, passive-, self-, and active-assisted exercises in the form of a 3-by-4-inch card—one designated for each exercise. This allows the therapist to select appropriate exercises for the client, compile them in a page format, photocopy (copyright provided with purchase), and then insert recommended intensity (repetitions and sets) to foster independence in the overall exercise program. See Figure 2-8 for a sample of this type of program.

Typical intervention strategies to facilitate increased AROM or AAROM can also include pulley exercises, wall-mounted shoulder wheels, arm ergometers, or the various attachments of work simulators such as the Baltimore Therapeutic Work Simulator (BTE) (Figure 2-9). Additional information about the BTE and other work simulators can be found in Appendix A. Though these techniques are not necessarily based in function, they are commonly employed as adjunctive methods and are proven strategies of remediation for addressing deficits in ROM. With more of an occupational emphasis, therapist may also employ activity analysis to foster these same biomechanical approaches in a functional context, such as having clients reach to hang clothes on a clothes line, replace dishes in upper kitchen cabinets, or even by engaging in a game of shuffleboard to address decreased glenohumeral flexion. Here the focus remains on remediation while employing creativity in the use of strategies that actively engage participation in personally meaningful activities.

PHYSICAL AGENT MODALITIES

Per state-specific guidelines, superficial heat modalities are frequently used as a precursor to techniques for ROM. The purpose here is to promote tissue elasticity in preparation for the stretch associated with range exercises. Moist heat packs, thermal (continuous) ultrasound, and fluidotherapy represent the most commonly-used methods for this purpose and, as indicated previously, are implemented for a duration of 15 to 20 minutes so as to achieve desired thermal effects

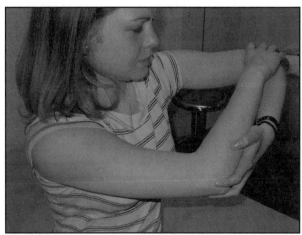

Figure 2-6. Demonstration of a self ROM exercise where the most mobile extremity supports and assists movement in the least mobile joints through the entire arc of horizontal abduction and adduction at the shoulder joint.

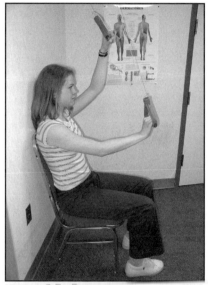

Figure 2-7. Demonstration of pulleys commonly considered either a technique of PROM or AAROM.

(Cameron, 2003). Again, careful attention must be paid to any conditions that may contraindicate the use of therapeutic heat. Refer to Table 2-24 for a review of indications and contraindications.

Techniques at a Glance

Refer to Table 2-11 and 2-23 for a general outline of remedial techniques commonly employed by the OT to address deficits in ROM.

Special Considerations

When remedial intervention strategies are implemented with the intent of increasing available range of motion at an affected joint or joints, the therapist must consider inherent precautions or contraindications specific to the underlying mode of injury or illness. An example can be found in weight-bearing precautions commonly put in place by the physician postacute fractures to allow ample and undisturbed time for the natural healing process. Also, the OT must be aware of any pre-existing range of motion limitations by prompting the client to report a history of prior injuries, fractures, or joint disorders, such as arthritis.

Clients should also be informed of the necessity for proper positioning. Here, OTs will provide education to clients emphasizing that a position of comfort may also lead to deformity via the shortening of soft tissues. Family members and caregivers should be oriented to proper positioning and the potential ramifications of prolonged immobility. This includes the use of splinting techniques, briefly described earlier in the pain and edema subsection of this chapter.

The efficient management of pain and edema are also critical components in optimizing ROM. Full ROM can be significantly impeded by the presence of pain and edema. Hence, it is of importance to ensure that these issues are addressed simultaneously, using the appropriate combination of aforementioned techniques, in order to optimize the ROM that a client is able to regain overall.

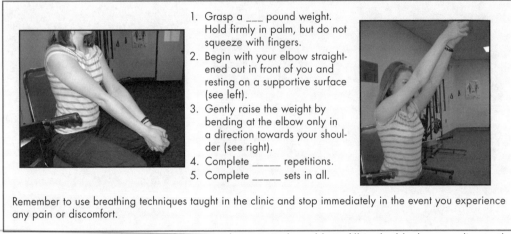

1. Grasp a ___ pound weight. Hold firmly in palm, but do not squeeze with fingers.
2. Begin with your elbow straightened out in front of you and resting on a supportive surface (see left).
3. Gently raise the weight by bending at the elbow only in a direction towards your shoulder (see right).
4. Complete _____ repetitions.
5. Complete _____ sets in all.

Remember to use breathing techniques taught in the clinic and stop immediately in the event you experience any pain or discomfort.

Figure 2-8. Sample card program for ROM. Therapist is then able to fill in the blanks according to the individual's needs and tolerance as part of the maintenance program.

Figure 2-9. Baltimore Therapeutic Work Simulator (BTE).

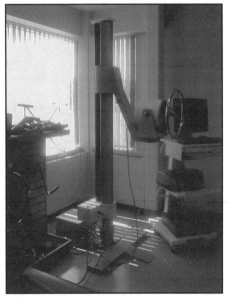

Maintenance Programs

An additionally important piece of remedial approaches for ROM is the creation and carryover of a client-specific maintenance program. Here, it is the role of the OT to create an individually meaningful exercise program that addresses client-specific needs, adheres to the condition-specific precautions, and is easily understood in both technique and importance to the healing process. With ROM, maintenance programs commonly consist of fostering active engagement in typical, everyday activity, such as dressing, grooming, washing, etc, as well as specific exercise programs to promote additional AROM, AAROM, or AROM. As mentioned earlier, the most commonly recommended maintenance programs recruit the use of readily available "card-style" systems, given the simplicity it provides for client understanding along with the ability for customization via recommended intensity of repetitions and sets. Typically, any well-rounded maintenance

---

Table 2-11

REMEDIAL TECHNIQUES FOR RANGE OF MOTION

- PROM: Pendulum exercises and therapist facilitated techniques.
- AROM: BTE, wall mounted shoulder wheels, card style programs, use of functional activity engagement.
- Physical agent modalities: Including moist heat, ultrasound, or fluidotherapy.
- AAROM: BTE, pulleys, shoulder wheels, card style programs.
- Self-ROM: Pulleys, dowel or cane exercises.

---

program includes emphasis on a balance between straightforward exercise and the engagement in meaningful activities that specifically recruit the targeted joint ROM.

REMEDIAL TECHNIQUES FOR STRENGTH

Strength is of critical importance and priority in reassuming independent engagement in meaningful activity following injury or illness. Of significance to note is the interrelationship between ROM and strength against gravity. Without strength, one will not be able to achieve full active ROM against the force of gravity.

The significance of gravity within the physical environment is often overlooked until one is faced with an injury or illness limiting strength capacity. It then becomes more evident that active motion can be limited by decreased strength alone. For example, a manual muscle test of the bicep muscle in elbow flexion yields a "Fair" rating of strength. This indicates the client is unable to achieve full active ROM in a gravity plane, however, is able in a gravity-eliminated plane. Hence, without the required strength from the muscle to move the limb segment into flexion against gravity, the client then too has limits in ROM. Therefore, remedial approaches for addressing strength vary greatly depending on the degree of limitation. In the aforementioned "Fair" elbow flexion example, simply to promote full active range against gravity alone would be an efficient remediation technique. Resistance would then be graded, beyond that of the gravitational force, once improvement is noted. Conversely, a client exhibiting full range of motion in all planes could then move to more aggressive remedial methods such as progressive resistive exercise (PRE) programs.

Definitional Analysis

Per the *Framework* (AOTA, 2002), strength is defined as a foundational skill or client factor specific to "neuromusculoskeletal and movement-related functions" of the body (p. 625). It is further categorized as a function of muscle power. With attention paid to general performance, strength is required to execute motor skills such as mobility, posturing, transporting, lifting, and calibrating, which collectively allow for "effective interaction with task objects" (AOTA, 2002, p. 621). Strength is also required to convey intentions and needs through the physicality of communication skills. In all, this foundational skill is paramount for the ability to successfully engage in many aspects of meaningful activity.

Modes of Injury or Illness

Strength, as a foundational skill, is affected by a wide array of health conditions. Primary modes of injury or illness, as they relate to strength, include those directly affecting the integrity

Table 2-12

REMEDIAL STRENGTH TECHNIQUES OF THE BIOMECHANICAL THEORY ACCORDING TO HEALTH CONDITION

Health Condition	Remedial Technique
Soft tissue injuries including tears, sprains, tendon lacerations, etc.	Therapeutic exercise programs designed to address the client's specific needs and interests, progressive resistive exercise (PRE), neuromuscular electrical stimulation, work simulators, aquatic rehabilitation techniques.
Prolonged immobility	
Degenerative diseases including MS, ALS, Guillane-Barré, and MG	

of the soft tissue and include conditions of muscle tearing or tendon evulsions. These conditions directly compromise the length-tension relationship of musculature and therefore, the ability to produce maximal force (Neumann, 2002).

Secondary causes are far more commonly seen and frequently are characterized by conditions that result in prolonged immobility. Here, the lack of physical movement creates an opportunity for muscle wasting and/or the formation of contractures and adhesions among muscular structures. Examples can be found in degenerative conditions including MG, ALS, Guillain-Barré, MS, or even conditions resulting from major multiple trauma to the body as is seen often in high velocity collisions. It is additionally important to note the significance of prognosis for the underlying condition. For example, ALS causes a progressive decline in strength with a poor prognosis, while Guillain-Barré also results in progressive weakness, yet with a more optimistic prognosis. The OT must consider each of these facts so as to create an intervention plan that is both individualized and effective in achieving the optimal outcome.

Remedial Techniques: Biomechanical Theory

As was the case with remedial ROM techniques, the intervention strategies used to address the underlying causes of decreased strength also are fundamentally based in the Biomechanical Theory. These commonly implemented techniques are summarized in Table 2-12 and Table 2-24.

THERAPEUTIC EXERCISE PROGRAMS

The most commonly implemented remedial technique for addressing strength is the use of therapeutic exercise programs designed specifically to meet a client's needs. This technique offers much flexibility based upon the degree of strength limitation each client experiences. This method has been viewed as controversial in the occupational therapy community who ascribes to functional activity engagement (Pedretti & Early, 2001) over traditional strengthening programs. However, given strength is a foundational skill to successful engagement in functional activity, OTs must address this specifically in order to assist the client in regaining overall indepen.

All clients must be physically able to endure a therapeutic exercise regime or deemed medically stable with regard to respiratory and cardiovascular functions prior to engaging in a strengthening program (refer to Special Considerations section). Given this point, the OT should have immediate access and ability to handle a stethoscope, blood pressure cuff, and a pulse oximeter (oxygen saturation measurement device) so as to monitor a client's tolerance closely.

OTs create therapeutic exercise programs to improve strength specifically using items such as free weights or barbells, BTE, wrist weights, hand grippers, Thera-Putty (North Coast Medical, Morgan Hill, Ca), and/or Thera-Band (Hygenic Corp, Akron, Ohio), while also infusing skills of

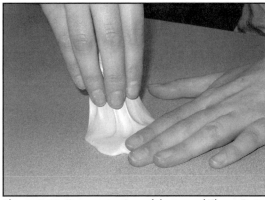

Figure 2-10. Demonstration of the use of Thera-Putty as a resistive exercise to promote increased strength in the finger flexors.

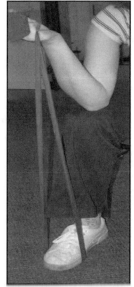

Figure 2-11. Demonstration of the use of Thera-Band as a resistive exercise to promote strength in the elbow flexor musculature.

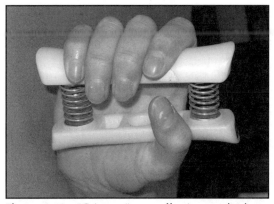

Figure 2-12. "Grippers" are effective methods to increase gross grasping strength of the hand.

gradation to provide enough challenge, yet avoid over-fatigue of the muscle tissue. This is achieved with the use of varied repetitions and sets of exercise unique to the capabilities of each client as well as with the use of graded resistance items. For example, Thera-Band, Thera-Putty, or hand grippers can be purchased from manufacturers as color-coded sets, illustrating for the therapist and client alike, the idea of graded resistance (Figures 2-10 through 2-12). For example, Thera-Putty is available in yellow as the least resistive compound, followed by red, green, and blue respectively. This same progression is available in Thera-Band products. A more current product on the market is Progressive putty (Sammons Preston Roylan, Bolingbrook, Il). With this product, additives are provided allowing the therapist to increase the resistive qualities of the same compound rather than purchasing various different compounds. Refer to Appendix A for more information on obtaining catalogs that offer an array strengthening tools.

Another technique for grading the resistance of strength exercises is to adjust the required type of muscle contraction that the client is asked to perform. Isometric muscle contractions do not produce limb movement, for example. This type of static contraction is commonly the first in the progressive exercise regime for cases of maximally compromised strength; contraction without movement eliminates the need to produce force against gravity. This technique is also implemented in cases where joint structure is compromised since strengthening can be fostered without eliciting potentially damaging movement among the joint structures. Isometric exercise, however, are contraindicated in cases of cardiac compromise due to the increase demand this type of contraction places on the heart.

Isotonic or concentric muscle contractions are facilitated by promoting a shortening in the length of a muscle against gravity. For example, an isotonic or concentric contraction of the bicep muscle would produce a shortening of that muscle and, therefore, elbow flexion. This exercise is commonly referred to as a bicep curl. With isotonics, motion against the force of gravity is recruited in an upright position further increasing the demands for muscle strength. This can be graded to meet individual needs by adjusting the direction of movement produced, the weighted resistance, the number of repetitions, and number of sets including in the exercise program.

Conversely, the therapist may choose to foster eccentric muscle contractions or activation of muscle fibers as the muscles lengths rather than shortens. This type of contraction can be achieved by using simple free weights. For example, a client with his or her arm fully extended overhead and grasping a 2-pound weight in their hand is then asked to bend at the elbow so as to "touch" the top of their head. This would then facilitate a lengthening contraction or eccentric contraction of the triceps muscle as the limb moves downward with gravity. For eccentric contraction, the therapist often recruits the assistance of a mini-gym or workout station as resisted lengthening is inherently difficult to achieve in a gravity environment.

Finally, the therapist may choose to foster isokinetic contraction of muscles. This technique allows for a more functional approach by eliciting reciprocation among the agonist and antagonistic muscles similar to that of movement required to interact with one's environment. Tools of isokinetics are often equipment-based and employ technology to simplify the process of providing graded resistance. An example is found in the use of arm ergometer that allows the speed of revolution to be mechanically controlled (Figure 2-13). This equipment requires the strength of reciprocating muscles, yet more importantly, allows ease of gradation via limits placed on duration or speed of movement. Regardless of the amount of effort applied by a client, the ergometer will only allow the preset number of revolutions. .

It is important to note that many OTs will choose to address strength in the context of meaningful activity engagement over that of pure biomechanical exercise. For example, the therapist may engage the client in a desired leisure task while wearing 1-pound wrist weights. This is a beneficial approach in working with individuals who do not typically engage in, nor find purpose from, engaging in a traditional weight-lifting program. This then offers occupational engagement while also creating enough resistance to foster muscle strength.

Neuromuscular Electrical Stimulation: A Physical Agent Modality

"The efficacy of electrical stimulation for the purposes of strengthening has been exclusively studied and is well established" (Bertoti, 2004). Neuromuscular electrical stimulation (NMES), also referred to as functional electrical stimulation (FES), is a method used to externally elicit active muscle contraction and, therefore, secondarily promote muscle strength. With this technique, electrical stimulation is provided via electrode placement over given motor points located along a weakened muscle's length. The electrical impulse causes a concentric contraction of the designated musculature and is considered remedial in nature when implemented in cases of temporary muscle weakness. This includes health conditions such as incomplete SCI, acquired brain injury, and in cases of shoulder subluxation. NMES is a physical agent modality that requires additional training in order to safely and effectively administer. Again, regulations on the use of PAMs vary from state to state and it is the responsibility of the therapist to be aware of governing legislation.

Work Simulators

Work simulators, such as the BTE (discussed previously) and the ERGOS Work Simulator (Simwork Systems, Tucson, Az), present another option for providing muscular resistance to

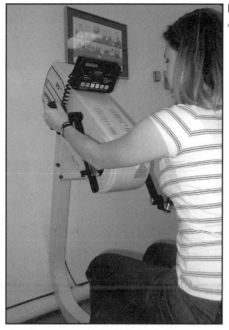

Figure 2-13. Demonstrations of the therapeutic use of an Arm Ergometer.

develop strength (Crepeau et al., 2003). These equipment-based options offer greater control in grading resistance provided to muscle groups during simulated functional activity. For example, the BTE Work Simulator offers an array of attachments designed to simulate particular movements required of a given activity including driving, golfing, or opening a jar. Resistance is graded via the simple twist of a knob that then adjusts the system's software program accordingly. The simulator also electronically records all pertinent data for both documentation and illustration to clients of the gains being made throughout the intervention process.

PROGRESSIVE RESISTIVE EXERCISE

PREs are derived from the DeLorme method (Trombly & Radomski, 2002). According to DeLorme, muscles must be taxed beyond everyday activity in order to promote the remediation of strength. Hence, the therapist must first identify the maximal capacity of a client, or the "maximum weight a person can lift with coordination through full ROM 10 times" (Trombly & Radomski, 2002). Once identified, the therapist will then prescribe resistive exercise: 10 repetitions at 25% the determined maximal capacity, 10 repetitions at 50%, and 10 repetitions at 100% capacity. The program is completed 1 time per day, 4 to 5 days of per week. As maximal capacity increases, resistance should too be increased. This is a formal program designed to increase strength; often times the OT will employ less formal variations of this original program. Refer to Table 2-24 for an outline of the PRE method.

AQUATIC REHABILITATION TECHNIQUES

Aquatic rehabilitation approaches may also be employed for the remediation of strength. Though aquatic rehabilitation does not currently require specific certification, continuing education is recommended prior to implementing intervention within a water environment. Water inherently provides an environment that is free of gravitational force. The simple elimination of this force, often taken for granted by individuals without strength limitations, presents an ideal opportunity to foster strength while also engaging in a leisure activity. Strength is fostered directly by the viscous properties of water, or the tendency of water molecules to adhere to one another.

Table 2-13
REMEDIAL TECHNIQUES FOR STRENGTHENING
• PREs • Work simulators • PAMs: NMES • Aquatic rehabilitation techniques • Traditional Exercise: Thera-Putty, Thera-Band, grippers, free weights

The force required to separate molecules of water far exceeds that of air molecules. Therefore, resistance to the simple activity of walking in water requires greater muscle strength than when walking on ground and without the application of additional weights. The resistance is upgraded by increasing depth of water or by the strategic incorporation of floatation devices that further enhance the resistive properties of water. Though an incredibly valuable option, the OT must again use his/her skills in client-centered intervention to ensure the successful use of an aquatic technique; not all individuals enjoy the thought of swimming and precautions must be taken in situations of open wounds, conditions of heat or fatigue sensitivity, and cardiac or respiratory compromise.

Techniques at a Glance

Refer to Table 2-13 and Table 2-24 for a summary of remediation techniques commonly used to address issues of strength.

Special Considerations

When using remedial techniques to address strength, the OT must be readily aware of the client's medical status and the presence of any possible contraindications or precautions. For example, physicians may contraindicate the use of exercise for clients with certain cardiac conditions or may put in place precautions, such as avoiding resistive exercise above 90 degrees of shoulder motions. Other common contraindications include conditions of general debility or acute exacerbations of disease. When implementing therapeutic exercise with any client it is imperative the OT be able to recognize signs of not only fatigue, but also of distress such as: excessive perspiration, labored or rapid breathing, or changes in face skin color (very pale or red). As to minimize the potential for these events, the OT should observe all governing guidelines for the use exercise as a therapeutic intervention. These guidelines are summarized in Table 2-14 and emphasize the use of a phased approach including warm up, stretching, strengthening, and relaxation portions during every exercise session.

As mentioned earlier in this section, the OT also must be considerate to the underlying cause for muscular weakness. For example, an individual with a progressive degenerative health condition would be particularly sensitive to over-fatigue of muscle tissue. Such a circumstance may even potentially set the client's progress back in the continuum of recovery. Therefore, this point is repeated to emphasize the attention a therapist must pay to both diagnostic and prognostic indicators in effort to foster maximal recovery of muscle strength.

Maintenance Programs

So as to achieve an overall increase in strength, the frequency in which the program is completed often warrants execution both within and outside the occupational therapy clinic (i.e., 2 to 3 times

Table 2-14

GENERAL GUIDELINES FOR ENGAGEMENT IN THERAPEUTIC EXERCISE PROGRAMS: A PHASED APPROACH

1. Request that the client report how he/she is feeling in general. Is there any report of pain or discomfort or other contraindicating symptoms such as nausea, dizziness, excessive fatigue, or shortness of breath (SOB)? Outside of the initial therapeutic exercise session, always request that the client report the tolerance of exercises performed in the previous session.

2. Obtain a baseline pulse rate, blood pressure reading, and baseline oxygen saturation, if indicated. Normal pulse rates at rest generally lie within the range of 60 to 100 beats per minute (bpm). Normal blood pressure at rest is under 140/90 and normal oxygen saturation is 90 to 100.

3. In the absence of any abnormalities previously identified, exercise should begin with a general warm up activity such as taking three deep, cleansing breaths followed directly by AROM, as tolerated, among all joints of focus for that sessions exercise elements.

4. Proceed to verbally instruct and demonstrate to the client elements of stretching muscles fibers as a preparatory technique for resistive exercise. Again, focus on muscle groups intended to be active during the session.

5. Provide the client with clear directions and demonstration as to the exercises he/she is expected to perform. For example, to activate the biceps, the therapist should demonstrate a traditional biceps curl while also pointing out proper positioning and joint alignment throughout each repetition.

6. Walk the client through each set of exercises. For example, have the client complete one set of five repetitions of bicep curls with a 1-pound weight. Re-evaluate client tolerance as outlined in guideline #1. This is the step where the OT will individually upgrade or downgrade the exercise itself by adjusting expected repetitions or sets. At the client's initial exercise session, expectations should be minimal so as to have the opportunity to evaluate tolerance not only during the exercise program, but also at the following session.

7. Monitor the client as he/she performs the recommended repetitions and sets at each of the designated joints. Be attentive to any signs or symptoms of poor tolerance as outlined briefly in guideline #1. In the event that poor tolerance is questioned, cease all exercises and obtain a pulse and blood pressure reading. Clients who have been inactive as a result of illness or disability should not have greater than a 20 to 30 bpm increase with the systolic blood pressure reading remaining relatively stable with the established baseline and no more than a 10 mm Hg increase from resting in the diastolic reading. In the presence of SOB, the occupational therapist may also obtain a pulse oximetry reading. These readings should then be shared with medical personnel or emergency services (911) who can further assess the client. Always err on the side of caution and ask for assistance to evaluate a client when any suspicion arises.

8. Given good tolerance, also provide the client with ample rest opportunities, particularly in the initial session. This may be as frequent as between each set of exercise completed. Ensure that the client has access to hydration and aware of any potential swallowing precautions such as those seen in acquired brain injuries and some degenerative diseases.

9. Following completion of recommended exercise program, take a pulse reading and guide the client through a relaxation exercise. For example, client may be requested to again take deep, cleansing breaths or the therapist may facilitate a simple guided imagery technique. This allows the body system with the time required to calm back to the resting point.

continued

Table 2-14, continued

GENERAL GUIDELINES FOR ENGAGEMENT IN THERAPEUTIC EXERCISE PROGRAMS: A PHASED APPROACH

10. Following relaxation, obtain a pulse reading. The client should have returned to the resting pulse level following the relaxation phase. Monitor the client until pulse returns to normal relative to the initial reading.

11. Within a short time period, clients are generally able to demonstrate independence with safely and effectively executing many aspects of the individualized program. The OT should always monitor the client's participation directly so as to assess tolerance levels.

12. All exercises should be immediately ceased and medical assistance called for any clients complaining of "chest pain or pain referred to the teeth, jaw, ear, or arm; excessive fatigue; light-headedness or dizziness; nausea or vomiting; SOB; or unusual weight gain of 3 to 5 pounds in 1 to 3 days" (Trombly & Radomski., 2002, p. 1078).

Adapted from Huntley, N. (2002). Cardiac and pulmonary diseases. In C.M. Trombly and M.V. Radomski (Eds.). *Occupational therapy for physical dysfunction* (5th ed.) (p. 1078). Philadelphia, PA: Lippincott Williams & Wilkins.

per day). Therefore, the therapist may initiate the actual program in the clinic, train the client as to proper completion of each component, and then recommend completion as part of the home program. Figure 2-14 provides a sample of this type of program. Frequently, clients are instructed to substitute traditional free weights or hand grippers with more common everyday items such as canned vegetables, a foam "squish" ball (often marketed for stress relief or in the children's section of local retail stores), or even by carrying everyday weighted items such as bags of groceries or baskets of laundry. In addition, OTs who have successfully integrated the use of aquatic techniques and established safe independence in pool-based exercise may consider encouraging client's to actively participate at community-based pools and aquatic centers. This allows the therapist to foster engagement in meaningful activity while still focusing on the remediation of strength.

REMEDIAL TECHNIQUES FOR ENDURANCE

Definitional Analysis

Endurance is categorized as a client factor per the *Framework* (AOTA, 2002), and is further defined as a function of the neuromusculoskeletal, cardiovascular, and respiratory systems. It is also considered a function of the muscles and of exercise tolerance, the later including aerobic capacity, stamina, and fatigability.

Jacobs & Jacobs (2004), reflects the above definition as "Sustaining cardiac, pulmonary, and musculoskeletal exertion over time; ability to sustain effort over time" (p. 76). This is a crucial aspect of endurance; without the ability to sustain effort overtime, a client's engagement in meaningful occupation is left seriously compromised.

Modes of Injury or Illness

In essence, any and all events of injury or illness can potentially affect one's level of endurance. A simple bout with the 24-hour flu can cause one to feel tired for a few days following. Magnify those consequences with such events as pneumonia, respiratory failure, or having sustained an

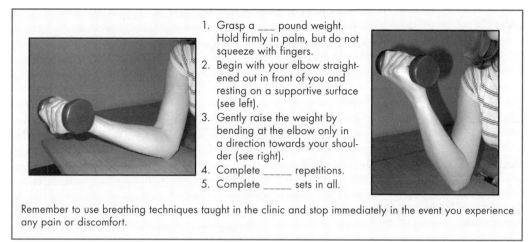

1. Grasp a ___ pound weight. Hold firmly in palm, but do not squeeze with fingers.
2. Begin with your elbow straightened out in front of you and resting on a supportive surface (see left).
3. Gently raise the weight by bending at the elbow only in a direction towards your shoulder (see right).
4. Complete _____ repetitions.
5. Complete _____ sets in all.

Remember to use breathing techniques taught in the clinic and stop immediately in the event you experience any pain or discomfort.

Figure 2-14. Sample card program for strength. The therapist then simply fills in the blanks to create an individualized program that best meets the needs of the client as part of the maintenance program.

acquired brain injury, which are all commonly associated with prolonged immobility and bed rest. This analogy allows us to better illustrate the wide expanse within which a decrease in endurance can impede functional performance and outlines the most evident reason or mode for it—a lack of engagement in everyday physical activity.

Any condition resulting in the inability to engage in daily activity for a prolonged period of time will result in debility, also known as decreased endurance. In its simplest form, endurance is then better categorized by the degree of impairment rather than mode of injury or illness. Many situations of mildly compromised endurance go without formal intervention and are addressed simply be re-engaging in normal daily routine as tolerated. These also tend to be situations characterized by short hospital stays of a few days or less with discharge back to the home setting. In the event that occupational therapy is required following discharge, intervention is commonly preformed in the outpatient clinic or in the home with a focus on the primary diagnosis, not the limitation of endurance. On the contrary, a client requiring a lengthy hospital stay, complicated by a subsequent visit to a subacute care or rehabilitative hospital setting represents the most common scenario associated with a moderate to maximal compromise in endurance level.

Modes of moderate to maximal level of impairment in endurance may include a client recovering from a fractured hip complicated by a deep vein thrombosis requiring anticoagulation therapy and bed rest for the period of several days to a week. It may include a client with Guillain-Barré syndrome resulting in temporary paralysis for weeks or possibly a client who has sustained an acquired brain injury or exacerbation of chronic obstructive pulmonary disease (COPD) resulting in the need for mechanical ventilation. Each plausible scenario presented will certainly yield significant impairment on a client's ability to endure personally meaningful activity engagement.

Remedial Techniques: Biomechanical Theory

As is the case with most remedial strategies for addressing physically-based foundational skills, the Biomechanical Theory outlines the most diverse array of methods commonly employed by the OT to address compromised endurance and are summarized in Table 2-15.

PROMOTION OF ACTIVITY ENGAGEMENT

As OTs, we historically embrace the therapeutic value of engagement in purposeful activity as well as the power of motivation and interest on the healing process. Therefore, OTs will interview

> **Table 2-15**
>
> ## REMEDIAL ENDURANCE TECHNIQUES OF THE BIOMECHANICAL THEORY
>
> - Active engagement in graded functional activity engagement designed to address the client's specific needs and interests.
> - Exercise programs with no or low weight, low repetitions and high number of sets.
> - Arm ergometers at a client specific frequency and duration.
> - Pulley programs at a client specific frequency and duration.

the client as to their interest, leisure pursuits, or hobbies and infuse those identified as methods for addressing issues of endurance. The OT implements his/her skills in gradation to provide the ideal challenge in completing the identified activity while avoiding over fatigue and minimizing frustration. These measures can take any form depending on the level of impairment presented by the client. For example, a session may be conducted where a client engages in painting while seated in a high back chair with arm rests and using a lap tray for 10 minutes. The sessions would then progress to standing at an upright easel for 30 minutes thereby fostering sustained activity over time. An additional technique commonly employed is *chaining*—forward or backward chaining. The OT may also elicit chaining as a means of ensuring motivational success for clients. As was detailed in Chapter 1, the OT will break down a functional task into its component parts and then grade the level of assistance provided in completing the task with the client. In backward chaining, the OT begins the task and the client completes it. This technique then promotes client confidence in his/her skills by avoiding a sense of failure inherent of being unsuccessfully in attempt. The therapist then decreases the assistance while the client continues to gain skill and confidence, eventually becoming independent with the entire task (Pedretti & Early, 2001). If the therapist is unable to decrease assistance, then remediation is no longer an appropriate approach. An example can be found by using cooking as a method of improving endurance levels. With backward changing a cooking task, the OT will begin the task by setting out all of the required supplies while the client is responsible for preparing only. This would then be graded accordingly to the point where the client completes all facets of the task independently. In general, clients tend to truly enjoy activity-based interventions and with infusing personal interest, are better motivated to actively participate and improve their level of endurance.

TRADITIONAL EXERCISE PROGRAMS

An additionally popular approach for remediating endurance is exercise with no or low weights and high repetitions, thereby fostering endurance rather than muscle strength. Examples of these include the use of pulley exercises, work simulators, and arm ergometers all previously described in further details amid the ROM and strength subsections of this chapter.

Techniques at a Glance

Table 2-15 outlines the most implemented remedial techniques for issues of endurance.

Special Considerations

Again, as was the case with strength, the OT must pay close attention as to how the client is tolerating intervention. Frequently, clients underestimate the effect that decreased endurance has on their ability to engage in daily activity. The signs and symptoms requiring the attention of the OT include diaphoresis, shortness of breath, pallor of skin, and/or client complaint of feeling faint or dizzy. For some, endurance has been so significantly impacted the process of sitting at the edge of the bed will bring on these symptoms. It is a responsibility of the OT to make steady gains in the client's ability to tolerate engagement in upright activities following through the efficient use of gradation skills as tolerated overtime.

An additional consideration for this foundational skill area is the likelihood for depression. The most common mode for decreased endurance is prolonged immobility and is most often due to the onset of complications resulting secondary to the initial injury or illness. It is within these often-severe illnesses and injuries that the likelihood for depression becomes evident and, therefore, specifically warrants the direct attention of the OT. It is important that the OT acknowledge a client's feelings, provide facts to enable clients to make educated decisions as to their level of participation in intervention, and make referrals for ancillary services within the treatment team as necessary.

Maintenance Programs

Overall, a maintenance program designed to foster optimal endurance should emphasize graded re-engagement in those activities a client would characterize as constituting a typical daily routine prior to the onset of the illness or injury. Careful attention should also be placed on the active and independent execution of work simplification and energy conservation techniques during the tasks of everyday living and are explained in further detail within Chapters 3 and 4 of this text.

REMEDIAL TECHNIQUES FOR COORDINATION

Definitional Analysis

Coordination is defined most specifically by the *Framework* document (AOTA, 2002) as a performance skill. Coordination "relates to using more than one body part to interact with task objects in a manner that supports task performance" (AOTA, 2002, p. 621). This classification of coordination illustrates its complexity as an integrated skill or product requiring an array of client factors. These client factors include functions of the sensory system, such as the vestibular sense, and neuromusculoskeletal systems in the form of movement-related functions. Movement-related functions require the subconscious integration of reflexes and righting reactions, as well as the interpretation of sensory information, so as to produce smooth movement of "two or more body parts together (for stabilizing and manipulating) task objects during bilateral motor tasks" (AOTA, 2002, p. 621).

Omitted from the *Framework* document, yet commonly used in clinical practice, is the delineation among fine motor coordination and gross motor coordination. Fine motor skills are commonly thought of as those movements controlled by smaller or more precise joints and musculature (Watson & Llorens, 1997). Conversely, gross motor skills refer to those movements generated by larger musculature and promote larger range movement such as the shoulder and hip joints (Watson & Llorens, 1997). The ability to coordinate both fine motor and gross motor movement relies heavily on accurate interpretation of sensory information and the ability to control resulting movement. "Coordinated movement involves multiple joints and muscles that are activated at the appropriate time and with the correct amount of force so smooth, efficient, and accurate movement occurs" (Shumway-Cook & Woollacott, 2001, p. 141). As a result, an array of illnesses and injuries may impede coordination through inadequate sensory input that then produces inaccurate motor output.

Modes of Injury or Illness

Neurologically based impairments of coordination, otherwise known as ataxia, are seen typically as secondary symptoms of an illness or injury. As is the case with many other foundational skills covered within the contents of this chapter, ataxia can occur as a result of a wide array of neurological conditions.

Acquired brain injury encapsulates many of these conditions. Injuries to the brain, and specifically to the cerebellum, include trauma by means of an external force (TBI), CVA caused by hemorrhage, ischemia, or infarct, meningitis, abscesses, or tumors. Each of these injuries may potentially affect the coordination centers of the brain and result in ataxic or uncoordinated movement patterns.

Degenerative disorders of the central and/or peripheral nervous systems may also represent the underlying cause for ataxia, dystonia, or dyskinesia. Dystonia is defined as "prolonged muscle contractions that may cause twisting and repetitive movements or abnormal posture" (Thomas, 1997, p. 592). This symptom is commonly seen in illnesses such as Parkinson's, Huntington's, and Creutzfeldt-Jakob diseases as well as in disease-related dementias. Dyskinesia is defines as "a defect in the ability to perform voluntary movement" (Thomas, 1997, p. 588), thus directly affecting the ability to perform coordinated movement. Some illnesses causing dyskinesia can include MS, post-polio syndrome, MG, ALS, or even peripheral neuropathies in general.

Therefore, overall, the mode of illness or injury responsible for a deficit in coordination can be quite inclusive, ranging from acute trauma to degenerative disease processes. However, the mode of injury or illness is of significance due to the impact it has on the choice of intervention strategy. This concept will be explored further in the Special Considerations portion of this subsection.

Remedial Techniques: Motor Learning and Neurodevelopmental Theories

When addressing coordination issues, remedial strategies applied tend to be grounded in Motor Learning and Neurodevelopmental Theories and are summarized in Table 2-16. The shared basic tenet of these theories is found in the concept of the brain's ability to reorganize following neurological insult, commonly referred to as the principle of neural plasticity. Due to this strong, shared belief, these theories they can also be grouped under a single title, the *Neurodevelopmental-Motor Learning Theory* (Trombly, 1995).

"Plasticity or neural modifiability, may be seen as a continuum from short term changes in the efficiency or strength of synaptic connections to the long term structural changes in the organization and numbers of connections among neurons" (Shumway-Cook & Woollacott, 2001, p. 92). Essentially, this principle asserts that the brain is able to regenerate neural pathways damaged by illness or injury through sprouting or regrowing alternate pathways that then allow for the recovery of motor control. An analogy can be found in the image of a collapsed interstate highway bridge. Immediately following the "collapse," traffic may be backed up for miles and chaos ensues as vehicles scramble to locate alternate routes to their ultimate destinations. Though the alternate route may not be the most efficient means to get where one needs to go, it does serve an important purpose in allowing the required time for "reconstruction" at the bridge site. Once reopened, the repaired bridge will again allow for the passage of vehicles as it did in the past, though never at it once had prior to the event. This is the same premise when considering the effect of injury or illness on the neural pathways of the brain. In neural plasticity, the collapse of one pathway will cause the diversion of impulses to alternate routes so as to reach their final destination. Though the diverted routes may never be as efficient as the original paths, nonetheless, they meet an important purpose for the interim. To enhance the efficiency in rebuilding neural pathways, repetition is believed to have significant value. Hence, this principle also emphasizes the repetition of normal movement patterns as a means of shaping the regeneration process.

The most contemporary theories for remediating motor performance are grounded in the Motor Learning Theory, where emphasis is placed upon the repetitive engagement in functional activity to foster recovery (Trombly & Radomski, 2002). With this theory, the guided practice of context-specific activities, within the naturally occurring environment, yield the remediation of coordinated movement (Trombly & Radomski, 2002).

Though the neurodevelopmental approaches share in the principles of neural plasticity and with emphasis on repetition, it additionally ascribes to the foundations of movement as reflexive and developmental in nature (Trombly, 1995). This premise dictates that intervention follows the human developmental sequence so as to facilitate remediation of coordinated movement. Very popular in use historically among the occupational and physical therapy domains, this theory prevailed as the strategy of choice for many years in the remediation of normal movement patterns following neurological impairment.

In the rehabilitative era of today, Ashwinik (2004) brings eloquent clarity to the shift from the use of traditional neurodevelopmental approaches to that of the contemporary motor learning approaches. Describing the phenomena as "...paradigm shifts related to the treatment of neuro-logic dysfunction" (Ashwinik, 2004, p. 94), the author concludes that, "The evidence reviewed... based on the results of randomized controlled trials, clearly demonstrates (at a grade A level) (supported by at least one level 1 study) that neurotherapeutic (neurodevelopmental) approaches are at best no more effective than traditional therapy and in fact are inferior to training based on a task-oriented approach" (Ashwinik, 2004, pp. 95 & 100). Therefore, the task-oriented techniques of the Motor Learning Theory will be reviewed first, and followed by those of the Neurodevelopmental Theory. Although lacking in evidence-base, as is summarized by Ashwinik (2004) and reproduced with permission in Tables 2-17 through 2-19, neurodevelopmental approaches do harbor historical significance in the shaping of the profession as it stands today and are, therefore, included in the text of this subsection.

THE MOTOR LEARNING THEORY: A REVIEW OF THE TASK-ORIENTED, CARR AND SHEPHERD, AND CONSTRAINT-INDUCED MOVEMENT APPROACHES

The Task-Oriented Approach

The *Task-Oriented Approach* was first coined by Horak in 1991 on behalf of a variety of multidisciplinary specialists working to "understand motor control and learning from the perspectives of neurophysiology, biomechanics, and behavioral science" (Ashwinik, 2004, p. 100). The Task-Oriented Approach also shares a foundation in neural plasticity, but uniquely recognizes the significance of client-centered intervention or the individual with unique interests, experiences, desires, and motivators. Hence, the return of coordinated movement within this approach is a result of repetitive engagement in personally preferred movement patterns occurring within the natural environment.

The onset of illness or injury disrupts the preferred motor patterns that enable successful activity engagement. This approach requires the OT to analyze the component parts of completing the preferred task, identify the physical barriers to engaging in those tasks (such as a lack of coordination), and facilitate successful re-engagement in that task by means of grading and chaining the client's participation accordingly. Therefore, the OT acts as a "teacher of motor skills" (Ashwinik, 2004, p. 100) and, just as any teacher, modifies the demands a task presents so as to allow for the appropriate challenge and ultimate success for the client. Ashwinik (2004), in review of current efficacy studies, states that some evidence has been demonstrated in the use of this relatively new approach when compared with that of a control group, but also notes that additional studies are required to develop a evidence base for the Task-Oriented Approach.

Table 2-16	
REMEDIAL COORDINATION TECHNIQUES OF THE MOTOR LEARNING AND NEURODEVELOPMENTAL THEORIES ACCORDING TO HEALTH CONDITION	
Mode of Injury	*Remedial Technique*
Acquired brain injuries including TBI, stroke, meningitis, abscesses, and tumors.	**Motor Learning Approaches**: • Task-oriented approach • Carr & Shepherd approach • Constraint induced approach • Graded, functionally-oriented tasks • Backward chaining of functionally-oriented tasks OR
Degenerative Diseases including Parkinson's, Huntington's, MS, ALS, Postpolio, etc.	**Traditional Sensorimotor Approaches** of… • **Bobath/NDT**: Weight-bearing, weight shifting, key points of control • **Proprioceptive Neuromuscular Facilitation (PNF)**: Diagonal movement patterns, multisensory cueing, kinesthetic feedback • **Rood**: Muscle cocontraction, multisensory cuing

The Carr and Shepherd Approach

Carr and Shepherd, Australian physical therapists, have applied motor control and learning principles to occupational therapy interventions for motor difficulties occurring secondary to CNS dysfunction. This approach, referred to as the *Motor Relearning Programme (MRP)*, very closely resembles that of that the Task-Oriented Approach given the emphasis of clients to engage in personally-preferred tasks, but differs in that intervention is implemented with the goal of motor recovery and not actual completion of the task itself (Shumway-Cook & Woollacott, 2001). Carr and Shepherd, therefore, use the engagement in functional activity for the powerful motivating factors it elicits within a client alone. Here, it is through engaging repetitively in motor tasks, that neural plasticity can be best facilitated.

The Carr and Shepherd Approach uniquely harbors a biomechanical component given a foundations in human kinesiology and specifically, the analysis of kinematic and kinetic requirements for completing functional tasks. This approach sees the therapist as a coach whose primary role in intervention is to provide education to clients by means of verbal and nonverbal communication techniques (Shumway-Cook & Woollacott, 2001), again similar to that of the Task-Oriented Approach. The secondary role is then to manually guide normal movement patterns and/or minimize abnormal movement patterns during activity engagement that arise commonly following neurological insult. Like other Motor Learning theories, Carr and Shepherd also place much emphasis on the use of repetitive practice to elicit the efficient return of coordinated motor performance. Overall, the method is one where the client is actively learning principles to optimize normal movement patterns, as guided by the therapist, during engagement in a preferred personal activity. In August 2000, Langhammer and Stranghelle published the results of a study designed to compare the efficacy of the Carr and Sheppard's *MRP* approach versus that of the Bobath Approach (also coined the neurodevelopmental [NDT] approach). After a review of the outcome measures, Langhammer and Stranghelle (2000, p.369) found that clients who received *MRP* techniques stayed fewer days in the hospital and achieved significantly better motor function when compared with that of the group who received the traditional techniques of the Bobath (NDT) approach.

Table 2-17

EVIDENCE FOR EFFECTIVENESS OF NEUROTHERAPIES

Authors and Year	Aims/Rationale	Design and Subjects	Intervention and Outcome Measures	Results	Comments	Rating
Basmajian et al. (1987)	Compare two PT approaches: Behavioral (including biofeedback) and Bobath in subacute stroke stage.	RCT. 29 subjects. Training 3 times a week for 5 weeks. Pretesting and posttesting; 9-month follow-up. Subjects with first MCA infarcts.	*Behavioral group:* Electromyographic biofeedback through conceptualization, skill learning, rehearsal, and transfer. *Bobath group:* Facilitation with controlled sensory input. 1. Upper Extremity Function Test 2. Health Belief System 3. Beck's Depression Inventory 4. 16 PF (for mood and affect)	Both groups improved; no differences were seen between groups. Bobath treatment was not superior to behavioral treatmen.	Small sample size. Good study.	II
Mudie et al. (2002)	Compare task-related, Bobath, and feedback approaches for training weight symmetry in subacute stroke stage.	Double-blind RCT. 40 subjects. Training 5 times a week for 2 weeks; assessment 1 week before study and 2 and 12 weeks after study.	*Feedback group:* Provided visual feedback of symmetry via monitor during reach. *Task-related group:* functional reach in various directions and distances. *Bobath group:* Increasing range of motion, normalize tone, improve balance during reach. *Control group:* Standard occupational therapy and PT. 1. Weight distribution in sitting 2. Weight distribution in standing 3. Barthel index	Bobath group was better at sitting symmetry at 2 weeks; feedback and task-related groups were better at 12 weeks; feedback group was better at standing symmetry at 2 weeks; task-related group was better than Bobath group; and task-related group was better in functional gains.	Good study. Small sample size.	II

continued

Table 2-17, continued

Evidence for Effectiveness of Neurotherapies

Authors and Year	Aims/Rationale	Design and Subjects	Intervention and Outcome Measures	Results	Comments	Rating
Pollack et al. (2002)	Test effect of independent sitting balance as adjunct to standard therapy based on Bobath approach in subacute stroke stage.	RCT with blocked randomization with 2:1 ratio 28 subjects. Training 5 times a week for 4 weeks; assessment at start at end of training and 2 weeks after training.	*Experimental group:* Construction tasks that encouraged balance. 1. Proportion of patients achieving normal symmetry of weight distribution during standing, sitting, rising to stand, sitting down, and reaching.	No differences were seen across groups.	Unequal groups. Small sample size. One outcome measure.	II
Lord and Hall (1986)	Compare NDT to traditional therapy.	Retrospective study of 39 subjects.	ADL scale.	No differences across groups.	Unequal groups.	IV
Wagenaar et al. (1990)	Compare NDT and Brunnstrom approaches in acute stroke stage.	Case series. Alternating treatment design. 7 subjects with MCA stroke. Training for 5 times a week for 21 weeks; each phase lasted 5 weeks.	1. Action Research Arm Test 2. Walking velocity over 8 m 3. Barthel index 4. VROPSOM List (Dutch version of the Depression Adjective Checklist) 5. Neuropsychologic tests	Walking speed was better for only one patient during Brunnstrom treatment; all patients showed some recovery in the first 8 to 10 weeks.	Small sample size. No true control group.	V

continued

Table 2-17, continued

EVIDENCE FOR EFFECTIVENESS OF NEUROTHERAPIES

Authors and Year	Aims/Rationale	Design and Subjects	Intervention and Outcome Measures	Results	Comments	Rating
Hesse et al. (1994)	Test the effect of an NDT-based inpatien program on gait in subacute stroke stage.	Case series. 148 subjects who could walk 20 m independently. Training 5 times a week for 4 weeks; assessment at beginning and at 4 weeks.	All patients received occupation therapy, speech therapy, and neuropsychologic training as needed. 1. Gait measures (peak vertical ground reaction force, loading and deloading rates, time to peak force) 2. 10-m walk 3. Walking endurance 4. Stair climbing	Time for walking and climbing improved, but no endurance; stance duration and symmetry improved.	No control group.	V

Reprinted from *Stroke Rehabilitation*, 2e, Gillen G., pp 96-99, ©2004 with permission from Elsevier.

Table 2-18

EVIDENCE FOR TASK-ORIENTED APPROACH

Authors and Year	Rationale	Design and Subjects	Intervention and Outcome Measures	Results	Comments	Rating
Kwakkel et al. (1999)	Test effect of different intensity of task-related leg and arm training in acute stroke stage; test whether training produces task-specific improvement.	Single-blind RCT. 101 subjects randomized in three groups (leg, arm, and control). Training for 5 days/week for 20 weeks. Follow-up until 26 weeks.	*Leg group:* Sitting, standing, and weight-bearing. *Arm group:* Leaning ball pinching, grasping (forced use). *Control:* Leg and arm immobilized. 1. Barthel index 2. FAC 3. Action Research Arm Test	Training influenced task-specific improvement. Experimental groups did better than control group on ADL scores, walking ability, and dexterity; leg training generalized better than arm training.	Very good study.	I
Kwakkel et al. (2002)	Test effect of different intensity of task-related leg and arm training 1 year after stroke.	RCT. Follow-up of 1999 study. 86 subjects from original group tested at 6 and 12 months.	1. Barthel index 2. FAC 3. Action Research Arm Test	No differences seen between groups at 6 months and 1 year; improvement was maintained at 1 year. Greater intensity of treatment improved speed of functional recovery in the first 6 months.	Very good study.	I

continued

Table 2-18, continued

EVIDENCE FOR TASK-ORIENTED APPROACH

continued

Authors and Year	Rationale	Design and Subjects	Intervention and Outcome Measures	Results	Comments	Rating
Richards et al. (1993)	Test effect of early gait-focused therapy.	RCT. 27 subjects. Experimental group: Early task-based therapy (1.74 hours/day). Control group 1: Early conventional PT (1.79 hours/day). Control group 2: Conventional PT (0.73 hours/day).	*Experimental group:* Early standing, weight-shifting, iso-kinetic exercises, and tread-mill training. 1. Fugl-Meyer Assessment 2. Barthel index 3. Berg Balance Scale 4. Gait velocity 6-month fol-low-up	Gait velocity was higher for experimen-tal group.	Benefit in only one variable.	II
Dean & Shepard (1997)	Test effect of a 2-week program on sitting balance.	RCT. 20 subjects. Experimental group: Reaching tasks. Control group: Sham cognitive tasks. 10 sessions over 2 weeks. Post-test at 10 weeks.	Training sitting balance dur-ing reaching tasks. Distance, direction, speed, seat height, and thigh support varied. 1. Ground reaction forces 2. Electromyography 3. Reaching distance 4. Movement time	Experimental group performed better on reach distance, reach time, and ground reaction force.	Good treatment and study design. Small sample size, few clinical tests given.	II

Table 2-18, continued

EVIDENCE FOR TASK-ORIENTED APPROACH

Authors and Year	Rationale	Design and Subjects	Intervention and Outcome Measures	Results	Comments	Rating
Dean, Richards, & Malouin (2000)	Test the effect of task-related circuit training.	RCT pilot study. 2-month follow-up. 9 subjects. Exercise for 1 hour, 3 times a week for 4 weeks.	Experimental group: Strengthening and functional activities. Control group: Functional activities. 1. Walking speed and endurance 2. Vertical ground reaction force 3. Step test	Experimental group performed better on walking speed and endurance and on force production.	Small sample size. Study only tested added influence of strength training.	II
Nelles et al. (2001)	Test brain plasticity after task-related training in early stroke stage.	RCT. 10 subjects after first stroke; early subacute stroke stage. Training 4 times a week for 3 weeks.	Task oriented functional reach in different directions and distances. Control group: Stretching, ROM. 1. Positron emission tomography scan.	After training, task-oriented group showed activation of contralateral sensorimotor cortex and bilateral activation of the inferior parietal cortex; control group showed weak activation of only the inferior parietal cortex.	Good study. Small sample size.	II
Malouin et al. (1992)	Test application of a task-oriented treatment in improving gait after acute stroke stage.	Case series design. 10 subjects. 2 sessions/day, 5 days/week for 8 weeks.	Early standing, weight-shifting, isokinetic exercises and treadmill training. 1. Treadmill velocity 2. Training duration	Treadmill velocity and training duration increased.	Small sample size. No control group. Double the typical treatment time in PT.	V

continued

Table 2-18, continued

EVIDENCE FOR TASK-ORIENTED APPROACH

Authors and Year	Rationale	Design and Subjects	Intervention and Outcome Measures	Results	Comments	Rating
Smith et al. (1999)	Test a task-oriented treadmill exercise program in chronic stroke stage.	Case series. 14 subjects. Training 3 times a week for 3 months.	Reflexive and volitional torque generated by dynamometer at different velocities.	Torque production for concentric and eccentric contractions increased.	Small sample size. No control group.	V
Monger, Carr, & Fowler (2002)	Test a task-specific home exercise program in chronic stroke stage.	Pretest, post-test case series design. 6 subjects, 1 year after stroke. 3-week home exercise program.	Intervention was based on motor learning; sit-to-stand and stepping was practiced at different seat heights, speeds, and repetitions. 1. Motor Assessment Scale (MAS) 2. Vertical ground reaction force 3. Walking speed over 10 m 4. Grip strength	Scores on the MAS, vertical ground reaction force, and walking speed improved for experimental group; grip force did not improve.	No control group; small sample size. Good pilot study.	V
Bassile et al. (2003)	Test effect of a task-related obstacle training program in chronic stroke stage.	Case-series. Pretraining and post-training; 1 month follow-up. 5 subjects. Training 2 times/week for 5 weeks.	Subjects walked along a 10-m walkway over obstacles on two thirds of the trials. 1. MAS walking section 2. 6-minute walk distance 3. Walking velocity 4. SF-36	Improvements seen in walking velocity, 6-minute walk distance, MAS, and SF-36.	Good pilot study. Small sample size. No control group.	V

Reprinted from *Stroke Rehabilitation*, 2e, Gillen G., pp 96-99, ©2004 with permission from Elsevier.

Table 2-19

Evidence Table for Constraint-Induced Movement Therapy

Authors and Year	Rationale	Design and Subjects	Intervention and Outcome Measures	Results	Comments	Rating
Van der Lee et al. (1999)	Evaluate the effectiveness of forced use therapy; compare CIMT with Bobath therapy in chronic stroke stage.	RCT. 60 subjects. Experimental group: immobilization and training. Control group: bimanual training based on NDT. Training was 6 hours/day 5 days/week for 2 weeks. Follow-up for 1 year.	Experimental group: Splint worn for most of the day; training of functional activities. Control group: Bimanual activities. 1. Rehabilitation Activities Profile 2. Action Research Arm Test (ARAT) 3. Fugl-Meyer Assessment 4. Motor Activity Log (MAL)	CIMT group performed better on ARAT and arm use 1 week after training; gains on ARAT were maintained after 1 year. CIMT group had greater amount of arm use, but did not maintain in the long term.	Good study. CIMT group performance better at start of training. Modest benefit of CIMT over Bobath approach.	I
Taub et al. (1993)	Test whether forced use of the impaired limb counteracts learned nonuse in chronic stroke stage.	RCT. 9 subjects in chronic stroke stage. Experimental group (4): restraint of the unimpaired limbs for 23 hours; therapy for 6 hours/day 5 days/week for 2 weeks.	Limb restrained for 23 hours/day for experimental group. Control group asked to focus on use of impaired limb. 1. Emory Motor Function Test 2. ARAT 3. MAL 4. Passive range of motion	Performance time was quicker for restraint group; quality of movement and functional ability were better for restraint group.	Small sample size. Experimental group had much more training. Training massed over 2 weeks. No comparison with traditional rehabilitation.	II

continued

Table 2-19, continued

EVIDENCE TABLE FOR CONSTRAINT-INDUCED MOVEMENT THERAPY

Authors and Year	Rationale	Design and Subjects	Intervention and Outcome Measures	Results	Comments	Rating
Dromerick, Edwards, and Hahn (2000)	Compare CIMT with OT in the acute stage.	RCT. 20 subjects. Experimental group (11): Mitten worn 6 hours/day, plus OT and CIMT training 2 hours/day for 5 days/week for 2 weeks. Control group (9): Standard OT and circuit training.	Mitten worn 5 hours/day for 14 days. 1. ARAT 2. Barthel index 3. Functional Independence Measure (FIM)	CIMT group had better total ARAT scores and upper extremity FIM scores. No other differences were seen.	Little support for benefit of CIMT approach. Small sample size.	II
Page et al. (2002)	Test the efficacy of a modified CIMT protocol in subacute stroke stage.	RCT. 14 subjects. Modified CIMT group: half hour PT and OT 2 times a week for 10 weeks.	*Modified CIMT group:* Restraint for 5 hours/day; training 1 hour/day. *Traditional group:* PNF therapy. 1. Fugl-Meyer Assessment 2. ARAT 3. MAL	No change was seen in traditional and control group. Modified CIMT group improved on Fugl-Meyer Assessment, ARAT, and MAL.	Small sample size.	II
Wolf et al. (1989)	First study to test CIMT in chronic stroke age.	Case series. Pretreatment and post-treatment 21 subjects. Restraint and training, 3-month follow-up.	14 days of restraint and 10 days of training. 1. Wolf Motor Function Test (WMFT)	Arm function improved following restraint and training.	No control group. Small sample size, limited outcome measures.	V

continued

Table 2-19, continued

Evidence Table for Constraint-Induced Movement Therapy

Authors and Year	Rationale	Design and Subjects	Intervention and Outcome Measures	Results	Comments	Rating
Kunkel et al. (1999)	Replicate findings of Taub et al.	Case series design. Pretreatment and post-treatment 5 subjects in chronic stroke stage 3-month follow-up.	Limb restrained for 23 hours a day for 14 days. 1. MAL 2. WMFT 3. ARAT	Restraint improved MAL, WMFT, and quality of movement.	No control group. Small sample size.	V
Blanton and Wolf (1999)	Test the effectiveness of CIMT in subacute stroke stage.	Case report. Pretreatment and post-treatment. 3 month follow-up 14 days of restraint and 10 days of training.	Hand constrained in a mitten for 23 hours a day. 1. WMFT 2. MAL	Completion time improved on the WMFT; improvement seen on self-report (MAL).	Single patient; limited generalizability.	V
Miltner et al. (1999)	Replicate earlier findings on the benefit of CIMT.	Case series 15 subjects in chronic stroke stage. Sling on arm for 90% of waking time for 12 days. Training for 7 hours/day for 8 days 6-month follow-up.	Restraint and shaping with familiar household objects. 1. MAL 2. WMFT 3. ARAT	Actual amount of use and quality of movement; functional ability improved and was retained over 6 months.	No control group. Small sample size. Massed practice.	V

continued

Table 2-19, continued

EVIDENCE TABLE FOR CONSTRAINT-INDUCED MOVEMENT THERAPY

Authors and Year	Rationale	Design and Subjects	Intervention and Outcome Measures	Results	Comments	Rating
Page et al. (2001)	Test the efficacy of a modified CIMT protocol; compare CIMT embedded in therapy with therapy and no therapy in a sub-acute outpatient setting	Case series 6 subjects. 2 subjects: OT/PT 3 times/week for 10 weeks plus sling and mitt for 5 hours/day 5 days/week. 2 subjects: OT/PT for 10 weeks. 2 subjects: no therapy 10-week follow-up.	CIMT and traditional group received 30 minutes of training 3 times a week. 1. Fugl-Meyer Assessment 2. ARAT 3. WMFT 4. MAL	CIMT group performed better on Fugl-Meyer Assessment, ARAT, WMFT, and MAL.	Small sample size. No statistical analysis of useful modification CIMT approach to out-patient therapy.	V

Reprinted from *Stroke Rehabilitation*, 2e, Gillen G., pp 96-99, ©2004 with permission from Elsevier.

The Constraint-Induced Movement Therapy Approach

Recently, more attention is being drawn toward the Constraint-Induced Movement Therapy (CIMT) Approach as the rehabilitative field moves toward evidence-based practice models. With related publications dating back to the 1960s, E. Taub and coworkers began by conducting experiments on primates where a single forelimb was deafferented surgically through dorsal rhizotomy (Ashwinik, 2004). Following the procedure, observations found that the primates tended to disuse the affected (deafferent) limb. Taub, Uswatte, & Pidikiti (1999) suggested that this was a learned behavior where the primates preferred the positive reinforcement obtained through coordinated use of the unaffected limb over the negative experiences resulting from the attempted use of the affected limb.

As the studies of Taub et al. (1999) continued to analyze this "learned nonuse" (p. 239) of the affected limb, the group discovered that by applying a device that physically constrained the movement of the unaffected or intact limb, the primates then resorted back to the use of the affected limb to perform essential activities such as grooming and feeding. These findings provided the foundation for the Constraint-Induced Therapy (CIT) approach, also referred to in literature as the CIMT or Forced Use Therapy approaches.

In occupational therapy intervention, the CIT approach requires the use of a constraint device, such as a mitt or sling, applied to the unaffected extremity of a client with hemiparesis, 14 hours per day for 2 weeks (Page, Sisto, Levine, Johnston, & Hughes, 2001, p. 584) while promoting active engagement in daily routines. Though evidence supports functional improvement in the coordinated use of the affected extremity, particularly in clients with chronic cardiovascular accidents, several barriers to the successful integration of the approach in intervention have been identified. The chief barrier includes the investment of time required by the client (and therapist) over the 2-week interval. This duration of 14 hours per day can quickly lead to frustration and poor compliance, therefore, negative results. As a result, Page, Sisto, & Johnston (2000) adapted the CIT approach, decreasing intensity to 5 hours per day, 5 days per week for a duration of 10 weeks. Results of studies on this modified CIT protocol have yielded similarly positive findings, "is effective in reducing upper limb impairment and improving upper limb use and function" (Page et al., 2001, p. 589).

Given the evidence in support, the CIT approach will continue to gain visibility into the foreseeable future. However, the method is not one suitable for all clientele. A client must be able to demonstrate specific degrees of active range (average of 10 degrees) in the digits and wrist to be considered eligible for success with this technique and certainly, attention must be paid to the potential safety risk posed by constraining the unaffected extremity of a client who has sustained a neurological injury.

THE NEURODEVELOPMENTAL THEORY: A REVIEW OF NDT, PNF, ROOD, AND BRUNNSTROM APPROACHES

Per the Neurodevelopmental Theory, the four most traditionally popular and commonly implemented approaches for coordination are the Bobath or NDT Approach, Kabat's Proprioceptive Neuromuscular Facilitation (PNF) Approach, the Rood Approach (Stroup & Snodgrass, 2005), and the Brunnstrom Approach. As mentioned above, each of these approaches share in the principles of neural plasticity further enhanced by the promotion of repetition. However, these approaches differ in that they also harbor a shared belief that it is through eliciting reflexive movements along the developmental continuum, that coordinated movement will be restored. Given the complexity of this belief, the use of these approaches often warrants continuing education on behalf of the therapist. Additional information regarding continuing education opportunities in these areas may be found in Appendix A.

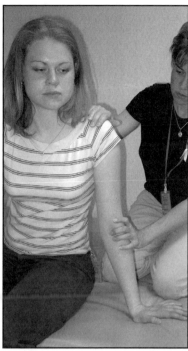

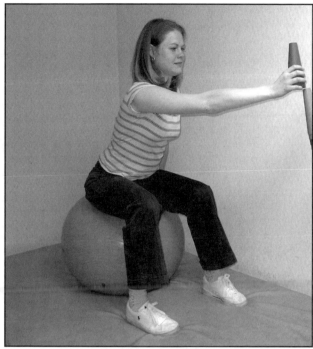

Figure 2-15. Demonstration of a typical weight-bearing position throughout the UE. Support and stability is provided by the therapist at the elbow and shoulder joint structures as the client leans towards the positioned extremity to bear body weight through shoulder, elbow, and wrist joints of the UE.

Figure 2-16. Demonstrated in this figure is an example of how weight-bearing can be promoted throughout the trunk and LE while also challenging postural control by reaching out of the base of support. Though an OT's primary focus is on engagement in functional activity, at times the use of cones is adopted. This procedure minimizes distraction, redirecting attention to the challenge demanded by both balancing and weight shifting in the presence of compromised proximal stability.

The NDT (Bobath) Approach, developed by a Dr. Karel and Berta Bobath, a 1940s husband and wife team (one a neurologist and the other, a physical therapist) places emphasis on the accurate interpretation of sensory input to produce refined motor output (Luke, Dodd, & Brock, 2003). Dysfunction in coordination is a result of abnormal sensation and, specifically, abnormal sensations of the upright posture. Without postural control in the core musculature, a client is unable to produce coordinated motion in the distal extremities. Therefore, much of the approach emphasizes the establishment of postural stability and alignment by employing techniques of weight-bear and weight shift (Bertoti, 2004). Here, the OT is fostering exaggerated sensory input by means of bearing weight directly through affected extremities to improve both interpretation via feedback and resulting motor output (Figure 2-15). With regard to weight shift, the OT promotes reaching, either in a functional capacity or with the use of a therapeutic ball, out of the base of support to introduce graded opportunities for challenging the core stability or underlying postural control. Figure 2-16 is an illustration of this technique. These remedial methods, guided by specific handling techniques designed to inhibit reflexive movement (key points of control), secondarily improve distal mobility or coordination of the extremities. Of note, though NDT is a historically popular remedial approach, "there is little evidence to show its effectiveness" (Stroup & Snodgrass, 2005, p. 49) when compared and contrasted with other methods of intervention. In a recent study conducted by the Dutch NDT group, Hafsteinsdottir, Algra, & Grypdonck (2005) reported that the NDT approach was not effective for clients diagnosed with a stroke in a hospital setting.

Figure 2-17. Movement in a diagonal or curvilinear pattern integrated into the execution of a functional activity.

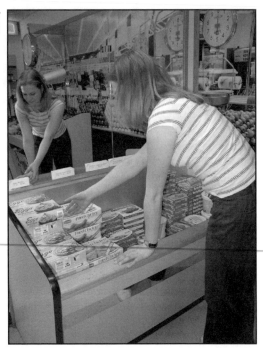

Herman Kabat, a neurophysiologist, developed the PNF Approach in the 1940s that again focuses on the developmental sequence of motor performance, yet with a strategic focus on agonist and antagonist muscle relationships (Pedretti & Early, 2001). The foundation of this approach is found in the belief that human motion occurs in a curvilinear plane and is requiring of the entire system to execute accurately. Function is a result of the fine orchestration, by the central nervous system, among antagonist and agonist muscle contractions. Remedial techniques of PNF foster gross motor motions in diagonal or curvilinear (Figure 2-17) patterns to best simulate functional motion and progress as dictated by typical motor development. Emphasis is placed heavily on repetition as the manner of retraining the motor control centers to specific sensory input and facilitated by way of verbal or tactile cuing. Upon regaining a cooperative relationship among the muscular system as a whole, coordination is, therefore, improved. As for efficacy of this approach, research is limited (Shimura & Kasai, 2001). In support, Godges, Mattson-Bell, Thorpe, and Shah (2003) found a single intervention of soft tissue mobilization and PNF was effective in improving glenohumeral external rotation and overhead reach in clients with shoulder dysfunction. Conversely, Kraft, Fitts, and Hammond (1992) found PNF to be the least effective method of intervention with clients who had a chronic stroke when compared to techniques of electrical stimulation.

Margaret Rood, who was versed in both occupational and physical therapy professions, developed the Rood Approach in the 1950s (Pedretti & Early, 2001). This approach addresses coordination deficits secondarily by prioritizing remedial techniques used to normalize muscle tone. Tone will be specifically addressed in a later subsection, while coordination remains the focus here, thus only a portion of the Rood Approach is directly applicable. Rood also, as does the NDT and PNF Approaches, emphasizes the developmental nature of motor control and the importance of postural alignment or stability. Like PNF, these techniques foster unison between agonistic and antagonist musculature, and like both PNF and NDT, repetition of normally coordinated movement patterns fosters remediation.

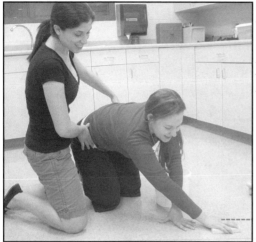

Figure 2-18. This demonstration illustrates the use of ontogenic positioning as a technique of weight-bearing in the remediation of coordinated movement. Here, challenge is provided along the developmental sequence, specifically, the quadruped position. To increase meaningfulness, cones can be replaced with cleaning the floor once the client has established improvement with coordinated movement.

With the Rood Approach, clients are placed in positions reflective of typical development, referred to as ontogenic positions. These include prone on elbows and/or quadruped, which require the subconscious cocontraction of heavy work or large proximal and stabilizing musculature. Clients are then requested to engage in meaningful activity using consciously controlled light work or distal mobilizing musculature while maintaining the ontogenic position. Figure 2-18 is an illustration of this technique. There is a lack of literature identifying the efficacy of the Rood Approach. However, Stroup and Snodgrass (2005) have stated that although "her work is of interest, it is not as widely accepted as NDT or PNF" (p. 49).

The Brunnstrom Approach, developed by Signe Brunnstrom in 1970, is not as commonly seen as NDT or PNF treatment approaches. Per Bertoti (2004), "the actual approach to intervention is considered outdated and inappropriate today, [although] Brunnstrom is credited with two main contributions which are still valuable: a description of the stereotypical synergy patterns and recovery stages of ...[clients] seen following a cerebrovascular accident (CVA)" (p. 189). It is, therefore, only these two concepts that will be discussed further in this chapter.

Brunnstrom, following observation of "thousands of stroke survivors" (Bertoti, 2004), documented the similarities in movement patterns and commonly seen phases of recovery. The patterning of the upper and lower extremity where characterized by dominating flexion or extension positions in the affected limbs—typically flexion of the upper and extension of the lower. Brunnstrom found that these synergistic patterns, occurring along a recognizable pattern of recovery, could be recruited to produce normal movement experiences for clients by way of associated reactions or brainstem reflexes (Katz, Alexander, & Klein, 1998). Because synergies are the result of tonal abnormalities, they are only introduced here and will be discussed in further detail within the "Remedial Techniques for Tone" section of this chapter. In brief, tonal abnormalities directly affect coordination.

Per Brunnstrom, the goal of occupational therapy intervention lies within managing the characteristics at each stage of recovery and by facilitating techniques that progress the client to the next stage. Techniques progress from postural or proximal trunk control to distal hand and wrist control by first using reflexive movements, which are also known as associated reactions. Progress is made to the point of using only verbal cuing to promote voluntary motor control of the affected limb. Again, Brunnstrom's findings are of most clinical significance in the descriptions provided by the patterning and stages of recovery and that the approach continues to hold meaning as a tool of remediation in common day practice (Katz, Alexander, & Klein, 1998).

Figure 2-19. Samples of weighted utensils employed to exaggerate sensory input and refine motor output, specifically here, for in the task of feeding.

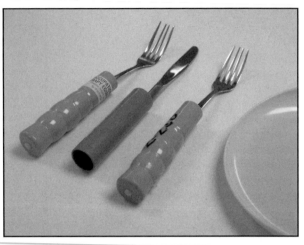

Finally, some OTs may use the simple principle of exaggerated sensory input to directly modify motor output when addressing issues of coordination. This technique is illustrated by the use of weighted everyday items such as utensils (Figure 2-19) to amplify typical sensory input and, therefore, refine motor output. This is a common technique in the presence of tremors such as is seen in Parkinson's disease, for example. These types of weighted items are readily available for purchase through the manufacturers listed in Appendix A. Additionally, the use of weighted cuffs placed upon extremities during engagement in personally meaningful and functional activity produces similar effects. Efficacy studies regarding this modified technique are limited and in need further exploration.

Special Considerations

The foremost consideration that must be made on behalf of clients with issues of coordination are those of personal safety. A lack of coordination increases the incidence of both orthopedic and various soft tissue injuries including sprains and strains. The likelihood for falls, cuts (such as with a knife or shaver), and even burns as a result of involuntary movements are significant and must be addressed with proactive educational measures, provided by the OT, as they relate to everyday routines. Low-tech adaptive equipment may also be recommended so as to ensure client safety. These techniques will be further explored in Chapters 3 and 4 of this text.

It is also important to reiterate here the nature of the underlying cause of coordination deficits—injury or illness to the brain or CNS. With this in mind, the OT must evaluate the client's cognitive status so as to appropriately adjust the remedial methods selected to address coordination. For example, a client with limited attention may not be able to participate in a structured activity for greater than 5 minutes. However, as a retired farmer, the same client is able to attend to the task of simple tabletop gardening for up to 20 minutes. Selecting appropriate methods for clients with cognitive issues will greatly increase the likelihood for successful remediation and will be discussed further later in this chapter.

"A question that frequently arises during the course of rehabilitating the patient with a CNS lesion is how much emphasis should be placed on promoting recovery of normal strategies versus teaching compensatory strategies for performing a task" (Shumway-Cook & Woollacott, 2001, p. 92). Shumway-Cook and Woollacott point out here the therapeutic significance of time; time that appropriately reflects the onset of injury or illness as well as the nature of the injury or illness. For example, Parkinson's diseases and MS are progressively degenerative, yet over a lengthier period of time than Huntington's or Creutzfeldt-Jakob diseases. Some, such as peripheral neuropathy, are caused by a loss in sensory input, while others result in loss of strength (as seen in MG or amyotrophic lateral sclerosis). Again still, some are chronic and progressive in nature while others are not. These are all critical considerations the OT must attend to while developing an individualized intervention plan with a client and specifically, as to whether they would benefit most from remedial or compensatory strategies to address issues of coordination.

Maintenance Programs

As with previously reviewed foundational skills, maintenance programs for coordination issues should also emphasize the infusion of the skills of everyday living. The OT should encourage those activities and tasks the client identifies as daily routine and naturally infuse concepts of motor learning, such as repetition and postural stability. Tying shoes, buttoning a shirt, applying toothpaste to a toothbrush, using the telephone or a television remote, typing on a computer keyboard, or having a game of bridge or bingo all require motor coordination and represent excellent tools for the OT to enforce as part of the individualized maintenance program. Emphasis should be placed not on the activity itself, but rather repeated practice overtime to facilitate improved coordination overall.

REMEDIAL TECHNIQUES FOR TONE

Definitional Analysis

Tone is defined by the *Framework* (AOTA, 2002) as a client factor relative to functions of the neuromusculoskeletal system. More specifically, it is categorized as a function of muscles. However, it is important to note that tone also directly affects the functions of joints and, therefore, movement in general. This concept is less obvious in the categorizations and definitions provided by the *Framework* document.

Again, additional definitions from other sources are included here to better illustrate the functional significance of tone as a foundational skill for engagement in meaningful occupation. Tone is defined by Thomas (1997) as "the resistance of muscles to passive elongation or stretch" (p. 1965). Muscle tone specifically is defined as, "The state of slight contraction usually present in muscles which contribute to posture and coordination..." Shumway-Cook and Woollacott (2001) elaborate with, " (a) certain level of tone is present in a conscious and relaxed person" (p. 169), which is not apparent using electromyography (EMG) or a record of muscle activity. Therefore, electrical impulses of the skeletal muscle are not required to maintain an individual's level of tone or quite simply, tone is not a function of consciousness (Shumway-Cook & Woollacott, 2001).

Notoriously, tone harbors ambiguity when presented by definition alone. Further discussion is required to gain more insight as to how a change in tone can be responsible for such an array of biomechanical limitations within the client's experience. For purposes of illustration, it is plausible to liken tone to the "electricity" that runs through the human body, just as electricity runs through the walls of a house. When electricity in a house is either lowered or increased, an effect is produced on each and every item plugged into the wall sockets. Recall conditions of periodic "brown outs" during hot summer days when many residents of the neighborhood were using their air conditioners. The demand for electricity exceeds the supply and the appliances are no longer produced their expected functions or desired effects. This case is the same when speaking of tone as the "electricity" running through the human body.

Tone is, in essence, the "electricity" that continuously runs through the body at a relatively static rate. Tone, therefore, allows a client to produce movement on demand just as plugging a lamp into a socket would allow for light on demand. Yet, similar to the "brown out" analogy, the level of tone within the human body may not always allow for optimal movement. Too little tone, or *hypotonia,* would then produce slowed, uncoordinated movement with hyperflexibility noted at the joint structures; too little tension or resistance to movement is produced by the muscles (Bertoti, 2004). The extreme of this is characterized as flaccidity or a condition where tone is completely absent (Bertoti, 2004). Conversely, high tone—also referred to as *hypertonia*—may produce fast, jerky, equally uncoordinated movement with limited flexibility noted at the joint structures and too much tension or resistance to movement produced in the muscles (Bertoti, 2004). The extremes of hypertonia are further categorized as either *spasticity* (an increase in tone dependent upon the velocity or movement) or *rigidity* (not directly related to the velocity of movement and typically involving only the flexor musculature) (Shumway-Cook & Woollacott, 2001). Various other categorizations of tonal abnormalities exist, yet with these most prevalent examples, we are better able to visualize the functional implications changes in muscle tone may cause on the successful engagement in occupation.

In concluding the definitional analysis of tone, it is also important to note that an individual's level of tone may vary from moment to moment or day to day. Common illustrations of this phenomenon include walking outside on a brisk winter day, as compared to a warm summer's one, or even having an unexpected visitor enter a room and startles its occupants. These situations cause a temporary increase in your body's level of tone or readiness to respond (Bertoti, 2004). What is significant is the spike in tone is temporary. Occupational therapy intervention becomes necessary when the fluctuations in tone are long-standing and, therefore, impede functional performance as is seen in a variety of neurologically-based health conditions.

Modes of Injury or Illness

Muscle tone is a function of neuromusculoskeletal system as outlined by the *Framework* (AOTA, 2002) and, therefore, is directly affected by illness or injury to the CNS. An array of health conditions may cause fluctuations in tone that, in turn, cause an individual to experience dysfunction. Many of these conditions lie in the categorizations of acquired brain injuries and spinal cord injuries. Either a result of external force inflicted upon the central nervous system itself, as seen in traumatic brain injury and traumatic spinal cord injury, or internal mechanisms, as seen by degenerative diseases, vascular abnormalities and infections, each can cause disruptions or alterations in the nerve impulses to the area of the brain responsible for the production of smooth, voluntary movement.

Hematomas, or tumors of blood, are commonly seen in both traumatic and nontraumatic injury (Beers & Berkow, 1999). Whether formed as a result of external trauma or internal bleeding from a vascular hemorrhage, this also presents an example of injury that may result in tonal abnormalities. Arteriovenous malformations, characterized by an abnormality in the junction between arteries and veins within the brain (Beers & Berkow, 1999), tumors of the brain itself, or even ischemic circumstances, may also disrupt tonal impulses and potentially impede volitional movement.

Tonal abnormalities are also associated with a variety of degenerative disease processes. With Parkinson's disease, clients may exhibit rigidity or an "increase in muscle tone of the agonist and antagonist muscles simultaneously" (Pedretti & Early, 2001, p. 366). In MS, spasticity may be present in one case, yet absent in another. Further more, with Huntington's disease, chorea-type tonal patterns may be observed as involuntary, irregular movements of the extremities that are exacerbated by stress, absent during sleep, and spastic in cases of early onset (Pedretti & Early, 2001).

The previous represents only a few examples of conditions that commonly disturb muscle tone within the body. Just as tone presents a challenge in defining, it also presents the same challenge in identifying all possible modes of injury or illness. Some clients with acquired brain injury may present with hypertonia, while others, spasticity, some clonus, others chorea, while even others may be spared tonal abnormalities altogether. Additionally, clients may still, and commonly do, experience fluctuations from hypotonia to hypertonia over the period of recovery from illness or injury. In all, any approaches the OT may choose to address tone must be client-specific and case-specific, changing in focus along with the healing process and sensitive to the prognosis of the injury or illness causing the disturbance itself.

Remedial Techniques: Biomechanical and Neurodevelopmental Theories

Foremost, prior to discussing the remediation of tone specifically, it is important to reemphasize the symbiotic relationship that exists between tone and coordination. Each skill relies heavily upon the other to successfully produce the functional movement that is necessary to engage in personally meaning activity. As a result, various techniques for the remediation of coordination will appropriately overlap with those used to address tonal abnormalities. In illustration of this point, the discussion of tone immediately follows that of coordination in sequence of this chapter.

Per the *Framework* (AOTA, 2002), which classifies muscle tone as a neuromusculoskeletal function, the majority of traditional techniques for the remediation of tone are grounded in the Neurodevelopment Theories. However, a current review of literature reveals that most often, OTs choose to incorporate the techniques of the Biomechanical Theory, in conjunction with those of the traditional neurodevelopmental approaches, to arrive at the desired outcome (Cameron, 2003). The approaches of both theories will be described in the following section and are categorized for the purpose of clarity as those with the explicit purpose of decreasing excessive tone (techniques of inhibition) versus those with the goal of increasing conditions of low tone (techniques of facilitation). An exception to this is found in the Saeboflex (Saebo, Charlotte, NC) technology in that this contemporary technique addresses issues of tone in general, and not to conditions of high or low tone specifically. Due the generalized nature of Saeboflex as a technique for addressing tone overall, in combination with the evidence-base it has begun to establish, it will be reviewed foremost and followed by those categorized as either inhibitory or facilitory.

Tone is notoriously resistant to corrective measures or techniques of remediation, and, therefore, presents the OT with great challenge at times. Most often, issues of tone are thought to be managed, rather than remedied, by a comprehensive team of rehabilitation specialists working together to preserve function and prevent deformity. Efficacy studies reviewed on the traditional approaches for tone show "little evidence to support their application" (Gallichio, 2004, p. 973), rather placing emphasis on the longevity of results over remediation of dysfunction. Overall, additional studies are needed to decipher which of the traditional approaches, or combination of, hold the most promise for the effective management of tonal abnormalities over time.

A Contemporary Approach: The Saeboflex

Developed by brothers John Farrell, OTR/L and Henry Hoffman, MS, OTR/L, the *SaeboFlex* is a custom-fit, dynamic orthotic device that allows a client with moderate tonal abnormalities resulting from neurological injury to produce functional grasp and release patterns of the wrist and hand (Northwest Hospital & Medical Center, 2005). Refer to Appendix A for additional resources on the *SaeboFlex*. The device places the wrist and fingers into extension. It is from this position that the client actively produces grasp, while the dynamic, spring-loaded outriggers assist in the extension for required to release. These patterns are repeated in 45-minute sessions, 3 times per week over 4 weeks with a trained OT (see Appendix A for additional information on training opportunities) and are supplemented by a home-based program designed to foster greater use of the device over the period of time (Northwest Hospital & Medical Center, 2005). Hoffman & Snyder (2003) measured significant improvements in the functional range of the affected extremity in chronic poststroke individuals. In an attempt to broaden this evidence-base, Farrell has reported that additional studies are currently being conducted at the University of Maryland and at the Kessler Institute for Rehabilitation in East Orange, New Jersey to further analyze what has been observed as "tremendous results with the acute population..." (Brachtesende, 2005, p. 11). With a shift towards the use of methods that demonstrate efficacy in use, the SaeboFlex shows a promising future within the field of occupational therapy for addressing tonal abnormalities that impede functional performance.

TRADITIONAL APPROACHES OF INHIBITION

Electrical Modalities

EMG biofeedback is a technique employed by the OT with advanced training (see Appendix A) to elicit the desired inhibition of tone. With this modality, a recording of muscle activity is transcribed into visible data along a computer screen by way of electrodes that have been placed strategically along the affected musculature. The therapist manually sets an audible alert at a pre-determined level of resting muscle activity. The client is then instructed to attempt to relax and once the preset level of resting muscle activity is achieved, the alert then sounds to provide auditory feedback and reinforcement to the client identifying measures effectively taken to decrease muscle tone. Research has demonstrated that the EMG biofeedback method holds statistically significant results in the effectiveness of decreasing hypertonia following cases of CVA specifically (Trombly & Radomski, 2002).

TENS has also been suggested as an inhibitory technique by Watanabe (2004). The theory behind the use of TENS directly relates to the function it holds as an effective modality in the management of chronic pain. Wntanabe (2004) suggests, "...pain can increase reflex afferent activity, so a modality which inhibits this input could [also] decrease spasticity" (p. 48).

In review of efficacy studies conducted in the area of electrical modalities as tool for inhibiting spasticity, Barnes (1998) points out that "None of these appear to have much long-term benefit but can have useful short-term effects, particular when used as an adjunctive treatment in combination with other measurements..." (Barnes, 1998, p. 239).

Positioning Techniques

Barnes (1998) describes *proper positioning* as a cornerstone approach to the effective management of spasticity, highlighting that a failure to promote biomechanically sound postures further exacerbates the tonal abnormality. Whether in supine or sitting, the therapist will promote positions of bilateral symmetry among joints to provide both stretch to involved musculature and the appropriate length tension to uninvolved musculature (Barnes, 1998). This is often fostered by application of positioning items such as foam wedges, strapping, or pillows to achieve the most optimal posture for a client with spasticity, while also minimizing the possibility for permanent muscle fiber shortening or contracture formation.

Serial casting is a relatively common, aggressive technique employed by OTs as a tool for the remediation of spasticity (Vandyck & Mukand, 2004, p. 11). With this approach, one therapist passively places the affected extremity in a position of stretch, which is often only possible through applying *direct pressure* to the tendon insertion of the affected muscle. Direct pressure mechanically causes the spastic muscle to relax at the level of the Pacinian corpuscles (Trombly & Radomski, 2002), thereby allowing for maximal passive range to be achieved. At this point a second therapist applies a protective barrier on the skin, additional padding at boney prominences of the limb to minimize pressure areas, and finally, the casting material. Once dry, the cast is then cut longitudinally using a cast cutter along both the medial and lateral aspects to create a "bi-valve." The bi-valve construction allows for maximal ease in application of the cast. An individualized wear schedule is devised according to tolerance and with close monitoring to prevent skin breakdown at areas of increased pressure (i.e., the styloid processes or olecranon process of the upper extremity). As a complement to the wear schedule, the client is also prescribed a *PROM* program designed to promote the appropriate length-tension relationship among involved musculature, minimize disuse, and prevent contractures or adhesions of the soft tissue. With noted improvement in the passive range at the affected joint, the casting process is repeated at the newly achieved length of prolonged stretch and the wear schedule modified accordingly.

Although this approach is widely used, it is "labor intensive and relatively expensive" when compared with implementing a prefabricated, low-load, prolonged stretch device designed to achieve the same desired effect (Vandyck & Mukand, 2004, p. 13). Refer to Appendix A for manufacturers of low-load, prolonged stretch devices Efficacy studies yield positive correlation among the PROM available at affected joints following the implementation of serial casting. However, Mortenson (2003), points out that additional research is required to analyze whether the actual mechanism of change is due to the prolonged stretch provided by the cast or as a result of muscle atrophy secondary to the prolonged immobility an aggressive wear schedule inherently promotes.

Thermal Modality Techniques

Trombly & Radomski (2002) describe using cold pack application (*cryotherapy*) at the temperature of 10° C as an additionally effective means of inhibiting tone achieved by directly decreasing "the monosynaptic stretch reflex excitability" (p. 579). To achieve this effect, the cold application must be provided at the duration of 20 minutes with careful attention to indications and precautions outlined for the use of this physical agent modality (see Table 2-21). Price, Lehmann, Boswell-Bessette, Burleigh, and deLateur (1993) studied the efficacy of cryotherapy on hypertonicity and concluded that statistically significant reduction can measured up to 1 hour postapplication. Therefore, this technique produces relatively short-term effects in reducing muscle spasticity.

Neurodevelopmental/Sensorimotor Techniques

Neurodevelopmental techniques (also referred to as sensorimotor techniques) of NDT, PNF, and Rood all ascribe to be methods of addressing hypertonia. This area of techniques harbor little evidence to support the claim and are in need of further study to validate efficacy. However, traditionally, OTs have implemented these techniques to address conditions of hypertonia and, therefore, are included in this discussion.

NDT (Bobath), PNF, and Rood Approaches mutually share a foundation in techniques that are *slow in speed* as tools to foster tone inhibition. Whether slow stroking along the spine outlined by Rood (Pedretti & Early, 2001, p. 584), promoting of slow, controlled movement patterns outlined by NDT (Pedretti & Early, 2001, p. 632), or using the slow relaxation methods outlined by PNF, these all share the common emphasis on the speed of implementation to provide necessary sensory and vestibular input that then relaxes the system and decreases the heightened level of muscle tone.

With NDT specifically, upright positioning of the body, or the facilitation of *postural control*, holds significant importance in normalizing tone. Per NDT, dysfunction is housed in the abnormality of core posture and is commonly seen following neurological insult. For example, as a result of sensory loss, a client may avoid weight-bearing on the affected side due to a fear of falling. "Fear is a major contributing factor in spasticity" (Pedretti, 2001, p. 626). Hence, remediation must begin by re-establishing security for the client in core stability, which is a precursor to distal mobility. Therefore, the techniques of NDT are executed to facilitate postural control and promote normal weight-bearing experiences. This then secondarily addresses the tonal abnormality via inhibiting the emotion of fear.

The NDT approach also specifies the use of trunk rotation, scapular retraction, and a forward pelvic position (or, in general, the proper positioning and length of proximal musculature) as cornerstones to promote the normalization of tone (Pedretti & Early, 2001). Emphasis is placed on deep pressure applied by the therapist and at proximal key points of control (as described earlier in remediation of coordination) so as to elicit the necessary lengthening of affected musculature (2001) and/or achieved by techniques of *weight-bearing* through the affected extremity. Whether by promoting through engagement in functional activity (Figure 2-20) or in isolation, the NDT

Figure 2-20. Weight-bearing through the UE, promoted by functional reaching during the engagement of meaningful occupation.

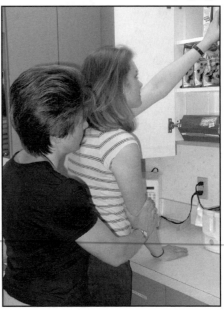

weight-bearing technique promotes a prolonged stretch to affected muscles and presents an additional tool of inhibition for the OT (Pedretti & Early, 2001).

Margaret Rood also describes position-specific techniques to address muscle spasticity. With this approach, emphasis is placed on positions of the traditional developmental sequence or *ontogenic positions*, described earlier in coordination. An example can be seen in the ontogenic position of quadruped coupled with the technique of *slow rocking*. The movement in this position is found to provide light compression of joint surfaces, as well as rhythmically stretch to spastic musculature (Pedretti & Early, 2001). *Neutral warmth* is also identified by Rood as a method of inhibition. With this technique, the client is provided a warm blanket and asked to assume a comfortable position for the period of 5 to 10 minutes allowing a sense of relaxation and in turn, a decrease in tone (Pedretti & Early, 2001).

With the PNF Approach, muscle contraction and hold patterns are outlined as effective means for normalizing spasticity. Trombly & Radomski (2002) describe that the facilitation of these cyclical movements—such as the PNF hold-relax or contract relax techniques—cause the activation of multiple Glogi Tendon Organs (GTOs) located within the muscle itself, resulting in "overriding autoinhibition" of the sustained contraction observed in cases of hypertonia. Generally termed *repeated contractions* in the PNF approach, other theorists have outlined the use of the same technique for inhibition of tone, coining the process as techniques of *reciprocal innervation* (Ivanhoe and Reistetter, 2004).

Pharmaceutical Techniques

It is significant to note the growing evidence in support for using medically-prescribed pharmacological agents as the primary effective method in managing conditions of hypertonia. Gallichio (2004) reported that the use of medications, such as baclofen, diazepam, or tizanidine, represent the most comprehensively studied area of spasticity management due to the longevity of results produced in comparison with any of the aforementioned techniques reviewed above.

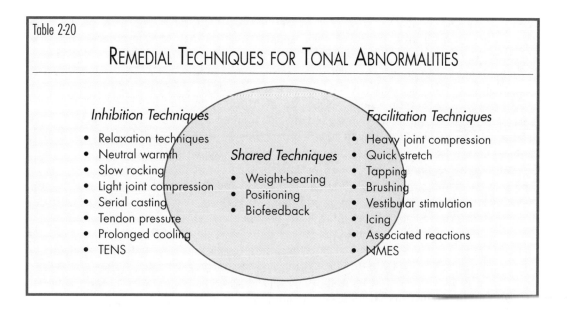

Table 2-20

REMEDIAL TECHNIQUES FOR TONAL ABNORMALITIES

Inhibition Techniques
- Relaxation techniques
- Neutral warmth
- Slow rocking
- Light joint compression
- Serial casting
- Tendon pressure
- Prolonged cooling
- TENS

Shared Techniques
- Weight-bearing
- Positioning
- Biofeedback

Facilitation Techniques
- Heavy joint compression
- Quick stretch
- Tapping
- Brushing
- Vestibular stimulation
- Icing
- Associated reactions
- NMES

TRADITIONAL APPROACHES OF FACILITATION

Electrical Modalities

"*Electrical stimulation* has been clearly demonstrated to be a valuable facilitation tool for ...[clients] with primary movement disorders" (Bertoti, 2004). Bertoti (2004) goes on to report that with augmentation of muscle activity via NMES, the degree of hypotonia is temporarily found to normalize. Faghri, Rodgers, Glaser, Bors, Ho, & Akuthota (1994) further support this conclusion in their study on the effects of electrical stimulation in cases of shoulder subluxation—a common complication of excessively low tone or flaccidity. In this study, clients who received electrical stimulation to the hypotonic, posterior deltoid muscle were found to have improved arm function and a decrease in the severity of the subluxation when compared with that of the control group. As a PAM, continuing education is required to implement this technique both safely and effectively. Refer to Appendix A for additional information and resources on the use of PAMs by an OT and Table 2-24 for an outline of indications and contraindications for the use of NMES. Additional benefits have also been found in the use of *biofeedback* as a modality to facilitate increased muscle tone (Bertoti, 2004), opposite than described earlier as a technique for inhibition. For facilitation, the client's attention is directed to effective measures taken in efforts to increase hypotonic muscle activity.

Neurodevelopmental/Sensorimotor Techniques

As depicted in Table 2-20, the same sensorimotor approaches outlined earlier as techniques of inhibition, also prescribe strategies for the facilitation of low tone.

As mentioned earlier in this segment, NDT outline techniques used in general to normalize tone, whether hyperactive or hypoactive, as they present in typical or synergistic patterns. Therefore, the methods presented by NDT are the same in both cases of inhibition and facilitation. Trunk rotation, scapular retraction and forward pelvic position are promoted to normalize low tone in the proximal musculature and through the use of handling techniques at identified key points of control. Weight-bearing is intended to assist in regulating overall abnormalities in tone throughout the body, just as was discussed in the inhibitory section. Recently, evidence is lacking in the use of the NDT approach postneurological insult. Hafsteindottir, Algra, Kappelle, & Grypdonck (2005) reported, in a study designed to measure the efficacy of NDT, that the "...approach was not found effective in the care of stroke patients in the hospital setting" (p. 792), going on to recommend that therapists reconsider the implementation of these traditionally popular techniques.

In both the PNF and Rood approaches, *heavy joint compression or approximation* is emphasized as a technique of facilitation. The Rood approach specifically defines heavy joint compression as pressure applied, greater than body weight, directly through the affected extremity (Pedretti & Early, 2001). This is contrasted from the use of light compression, or less than body weight, which is identified by Rood as a technique of inhibition. Hence, promoting full body weight-bearing through the affected extremity is therefore, considered a technique of facilitation.

Various other facilitory techniques are outlined by the Rood Approach including quick stretch, brushing, vestibular stimulation, vibration, light touch, and icing (cryotherapy) as tools in normalizing low tone. A quick stretch to the affected muscle fibers, followed by rapid and repetitive tapping along the same muscle belly during an attempted movement, is believed to both inhibit the antagonistic muscle and activate the reflexive stretch response of the agonistic, or affected muscle (Trombly & Radomski, 2002). This is the same principle illustrated in the use of high intensity vibration applied directly to the affected and slightly stretched muscle belly; however, caution is advised here due to the secondary heat (friction) produced at the skin's surface. *Brushing* the hair receptors of the skin at the coinciding dermatome level with either a high intensity, battery-operated, soft-haired brush or by manual stroking at the rate of twice per 10 second interval (repeated 3 to 5 times), also elicits increased muscle tone through stimulation of the reflexive withdrawal response (Trombly & Radomski, 2002). Quick, vestibular stimulation in an anterior-posterior or medial-lateral plane has also been found to elicit protective reflexes and, therefore, assist in promoting an increase in tone. *Quick icing* or quickly swiping the skin surface with ice similarly produces a protective withdrawal reflex, again acting as a technique to increase the level of tone.

The Brunnstrom Approach describes specific patterns of recovery, each characterized by alterations in tone, which occur following CVA. Brunnstrom emphasizes that recovery follows a developmental sequence: proximal to distal musculature, flaccid to spastic tonal patterns, and followed by the return of normal movement patterns. Intervention is focused on facilitating and managing the underlying patterns of tone, also known as synergies, which present in varying degrees along each stage of the recovery process. Brunnstrom recruits the use of *associated reactions*, otherwise described as brainstem reflexes (e.g., asymmetrical tonic neck reflex [ATNR]), to evoke movement where it was otherwise nonexistent due to the lack of sufficient muscle tone (Trombly & Radomski, 2002). Hence, resistance to movement in the unaffected extremity will elicit a synergistic pattern of heightened tone in the affected extremity and potentially allow for the production of movement. For example, resisted grasp in the unaffected hand will cause a grasping pattern of movement in the affected hand allowing for potentially functional use (Trombly & Radomski, 2002). This movement is then physically experienced by the client and practiced readily in order to achieve normal movement patterns. The Brunnstrom Approach also outlines the use of repetitive tapping, quick stretch, and brisk stimulation or brushing, to facilitate tone similar to that of the Rood Approach described above.

Special Considerations

Clients presenting with tonal abnormalities are also susceptible to an array of secondarily harmful conditions that warrant the attention of the OT. As a normal level of tone within the musculature allows for optimal movement, too little or too much tone hinders movement and may also cause the potential for further disability. This principle can be best illustrated in situations of joint subluxation and contracture formations.

In the absence of tone, the joint structures and the capsule specifically become laxed or stretched due to the overpowering, unopposed force of gravity on extremities in the upright position. This

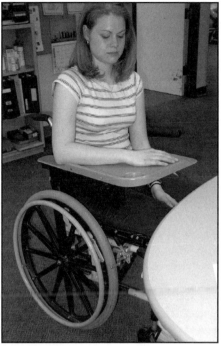

Figure 2-21. Demonstration of the use of a hemi-tray to provide proper positioning of the upper extremity.

allows for of the humeral head from the glenoid fossa, know formally as *shoulder subluxation*, and is commonly observed in clients having sustained CVAs. Shoulder subluxations are not only painful for clients, but also potentially harmful due to the excessive stretch on nerves and blood vessels that can secondarily lead to complicating conditions such as complex regional pain syndrome (CRPS) or adhesive capsulitis. It is the responsibility of the OT to be attentive to joint laxity so as to minimize the likelihood for complications. Intervention strategies include proper positioning and support against gravity that can be achieved by adding a hemi-tray (Figure 2-21), arm trough, lap tray, or, though controversial for fostering further disuse, a shoulder sling. It should be noted that a lap tray is considered a restraint unless the client can remove it independently. Regardless of which equipment is being incorporated, the therapist must attend to a careful wear schedule that minimizes disuse while also providing necessary protection from excessive joint distraction or severity of subluxation (Gilmore, Spaulding, & Vandervoort, 2004).

In cases of spasticity, sustained contraction of the muscle tissue can produce damaging contractures within muscle fibers themselves. The prevention of contractures, or permanent shortening of muscle fibers, is routinely a focus of intervention that employs such aggressive measures as serial casting and low load, prolonged stretch devices, both described earlier on in this subsection.

It is also important to note the significance of the scapulohumeral rhythm (Neumann, 2002) when remediating tonal issues of the UE. The OT must attend to the collaborative relationship between the scapula and the humerus (scapulohumeral rhythm) so as to foster a return of normal movement patterns throughout the entire upper extremity. In cases of low tone, the scapula may become malaligned in its orientation to the thorax, commonly referred to as scapular winging. Likewise, in cases of high tone, the scapula may become fixed relative to the thorax. Each condition directly impedes of scapular mobility and, therefore, biomechanically prevents the ability for full shoulder movement in the upper ranges of motion.

When addressing tone, the underlying significance of an individual's preferences (his or her adversities) and fears are of additional importance to the OT. A proven and strong correlation exists among a client's emotional status and their level of muscle tone. For example, a client who is particularly adverse to cold will not find prolonged icing or cryotherapy to be an effective technique of inhibition. Similarly, a client who is particularly fearful of anticipated pain with movement will be less likely to benefit from the technique of prolonged stretch. It is critical that the OT openly communicate with the client and establish trusting, therapeutic rapport so as to ascertain which options may present as most effective in managing his or her individual tonal issues.

As a final note, consideration should also be paid to the therapeutic benefits of aquatic therapy interventions to address issues of tone. For example, supported floating using assistive floatation devices in a warm water pool may be found particularly relaxing for a client and, therefore, an effective technique of tonal inhibition. In a study conducted by Kesiktas, Paker, Erdogan, Gulsen, Bicki, and Yilmaz (2004) entitled, *The Use of Hydrotherapy for the Management of Spasticity*, water-based intervention programs were found to be "helpful in decreasing the amount of medication required" (p. 273) to decrease conditions of spasticity and "when compared to the control group, the use of hydrotherapy produced a significant decrease in [muscle] spasm severity" (p. 272). Alternately, exercise in a cool water environment may have a facilitory affect on muscle tone. A specialized aquatic technique, entitled Watsu or Water Shiatsu, specifically uses slow rocking movements provided passively by the therapist with the goal of inducing a deep state of relaxation. The primary purpose of this relaxed state is to allow for rotational movements of the limbs and trunk with the goal of equalizing the body's meridians or pathways of energy as described in Eastern medical philosophies (Ruoti et al., 1997). This deepened state of relaxation also promotes a reduction of spasticity. As a precaution, clients who are fearful of water would not benefit from aquatic intervention strategies since emotion directly affects one's degree of muscle tone. Additional training is recommended for aquatic intervention, particularly in the use of Watsu techniques. Refer to Appendix A for more information on aquatic rehabilitation.

Techniques at a Glance

See Table 2-20 for an outline that illustrates the most commonly employed techniques for the inhibition of tone, the facilitation of tone, and those that are shared effectiveness in either case of tonal abnormality.

Maintenance Programs

Due to the specialized nature of remediation techniques for tone, they are not traditionally carried over into client-facilitated maintenance programs. Rather, these techniques are an integral component of the clinic-based therapy sessions themselves. This is not to say that with demonstrated safety and independence in the use of weight-bearing, for example, a client and his or her caregivers would not be supported in the desire to continue the use of techniques outside of the therapy session. This may also include simplified strategies of prolonged stretch, neutral warmth, or modified associated reactions.

Techniques of proper positioning, including casting and splinting applications, are traditionally seen as maintenance approaches for affected extremities. The goal for such methods is to maintain the ideal length of the connective tissue's that underlie the production of movement. For example, a wrist cock up splint would provide the ideal length of stretch for finger flexors in the absence of active wrist extension. Again, as is always the case with positioning tools, a client-specific wear schedule must be created to minimize the disuse of the area affected and preventing further disability. For illustration, this may include only nighttime application followed by an early morning AROM program designed to restretch the immobilized soft tissues. Independence with application of all required positioning devices must also be established prior to execution as part of a maintenance program.

REMEDIATION OF THE PRIMARY FUNCTIONAL SKILLS AT A GLANCE

The remedial techniques discussed in this chapter are summarized in Table 2-21 (pain and edema), Table 2-22 (sensation: hyposensitivity and hypersensitivity), Table 2-23 (range of motion), and Table 2-24 (strength).

Remedial Techniques for Cognition and Perception

DEFINITIONAL ANALYSIS

Per the *Framework* (AOTA, 2002), both perception and cognition are categorized as mental functions. This is a broad categorization for these skill areas, each considered very comprehensive and influential in the execution of performance and active engagement in meaningful activity. Mental functions in general are then further subdivided into categories of global mental functions and specific mental functions.

Global mental functions include a general overview of those skills most commonly associated with cognition and affect or the ability to express emotion congruent with facial expression (AOTA, 2002). Examples include a client's level of arousal, awareness of self, time, place, amount and quality of sleep, degree of emotional stability, level of motivation, awareness of values and interests, as well as the ability to control impulses. Though not formally defined by the *Framework*, "the ability to control impulses, use feedback to control behavior [level of insight] and to evaluate the consequences of his [or her] behavior" (Zoltan, 1996, p.149) define a client's skills of *executive functioning*. These functions are of equal importance when considering the remediation of cognition specifically and will be discussed further in this subsection.

Specific mental functions continue to elaborate upon skills commonly associated with cognition with emphasis on the relationship among one's perceptual functions and the thinking process. These include such cognitive skills as attention, memory, thought process, judgment, problem solving, and time management as illustrations. The significance of perception and its impact on cognition is reflected by further including visuospatial relations, interpretation of sensory input from tactile, visual, auditory, olfactory, and gustatory senses, as well as interpretation and execution of language, calculation functions, and skills of motor planning in general. Subtitles within this category also include psychosocial and psychomotor skills, such as the perception of self, in addition to one's ability to adequately regulate emotion and "motor responses to psychological events" (AOTA, 2002, p. 625).

In the absence of more formal definitions from the *Framework* document, those provided by Jacobs and Jacobs in *Quick Reference Dictionary for Occupational Therapy* are included as they apply to cognition and perception. Jacobs and Jacobs (2004) define *cognition* as "mental processes that include thinking, perceiving, feeling, recognizing, remembering, problem solving, knowing, sensing, learning, judging, and metacognition" (p. 44). *Perception* is defined specifically as the "ability to organize and interpret incoming sensory information" (Jacobs & Jacobs, 2004, p. 172). Again an overlap in terminology is obvious. In essence, the ability to purposefully interact within all facets of the world requires not only the accurate interpretation of all that is seen, felt, heard, touched, and smelled, but also, how one reacts to that sensory information (i.e., cognitive-perceptual skills).

continued on page 112

Table 2-21

REMEDIAL TECHNIQUES FOR PAIN AND EDEMA

Pain and Edema Modality or Intervention Techniques	Cold pack	Ice bath Gillen & Burkhardt, 2004	Contrast Bath Cochrane, 2004	Vapocoolant Spray
Rationale/Indications for Use	Desensitize pain receptors and decrease pain. Typically, 24-48 hours postinjury to address edema, pain exacerbations of arthritis, acute bursitis or tendonitis, spasticity, acute or chronic pain secondary to muscle spasm.	Desensitize pain receptors as well as quick vasomotor restriction.	Desensitize pain receptors as well as create rapid vasoconstriction and vaso-dilation.	Decrease muscle spasms and trigger point discomfort for a short period of time (10-15 min) (Bracciano, 2000).
Average Length of Time per Session	10-20 minutes	3-5 seconds and repeated 2-3 times	6-10 seconds repeated 2-3 times	2-3 sprays (Micholovitz, 1990)
Process	• One layer of towel between the client and the cold pack. • Cold pack is placed over or around the area of pain/edema	• Ice bucket is placed on the floor • Arm is placed in the ice water for 3-5 seconds and then removed • Repeat 2-3 times	• Ice and warm water buckets are placed on the floor • Arm is placed in the ice water for 3-5 seconds • Arm is placed in the warm water for 3-5 seconds	• Position client with identified muscle on passive stretch • Spray bottle is inverted at 30 degree angle, about 45 cm from skin • Muscle or trigger point sprayed in unidirectional sweeping motion 2-3 times
Precautions (With all physical agent modalities, always monitor and protect underlying skin)	Avoid use with clients having significantly impaired circulation or hypersensitivity to cold; avoid application over wounds, prolonged placement over superficial nerves, compromised cognitive status. Vapocoolant spray cannot be used if client or therapist is pregnant.			

continued

Table 22-1, continued

REMEDIAL TECHNIQUES FOR PAIN AND EDEMA

Pain and Edema Modality or Intervention Techniques	Moist Heat Pack	Paraffin Wax	Fluidotherapy Thermal Mode
Rationale/Indications for Use	Stiff joints, subcutaneous adhesions, contractures, chronic arthritis, subacute or chronic cumulative trauma, neuromas, spasms.	Circumferential heating for stiff joints, subcutaneous adhesions, contractures, chronic arthritis, subacute or chronic cumulative trauma.	Programmable and adjustable heat, adjustable fan for stiff joints, subcutaneous adhesions, contractures, chronic arthritis, subacute or chronic cumulative trauma, neuromas, spasms.
Average Length of Time per Session	15-20 minutes	15-20 minutes	15-20 minutes
Process	• Six to eight layers of towels between the client and the moist heat pack. • Moist heat pack is placed over or around the area of pain/edema.	Hand is dipped into paraffin five times, wrapped in plastic and then wrapped in a towel.	Machine is preheated. Extremity is placed into the heated corn husks and the "sleeve" is wrapped around the client's extremity.
Precautions (With all physical agent modalities, always monitor and protect underlying skin)	Acute injury, diminished sensation, decreased circulation, compromised cognitive status, tumors or cancers, acute edma, deep vein thrombosis, pregnancy, bleeding abnormalities, infection, advanced cardiac disease, underlying skin, some case of rheumatoid arthritis where client may experience exacerbation following heat (Shankar & Randall, 2002).		

continued

Table 2-21, continued

REMEDIAL TECHNIQUES FOR PAIN AND EDEMA

Pain and Edema Modality or Intervention Techniques	Iontophoresis (see Figure 2-1)	Transcutaneous Electrical Nerve Stimulation (TENS)
Rationale/Indications for Use	Promotes healing and decreases pain and edema through using electric currents to deliver transcutaneous prescription medications such as cortico steroids and analgesics.	Interrupts the pain cycle at the spinal level (Cameron, 2003).
Average Length of Time per Session	Typically 20-30 minutes depending upon client tolerance (Bracciano, 2000).	Time can vary from 15-45 minutes depending upon the condition and other chosen parameters (Bracciano, 2000).
Process	• Medication is injected into the iontophoreis pad • Medication pad is placed over the area of pain/edema • Disbursive pad is placed on the same side of the body at any location (typically low back, shoulder, or thigh) • Parameters should be set at a low current density to prevent irritation such as 0.5 mA/cm^2	• Stimulation sites selected based upon the condition and client goals. • 3 areas to facilitate current flow are motor, trigger, and acupuncture points (Bracciano, 2000). Further training is required to become competent in the different protocols utilized with TENS.
Precautions (With all physical agent modalities, always monitor and protect underlying skin)	Pregnancy, skin lesions or sensitivity, allergy to medications used, cardiac pacemaker or arrhythmias, placement over the carotid sinus, blood clots, impaired sensation, malignant tumor.	Presence of cardiac pacemakers, pregnancy, tumors/malignancy, epilepsy, over the ocular orbits or carotid sinus, active infection, peripheral vascular disease, cardiac disease, muscosal surfaces, compromised cognitive status. Caution must be used in clients experiencing acute pain symptoms or undiagnosed pain (Shankar, 2002).

continued

Table 2-21, continued

REMEDIAL TECHNIQUES FOR PAIN AND EDEMA

Pain and Edema Modality or Intervention Techniques	Compression
Rationale/Indications for Use	Decreases edema through facilitation of the return of edematous fluids to the heart for efficient removal from the system (Cameron, 2003).
Average Length of Time per Session	Time varies with form of intervention and the degree of edema.
Process	• Positioning of an affected area in elevation above the heart allows for gravitational forces to engage in removing excess fluids • Aquatic rehabilitation techniques recruit the principles of hydrostatic pressure to circumferentially compress affected areas (Salzman, 1998) • Wrappings, garments such as Isotoner gloves (see Figure 2-3) • Electric pumps which provide timed, intermittent compression via filling a sleeve surrounding the area with air
Precautions (With all physical agent modalities, always monitor and protect underlying skin)	Extensive/overly prolonged compression that can cause further circulation problems, decreased sensation, presence/risk of blood clots, open wounds/infections/cellulitis, systemic febrile illness malignancy, fragile skin, acute cardiac disease, pregnancy (Shankar & Randall, 2002).

continued

Table 2-2), continued

REMEDIAL TECHNIQUES FOR PAIN AND EDEMA

Pain and Edema Modality or Intervention Techniques	Massage: • Retrograde massage through manual compression (subacute) • Manual lymph drainage (chronic conditions)
Rationale/Indications for Use	• Retrograde massage: Decreases edema through providing compression to the affected tissues • Manual lymph drainage: Decreases edema through use of specialized techniques to elicit a release of "trapped" lymph within the circulatory system (Cameron, 2003)
Average Length of Time per Session	• Retrograde massage: 10-20 minutes • Manual lymph drainage gradual increase from 20 minutes to a maximum of 60 minutes.
Process	Retrograde massage: 1. Place the client in a position which is respectful of comfort, yet also considerate to elevation above the heart. Pillows, etc. should be used to maximize client's level of comfort 2. Clarify with the client any possible allergies to skin lotions or creams 3. Ideally, a lanolin-based or vitamin E cream is applied to all surfaces of the skin in the area where massage will be applied to decrease friction produced by massaging technique 4. Therapist begins to provide pressure sensitive to the client's discomfort and moving in a direction towards the heart. Pressure should be circumferential, or provided to all surfaces of the skin simultaneously (see Figure 2-4.) 5. This "mechanical pumping", in the distal to proximal direction and using the lanolin-based cream to decrease friction between surfaces, is a frequently used remedial technique in addressing subacute edema for 3-5 minutes at the intensity of 4-6 times per day (Prosser & Conolly, 2003) Manual lymph drainage: Lymphedema is a specialty area within occupational therapy and requires additional training for proficiency
Precautions (With all physical agent modalities, always monitor and protect underlying skin)	*See Compression.

continued

Table 2-21, continued

REMEDIAL TECHNIQUES FOR PAIN AND EDEMA

Pain and Edema Modality or Intervention Techniques	
	ROM: • AROM • AAROM • PROM	Manual therapies (therapeutic touch): • Crainio-sacral • Myofascial release • Strain counter strain (subacute or chronic)
Rationale/Indications for Use	Promotes movement to limit the accumulation of fluids and the pain/adhesions associated with guarding or misuse of an extremity (Cameron, 2003).	Though each has its own unique approach, collectively, these techniques are founded on the belief dysfunction arises from tensions occurring throughout the body and techniques implemented are intended to restore uniformity throughout the system.
Average Length of Time per Session	Time varies with particular technique.	Time varies with particular technique.
Process	Example of AROM exercise for edema/pain: • Tendon gliding (see Figure 2-4) completed five repetitions twice daily until edema is effectively diminished (Prosser & Conolly, 2003).	Due to the specialized nature of these techniques, continuing education is required to ensure safe and successful implementation. Refer to Appendix A for additional information and resources on these specialized technique options.
Precautions (With all physical agent modalities, always monitor and protect underlying skin)	See Table 2-24.	Due to the fact that these are specialized areas, precautions are dependent and individualized for each technique.

Table 2-22

REMEDIAL TECHNIQUES FOR SENSATION: HYPOSENSITIVITY AND HYPERSENSITIVITY

Sensation: Hyposensitivity	Sensory retraining: Direct sensory input	Sensory retraining: Functional activities
Modality or Intervention Techniques	• Buckets • Wands • Textures	
Rational/Indications for Use (For complete descriptions see narrative information)	Direct sensory input applied to re-educate the client of these sensations.	"...therapy aimed at enabling a person to regain contact with his or her environment; (via sensory input and) includes... body awareness exercises and sensory activities utilizing objects (Jacobs & Jacobs, 2004, p. 213).
Average Length of Time per Session	Time varies.	Time varies.
Process	Intervention is initiated by having the client organize the sensory stimulation bins or dowels in a sequence of least to most abrasive, then begin with stimulation via the texture which is tolerated, applied directly to the affected area (Waylett-Rendall, 2002). Graded progression to less abrasive textures is then guided by the therapist with particular attention to the client's ability to feel the texture. Vibration can also be added post intervention with dowels/textures.	• Provide clients with an array of opportunities that provide engagement in familiar sensory experiences of all kinds • Retraining activities may include an array of activities such as a fine motor task in identifying coins to those of a gross motor nature such as moving the arm above the head so as to successfully brush hair. Emphasis is not so much placed on the type of item or movement, but rather to recruit other perceptions, such as vision, in retraining the "sense" the item or movement provides
Precautions	Do not allow client to begin with a texture which is abrasive and can cause undetected irritation to the skin. Avoid any sharp objects.	See direct sensory input.

continued

Table 2-22, continued

REMEDIAL TECHNIQUES FOR SENSATION: HYPOSENSITIVITY AND HYPERSENSITIVITY

Sensation: Hyposensitivity Modality or Intervention Techniques	*Rational/Indications for Use* (For complete descriptions see narrative information)	*Average Length of Time per Session*	*Process*	*Precautions*
Desensitization: Direct sensory input. • Buckets • Wands • Textures • Vibration	Desensitization of sensory receptors.	10 minutes, 3-4 times per day.	Intervention is initiated by having the client organize the sensory stimulation bins or dowels in a sequence of least to most abrasive, then begin with stimulation via the texture which is tolerated, applied directly to the affected area (Weylatt-Rendall, 2002). Graded progression to increasing more abrasive textures is then guided by the therapist with particular attention to the client's level of comfort. Vibration can also be added post intervention with dowels/textures.	*Do not over stimulate as this may result in pain.
Fluidotherapy: Nonthermal or thermal effect depending on client's tolerance and preference.	Corn husk contact can be graded by fan control allowing progressive input. Temperature can also be graded.	15-20 minutes.	• If thermal, machine is preheated • Client's extremity is placed in the fluidotherapy machine and the "sleeve" is wrapped around the client's extremity • Fan setting begins low and is increased as tolerated • Heat setting begins low and is increased as tolerated within therapeutic range of 38°C to 50.6°C • If open wound/skin lesions/infections, cover prior to placing hand into machine	If thermal, please see precautions under Pain and Edema table. If nonthermal, no further precautions.

Table 2-23

REMEDIAL TECHNIQUES FOR RANGE OF MOTION

Sensation: Hyposensitivity Modality or Intervention Techniques	PROM • Completed by caregiver • Pendulum exercises (Codman) • Self ROM	AROM/AAROM • Pulleys • Shoulder wheel • Arm ergometer • ROM arch • Wall ladder • Work hardening equipment, such as BTE (Figure 2-9)
Rational/Indications for Use (For complete descriptions see narrative information)	Maintain ROM, prevent contractures, adhesions, and joint deformities (Pedretti, 1990).	Increase ROM, prevent contractures, adhesions, and joint deformities (Pedretti, 1990).
Average Length of Time per Session	Completion requires approximately 15 minutes, 3 times per day.	Completion requires approximately 15 minutes, 3 times per day.
Process	• Caregiver: move extremity through entire range of joint • Pendulum: Client bends forward at the waist using the unaffected arm as support on a stable surface • All the affected arm to hang down to the floor • The body is moved so that the momentum of the body causes the arm to move in a straight line for ward/back and side to side, as well as clockwise/counter-clockwise in a circle (www.Draubreysmith.com) • Self ROM: See Figures 2-6 and 2-7	See Figure 2-8 for a sample AROM program.
Precautions	Dislocation of a joint, myositis ossificans, infection or inflammatory conditions within the joint, recent surgical procedure, unhealed fracture, marked osteoporosis, carcinoma of the bone or any fragile bone condition, significant hypermobility, significant pain, hemophelia, hematoma in the joint.	See PROM.

continued

Table 2-23, continued

REMEDIAL TECHNIQUES FOR RANGE OF MOTION

Sensation: Hyposensitivity Modality or Intervention Techniques	Moist Heat Packs	Fluidotherapy Thermal mode	Ultrasound (continuous setting: thermal) (see Figure 2-2)
Rational/Indications for Use (For complete descriptions see narrative information)	To promote tissue elasticity in preparation for the stretch associated with range exercises as well as to minimize the perception of pain at the session start.	To promote tissue elasticity in preparation for the stretch associated with range exercises as well as to minimize the perception of pain at the session start.	Promotes tissue healing and removal of waste products generated by the healing process.
Average Length of Time per Session	15-20 minutes.	15-20 minutes.	15-20 minutes, 3x/week, alternating days, approx. 10 treatments.
Process	• Six to eight layers of towels between the client and the moist heat pack. • Moist heat pack is placed over or around the area of pain/edema	Machine is pre-heated. Extremity is placed into the heated corn husks and the "sleeve" is wrapped around the client's extremity. Heat setting within therapeutic range of 38 degrees Celsius to 50.6 degrees Celsius. If open wound/skin lesions/infections, cover prior to placing hand into machine.	• Parameters vary from: 1.0-2.0 W/cm² for 5-8 mins, 1 or 3 MHz • Ultrasound coupling gel is placed on the site of injury. • Wand is moved slowly and without stopping (Bracciano, 2000)
Precautions	• See fluidotherapy and thermal ultrasound	Acute injury, diminished sensation, decreased circulation, compromised cognitive status, tumors or cancers, acute edema, deep vein thrombosis, pregnancy, bleeding abnormalities, infection, advanced cardiac disease, some case of rheumatoid arthritis where client may experience exacerbation following heat.	

Table 2-24

REMEDIAL TECHNIQUES FOR STRENGTH

Strength: Modality or Intervention Techniques	Strength training • Hand grippers • Thera-Putty/Thera-Band • Free weights/wrist weights • BTE	Isometric exercises
Rationale/Indications for Use (For complete descriptions see narrative information)	Given that strength is a remedial skill for successful engagement in functional activity, occupational therapy practitioners commonly must address strength specifically in order to assist the client in regaining independence in desired occupations.	Static strengthening in which muscular contraction/tension occurs without shortening or lengthening of the muscle. Typically used postinjury rehabilitation or postsurgical procedures as the first stage of strengthening. (Robergs & Roberts, 2000).
Average Length of Time per Session	Used as a precursor to functional activity, therefore no more than 15 minutes.	Hold each attempt for 5-10 seconds, 10 times, 1-2 times per day, daily, pending level of tolerance and progress. (Caution: Do not hold breath! Contraindicated for clients with cardiac and hypertension as isometrics can increase blood pressure.)
Process	Thera-Band, Thera-Putty, or hand grippers are generally color-coded by the manufacturer to illustrate for the therapist and client alike, the idea of graded resistance (see Figures 2-10, 2-11, and 1-12).	Exercises may be performed lying, sitting, or standing depending upon client's abilities and body part being strengthened. The client tightens and holds the contraction or may hold the body part against a resistance such as a wall or table. Example: Tightening the quadriceps muscle in a sitting position or holding the wrist into extension against the side of a table. (Caution: Do not hold breath! Contraindicated for clients with cardiac and hypertension as isometrics can increase blood pressure).
Precautions	*See isometric/isokinetic exercises	Inflammation, significant pain, recent fracture, bone carcinoma or any fragile bone condition, significant spasticity, cardiovascular conditions, hypertension, chronic obstructive pulmonary disease, any condition where fatigue might exacerbate the condition, and arthritis.

continued

Table 2-24, continued

REMEDIAL TECHNIQUES FOR STRENGTH

Strength: Modality or Intervention Techniques	Isokinetic exercise	Isotonic exercises • Concentric • Eccentric
Rationale/Indications for Use (For complete descriptions see narrative information)	Achieved through the use of exercise machines designed to strengthen muscles while working at a regulated speed and resistance (Robergs & Roberts, 2000).	Strengthening exercises which involve a shortening and lengthening contraction of the involved muscle against a constant load or resistance. Typically used in the subacute stages of healing (Robergs & Roberts, 2000).
Average Length of Time per Session	Repetitions can vary from 8-20 times depending on client goals. Sets will vary from 1-3, depending upon client tolerance and progress. Typically performed on alternating days.	Repetitions can vary from 8-20 times depending on client goals. Sets will vary from 1-3, depending upon client tolerance and progress. Typically performed on alternating days.
Process	Exercise machines are used in therapy clinics to achieve the desired resistance and velocity. Examples include: • Cybex • BTE PrimusRS • Biodex • Lido • KinCom • Isocom	Exercises may include calisthenics, weight training with free weights or machines or progressive resistance exercise (PREs). This involves the use of gradually increasing resistance over time and progress.
Precautions	Inflammation, significant pain, recent fracture, bone carcinoma or any fragile bone condition, significant spasticity, cardiovascular conditions, hypertension, chronic obstructive pulmonary disease, any condition where fatigue might exacerbate the condition, and arthritis.	*See isometric/isokinetic exercises.

continued

Table 2-24, continued

REMEDIAL TECHNIQUES FOR STRENGTH

Strength: Modality or Intervention Techniques	Progressive Resistive Exercises (PREs)	Work Simulator • BTE • ERGOS
Rationale/Indications for Use (For complete descriptions see narrative information)	Uses a specific method based on outlined parameters to strengthen.	This equipment option offers greater control in grading the resistance provided to muscle tissue as well as the unique capacity to simulate of planes of motion related to functional activity.
Average Length of Time per Session	Time is dependent on number of repetitions/sets completed, however a recommended frequency is to complete each of the above 1 time per day over 4-5 days per week.	Movements or activities are simulated through the use of tool/equipment choices and body positioning. Repetitions can vary from 8-20 times depending on client goals. Sets will vary from 1-3, depending upon client tolerance and progress. Typically performed on alternating days.
Process	1. Assess the client's overall maximal strength level within the defined area (i.e., right upper extremity) or the maximal weight through which the client is able to complete a full ROM with coordinated movement. 2. Foster 10 repetitions of muscle contraction within the defined area using weights equal to 50% of the determined maximal capacity 3. Follow with 10 repetitions of muscle contraction within the defined area using weights equal to 75% of the determined maximal capacity 4. Complete with 10 repetitions of muscle contraction within the defined area using weights equal to 100% of the determined maximal capacity	For example, with the BTE Work Simulator, available attachments for are designed to simulate particular aspects of a given functional activity such as driving, golfing, or opening a jar. Resistance is increased, or decreased, via the simple, and even fractional, adjustment in the software programming.
Precautions	See isometric/isokinetic exercises.	Same as strengthening precautions listed earlier in this table.

continued

Table 2-24, continued

REMEDIAL TECHNIQUES FOR STRENGTH

Strength: Modality or Intervention Techniques	Neuromuscular Electrical Stimulation (NMES) or Functional Electrical Stimulation (FES)
Rationale/Indications for Use (For complete descriptions see narrative information)	"The efficacy of electrical stimulation for the purposes of strengthening has been exclusively studied and is well established" (Bertoti, 2004). Used to externally elicit active muscle contraction, and therefore, secondarily addresses issues of strength.
Average Length of Time per Session	Time varies with chosen protocols and the tolerance of the clients.
Process	Electrical stimulation is provided via electrode placement over given motor points located along a weakened muscle's length. The electrical impulses then elicit contraction of the designated musculature and produce an active concentric contraction. Depending on the client, a variety of wave amplitudes, duty cycles, and frequencies will be appropriate. Further training in electrical stimulation is required.
Precautions	Presence of cardiac pacemakers, pregnancy, tumors/malignancy, epilepsy, over the ocular orbits, carotid sinus, or heart areas, blood pressure abnormalities, obesity, active infection, peripheral vascular disease, cardiac disease, mucosal surfaces, skin conditions such as eczema, impaired sensation, compromised cognitive status. Caution should be taken in case of compromised circulation due to clotting or thrombus, in cases of prosthetic implants, and in the presence of degenerative disease processes. Caution must be used in clients experiencing acute pain symptoms or undiagnosed pain.

Continued from page 97

Modes of Injury or Illness

The modes of injury or illness related to cognition and perception are rather broad in nature. These include acquired brain injuries of any type and level of severity and those of a degenerative nature such as Huntington's disease, MS, Alzheimer's disease, and other dementia-related conditions.

A client with any of the above health conditions may present with cognitive deficits, perceptual deficits, or, most commonly, cognitive and perceptual deficits. It is not the mode of injury or illness that is of importance to the OT, but rather the presentation of individually-manifested cognitive and/or perceptual deficits, directly related to the extent of injury to the brain itself, and represent the focus for selecting appropriate intervention strategies.

An Overview of Cognitive Perceptual Remediation

A good deal of controversy exists regarding recovery following an insult to the brain. Does the client with cognitive and/or perceptual deficits actually benefit from remediation efforts and do these efforts directly affect the rate of recovery within the brain? Recently, methods of surgical tissue transplants and pharmacological interventions are dominating in popularity, specifically with degenerative diseases including Alzheimer's and Parkinson's, however not among the acquired brain injury population. Rather, similar to sensory remediation, direct retraining of skills represents the technique of choice in facilitating recovery at the current time. "Direct retraining of cognition is, perhaps, the most controversial model of neurotraining because there is little evidence it improves functioning more than one would expect due to the passage of time alone" (Parenté & Herrmann, 2003, p. 58). For example, acute injury to the brain results in edema. This edema causes further increases in intracranial pressure or compression of the brain tissue that is confined within the defined borders of the skull. The pressure alone is enough to cause additional injury to the CNS, further impeding functional performance. Hence, are remedial techniques responsible for improved cognitive perceptual function or it is merely a result of the decrease in edema as the tissues of the brain begin to heal? Ongoing and future research is required to more accurately assess to what degree remediation efforts are effective.

Regardless of this debate, the OT does dedicate efforts of remediation for working with clients demonstrating cognitive and/or perceptual deficits. To do so, it is essential that the therapist understands the nature of the functional impact caused by the impairment in either of these skill areas. Cognition allows an individual to process, store, and manipulate information while perception refers to the integration of senses into meaningful information (Shumway-Cook & Woollacott, 2001, p. 156). Though interrelated, each holds vital importance in one's ability to purposefully and successfully interact with his or her environment. Perception is not sensation alone; rather sensation must be intact to address issues arising from perceptual deficits. Likewise, the degree of success with cognitive retraining is dependent upon the client's ability to learn through concept formation and generalization (e.g., each are underlying skills of cognition).

Engagement in functional activity represents the most efficient means of fostering remediation. These represent the very same tools used as compensatory or adaptive methods as well with variation only among the goals underlying implementation. With a remedial focus, the OT promotes active participation in meaningful activity so as to improve the perception of and responses to task demands. With a compensatory focus, the OT may use the very same functional activity however, has the ultimate goal of deciphering what techniques or equipment will promote optimal safety and independence in function alone. Refer to Chapters 3 and 4 for discussion of adaptive and compensatory techniques. Regardless of the intent, the client is certain to have more success with activities that are personally meaningful and part of the individual's daily routine, particularly in the presence of cognitive or perceptual compromise. Many clients may have significant difficulty with new situations while those that were part of the premorbid routine remain intact. Hence, it is optimal for the OT to gather information about a client's previous interests and daily engagements prior to deciding on strategies for addressing the remedial goals of cognition and/or perception. At times, it may even be necessary to interview families in order to accurately obtain these facts in cases where a client may be unable to accurately recall or report this information secondary to cognitive impairment.

In all, cognitive perceptual remediation is a complex area of expertise and is only summarized for means of introduction and illustration in the context of this chapter. This subsection is divided into components of perception and components of cognition separately for the purpose of simplicity. Focus is, therefore, placed on methods typically used to address the specific subcomponents rather than the combined skill area in general.

Perception

A REVIEW OF PERCEPTUAL TERMINOLOGY

In order to best outline remedial strategies for perceptual deficits, an overview of the coinciding subskills and related terminology is provided with priority below.

Visual Processing Skills

Visual processing is a term used to describe the act of physically viewing the environment, integrating that information with those of other sensory signals, and then to accurately and effectively create a visuo-motor response. Per Zoltan (1996), this process is two-fold, integrating both focal and ambient vision. "Focal vision provides attention to important features of an object" (1996, p. 27), while ambient vision "works in connection with proprioceptive, kinesthetic, tactual, and vestibular systems and acts as a feed-forward system" (1996, p. 27). The subskills required of visual processing include acuity, ocular alignment, visual fields, visual fixation, oculomotor control, and visual spatial attention. Only those of the aforementioned subskills considered appropriate for efforts of remediation will be further discussed below.

Ocular alignment includes the ability to coordinate the movements of the two eyes simultaneously. Impairment of alignment can cause clients to experience "diplopia (double vision), vertigo, confusion, clumsiness, motion sickness, and/or poor spatial judgment" (Zoltan, 1996, p. 32) and, therefore, impede the client's attempts to interact with their environment.

Visual field refers to the scope of our visual sense or degree one is able to physically see upward, downward, to the left and the right. This subskill is commonly affected by injury or illness of the CNS. Clients may describe a haze or even darkness in the center of the visual field, while others experience this symptom in left, right, upper, lower, inner, or outer hemispheres of the visual field. This is often referred to as a visual field cut. Others may experience symptoms bilaterally, characteristic of hemianopsia, and often indicative of right-brain involvement. These symptoms may be bothersome to the client or not even noticed at all (see visual spatial inattention). Regardless, impairments to the visual field present a direct barrier to active engagement in meaningful occupation via the incomplete representation of ones surrounding environment.

Visual fixation describes the ability to sustain focus on an object within the environment. It is important to note difficulty in this sub-skill can be either primary in nature or can secondary to other issues, such as a cognitive inability to attend.

Oculomotor control groups various subskills that together allow for the fluent movement of the eyes. These include aspects of the aforementioned skill, visual fixation, as well as saccadic eye movements (scanning) and smooth eye pursuits. In essence, so as to visually attend to one object within the visual field, a client must be able to fix (fixation) their vision on the object, make necessary fractional adjustments in eye position to maintain the object within the line-of-sight (saccades), and follow the object, while sustaining focus, as it moves through space (smooth eye pursuits). These skills collaborate to allow the observation of movement through all visual fields and without the need to reposition the head. Deficits within this area can prevent a client from engaging in the activity of reading.

Visual spatial inattention is most commonly the result of a CNS lesion that disrupts the ability to visually attend to each and all visual fields spontaneously. In most circumstances, the impairment is seen with right-brain lesions resulting in a disruption of visual attention to items in the left visual hemisphere. Clients presenting with inattention may appear with a rightward-gaze preference that also are often further complicated by concurrent visual field cuts, discussed previously, or body neglect, to be further discussed later in this subsection. In isolated visual inattention, a client will respond to cues of redirection, however, this is not the case when field cuts and/or body neglect are additionally present. Again, the ability to accurate view the environment around them impedes successful engagement in an array of functional tasks ranging from activities of daily living to leisure and social pursuits.

Praxis

Praxis is a component of motor planning and refers to one's ability to create and execute a motor response so as to effectively interact within his/her environment. Apraxia (or literally *without praxis*) further describes the inability to create or execute a motor plan in the absence of any other underlying sensory, strength, or coordination deficit. Apraxia is further categorized into two separate types based upon the manifestation of the actual deficit: ideomotor apraxia and ideational apraxia.

Ideomotor apraxia describes "the inability to imitate gestures or perform a purposeful motor task on command even though the ...(client) fully understands the idea or concept of the task" (Zoltan, 1996, p. 54). Conversely, *ideational apraxia* describes the inability to conceptualize the sequence of a motor plan and therefore, affects the execution of a purposeful motor task. The functional implication of the later type manifests with greater severity when compared to that of an ideomotor origin due to the absence of the client's ability to understand the concept of movement itself. For illustration, a client with ideomotor apraxia may not be able to mimic the task of brushing his or her teeth regardless of verbal prompts provided, yet is observed doing so successfully on his or her own during their regular morning routine. With ideomotor apraxia, the client may attempt to comb his/her hair when presented with the toothbrush, demonstrating a deficit in the conceptualization of the use for this tool.

Dressing apraxia is a term used to describe the inability to dress oneself due to underlying deficits in body scheme. As noted by Pedretti & Early (2001) and Gillen (2005), this classification has been refuted in recent years reflective of the isolated nature in which the apraxia presents only with dressing tasks. For this reason, many believe this deficit to be related more closely to a body scheme disorder than apraxia.

Additionally, the term *constructional apraxia*, may also be categorized here however, "*constructional disorder* is now favored over the previously used term... since the deficit does not clearly fall within the definition of apraxia" (Pedretti & Early, 2001, p. 451). Here, Zoltan (1996) describes clients as having difficulty replicating or creating two to three dimensional designs, via copying or drawing, either spontaneously or upon command. She continues by outlining research studies performed that link this specific disorder directly with a client's ability to either prepare meals or perform the skill of dressing accurately.

Body Scheme Disorders

Body scheme is a general categorization of skills required to spatially orient one's own body parts. Deficits within this area include somatognosia, unilateral body neglect, anosognosia, and issues of distinguishing right from left or right-left discrimination. As a group, these deficits present significant functional impairment as is evident by the descriptions provided below.

Somatognosia classifies those deficits where a client may have difficulty recognizing his/her own body parts, and/or be unable to differentiate between the body parts of others verses his/her own. The client may be unable to follow a request to point to his or her nose or leg regardless of whether the request is made verbally or by imitation. Asking the client to draw a person on a sheet of paper may yield an arm in the place of a leg, two arms and no representation of legs, or even extremities in the absence of a trunk.

Unilateral body neglect describes a condition where the client lacks the integration of sensory input on one half of the body, resulting in a lack of awareness for the existence of that side of the body. For example, a client may only draw one half of the body when asked to draw a person, may only dress one half of their body during the morning routine, or comb only one half of the hair on his or her head. Typically, neglect of the left half of the body is again, indicative of right-brain involvement and may or may not be accompanied by visual field cuts or visual inattention of the same side. *Anosognosia* represents an extreme form of unilateral body neglect characterized by a lack of acceptance or even denial of paralysis experienced within the body. Confusion and confabulation may also accompany this disorder as illustrated by the client who exclaims his or her paralyzed limb has simply, "always had a mind of its own" or who falls from the bed when attempting to stand stating, "It's just asleep." This deficit is commonly associated with a concurrent cognitive impairment, yet, is not always the case (Zoltan, 1996).

Deficits resulting in impairment of *right-left discrimination* are characterized by a client's inability to follow therapist commands such as "point to your left knee" or "raise your right hand." Impaired right-left discrimination is "considered by some to be a rare, but striking disorder" (Zoltan, 1996, p. 83).

Finger agnosia is a body scheme disorder causing difficulty in naming fingers, identifying the finger touched and a decreased ability to imitate gestures. Clients often present with bilateral involvement resulting in poor manipulation skills involving coordination of the fingers. Because the hand and fingers represent the cornerstone of function, finger agnosia can pose significant limitations in one's ability to perform functional, everyday tasks (Zoltan, 1996).

Agnosias

Agnosias related to perceptual deficits (but not specifically to body scheme disorders mentioned previously) include visual agnosia, visual object agnosia, prosopagnosia, simultagnosia, visual-spatial agnosia, tactile agnosia, auditory agnosia, and apractognosia. These types of agnosias result in the lack of recognition of familiar items or people due to the perceptual misinterpretation of input from visual, tactile, proprioceptive, and auditory systems alone (Zoltan, 1996). Because these occur infrequently and because intervention is similar as for body scheme disorders, intervention for these particular disorders will not be specifically addressed.

Visual Discrimination Skills

Visual discrimination refers to the ability to distinguish characteristics among items physically viewed. Visual discrimination is further classified to include five separate subtypes; form discrimination, depth perception, figure ground, spatial relations, and topographical orientation (Zoltan, 1996).

Form discrimination involves visual recognition of objects, shapes, color, and edges regardless of the context in which they are presented. When form discrimination is affected by injury or illness, clients may not be able to recognize subtle changes in form and therefore, properly adjust the motor response. Zoltan (1996) cites the classic example of a client attempting to use a water pitcher as a urinal.

Depth perception involves the ability to judge distance within the environment such as is needed for reaching to grasp a container of milk in the refrigerator. It is a skill that demands accurate visual input to produce accurate motor output. Deficits in this area may present as "undershooting" or "overshooting" when attempting to retrieve common everyday items needed to engage in daily occupations (Zoltan, 1996).

Figure ground involves the ability to perceive the foreground from the background. Though similar to depth perception and form discrimination, this skill specifically requires the ability to distinguish items that are closest to or furthest from oneself based on variations in color, texture, shape, and/or shadow. For example, a deficit in figure ground may hinder a client's ability to locate a white shirt placed on the white bedspread, or for that matter, the white buttons sewed on a white shirt, thereby impairing the overall level of independence with the task of dressing (Zoltan, 1996).

Spatial relations refers to the ability to judge the relationship of items to oneself as well as each other. This includes the subconscious interpretation of what is seen, such as the control knobs of a water facet located to each side of the water spout itself. For instance, to use the water faucet, one must be able to gauge the distance between themselves and the faucet as well as the components of the faucet including the orientation of right versus left (hot/cold), above versus below (faucet/basin), and on versus off. A client experiencing deficits with spatial relations would have difficulty following requests such as, "can you hand me the dish towel hanging next to the refrigerator" (Zoltan, 1996).

The final subskill of visual discrimination is *topographical orientation*. Topographical orientation refers to one's ability to navigate the environment, both immediate and on a more global scope. This skill results from the ability to recognize familiar settings and conceptualize the relationship of one place to another. A deficit in this skill area may cause a client to unsuccessfully locate the hospital-based bathroom in relationship to their adjoining room or identify the route necessary to get from one point in the community to another. As outlined by Zoltan (1996), remedial techniques are not generally attempted in this subskill area, with preference given to strategies of compensation or adaptation.

COMMON THEORIES FOR PERCEPTUAL INTERVENTION

In general, the prevailing theory that dictates remedial intervention methods implemented by the OT is the Cognitive Perceptual Theory. With the Cognitive Perceptual Theory, dysfunction is described as faulty sensory experiences resulting in limitations in the performance of occupational tasks. Refer to Chapter 3 for a brief analysis of this theory. The theory is based on the concept that the brain has the capability of both healing and adapting for dysfunction or neural plasticity—a principle that is described with more detail within the coordination subsection of this chapter. Methods prescribed here foster the repetition of sensorimotor experiences that in turn, foster overall relearning for the system. Much of the methods implemented are too based from concepts of teaching-learning combined with the integration of routine, everyday task performance.

REMEDIAL TECHNIQUES FOR PERCEPTION

There exist several underlying techniques the OT must attend to as precursors to the specific methods implemented in promoting the remediation of perceptual skills. These most commonly employed techniques are summarized below and represented in Tables 2-25 through 2-28, which outline specific methods as they relate to the terminology previously reviewed.

The use of cuing and chaining (forward and backward) are frequently implemented as both remedial and compensatory approaches employed by the OT when addressing perceptual deficits. Cuing is provided as a form of graded assistance during the performance of functional activities. Cuing is graded not only by the quantity of cues offered by the therapist, but also the manner in which they are provided. For example, a client may be offered both tactile and verbal cues. With improved performance, the OT will then grade to the use of only verbal cues or only visual cues fostering increased independence with performance demands. For illustration, a client who has a visual field cut may be reminded to attend to the affected side during the morning routine by having the therapist tactilely rub the affected extremity in addition to verbal reminders to look to that

Table 2-25

REMEDIAL TECHNIQUES FOR VISUAL PROCESSING

Visual Processing Skill Area	Remedial Strategies
Ocular alignment	Use of eye patches with attention to a wear schedule that fosters strengthening of the affected eye while avoiding weakening of the nonaffected eye; table top worksheet tasks that promote ocular alignment such as reading or following moving targets.
Visual fields	Use of anchoring techniques (Figure 2-22) are common where the OT will place a yellow (for example) border to the affected side and then use graded tactile and verbal cues reminding the client until they are able to see the yellow anchor. This provides the client with an environmental cue indicating that they are seeing the full visual field. Frequently combined with acts of function, such as eating a meal, in table top worksheet tasks, or with computer generated tasks which foster improved attention to the affected side. If anchoring continues, it becomes an adaptive/compensation or maintenance technique, as seen in Chapters 3 and 4.
Visual fixation	Due to the nature of the close relationship among scanning and fixation, the most commonly implemented remedial technique used here is reading. Therapist will grade these tasks from letter identification to reading a paragraph (Zoltan, 1996).
Oculomotor control and scanning	Fostering functional engagement in tasks requiring the skill of scanning, saccades, and smooth eye pursuits (Figure 2-23). The client may be asked to locate various items within their room, home, or hospital environment; identify the price of grocery items by locating price tags; and locate various items within a newspaper. Table-top worksheets or computer generated programs that foster scanning, or even participation in crossword puzzles pending level of interest.
Visual spatial inattention	Most commonly, techniques described above in the visual field section are repeated here so many times that they occur simultaneously. The OT may also use external stimulus, such as bright colors and/or lights in the affected area along with graded cuing statements to promote attention to that side during any functional tasks. Table top worksheets, such as bisecting lines, as well as a computer generated program specific to inattention are also commonly used tools.

side during task execution. The OT may then grade the cues provided by eliminating the tactile cues and using only verbal (or even written) cues to remind the client to attend to the affected side, thereby promoting increased independent participation in the grooming task.

Finally, it is important to note the therapist must allow for ample processing and response time in the performance of functional activity for a client with perceptual deficits. Adjusting time constraints for the completion of a given task too becomes a potential method for remediation.

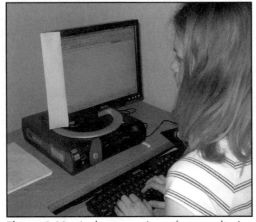

Figure 2-22. A demonstration of an anchoring technique. Here, while engaging in the functional task working at a computer, the OT will provide cues to guide the client's visual attention to the left side by placing a yellow strip along the left edge of the computer screen. Repeating this technique enables the individual to independently use the brightly colored strip as a cue that he/she is seeing all of what is placed in front of him/her whether it is a computer screen, a book, or a newspaper.

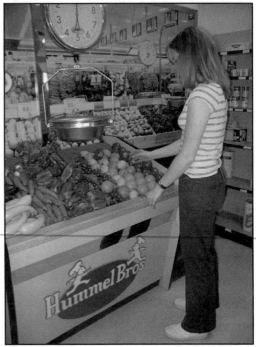

Figure 2-23. A sample of a functional environment where the OT is able to employ the remediation of oculomotor control and scanning.

Additionally, the therapist must be aware the return to function begins at the lowest skill level subsequently building upon those foundations so as to promote the overall remediation of the perceptual skill. As an illustration, a client must have good attention skills in order to have short-term memory and short-term memory to have topographical orientation. This again illustrates the complex inter-relationship among cognitive and perceptual skill execution.

Cognition

REVIEW OF COGNITIVE TERMINOLOGY

In order to best outline remedial techniques for cognitive deficits, a specific overview of the coinciding subskills and related terminology is again provided below with priority.

Orientation

Orientation is most commonly described in three facets: one's ability to recognize self, place, and time (Jacobs & Jacobs, 2004). A client experiencing disorientation may be unable to recall his/her name, birth date, family members (orientation to self), or location (orientation to place) and/or unable to state the present time, day, month, year, or season (orientation to time). Commonly, a state of disorientation will cause clients to become easily lost or frustrated due to repetitive prompting for what was once customary information, such as, "where are we now?" or "how old are you?" Clients may also be observed asking the same questions repetitively lacking the recall to realize it had already been asked previously.

Table 2-26	
REMEDIAL TECHNIQUES FOR APRAXIA	
Apraxias	*Remedial Strategies*
Ideational and ideomotor apraxias	Use of hand-over-hand techniques (tactile, proprioceptive and kinesthetic cuing) depicted in Figure 2-24 are most commonly implemented within the context of functional task engagement (such as dressing or washing) where the OT will physically move the affected body part for the client. Repetition is then promoted in the patterns of functional movement and frequently follow a developmental sequence. The OT may also use graded verbal cues as performance improves yet is seen mostly as a frustration to clients in the initial stages of recovery. Chaining is also implemented so as to ensure client successes.

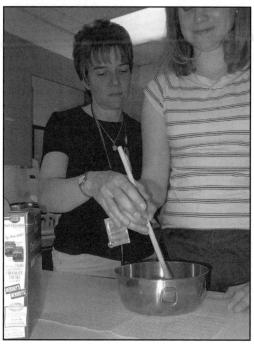

Figure 2-24. The hand-over-hand technique is implemented by the therapist to specifically provide exaggerated proprioceptive, kinesthetic, and tactile input as to normal movement patterns in the presence of apraxia.

Attention

Commonly, *arousal* is additionally considered as a component of attention due to the nature in which they are inter-related. One is unable to attend without first being aroused. Zoltan (1996) describes arousal as the level of alertness one displays or degree to which they are able to sustain a state of wakefulness and also notes that this level may fluctuate depending upon the state of one's CNS. Attention, therefore, is compromised in the presence of an altered level of arousal. *Attention*, or the ability to focus one's attention on a given task (Jacobs & Jacobs, 2004), is specifically considered a building block for an array of higher level specific mental functions including memory and problem-solving. Therefore, attention (and arousal) must be addressed with priority by the OT in a bottom-up approach with the goal of remediating overall cognitive functions.

Table 2-27

REMEDIAL TECHNIQUES FOR BODY SCHEME

Body Scheme Skill Area	Remedial Strategies
Somatognosia	Use graded tactile, verbal, and visual cues to increase awareness of body parts within the context of engaging in a functional task. In addition, the OT will frequently provide these cues in association with choices for the client and then grade this level of assistance (e.g., "is this your hand or your foot" while gently stroking the hand). Methods also include participation in body puzzles or computer generated programs fostering improved body orientation.
Finger agnosia	Fostering improved performance in functional tasks via repeated attempts, chaining, and cuing. The OT may provide nonadversive tactile stimulation (refer to sensation section) to isolated digits regularly requesting identification of the specific digit given added sensory input. A developmental progression is generally followed moving from gross grasp patterns to more precise movement of the fingers demanded in the engagement of functional activity
Unilateral body neglect/anosognosia	Use of hand over hand techniques to physically guide the client's attention to the affected extremity using the unaffected extremity. Fostering added sensory input to the affected extremity via rubbing with appropriate textures prior to engagement in functional tasks. Occasionally, aspects of the NDT, such as weight-bearing through the affected extremity, may also be implemented just prior to functional task participation to again, provide added sensory stimulation. Therapist cuing and chaining are regularly graded during these activities.
Right-left discrimination	Most commonly, the OT will initiate visual cuing techniques to foster success with functional tasks. This may include the use of a wrist weight on the dominant hand during functional activities and be graded to simply a colored wrist band as performance and accuracy improves. Again, common to see cuing, chaining techniques as well as the provision of choice to enable success.

Memory

Memory is defined as one's ability to successfully process, store, and retrieve information as required to engage and re-engage successfully in purposeful activity (Jacobs & Jacobs, 2004). This area is again contingent upon other areas including attention and perception. For example, without the ability to attend to a task, the client may be unable to create memory about an experience. Similarly, without having the ability to recognize various situations accurately, as is seen with perceptual disturbances, it becomes increasingly difficult to form the accurate memory of a given experience for future reference. In addition, there also exists varying types of memory; hence, one type may represent a barrier for a client while another, strength. Most frequently, memory is classified as *short-term* or *long-term*, reflective of the extent to which the information is stored within the brain.

Table 2-28

REMEDIAL TECHNIQUES FOR VISUAL DISCRIMINATION

Visual Discrimination Skill	Remedial Strategies
Form discrimination	Use of graded verbal, visual cues and the use of vision to foster improved performance are commonly implemented. Clients may be requested to repeat various functional tasks which require form discrimination such as sorting items, for example, a bag of bolts or a drawer of utensils (Zoltan, 1996).
Depth perception	Functional activity engagement requiring of reach and grasp (Figure 2-25), table top worksheets, and computer generated programs designed for remediation of this skill are frequently implemented. Heavy emphasis may also be placed on verbal guidance, or cues, through the act of reach so as to retrain the sense of depth during functional movement patterns.
Figure ground perception	Scattering of everyday common objects and requesting the client point to the requested item (Zoltan, 1996). Use of cuing and grading of size and degree of subtle qualities inherent of the objects provided and requested are common.
Spatial relations	Repetitive use of graded verbal techniques as well as provided choices to promote success. For example, "your shirt is on the shelf above your socks" or "the toothpaste is in the drawer beneath the sink." Hand-over-hand techniques may also be of assistance in guiding the client through the excursion of the required movement.

Short-term memory describes information that is stored for the purpose of immediate recall, either within seconds, minutes, or hours. Long-term memory characterizes those events one is able to recall after the period of days, and years following the initial event. Limitations in either category can significantly impede a client's ability to function safely and independently within the environment.

Executive Functions

The term *executive functions* is used to describe a variety of higher level, multistep cognitive skills combined (Jacobs & Jacobs, 2004). These skills include initiation, self-awareness and insight, planning and organization, problem solving, and mental flexibility.

Initiation describes the ability one has to begin engagement in a given task without hesitation (AOTA, 2002). A client with decreased initiation may have great difficulty starting tasks, regardless of any other comorbid, cognitive deficit. The client simply is unable to get started, however, once the activity has been initiated and has no issues with completing the task to its entirety. The converse of initiation is the skill of *termination*, or lack thereof, where a client is unable to cease engagement in the activity or task regardless of the fact it has been already been completed. This is also referred to as *perseveration* (O'Toole, 2003).

Self-awareness and insight are terms used to describe the degree to which clients are aware of their deficits. Compromise in this area presents the OT with a great challenge given the client's lack of awareness as to the existence of deficits and therefore, appropriately draws significant concern for the client's safety and well being in general. This lack of deficit awareness may be so

Figure 2-25. Again, using the grocery store as an illustration, having the client place items within the scale is a functional example requiring the integration of depth perception in addition to several other perceptual skills.

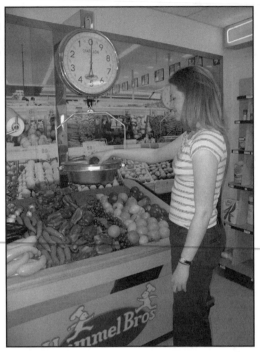

intense in some cases that attempts to foster insight into disability will yield aggressive rebuttal or uncharacteristic hostility towards the therapist.

Planning and organization are skills that enable one to formulate goals or objectives and the coinciding plan that allows for the achievement of those goals. It is arguable that all task participation on daily basis is a result of planning and organizing. For example, one must rise in the morning, decide upon what needs to be completed that day, apply priorities, assess time constraints, develop a plan, conceive potential barriers to success, and then execute the plan. Not only does this process call upon planning and organizing as executive functions, but also requires memory, orientation, attention, and mental flexibility to be intact (Zoltan, 1996).

Problem solving, as indicated above, is critical to carry out functional tasks successfully throughout the day. As was the situation with planning and organization, problem solving also represents a skill dependent upon others, such as insight, impulse control, reasoning skills, and mental flexibility (Zoltan, 1996). For example, the client may have planned a visit to the local grocery store so as to obtain supplies necessary to prepare a meal. In executing this plan, the client discovers he or she has missed the bus that would provide transportation to the grocery store or possibly, that the supplies required to prepare the meal are out of stock. The client must first identify the problem and then consider alternate plans that will continue to allow for success in the overall goal. These may include calling a cab, waiting on the next bus, or substituting ingredients required to prepare the planned meal. Each of these options will require additional consideration of time constraints, feasibility, cost, and overall foresight. This illustrates a classic example of the capacity to problem solve.

Mental Flexibility

Mental flexibility provides one with the ability to think conceptually, to generalize information and, overall, to think with abstraction (Zoltan, 1996). Clients who demonstrate impairment with mental flexibility may appear very literal or concrete in their thought process or contributions to conversation. They may be unable to shift their thinking from one topic to the next and back again (often referred to as multitasking) or are commonly observed to be perseverative (consumed by one thought) on superficial experiences in the immediate environment or those offering ease in association. As with most cognitive skills, mental flexibility is again dependent upon other skills including memory, attention, and problem solving; hence, deficits in any one or more of these areas may also manifest themselves in a similar manner.

Acalculia

Acalculia is a term used to describe difficulty with calculations. It is often taken for granted how frequently one uses their ability to perform calculations on a daily basis: to manage funds, complete simple money transactions, maintain a suitable budget, identify the costs of items necessary to purchase, use the telephone, or even to address mailing envelopes (Zoltan, 1996). Acalculia identifies a specific disorder in the processing of any numeric information. The deficit can result from perceptual or processing impairments as illustrated by a client who may see a 6 as a 9 (perceptual) versus one who may not conceive the concept behind the symbol + versus - or x. These types of deficits may present concurrently or in isolation.

THEORY OF COGNITIVE INTERVENTION

Toglia and Abreu's Theory of Cognitive Rehabilitation is predominately used to guide intervention when working with clients experiencing cognitive deficits. Originally based on learning theory, and now updated by Toglia to include metacognition (insight into own capabilities), this theory emphasizes the retraining of cognition in a hierarchical manner while embracing the principle of neural plasticity and specifically speaks to orientation, attention, visual processing, and motor planning (Cole, 2005).

REMEDIAL TECHNIQUES FOR COGNITION

Prior to outlining the specific approaches employed by the OT, it is paramount to discuss various key concepts critical to maximizing the success when working with clients experiencing issues with cognitive ability. The most commonly implemented techniques are summarized within Table 2-29, outlining specific method options as they relate to the terminology reviewed above.

Foremost, the therapist must always consider the benefits of a nondistractible environment to further enable success for a client with cognitive issues. Aspects considered most easily modified include the lighting, smells, and sounds typical of the area where intervention is planned to occur. A less stimulating environment may enhance results for a client who is distractible, while the opposite would be preferred when attempting to promote increased arousal.

Techniques of remediation should regularly coincide with the execution of everyday routines and habits. This is achieved by aggressively infusing a client's premorbid routines as inherently motivating methods for reestablishing independence. For example, a client who has just awaked may wander around his or her unfamiliar hospital room, seemingly anxious, irritable, and unable to self-engage in any task. Yet, when the client is verbally prompted to take his/her typical morning shower, they are then able to locate all necessary items and complete the task with only supervision as a means of ensuring safety.

Similar to the techniques reviewed for perception, the OT addressing cognition will also benefit from the use of repetitive and frequent verbal, tactile, and visual cuing; methods of chaining; and overall skills in gradation to facilitate the successful completion occupational tasks. Also of note is the OT who will, at specific times, avoid providing cues altogether so as to allow the opportunity for a client to plan, organize, and problem solve independently. This technique is commonly employed to assist a client in developing awareness or insight into their areas of weakness. For example, the OT may ask the client to make a simple meal, such as his or her regular morning breakfast choice, and provide only supervision for the purpose of ensuring safety. This client may forget to plug in the toaster or forget to place the coffee grinds in the coffee maker as a result of his

Table 2-29

REMEDIAL TECHNIQUES FOR COGNITIVE RETRAINING

Cognitive Skill	*Remediation Strategies*
Orientation	Regularly requesting client orientation responses that foster the use of graded cues for accuracy such as looking out windows for signs of season; adoption of a daily planner outlining important personal information with the use of regular prompting to promote automatic use.
Attention	Foster the active engagement in activities of premorbid interest such as playing a game of cards, knitting, or drawing for example, gradually increasing time constraints; use of computer generated programs designed to improve attention skills; implement reward system such as engagement in a preferred task for 5 minutes followed by 2 minutes of therapist-selected tasks; include activities that require physical activity as this often assists in promoting attention.
Memory	Provide verbal cuing via choice of two in prompting responses; implement regular structure into the daily routine; table top memory drills or games, where deemed age appropriate.
Initiation	Foster engagement in activities of premorbid interest and routine; provide incentives and client-specific rewards for goal attainment; provide multisensory environment with colors, light, and the use of graded verbal, tactile, and visual cuing.
Self awareness/insight	Videotaping, role playing, photo collages of premorbid activity engagement, self reflective questioning, engagement in activities of everyday living while allowing for feedback through self reflection, active participation of family members, and/or significant others within intervention so as to provide "nonthreatening" feedback regarding deficit areas.
Planning and organization	Techniques of preplanning and organizing through developing specific daily schedules; table top worksheet activities (Figure 2-26) and computer generated programs which require preplanning and organization; participation in a supervised community outing planned by the client.
Problem solving	Allow the client to engage in a functional activity such as a simple cooking task; use graded cuing and provide choices to assist in identifying errors and support in finding solutions for those errors.
Mental flexibility	Fostering engagement in an activity that requires both visual and auditory interpretation (e.g., participation in a group-based exercise program); implement the use of computer generated programs designed to foster improved mental flexibility skills.
Generalization	Provision of experiences that require generalization such as reading directional signs in the clinic as well as out in the community as a means of navigation or locating items in one pharmacy as compared to another.
Acalculia and calculations	Computer generated programs and/or table top worksheet tasks, assist the client in paying simple bills or placing a phone call.

Worksheet: Planning Your Day

You wake in the morning and spend a few minutes considering the tasks you must complete prior to a scheduled dinner reception at 6:00 pm. These tasks include...

1. Go to the gift store and purchase an item for the dinner reception you are attending this evening.
2. Go to the pharmacy to pick up your prescription and purchase a card to accompany the gift you are giving at the dinner reception this evening.
3. Attend your 9:00 am doctor appointment.
4. Your car has an empty gas tank.
5. Your outfit for this evening is at the dry cleaner that closes at 4:00 pm.
6. You will need to stop at the bank to withdraw money from your savings account. Your wallet is without cash and you do not possess any debit, credit, or checking accounts.
7. Your scheduled hair cut appointment is at 2:00 pm and generally takes about an hour.
8. You are in need of a quick stop to the grocery store for milk, orange juice, and deli meats.

You are being asked to sequence the events summarized above so as to manage your time efficiently and arrive to your dinner appointment on time (6:00 pm). Use the following space to rewrite the tasks in the order that will allow for you to meet this goal.

TIME:	TASK TO BE COMPLETED:
1.	
2.	
3.	
4.	
5.	
6.	
7.	
8.	

Figure 2-26. Sample cognitive worksheet.

or her inability to accurately sequence. When the bread is not toasted or the coffee remains merely water, an exaggerated opportunity has been provided for the client to identify a problem and find a solution, while also concretely illustrating that skills once executed with ease might now require more attention following the incidence of injury or illness.

Finally, it is important to reiterate that cognitive skills are hierarchical in nature—a concept embraced specifically by the Cognitive Rehabilitation theory. Fundamental cognitive skills represent the foundation for remediation so as to reestablish higher level, executive skill execution. As an illustration, without being cognitively alert, attention to task is not possible. Furthermore, without attention, completion of a given task may not be possible. The therapist must then follow a bottom-up approach that prioritizes those fundamental skills, so as to realistically plan methods of intervention.

Special Considerations for Cognitive Perceptual Intervention

There exists an array of special considerations for selecting occupational therapy intervention strategies for clients who have cognitive, perceptual, or cognitive and perceptual deficits. The most important are summarized in the following paragraphs.

Foremost, it is important that the OT engage the family, significant others, and potential caregivers in the carryover of techniques very early on so as to foster optimal intensity and repetition required the regain these skills. Training should be provided early on and modified as necessary so that they are also able to foster recall and independence with cuing. As many clients with cognitive or perceptual issues are hospitalized for the initial rehabilitation phase, families are often requested to adorn the hospital room with familiar items including typical items of their morning routine (e.g., hair brush), as well as blankets, pillows, and photos of loved ones. This also allows the therapist to infuse these familiar items into treatment sessions as an opportunity to promote success for the client.

The OT must also be considerate of the client's available support systems and their significance during the healing process. Working with clients that have sustained cognitive and/or perceptual deficits often requires the provision of education to those significant others wishing to provide this much needed support. Education is frequently provided by request in form of questions stemming from the observation of uncharacteristic behaviors demonstrated by the client. The therapist must use always use caution as the explicit sharing of client-specific information is restricted by federal legislation. The Health Insurance Portability and Accountability Act of 1996 (PL 104-191) was enacted, in part, to preserve the privacy of a client's health information (Pozgar, 1999).

Client safety is also of paramount importance when working with those who have impaired cognition and/or perception. As discussed previously, some clients with cognitive issues may experience bouts of hostility and frustration. This is a recognized level of the recovery process, outlined by the Rancho Los Amigo (RLA) Scale, as the RLA IV level. The RLA Scale is a measurement tool, devised at the Rancho Los Amigo Hospital in Downey, California, that defines eight distinct levels through which individuals generally progress during the healing process and for case of brain injury specifically. Each level is characterized by a set of observable behaviors. For example, RLA Level I is characterized by complete nonresponsiveness where Level VIII is defined by a return to purposeful and appropriate level of cognitive functioning (Pedretti & Early, 2001). Refer to Figure 2-27 for a brief summary of the Ranchos Los Amigo Scale, Levels of Cognitive Functioning. In cases of RLA IV, not only is client safety of importance, but also that of the treatment team, while always recalling that hostility is symptom of the injury in a given phase of recovery, and not necessarily the client's cognitive intent.

Maintenance Programs

With regard to maintenance programs for clients with cognitive and/or perceptual deficits, it must be emphasized that recovery can vary greatly from client to client. Some improve at a faster rate yielding discharge directly to the home with continued outpatient services while others require discharge to a more structured transitional living program prior to returning home. Often, it is this proposed discharge environment that will direct not only efforts of remediation, but also the specific maintenance program recommended for the client.

The maintenance program will typically emphasize the specific carryover of any and all techniques found to be successful for fostering maximal independence during treatment session. Careful consideration should also be paid to the societal acceptance of recommended techniques so as to enhance the probability it is carried over. For example, a client with memory issues would be most likely to actively adopt the use of a handheld organizer in assisting with the recall of daily routines over that of a cumbersome notebook filled with check lists.

Finally, the importance of local community-based resources should be formally identified and provided to clients and their caregivers. This may include a variety of support services including support groups, vocational rehabilitation programs, driving rehabilitation programs as applicable, or contact information regarding accessible housing, local means of transportation, or marketplaces for assistive technology needs, as examples. This notoriously individualized, comprehensive, and proactive approach often leads to a maximal level of independence for the lives of clients who have experienced cognitive perceptual impairments.

RANCHOS LOS AMIGOS SCALE OF COGNITIVE FUNCTIONING

RLA I: No Response
Client is nonarousable; no response to stimlus of any type.

RLA II: Generalized Response
Client can initiate gross reactions to stimuli in some manner.

RLA III: Localized Response
Client begins to respond with more appropriate gestures such as turning head to the sound of a familiar family member. May also respond to simple commands such as "squeeze my hand."

RLA IV. Confused-Agitated
Client gains alertness in state of confusion displaying heightened reactions to simple requests, such as aggressive outbursts or emotional lability. Behavior is often characterized as inappropriate and internally driven with respect to societal norms or expectations.

RLA V: Confused – Inappropriate – Nonagitated
Client is able to consistently respond to simple commands, requires prompting and structure in all tasks, incongruent, inappropriate, emotional responses may continue yet are less aggressive in nature.

RLA VI: Confused – Appropriate
Client is gaining ability to engage in goal oriented and purposeful behavior. Attention is improving along with the ability to follow commands with less structure provided. Remains confused, though appropriate in reaction to events leading up to injury and the characteristics of the injury (insight).

RLA VII: Automatic – Appropriate
Client is able to function in a structured daily routine without assistance though continues to require supervision for safety in multi-stepped tasks or in those lacking in definite structure. Behavior is considered automatic and rote in nature.

RLA VIII: Purposeful – Appropriate
Client is aware of remaining limitation as well as all events leading to injury. He/she is able to perform in all areas of occupation, however, may continue to require supports for higher level executive functioning skills such as work or money management, for example.

Figure 2-27. Original Scale, Levels of Cognitive Functioning, 1980. Acknowledgment of Ranchos Los Amigos Medical Center, Downey, California, Adult Brain Injury Service.

Summary Questions

1. Define remediation and discuss the "bottom-up" approach to intervention.

2. List and describe remedial techniques for pain management, sensation, ROM, and strength.

3. Discuss precautions and contraindications as related to techniques described in each subsection of this chapter.

4. Discuss the potential limitations to occupational therapy practice in terms of the use of PAMs.

5. Discuss the impact of modes of injury upon foundational skill areas.

Acknowledgments

A special thanks to Anne Albert, OTR\L, Supervisor of SCINO and Medical Rehabilitation Programs at Gaylord Hospital, Wallingford, CT and to Carolyn Matrian, a fieldwork level II student from Ithica College, NY on affiliation at Gaylord Hospital, for their demonstrations illustrated within this chapter's photographs.

Additional thanks are extended to the editors of this text, Catherine Meriano, JD, MHS, OTR/L and Donna Latella, EdD, MA, OTR/L, for their enduring vision, resourcefulness, contributions, and patience throughout the lengthy process of completing this chapter.

References

American Occupational Therapy Association. (2002). *Occupational therapy practice framework: Domain & process*. Bethesda, MD: AOTA.

Ashwinik, R. (2004). Approaches to motor control dysfunction: An evidence-based review. In G. Gillen & A. Burkhardt. *Stroke rehabilitation: A function-based approach* (2nd ed., pp.93-118). St. Louis: Mosby.

Barber, L. (1990). Desensitization of the traumatized hand. In J. Hunter, L. Schneider, E. Mackin, & A. Callahan (Eds). *Rehabilitation of the hand* (3rd ed., pp. 721-730). St Louis: Mosby.

Barnes, M. P. (1998). Management of spasticity. *Age and Aging, 27*(2), 238-245.

Beers, M. H., & Berkow, R. (1999). *The Merck manual of diagnosis and therapy* (10th ed.). Whitehouse Station, NJ: Merck Research Laboratories.

Bertoti, D. B. (2004). *Functional neurorehabilitation through the life span*. Philadelphia, PA: F.A. Davis.

Bracciano, A. G. (2000). *Physical agent modalities: Theory and application for the occupational therapist*. Thorofare, NJ: SLACK.

Brachtesende, A. (2005, November 21). Adventures in venture capital. *OT Practice*, 9-11. Retrieved June 10, 2006, from http://saebo.com/customers/104072910252887/filemanager/Careers_Nov21FINAL.pdf

Cameron, M. H. (2003). *Physical agents in rehabilitation: From research to practice* (2nd ed.). Philadelphia: Saunders.

Chattanooga Group. (2005). *Fluidotherapy*. Retrieved June 12, 2005, from www.fluidotherapy.com.

Cochrane, D. J. (2004, February). Alternating hot and cold water immersion for athlete recovery: A review. *Physical Therapy in Sport, 5*(1), 26-32.

Cole, M. B. (2005). *Group dynamics in occupational therapy: The theoretical basis and practice application of group intervention* (3rd ed.). Thorofare, NJ: SLACK Incorporated.

Crepeau, E. B. Cohn, E. S., & Schell, B. A. B. (2003). *Willard & Spackman's occupational therapy* (10th ed.). Philadelphia, PA: Lippincott, Williams & Wilkens.

Faghri, P. D., Rodgers, M. M., Glaser, R. M., Bors, J. G., Ho, C., & Akuthota, P. (1994). The effects of functional electrical stimulation on shoulder subluxation, arm function recovery, and shoulder pain in hemiplegic stroke patients. *Archives of Physical Medicine and Rehabilitation, 75*(1), 73-79.

Falvo, D. (2005). *Medical and psychosocial aspects of chronic illness and disability* (3rd ed.). Sudbury, MA: Jones and Bartlett Publishers.

Gallichio, J. (2004). Pharmacologic management of spasticity following stroke. *Physical Therapy, 84*(10), 973-982.

Gillen, G. (2005, June). *Cognitive-Perceptual Assessment: A functional based-approach.* Workshop presented June 11, 2005.

Gillen, G., & Burkhardt, A. (2004). *Stroke rehabilitation: A function-based approach* (2nd ed.) St. Louis: Mosby.

Gilmore, P. E., Spaulding, S. J., & Vandervoort, A. A. (2004). Hemiplegic shoulder pain: Implications for occupational therapy treatment. *Canadian Journal of Occupational Therapy, 71*(1), 36-47.

Glennon (2004).

Godges, J. J., Mattson-Bell, M., Thorpe, D., & Shah, D. (2003). The immediate effects of soft tissue mobilization with proprioceptive neuromuscular facilitation on glenohumeral external rotation and overhead reach. *Journal of Orthopaedic and Sports Physical Therapy, 33*(12), 713-717.

Hafsteindottir, T. B., Algra, A., Kappelle, L. J., & Grypdonck, M. H. (2005). Neurodevelopmental treatment after stroke: A comparative study. *Journal of Neurological Neurosurgical Psychiatry, 76*(6), 788-792.

Hoffman, H., & Snyder, J. (2003). The effects of the Functional Tone Management (FTM) arm training program on upper extremity motor control on chronic post-stroke individuals. *Journal or Stroke & Cerebrovascular Diseases,* 5. Retrieved June 10, 2006, from http://saebo.com/programresults.html.

Huntley, N. (2002). Cardiac and pulmonary diseases. In C. M. Trombly and M. V. Radomski (Eds.). *Occupational therapy for physical dysfunction* (5th ed., p. 1078), Philadelphia, PA: Lippincott Williams & Wilkens.

Ivanhoe, C. B., & Reistetter, T. A. (2004). Spasticity: The misunderstood part of the upper motor neuron syndrome. *American Journal of Physical Medicine and Rehabilitation, 83*(10 Suppl.), S3-S9.

Jamil, T. (1997). *Complimentary medicine: A practical guide.* Jordan Hill, Oxford: Butterworth-Heinemann.

Jacobs, K., & Jacobs, L. (2004). *Quick reference dictionary for occupational therapy* (4th ed.). Thorofare, NJ: SLACK Incorporated.

Katz, D. I., Alexander, M. P., & Klein, R. B. (1998). Recovery of arm function in patients with paresis after traumatic brain injury. *Archives of Physical Medicine, 79,* 488-493.

Kesiktas, N., Paker, N, Erdogan, N., Gulsen, G., Bicki, D., & Yilmaz, H. (2004). The use of hydrotherapy for the management of spasticity. *Neurorehabilitation and Neural Repair, 18*(4), 268-73.

Kraft, G. H., Fitts, S. S., Hammond, M. C. (1992). Techniques to improve function of the arm and hand in chronic hemiplegia. *Archives of Physical Medicine and Rehabilitation, 73,* 220-227.

Langhammer, B., & Stanghelle, J. K. (2000). Bobath or Motor Relearning Programme? A comparison of two different approaches of physiotherapy in stroke rehabilitation: a randomized controlled study. *Clinical Rehabilitation, 14*(4), 361-369.

Luke, C., Dodd, K. J., & Brock, K. (2003). Outcomes of the Bobath concept on upper limb recovery following stroke. *Clinical Rehabilitation, 18,* 888-898.

Michlovitz, S. (1996). *Thermal agents in rehabilitation* (3rd ed.). Philadelphia: F.A. Davis.

Mortenson, P. A. (2003, July). The use of casts in the management of joint mobility and hypertonia following brain injury in adults: A systematic review. *Physical Therapy, 83*(7), 648-658.

Neumann, D. A. (2002). *Kinesiology of the musculoskeletal system: Foundations for physical rehabilitation.* St. Louis: Mosby.

Northwest Hospital & Medical Center. (2005, June/July). What's new in rehab? Retrieved June 10, 2006, from http://www.saebo.com/customers/104072910252887/filemanager/NewsletterJune_July2005.pdf

O'Toole, M. T. (Ed). (2003). *Miller-Keane encyclopedia and dictionary of medicine, nursing, and allied health.* Philadelphia: Saunders.

Page, S. J, Sisto, S. A., & Johnston, M. V. (2000). Modified constraint-induced therapy in stroke: a case study. *Archives of Physical Medicine, 81*(12), 1620.

Page, S. J., Sisto, S. A., Levine, P., Johnston, M. V., & Hughes, M. (2001). Modified constraint-induced therapy: a randomized feasibility and efficacy study. *Journal of Rehabilitation Research and Development, 38*(5), 583-590.

Parenté, R., & Herrmann, D. (2003). *Retraining cognition: Techniques and application* (2nd ed.). Austin, TX: Pro-Ed.

Pedretti, L. W., & Early, M. B (Eds.). (2001). *Occupational therapy: Practice skills for physical dysfunction* (5th ed.). St Louis: Mosby.

Pozgar, G. D. (1999). *Legal aspects of health care administration.* Gaithersburg, MD: Aspen.

Price R., Lehmann, J. F., Boswell-Bessette, S., Burleigh, A., & deLateur, B. J. (1993). Influence of cryotherapy on spasticity of the human ankle. *Archives of Physical Medicine and Rehabilitation, 74*(3), 300-304.

Prosser, R., & Conolly, W. B. (Eds.). (2003). *Rehabilitation of the hand & upper limb.* Leith Walk, Edinburgh: Butterworth-Heinemann.

Reed, K. L. (2001). *Quick reference to occupational therapy* (2nd ed.). Austin, TX: Pro-Ed.

Robergs, R. A., & Roberts, S. (2000). *Fundamental principles of exercise physiology: For fitness, performance, and health.* Boston: McGraw-Hill.

Ruoti, R. G., Morris, D. M., & Cole, A. J. (1997). *Aquatic rehabilitation.* Philadelphia: Lippincott-Raven.

Salzman, A. P. (1998). *The teacher's manual of advanced aquatic therapy.* Oak Ridge, TN: Concepts in Physical Therapy.

Shankar, K., & Randall, K. D. (2002). *Therapeutic physical modalities.* Philadelphia: Hanley & Belfus.

Shimura, K., & Kasai, T. (2001). Effects of proprioceptive neuromuscular facilitation on the initiation of voluntary movement and motor evoked potentials in upper limb muscles. *Human Movement Science, 21*(1), 101-113.

Shumway-Cook, A., & Woollacott, M. H. (2001). *Motor control: Theory and practical applications* (2nd ed.). Baltimore: Lippincott Williams & Wilkins.

Smith, A. (2005). Codman's exercises, otherwise known as pendulum or tic-toc exercises. Retrieved July 15, 2007, from http://www.draubreysmith.com/codman.htm.

Spicher, C., Kohut, G., & Miauton, J. (1999). At which stage of sensory recovery can a tingling sign be expected? *Journal of Hand Therapy, 12*(4), 305.

Stroup, E. L., & Snodgrass, J. (2005). The motor control model: Treatment applications and research considerations. *Advance for Occupational Therapy Practitioners, 21*(3), 48-49.

Thomas, C. L. (Ed.). (1997). *Taber's cyclopedic medical dictionary.* Philadelphia, PA: F.A. Davis.

Trombly, C. A. (Ed.) (1995). *Occupational therapy for physical dysfunction* (4th ed.). Baltimore: Williams & Wilkins.

Trombly, C. A., & Radomski, M. V. (Eds.). (2002). *Occupational therapy for physical dysfunction* (5th ed.). Philadelphia, PA: Lippincott, Williams & Wilkins.

Taub, E., Uswatte, G., & Pidikiti, R. (1999). Constraint-induced movement therapy: A new family of techniques with broad application to physical rehabilitation—A clinical review. *Journal of Rehabilitation Research and Development, 36*(3), 237-251.

Vandyck, W. & Mukand, J. (2004). Reducing contractures after TBI. *OT Practice, 9*(19), 11-15.

Watanabe, T. (2004). The role of therapy in spasticity management. *American Journal of Physical Medicine and Rehabilitation, 83*(10 Suppl), S45-S49.

Watson, D. E., & Llorens, L. A. (1997). *Task analysis: An occupational performance approach.* Bethesda, MD: AOTA.

Waylett-Rendall, J. (2002) Desensitization of the traumatized hand. In E. J. Mackin, A. D. Callahan, A. L. Osterman, T. M. Skirven, L. H. Schneider, & R. R. Hunter (Eds). *Hunter, Mackin and Callahan's rehabilitation of the hand* (5th ed., pp. 693-700). St. Louis: Mosby.

Zoltan, B. (1996). *Vision, perception, and cognition: A manual for the evaluation and treatment of the neurologically impaired adult* (3rd ed.). Thorofare, NJ: SLACK Incorporated.

Zuther, J. E. (2003). Daily use of compression therapy for lymphedema. *Advance for Occupational Therapy Practitioners, 19*(17), 40-41.

3 Activities of Daily Living

Catherine Meriano, JD, MHS, OTR/L
Donna Latella, EdD, OTR/L

CHAPTER OBJECTIVES

- ☑ Define **activities of daily living (ADLs)** as it pertains to the *Occupational Therapy Practice Framework (Framework)*.
- ☑ Describe specific **models/frames of reference** as related to ADL.
- ☑ Comprehend **safety issues** as related to ADLs.
- ☑ Delineate between the role of the **occupational therapist** (OT) and the **occupational therapy assistant** (OTA) as they pertain to the occupation of ADLs.
- ☑ Comprehend and identify related **psychological implications** as related to decreased independence in ADLs.
- ☑ Describe the impact of **contextual factors** upon ADLs.
- ☑ Identify appropriate ADL intervention strategies based on various **performance skills and client factors**.
- ☑ Identify specific ADL **compensation/adaptation** strategies.
- ☑ Identify general ADL **remediation** strategies.
- ☑ Identify ADL compensation/adaptation intervention strategies related to **vision, perception, and cognition**.
- ☑ Identify general ADL **maintenance** strategies.

INTRODUCTION

ADLs are defined by American Occupational Therapy Association (AOTA) as "Activities which are oriented toward caring for one's own body (adapted from Rogers & Holm, 1994, pp. 101-202) also called basic activities of daily living (BADL) or personal activities of daily living (PADL)" (AOTA, 2002a, p. 620). This chapter will first discuss general aspects of all ADLs. These will include methods and frames of reference for intervention, safety, psychological issues, the role of the OTA, as well as the *Framework* definitions of context, performance patterns, and activity demands. Following these topics, interventions for ADLs are discussed in the categories of self-care (bathing, hygiene, dressing, feeding, and toileting skills), functional mobility, eating/dysphagia, and sexual activity. In each of these categories, different intervention approaches, as described in Chapter 1 will be discussed. These approaches are remediation, compensation/adaptation, and maintenance. In addition, compensation and adaptation interventions will be broken down even

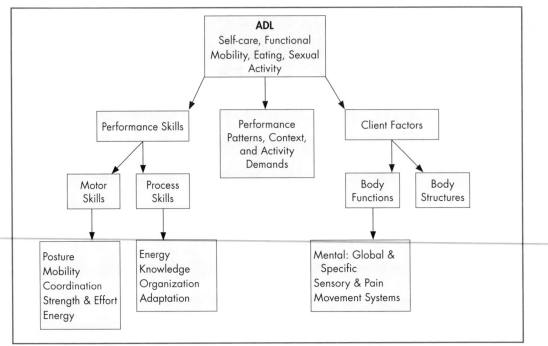

Figure 3-1. Components of ADLs (adapted from American Occupational Therapy Association. [2002a]. *Occupational therapy practice framework: Domain and process.* Bethesda, MD: AOTA).

further based on whether the compensation is "changing the task" or "changing the tools." Figure 3-1 depicts the areas of the AOTA *Framework* that will be addressed in this chapter. Similar charts are placed throughout the chapter in reference to the information within each area covered.

Because ADLs are often addressed in conjunction with other interventions and because occupational therapy intervention is a continuum of client care, references will be made to other sections of the book throughout this chapter. The earlier information regarding the AOTA *Framework* document from Chapter 1 and the client factors, motor skills, and performance skills discussed in Chapter 2, and later chapters will be referenced as appropriate.

METHOD OF INTERVENTION: BOTTOM UP VS TOP DOWN

As stated in Chapter 1, intervention for ADLs can follow one of two approaches. The first approach, according to Zoltan (1996) is called the *bottom-up approach.* If using the bottom-up approach, the OT would decide to provide intervention for foundational activities that impact ADLs. For example, if after the completion of a task analysis, the OT determines the client has limited ADLs as a result of fine motor coordination deficits, the intervention would be provided for the remediation of fine motor coordination deficits, as described in Chapter 2. The reasoning behind this approach is based on the idea that if fine motor coordination skills are remediated, then ADL skills would also improve.

The negative aspect of this approach is carryover/generalization to ADLs is not guaranteed by the fact that foundational skills are present in isolation. As discussed in Chapter 1, carryover includes completing the same task in a similar setting. Generalization is the ability to complete a similar task in a variety of settings. While some researchers have found that exercises completed by individuals on one upper extremity (UE) does demonstrate improved performance of the same exercise on the contralateral extremity (Nagel & Rice, 2001), this does not necessarily guarantee carryover to ADLs. One reason may be because rote exercise does not hold meaning to the individual as a purposeful activity would. Fasoli, Trombly, Tickle-Degnen, & Verfaellie (2002) found "motor actions during material-based occupation appeared to be strongly influenced by the added purpose and meaning derived from the use of tools and objects" (2002, p. 126). It is also interesting to note the reverse carryover from ADLs to foundational skills may be found. Nelson, Konosky, Fleharty, Webb, Newer, & Hazboun (1996) found despite the same amount of tone present in clients who had a cerebral vascular accident, those who completed functional tasks were found to have greater return of supination than those who completed rote exercise.

Because carryover to ADLs as well as foundational skills can be found when using functional activities, the second approach, called *top-down* as discussed by Zoltan and the Occupational Therapy Intervention Process Model (OTIPM) by Fisher, is generally preferred (Zoltan, 2007; Fisher, 2002). Using this approach, the OT would perform ADL skills incorporating remediation for functional activity deficits into the session. Using the same fine motor coordination skills as the deficit, the OT would be sure to include buttoning, opening of a small container such as toothpaste, and other fine motor tasks into the ADL session.

While the top-down approach is preferred, both of these approaches do have merit. The therapist must use clinical judgment to determine which approach works best for each individual client and each clinical setting. If a client is in an acute care hospital and clothes are not available, then the top-down approach is not realistic. On the other hand, if a client has significant cognitive deficits along with the fine motor deficits, the top-down approach will offer better carryover to ADLs. This section of the book will discuss primarily top-down approaches, as the bottom-up approaches were already addressed in Chapter 2.

FRAMES OF REFERENCE FOR ADL INTERVENTION

There are a variety of frames of reference that can be utilized when working on ADLs. Chapter 1 discussed the client-centered models such as the Person-Environment Occupational Performance (PEOP) Model, and the Person-Environment Occupation (PEO) Model, as well as systems models such as the Model of Human Occupation (MOHO) and the Ecology of Human Performance.

In addition to these, therapists using the top-down approach may also use frames of reference based on clients' specific situations. For a client who is aging, a developmental frame of reference, such as Jung's spiritual stages, Erickson's psychosocial stages, or Levinson's life transitions may be utilized (Cole, 1998).

For a client who has experienced a traumatic brain injury or a cerebral vascular accident where behavior changes are apparent, a behaviorist theory, such as behavior modification, may be employed. Behavior modification is based on environmental reinforcers in order to shape behavior (Cole, 1998). This same client may have cognitive deficits and will require a cognitive frame of reference such as Toglia and Abreu's cognitive rehabilitation frame of reference. Originally based on learning theory and now updated by Toglia to include metacognition (insight into own capabilities), this frame of reference emphasizes retraining cognition that occurs through hierarchical intervention and brain plasticity (Cole, 1998).

Because behavior modification is based on environmental feedback, better carryover should be demonstrated again with the use of functional activities rather than rote exercise. This is also true of cognitive rehabilitation. According to Cole, "cognitive strategies are always taught in the context of an activity" (1998, p.149).

SAFETY DURING ADL INTERVENTIONS

One of our primary concerns during any type of ADL is the safety of our client. Because ADLs include hot water, sharp objects, and other safety hazards, it is vital that therapists monitor these safety hazards and provide client and caregiver education. Safety concerns will be addressed throughout this section with specific tasks as examples.

IMPLICATIONS FOR PSYCHOLOGICAL IMPACT ON ADLS

The OT practitioner must not concentrate so heavily on the functional aspects of recovery that the psychological aspects are overlooked. Because ADLs are typically very personal experiences, there can be a significant psychological impact on a client when there are limited ADL skills. The roles of the individual and the impact of decreased ADLs on the family or work context can be significant. For example, when the family breadwinner is suddenly not only unable to support his family, but cannot even feed himself, his self-esteem and family interactions can be significantly changed. In addition, most clients are going to be uncomfortable or embarrassed when unable to perform personal tasks such as washing or cleaning themselves after using the toilet.

In general, the psychological issues that arise can be dealt with during the ADL sessions. There are times however, when these issues become too overwhelming for the client. For example, if a client is showing signs of significant depression and this is impacting his/her motivational level for ADLs, more time needs to be devoted to addressing the depression. Typically, even in settings where the main focus is on physical rehabilitation rather than psychological, these psychological interventions are reimbursable as long as these interventions relate back to the functional status of the client.

CONTEXT OF ADLS

Therapists often have thought of the context as the environment where ADLs take place. The importance of this context was underscored with the work of Gibson & Schkade (1997). Their study found that occupational therapy intervention that was focused on the roles and contexts identified as important by the clients resulted in higher levels of independence and less restrictive discharge environments (1997). According to the AOTA *Framework*, context goes beyond just the physical space, as "contexts can be cultural, physical, social, personal, spiritual, temporal and virtual" (2002, p. 613). These general definitions were explained in Chapter 1, but Table 3-1 describes examples of how some of these contexts can be related to ADLs. In order to work with clients in a holistic manner, all of these contexts must be considered and incorporated into the intervention plan of the individual client.

PERFORMANCE PATTERNS RELATED TO ADLS

Along with context, the performance patterns of the client's ADLs must also be considered when formulating an intervention plan. Performance patterns were discussed in Chapter 1. These patterns of behavior include habits, routines, and roles according to the AOTA *Framework* (2002a). When establishing an intervention plan, it is essential to determine the client's habits and routines regarding ADLs. For example, some clients prefer to sponge bathe, others shower, and still others soak in the tub. Each of these routines will certainly change the type of interventions provided.

Table 3-1	
CONTEXT AND IMPACT ON ACTIVITIES OF DAILY LIVING	
Context	*ADL Example*
Cultural	Cultural and societal beliefs regarding frequency of bathing
Physical (relates to space demands)	Accessibility to bathroom or bedroom layout
Social	Expectations of spouse to assist with ADLs even if the client has the skills
Personal	Socioeconomic status impacting ability to change the physical environment of ADL space
Temporal	Time of day when client prefers to complete certain ADLs

A client's role(s) within the family unit as well as society may also impact ADLs. An example of this would be if the role of the client is the caregiver. It may be difficult for others to step in to care for this client because they have never had to experience that role within the family. Another example would be if the expectation within a society is for the spouse to care for the ill family member, not health care professionals. These societal and family roles are often interdependent within the cultural context as described above.

ACTIVITY DEMANDS OF ADLS

The activity demands of ADLs include the required tools, space, time, foundational skills, and social skills to complete different ADL tasks (AOTA, 2002a). As with performance patterns, aspects of activity demands are also related to the client's context. Table 3-2 provides examples of activity demands and ADLs.

THE ROLE OF THE REGISTERED OCCUPATIONAL THERAPIST/ OCCUPATIONAL THERAPY ASSISTANT

Intervention for ADLs can be completed by occupational therapists (OTR) or occupational therapy assistants (OTA). Both have adequate training and knowledge regarding most ADL tasks. As stated in the introduction chapter of this text, the OTR and OTA create a team effort for providing intervention to each client. In this chapter, the term "occupational therapist" represents both of these professionals.

The information provided regarding ADLs is primarily entry-level information for both OTRs and OTAs. If further training is required beyond entry-level skills, this will be indicated with particular areas of intervention, such as dysphagia.

Table 3-2	
ACTIVITY DEMANDS AND THE RELATIONSHIP TO ADLs	
Activity Demands According to AOTA Framework (2002)	*Examples Related to ADLs*
Objects	ADL supplies or equipment
Space demands (relates to physical context)	Bathroom space available for ADLs
Social demands	Expectations of the individual to perform ADLs independently
Sequence and timing	Steps and proper sequencing required to complete ADLs properly
Required actions	Foundational skills required to complete ADLs
Body functions & structure	ROM and anatomical parts (hands) required for ADL completion

ACTIVITIES OF DAILY LIVING: REMEDIATION, ADAPTATION/COMPENSATION, AND MAINTENANCE

SELF-CARE: BATHING, HYGIENE, DRESSING, FEEDING, TOILETING

The definitions of these self-care activities according to the AOTA *Framework* (2002a) are as follows:

- "**Bathing, showering**: Obtaining and using supplies; soaping, rinsing, and drying body parts; maintaining bathing position; and transferring to and from bathing positions (p. 620)."

- "**Personal hygiene and grooming**: Obtaining and using supplies; removing body hair (use of razors, tweezers, lotions, etc.); applying and removing cosmetics; washing, drying combing, styling, brushing and trimming hair; caring for nails (hand and feet); caring for skin, ears, eyes, and nose; applying deodorant; cleaning mouth; brushing and flossing teeth; or removing, cleaning, and reinserting dental orthotics and prosthetics (p. 620)."

- "**Dressing**: Selecting clothing and accessories appropriate to time of day, weather, and occasion; obtaining clothing from storage area; dressing and undressing in a sequential fashion; fastening and adjusting clothing and shoes; and applying and removing personal devices, prosthesis, or orthoses (p. 620)."

- **Feeding**: "The process of (setting up, arranging, and) bringing food (fluids) from the plate or cup to the mouth (O'Sullivan, 1995, p.191; AOTA, 2000a, p. 620)."

- **Toilet hygiene**: "Obtaining and using supplies; clothing management; maintaining toilet position; transferring to and from toileting position; cleaning body; and caring for menstrual and continence needs (including catheters, colostomies, and suppository management) (p. 620)."

It should be noted that the AOTA *Framework* document also includes bowel and bladder management, personal device care, and sleep/rest as separate self-care activities. These definitions will be provided below; however, these tasks will be incorporated into toileting, bathing, hygiene, and dressing as they are typically incorporated into these interventions rather than completed in isolation.

The definitions of these ADLs, according to the AOTA *Framework* (2002a) are as follows:

- "**Bowel and bladder management**: Includes complete intentional control of bowel movements and urinary bladder and, if necessary, use of equipment or agents for bladder control (Uniform Data System for Medical Rehabilitation [UDSMR] as cited by AOTA, 2002a, p. 620)."

- "**Personal device care**: Using, cleaning, and maintaining personal care items, such as hearing aids, contact lenses, glasses, orthotics, prosthetics, adaptive equipment, and contraceptive and sexual devices (p. 620)."

- "**Sleep/rest**: A period of inactivity in which one may or may not suspend consciousness (p. 620)."

EVALUATION OF ADLS

While the focus of this text is intervention, evaluations will be discussed briefly because they are an important component of the intervention plan. The first step of any evaluation is the completion of an interview or an occupational profile with the client. This allows the therapist to gather information regarding the client's motivating factors, goals, discharge needs, etc. One tool that can quickly and easily be administered to assist in this process is the Canadian Occupational Performance Measure (COPM). This tool allows the client to identify areas of occupation in which he/she would like to improve. (Law, Baptiste, Carswell, McColl, Polatajko, & Pollock, 1998). Using a functional approach, therapist would then begin to evaluate specific ADLs that the client desires to work on and which are required for discharge planning. The COPM is available for purchase through AOTA. While there are many evaluations available, a few examples of formal evaluations include the Performance Assessment of Self-Care Skills (PASS), the Assessment of Motor and Process Skills (AMPS), the Arnadottir OT-ADL Neurobehavioral Evaluation (A-ONE), and the Functional Independence Measure: Guide for the Uniform Data Set for Medical Rehabilitation (FIM). These evaluations have been chosen because they all begin with function. This text is emphasizing the top-down approach, and these tools fit well with this approach. In addition, the AMPs and the A-ONE assess cognition and perception along with ADLs, allowing for a more holistic evaluation of the client.

The Performance Assessment of Self-Care Skills (PASS), developed by Rogers and Holm (1989), includes 26 activities that can be evaluated as a whole or individually. Eight of the 26 items are related to ADLs as defined by AOTA, and the client is scored based on independence in completing a task, safety during the task, as well as the appropriate completion or outcome of the task. This evaluation has two versions—clinic and home; therefore, it can be used in multiple settings. The tasks are the same for the two versions; however the materials are different so this evaluation can be utilized in the home even if it has previously been used in the clinic. Training is required prior to using the PASS, but once trained, the tool is available to the clinician for use.

The AMPS, developed by Fisher (2001), evaluates both motor and process skills through the use of ADLs. The clients are scored based on their "effort, safety, efficiency, and independence" (www.ampsintl.com). This tool has excellent validity and reliability as well as cultural sensitivity (a significant number of international subjects were included in the research of this tool). Unlike the PASS, the client is not asked to perform a task as he/she normally would, but rather is given a specific set of instructions. In general, however, therapists will be able to locate tasks that are appropriate for clients due to the large number of tasks available in the evaluation tool. Documentation of this tool is completed on the computer, and training is required. Information regarding training can be found at www.ampsintl.com and in Appendix A.

The A-ONE, developed by Arnadottir (1990), evaluates ADLs and correlates them to neurobehavioral deficits, such as apraxia, agnosias, and neglect. ADL tasks, when using this tool, are completed by the client without specific directions to complete the task in a particular way. Scoring is based on the client's independence as well as any neurobehavioral impairments noted during the ADL task. Training is required for use of this tool. Information regarding this evaluation tool can be found in *Brain and Behavior: Assessing Cortical Dysfunction Through Activities of Daily Living* (Gillen & Burkhardt, 2004).

While based on function, the Functional Independence Measure (FIM) is the most limited of the evaluation tools listed; however, it is one that is frequently used by rehabilitation facilities. One reason for the frequent use of this tool is the fact that training is cost effective and completed fairly quickly compared to the other tools above. A second reason is that the FIM is often used in an interdisciplinary format with speech, occupational therapy, physical therapy, and nursing filling out different sections. The FIM evaluates self-care, continence, mobility/locomotion, communication, and social cognition. The scores are simply 1 to 7 and there is no opportunity to explain why the level is below the 7 or independent score. One client may have perceptual deficits and another cognitive, but both could have the same score. Administrators like the FIM because the standardized results can be sent to the Uniform Data Systems for a fee, and the facility will receive "benchmark" outcome data comparing like facilities (www.udsmr.org).

In addition to standardized and formal evaluations, informal evaluations are also created by individual facilities. The advantage of these is the low cost; however, the reliability and validity of these tools is not tested. Examples of informal evaluations include self-care evaluations; home evaluations to address the context, safety, and function of the client in whatever environment is planned postdischarge; and table top cognitive/perceptual evaluations. Because table top activities are not generally directly related to function, and often not of value to the client, these are not recommended in favor of more functional assessments. For more information regarding specific evaluation tools, see Appendix B.

REMEDIATION OF SELF-CARE

Remediation of self-care skills using the "top-down" approach will typically include completion of an ADL session. By completing this session, the therapist can incorporate performance skill issues, such as decreased fine motor skills or decreased cognitive skills; however, the focus is on practicing the actual skills that the client will utilize on a daily basis. Remediation by definition is improving the skills, not adapting them; therefore, practice and training are the cornerstones of this approach. In addition, context, activity demands, performance patterns, and safety must be considered as discussed earlier in this chapter. For remediation to be most successful, the environment and activity demands must be as close as possible to the performance of this task in the client's actual environment. Simulation will not lead to remediation for most individuals (Trombly & Radomski, 2002).

One technique used for remediation is called "backward chaining." This technique, as described in Chapter 1, allows the client to finish the task, rather than start it and stop once he or she has "failed." By using this technique, the client gains confidence in his or her skills and a stronger rapport is established with the therapist. As the therapist decreases the assistance given, the client continues to gain skill and confidence, eventually becoming independent. If the therapist is unable to decrease assistance, then remediation is no longer an appropriate approach.

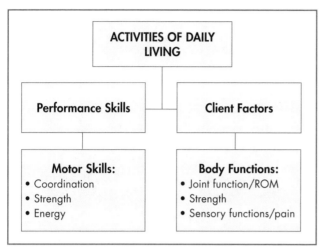

Figure 3-2. Components of performance skills/client factors related to ADLs (adapted from American Occupational Therapy Association. [2002a]. *Occupational therapy practice framework: Domain and process.* Bethesda, MD: AOTA).

COMPENSATION/ADAPTATION OF SELF-CARE DEFICITS FOR CLIENTS WITH PHYSICAL LIMITATIONS: PERFORMANCE SKILLS/CLIENT FACTORS

As stated in Chapter 1, the AOTA *Framework* uses the term "modify," as well as compensation and adaptation. Other resources will distinguish between adaptation and compensation by stating adaptation is that when the environment is changed and compensation is when the task or environment is changed (Zoltan, 2007). In practice, many therapists use these terms interchangeably. For these reasons, the compensation and adaptation sections are broken down into "Change of task" and "Change of tools" for maximum clarity.

Both compensation and adaptation can be used to achieve short- or long-term goals with clients. If a client will be quickly discharged from a facility, a therapist may use compensation/adaptation to allow the client to regain independence until further remedial therapy can improve the self-care skills. For other clients, remediation is not appropriate due to the underlying pathology; therefore, compensation/adaptation will be the best choice of intervention for a longer period of time. Once these compensations and adaptations become a permanent part of the self-care routine, they are considered "maintenance" according to the AOTA *Framework* (2002a) (Figure 3-2). Maintenance will be discussed later in this chapter.

Because the form of compensation/adaptation depends largely on the underlying pathology or symptoms of the pathology, the intervention strategies discussed below have been broken down into sections based on a grouping of symptoms. For self-care, these groupings are clients with motor skill deficits and clients with processing skill deficits.

Interventions for these groupings are not exclusive and overlap may exist. For example, a client may demonstrate hemiparesis, cognitive deficits, and perceptual deficits at the same time. In this situation, a therapist must utilize clinical judgment as to which combination of approaches will be appropriate for this particular client.

Other factors that will determine the form of compensation/adaptation include the context of the client upon discharge from therapy, the performance patterns of the client, the activity demands of the task, as well as the individual preferences of the client.

Figure 3-3. Relationship of ROM, strength, and coordination to ADLs (adapted from American Occupational Therapy Association. [2002a]. *Occupational therapy practice framework: Domain and process*. Bethesda, MD: AOTA).

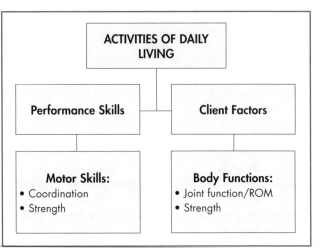

Compensation/Adaptation Interventions of Self-Care for Range of Motion, Strength, and Coordination Deficits

Range of motion (ROM), strength, and coordination are found in the AOTA Framework document under motor skills and body functions (2002a) (Figure 3-3). Definitions of these can be found in the "foundations" Chapter 2.

While modes of injury were discussed in Chapter 1, those related to ROM, strength, and coordination specifically will be reviewed again. The most common neurological pathologies leading to deficits in these three areas are CVA and head injury; however, clients with a variety of neurological pathologies could demonstrate deficits. In addition, many clients with orthopedic or traumatic injuries, burns, arthritis, or other joint dysfunction will demonstrate deficits in these areas. While some clients will experience bilateral deficits, it is more common for there to be unilateral injury. For this reason, the self-care section will more often refer to an "affected" versus "unaffected" extremity. In addition, the range of function within these categories is tremendous. One client could have mild weakness, allowing a great deal of function, while another client could have hemiplegia with no function or tone noted in the arm. Certainly, the intervention for these clients is markedly different. It is vital to understand the basic concepts of intervention for populations of clients, but to tailor each intervention plan to the unique characteristics, interests, and environment of the client sitting before the therapist.

For clients with motor deficits, many self-care tasks are generally impacted. It is best to first attempt to change the task, rather than add adaptive equipment, because there is less of a financial burden and often less to confuse an individual client. In addition, if the adaptive equipment is for some reason unavailable, the client's skills are significantly impacted.

However, there are times when tools, such as adaptive equipment and durable medical equipment (DME), will offer greater opportunities for the client. One approach to providing compensation/adaptation for the client with limited or no use of one side of the body is to provide tools that are available for the general population. Today a large number of self-care products are available in a pump dispenser for bathing and hygiene. These products can easily be used with one hand and their availability makes them easy to replace for the client when necessary. If liquid products are not desirable to the client, "soap on a rope" or a suctioned holder such as the "octopus" can be used. Other tools available to the general public are elastic pants to increase the ease of donning pants, shoes with hook/loop fasteners instead of laces, and button extenders created for shirt collars can be used for shirt cuffs.

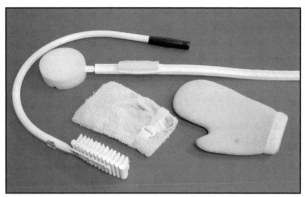

Figure 3-4. Sample bathing equipment: wash mitts, long-handled back brush, and long-handled sponge.

In addition to these commonplace tools, adaptive equipment is also available. Examples of these tools include: long-handled sponges, wash mitts, and adapted bath brushes (Figure 3-4). As discussed in Chapter 1, there are considerations that must be addressed prior to providing training with adaptive equipment. These considerations include cost, client preferences, and insurance coverage.

Another alternative to adaptive equipment is to change the environment, thus altering the task. Moving items within easy reach in cabinets, closets, and drawers will provide greater independence to the client without the need for reachers or other adaptive equipment.

Bathing

Changing the Task to Achieve Independence

During self-care, the client who does not have functional use of one UE needs to learn to function with the remaining extremity. For bathing, the clients are typically able to use the unaffected extremity to complete these tasks, particularly if the dominant arm is the unaffected arm. There may be some difficulty with washing related to standing to wash, but this will be discussed later under toileting.

Changing the Tools to Achieve Independence

Clients with motor deficits can use adaptive equipment throughout self-care activities. For example, during bathing, a client can be given a wash mitt that allows for the soap to be placed in the mitt. With this tool, a client will no longer drop the soap while trying to wash. (An alternative to this tool is for the client to buy any type of bath sponge and use pump soap to apply onto the sponge.) For clients with limited lower extremity (LE) ROM, a long-handled sponge will allow them to wash the LEs without leaning forward. After washing, a towel can be wrapped around the sponge to dry the LEs as well.

For information regarding bathroom equipment, such as raised toilet seats and shower seats, please refer to the section on functional mobility later in this chapter.

Grooming/Hygiene

Changing the Task to Achieve Independence

The majority of hygiene tasks can also be completed utilizing the unaffected extremity. Some bilateral tasks such as drying/styling hair, painting nails on the unaffected hand, and flossing teeth will be more difficult. In addition, "personal care devices" (AOTA, 2002a) often require bilateral use. It is difficult to put in a hearing aid battery or contact lenses with only one extremity. Some clients will eliminate these difficulties by changing the task completely—choosing to change their hairstyles to ones that require no styling, eliminating nail polish, or wearing glasses instead of contact lenses. While it is not generally recommended for the therapist to encourage clients to limit activities they enjoyed prior to an injury or illness, these activities may not hold a great deal of value to certain clients and still other clients may prefer the limitations over the frustration of attempting the activities. Of course, adaptive equipment, as discussed below, is another option.

Changing the Tools to Achieve Independence

A variety of tools are available to assist clients who demonstrate motor deficits. For the client with limited use of one extremity, there are hygiene tools that suction to the sink such as a denture brushes, nail brushes, or nail clippers. Again, mainstream items such as pump toothpaste or pump shampoo will also assist as well. There are even stands available to the general public that hold a hair dryer for individuals with limited arm strength or ROM. Other tools have extended handles and will hold toothbrushes, combs, brushes, etc allowing for function even with limited motor skills.

FEEDING

Changing the Task to Achieve Independence

Clients with limited motor skills will generally have difficulty holding utensils and cups to feed themselves. One way to change the task is to choose foods that allow greater independence. A sandwich or other finger foods may be easier for the clients to bring to their mouths than soup or peas on a spoon. This choice takes a great deal of coordination with the client, the family, and the dietary department. It is typically not a permanent solution because it would be too limiting to the client, however it does provide greater independence until the client regains functional skills for other foods.

Changing the Tools to Achieve Independence

As stated earlier, many clients with motor deficits will be fairly independent in feeding if the unaffected side is also the dominant side. The tasks that will cause difficulty for even this client are the tasks requiring two hands such as cutting food and opening containers. For clients who have use of the dominant arm, as well as those who do not, there are multiple pieces of adaptive equipment. Again, we first look for tools available to the general public. Cardboard milk and juice containers with screw-top openings rather than the traditional openings are one example. Once these possibilities have been examined, appropriate adaptive equipment is reviewed. Examples of equipment for feeding are rocker knives for one-handed cutting, swivel spoons to avoid spilling with tremors, adapted handled utensils for clients with limited grip, scoop dishes, nonslip mats to avoid plate slippage, and covered cups to avoid spilling. Examples of adaptive equipment for feeding are shown in Figure 3-5.

DRESSING

Changing the Task to Achieve Independence

Dressing is the most difficult task for the majority of individuals with motor deficits. One-handed dressing techniques do allow for independence; however, practice is required as these techniques are new to clients. In general, the client should dress the affected extremity first, and undress the affected extremity last. As stated earlier, there is a large range of function among individuals with motor deficits. This text will describe the methods that should be used for clients with the most severe deficits: hemiparesis or hemiplegia. If the client has some function of the affected side, he/she should always be encouraged to use it during dressing tasks. This may alter the methods described below, but these methods are only general guidelines that should be tailored to fit each individual client.

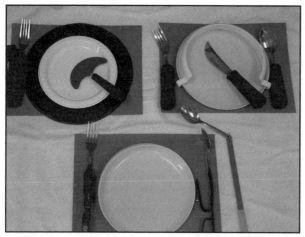

Figure 3-5. Sample feeding equipment: adapted utensils/dishes and dycem.

For dressing the upper half of the body, the client should be sitting either in a chair or at the edge of the bed, depending on sitting balance skills. If there is any concern regarding a client's sitting balance, a chair must be utilized for the safety of the client. In addition, the chair should have armrests to allow for greater support of the client, as well as a firm surface to assist in standing.

Generally, the first step for women is to put on a bra. There are a few methods available to change this task. The first is to hook the bra ahead of time and then put it on over the head as if it was a pullover shirt. The method for a pullover shirt is discussed below. This works well with women of smaller build. The second method is to use the unaffected arm to push the hook of the bra behind the body, followed by reaching across the front of the body to bring the bra hook to the front midline. The bra can then be hooked in front with the unaffected arm and rotated around the body until the cups are in the front. The bra strap is placed on the affected arm and pulled up the arm as far as possible. The unaffected arm is then place into the other bra strap and pulled up in place. Front closure bras or adapted bras can also be used; however, these will be discussed below as "changing the tools." Table 3-3 summarizes the different steps to putting on a bra.

Some women will chose to wear an undershirt rather than a bra, and many men will also wear undershirts. The undershirt, as well as any other types of shirts, sweaters, or sweatshirts that go on over the head, are put on using the "pullover" method. Again, the client dresses the affected arm first. This is often the most difficult part, particularly for clients with little to no function of the affected UE. Short sleeve shirts are easier to begin with because there is less length to pull onto the affected extremity. The first step is to gather the shirt sleeve of the affected arm using the unaffected arm. This gathered sleeve is placed on the lap in front of the affected arm so the unaffected arm can be used to place the affected arm into the gathered sleeve (Figure 3-6). The sleeve is then pulled up the affected arm as far as possible, at least over the elbow. If the shirt is pushed over the shoulder, this will allow greater ease when the shirt is brought over the head. Once the affected arm is in the sleeve, the client puts the unaffected arm into the other sleeve and brings the shirt over his/her head, or brings the shirt over the head first, and then places the unaffected arm into the sleeve (Figure 3-7). This will depend on client preference. Lastly, the client reaches behind the back to straighten out the shirt. It is often necessary to push the shirt over the affected shoulder with the unaffected arm as the shirt gets caught on the front of the shoulder. Table 3-4 summarizes the methods for donning a pullover type shirt.

Clients with severe motor impairments may have difficulty with this method because the weakened wrist and hand may flex as the shirt sleeve is being pulled up and can result in the shirt sleeve getting stuck. Some clients prefer to use an alternate method in order to get the affected extremity into the sleeve. These clients use the unaffected arm to enter the end of the sleeve of the

Table 3-3

STEPS TO DON A BRA

1. Keep bra hooked and put on as pullover shirt.
2a. Using unaffected arm, push hook behind the back.
2b. Using unaffected arm, reach across the body and bring hook to front.
2c. Using unaffected arm, hook bra in front and rotate bra around body until cups are in front.
2d. Bring strap onto affected arm and then unaffected arm.
3a. Using unaffected arm, front hook bra or adapted bra is hooked in front.
3b. Bring strap onto affected arm and then unaffected arm.

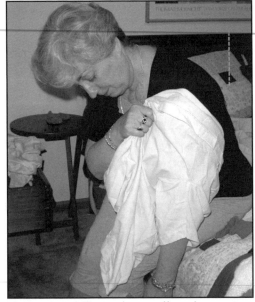

Figure 3-6. Client places affected arm into sleeve.

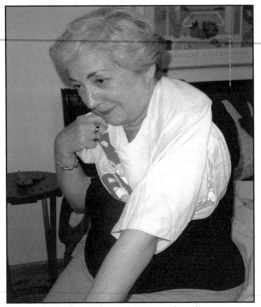

Figure 3-7. Client dons shirt over head.

affected arm. They reach through this sleeve and grab the affected hand. The sleeve is then pulled over the affected hand by either pushing against the lap or pulling with the teeth. Once the hand is out of the sleeve, the unaffected arm can be used to pull the sleeve up the affected arm. The remainder of the process is the same.

For clients who choose to wear a button-down shirt, the method is slightly different. The same methods described above are used to get the affected arm into the sleeve. Once the affected arm is in the sleeve, the client reaches across the body and holds the label of the collar or the end of the collar, depending on comfort, with the unaffected arm. The client then brings the collar around the back and places the unaffected arm into the sleeve. Once straightened with the unaffected arm, the client then buttons the shirt with the unaffected arm (Figure 3-8). If there are buttons at the cuffs, the client can button the cuff of the affected arm using the unaffected arm. For the affected arm, the client can either keep the cuff buttoned or add elastic buttons (which will be discussed later). In addition, a client can also chose to keep all buttons closed and put on a button-down shirt using the pullover shirt method. This works best with clients with smaller frames. Table 3-5 summarizes the method to don a buttondown type shirt.

Table 3-4

STEPS TO DON A PULLOVER SHIRT

1. Gather the shirt sleeve and place on the lap.
2. Use the unaffected arm to place the affected arm into the sleeve of the shirt.
3. Pull the sleeve up the affected arm as far as possible: at least over the elbow, preferably over the affected shoulder.
4. Place the unaffected arm into the sleeve.
5. Pull the head opening over the head.
6. Reach behind the back to straighten the shirt.

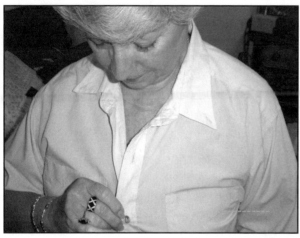

Figure 3-8. Client buttons shirt with unaffected arm.

LE dressing includes shoes, socks, underwear, protective garments (as needed), and pants. Underwear and pants are put on in the same manner. The affected leg is placed in the pant leg first, followed by the unaffected leg. There are different methods to get the affected leg into the pants based on the client's sitting balance skills as well as the function of the LE. If the client is able to safely bend forward and place the pants or underpants on the floor, he/she can then use the unaffected arm or leg to lift the affected leg into the pants/underwear. The client can then lean forward and pull the pants/underwear up onto the affected leg. This method works best if the client has enough strength in the affected leg to lift the heel off of the floor. If the affected leg has no function, the pants/underwear can be difficult to pull up. In addition, some clients prefer to put the affected leg onto a small foot stool (Figure 3-9). This provides a shorter distance to reach as well as a better angle to pull once the pants/underwear are being pulled up.

If a client does not have the ability to reach forward, the affected leg can be lifted with the unaffected arm and crossed over the unaffected leg. Once in this position, the client can use the unaffected arm to take hold of the affected ankle and pull the ankle/foot up so the affected foot is placed onto the unaffected thigh (Figure 3-10). With the affected foot now close to the client, it is not necessary to lean forward. The client can place the pants/underwear over the foot with the unaffected arm and then hold the pants while guiding the affected leg off of the unaffected leg. As the affected leg is lowered, it will automatically enter the pant leg or go through the leg hole of the underwear. At this point, the unaffected leg can be placed in the other pant/underwear leg. It should be noted that clients who have severe hemiparesis might have difficulty keeping the affected leg on the unaffected leg because it will fall forward too quickly. If this happens, the client

Table 3-5

STEPS TO DON A BUTTONDOWN SHIRT

1. Gather the shirt sleeve and place on the lap.
2. Use the unaffected arm to place the affected arm into the sleeve of the shirt.
3. Pull the sleeve up the affected arm as far as possible: at least over the elbow, preferably over the affected shoulder.
4. With the unaffected arm, reach across the body and hold the label or the end of the collar.
5. Bring the collar around the back to the unaffected side.
6. Place the unaffected arm into the sleeve.
7. Straighten the shirt and button.

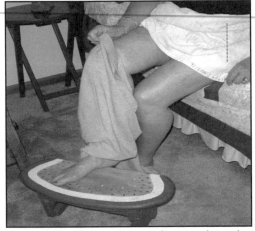

Figure 3-9. Client utilizes a foot stool to don pants.

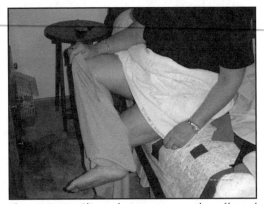

Figure 3-10. Client dons pants on the affected side.

and therapist need to problem solve how best to keep the foot in place long enough to get the pant leg on. If able, some clients pull the affected leg higher up the unaffected thigh, others place the unaffected leg on a foot stool to utilize the forces of gravity, and still other clients simply learn to move quickly to apply the pant leg. If these methods are unsuccessful or causing greater frustration to the client, then adaptive equipment may be a better choice.

Prior to standing, clients should check to see if the pants are still under either foot. If this has occurred, the client should pull up the pants so he/she is not stepping on them when standing and hiking the pants. If mobility is an issue, it is best to complete the above steps for both the underwear and the pants so the client will only be required to stand once to hike up both garments. If mobility is not an issue, then the client can be asked to stand each time a garment is put on. While standing, the client uses the unaffected arm to pull up both sides of the pants/underwear. Many clients also prefer to complete any closures while standing. This is beneficial for a few reasons. First, most of us complete this task while standing, so this will simulate a more traditional and ingrained method for clients. Second, closures are more likely to bunch up or become misaligned when sitting. Other clients prefer pants with an elastic waist so closures are not an issue. Note that if the client did not use this type of pants prior to the injury, this may be considered "changing the tools" of the task as discussed later. Table 3-6 summarizes the steps to don pants.

Table 3-6

STEPS TO DON PANTS

1a. Place garments on the floor and use the unaffected leg/arm to place the affected into the hole of the garments.
1b. Place the affected leg onto a foot stool and reach forward to put the garment over the foot.
1c. Cross the affected leg over the unaffected using the unaffected arm. Pull the affected foot onto the unaffected thigh and place the garment over the foot.
2. Once the affected leg is into the garment, place the unaffected leg into the other hole.
3. Pull up the pants until all material is free of the feet.
4. Stand and hike up the pants using the unaffected side.
5. Complete fasteners.

If a client requires a smaller protective garment in his/her underwear, this can be applied prior to standing up. These usually are pressed into the underwear with adhesive that can be used once strips of paper are removed from the protective garment. Larger garments, such as adult diapers, may be worn with or without underwear. Some of these protective garments are put on like underwear, and the methods described above can be used. Others are put on like a traditional diaper, which is a more difficult process for clients with hemiparesis. One method to don these adult diapers is to lightly fasten the side so they can be put on like underwear and then tightened once standing. This will only work if the fasteners can be readjusted after the first use. Some fasteners will rip the adult diaper if refastening is attempted. Another method is to partially place the adult diaper inside underwear. The underwear acts as a cradle to the adult diaper affording the client the opportunity to straighten and fasten the adult diaper using the affected arm without the diaper falling to his/her knees. This method is not well received at some facilities because it creates an extra step when the soiled adult diaper needs to be changed. Lastly, clients with better LE mobility are able to stand long enough to place the adult diaper between the legs. Once in place, these clients can hold the adult diaper between the legs long enough to fasten the diaper on the sides with the unaffected extremity. Ideally, clients will become continent again after an illness and will be able to function without adult diapers; however, for some clients, these will remain a necessity.

The last two items to be donned are shoes and socks. Some clients prefer to put on socks before pants, others after pants. In either case, the methods for donning socks are similar to putting on one's pants. Depending on the sitting balance skills of the client, he/she can either lean forward to put the sock over the affected foot or bring the affected foot up to the lap, as explained earlier, in order to put on the sock. The most difficult part of putting on socks is usually getting the socks over all the toes with one hand. Some clients prefer to hook the sock on one side of the foot and pull it over the other using the unaffected arm. Others prefer to place the unaffected hand into the top of the sock and then abduct all of the fingers (Figure 3-11). This causes the top of the sock to open wide enough for the client to then slip the top of the sock over all the toes at once. With the toes in the sock, the client can then use the unaffected arm to pull up the sock. Again, if the client is using the "lap" method, as the leg is lowered it will enter into the sock. Once the affected leg is completed, the same methods can be used for the unaffected foot in order to don the sock.

The last item is the shoes. For safety, it is best if clients wear shoes with rubber soles and good support. This often means wearing sneakers or another form of tie shoes. While donning shoes can be difficult, tying is often the hardest part. The method chosen to don the shoes will once again depend on the client's safety while leaning forward. If a client has good sitting balance, the shoe is placed on the floor with the tongue of the shoe pulled back as far as possible. The client then places

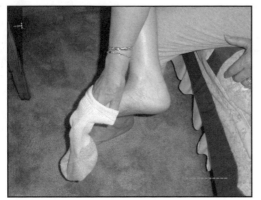

Figure 3-11. Client abducts fingers of unaffected hand to don socks.

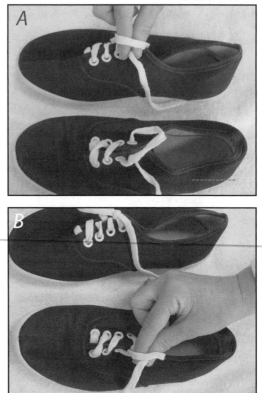

Figure 3-12. (A) One-handed shoe tying: steps 1 and 2. (B) One-handed shoe tying: steps 3 and 4.

the affected leg into the shoe using the unaffected arm. Once the leg is placed, the client will need to pull the back and/or the tongue of the shoe to get the foot properly placed in the shoe.

If the client does not have sufficient sitting balance to use this method, the affected leg should be placed on the unaffected thigh, as done earlier for pants and socks, and then the shoe is placed over the foot. In this position, the client can push the shoe on by holding the bottom of the shoe, or by pulling the back of the shoe.

If the client is able to get the shoes on with the shoes tied, this simplifies the method as it avoids the need to tie shoes. Certainly each new pair will need to be tied initially, but once tied in a double knot, the shoes can stay tied. If the shoes need to be tied each time, the client will need to learn to tie with one hand or use adaptive equipment such as elastic laces. (Elastic laces would be "changing the tool.")

To tie a shoe with one hand, the laces must be removed from the shoe and a knot is tied in one end. The lace is then put through the shoes from side to side. This allows a traditional look to the lace, but only one lace is left at the end. The client leaves the lace hanging to the side and forms a small loop by pulling up the lace between the last two lace holes. The client then reaches through this loop with the index finger and thumb grabbing the hanging lace closest to the last lace hole (Figure 3-12a). A second small loop is formed with this piece of lace, as the first loop is pulled tight around this new loop. This process is completed again with the client reaching through the second loop to pull the lace closest to the loops. This time the client pulls the third loop larger and tighter so the shoe will not untie (Figure 3-12b). If there is a great deal of lace left, this can be tucked into the side of the shoe. To untie the shoe, the client simply pulls the end of the lace and all of the loops will untie.

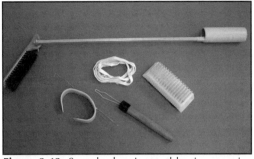

Figure 3-13. Sample dressing and hygiene equipment: long-handled hairbrush, elastic laces, button hooks and suction nail brush.

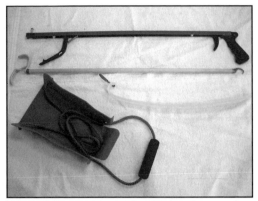

Figure 3-14. Equipment for LE dressing: reacher, dressing stick, long-handled shoehorn, sock aid.

The above methods are sufficient for most individuals with limited motor skills; however, one particular population requires different instructions. The clients who have had a total hip replacement cannot lean forward or cross the legs because of the "total hip precautions" postsurgery. For these clients, changing the task is not a possibility, but changing the tools is required and will be discussed on the following page.

Changing the Tools to Achieve Independence

During dressing, a client can utilize a variety of adaptive equipment such as button hooks for one handed buttoning, elastic laces for the shoes, sock aids to put on socks, reachers for donning and doffing pants/underpants, and long-handled shoe horns to limit leaning forward while donning shoes. Figure 3-13 depicts examples of dressing and hygiene tools.

For the clients with a diagnosis of total hip replacement, these pieces of adaptive equipment will be vital. The typical equipment provided consists of a reacher and/or a dressing stick, elastic shoelaces, and a long-handled shoehorn. These are shown in Figures 3-13 and 3-14. As stated earlier, total hip precautions will significantly limit the client's ability to dress the affected leg. These precautions depend on the anterior or posterior surgical intervention, but in general, clients should not flex the hip past 90 degrees, adduct the hip past neutral, or internally/externally rotate the hip until cleared by the physician to do so (Pierson, 1999). This clearance may not occur for several weeks to months, depending on the healing progress of the client. These clients will require a dressing stick or reacher to put on pants/underwear, a sock aid, and elastic laces. Some clients will also require a long-handled shoehorn. In addition, a raised toilet seat is typically required. This will be discussed later in this chapter.

TOILETING

Changing the Task to Achieve Independence

The aspects of toileting that cause the most difficulty for clients with motor deficits are the transfers on/off the toilet and the clothing management. Other issues can also cause problems such as toilet paper use, and the use of menstrual and bowel/bladder management tools.

Transfer skills will be addressed under "functional mobility" later in this section. The task of clothing management can be improved by having the client prepare prior to the transfer. If possible, the client should undo the belt and top button of the pants if present. This will allow the client to release the pant zipper once at the toilet and quickly lower the pants. Underwear can be pulled down with the unaffected extremity. It is important not to allow the pants to fall to the floor prior to the completion of the transfer. This may cause a hazard while transferring if the clothing becomes entangled in the client's feet.

To increase independence with cleaning and the use of menstrual and bowel/bladder management tools, it is important to place all necessary items in a location where the client can reach them with the unaffected extremity. This may require relocation of the toilet paper dispenser and the use of baskets near the toilet for supplies.

Changing the Tools to Achieve Independence

Adapted tools may be required if the client is unable to properly maintain personal care due to the his/her limited motor skills. Tools that can be provided include flushable wipes instead of toilet paper, lengthened suppository inserters to increase ease, and adapted catheter or colostomy bags to allow for emptying without full bilateral hand use. Some of these adaptations are available commercially, but some are created for the particular client by the therapist. An example of this would be removing the elastic bands typically provided with a catheter leg bag and replacing these with hook and loop fastener straps if the client is unable to fasten the elastic bands.

Compensation/Adaptation Interventions of Self-Care for Clients With Decreased Performance Skills/Client Factors: Sensation and Pain

Sensation and pain can be found in the AOTA *Framework* document under client factors (AOTA, 2002a) (Figure 3-15). While this area of the document covers all sensory issues, only sensation changes and pain will be addressed in this section. Changes in sensation can be a result of central nervous system damage, such as CVA or head injury, or peripheral nervous system damage, such as nerve lacerations. These forms of injury typically cause *hyposensitivity*, or a decrease in sensation (Jacobs & Jacobs, 2004).

Sensation changes can also lead to *hypersensitivity*, an increase in sensation (Jacobs & Jacobs, 2004). Some clients can interpret hypersensitivity as pain. Typically, hypersensitivity occurs with trauma, such as an amputation, or surgical repair, such as carpal tunnel surgery, but some clients with central nervous system and peripheral nervous system injuries also experience hypersensitivity, such as clients with chronic regional pain syndrome (previously referred to as reflex sympathetic dystrophy). For additional information regarding modes of injury, refer to Chapter 1.

While it is important to understand a client's diagnosis and prognosis, this section will discuss only the hypersensitivity and hyposensitivity symptoms resulting from these varied diagnoses. Because these two areas of sensation are opposites by definition, they are also treated differently. Pain management will be addressed briefly in this section, but more in-depth in the maintenance section.

HYPERSENSITIVITY

Clients experiencing hypersensitivity, will often be fearful of interventions because they may experience pain. It is vital to provide only as much sensory input as the individual client can tolerate. While remediation may center on decreasing the hypersensitivity through input, compensation/adaptation interventions will attempt to keep the client independent while the hypersensitivity is still present. Remediation is preferred to compensation/adaptation because it encourages use of the affected extremity; therefore, the techniques below should generally not be employed as long-term strategies.

Changing the Task to Achieve Independence

The primary way to change the task when hypersensitivity is present is to utilize the unaffected extremity to "check" situations first, such as water temperature. This will allow the client to use both extremities without overstimulating the hypersensitive extremity.

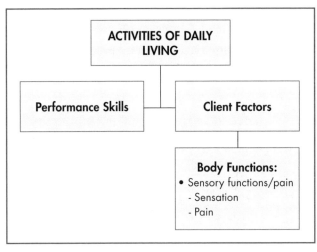

Figure 3-15. Relationship of sensation/ pain to ADLs (adapted from American Occupational Therapy Association. [2002a]. *Occupational therapy practice framework: Domain and process.* Bethesda, MD: AOTA).

- *Bathing example*: Water should always be checked with the unaffected hand to ensure proper temperature. Water pressure on showers may need to be lowered to offer less stimulation. Some showers allow this adjustment at the shower controls or showerhead.

- *Grooming/hygiene example*: Electric razors or toothbrushes may provide too much stimuli to the affected extremity; therefore, the client may need to hold the grooming tool with only the unaffected extremity until increased stimulation is tolerated.

- *Feeding example*: The pressure required to cut certain harder food items may aggravate the client's affected extremity. The client can either reverse hands, which many find difficult, or use repeated lighter cuts with a knife rather than apply heavy pressure.

- *Dressing example*: For some, simply pulling clothes over the affected extremity is too much stimulation. Sleeves should be left unbuttoned and preferably should be without a taper on the end. This will allow the extremity to be placed through the sleeve with minimal contact.

- *Toileting example*: Generally, there will be little impact on toileting; however, if the affected extremity is the dominant side, the client may need to learn to clean him/herself with the nondominant hand. Women will also need to learn to apply feminine products with the nondominant hand.

Changing the Tools to Achieve Independence

The majority of tools provided in all areas of ADLs are intended to protect the hypersensitive area of the extremity, typically the hand.

- *Bathing example*: A glove can be worn during bathing if the temperature of the water aggravates the affected extremity. Often, warm water is soothing; however, certain clients may find this aggravating to the injury. If water pressure adjustments are required, as mentioned above, and controls are not adjustable, a new showerhead or a hand-held shower may be required.

- *Grooming/hygiene example*: As stated earlier, electric razors and toothbrushes may cause overstimulation; therefore, regular razors and toothbrushes may be required until the client can tolerate the vibration of the electric tool. If grasping any grooming/hygiene tools is painful, handles can be built up to allow larger grasp.

- *Feeding example*: If the pressure of cutting is not tolerable to clients, they can utilize rocker knives to spread out the pressure, or utilize one-handed cutting boards with the unaffected extremity. If grasping utensils is painful, handles can be built up to allow a larger grasp.

- *Dressing example*: Shirts with elastic at the sleeves should not be worn and gloves can be purchased one size larger in order to allow less stimulation when donning and doffing.

- *Toileting example*: As stated earlier, generally toileting is not impacted by hypersensitivity to the extent where introduction of tools is required.

HYPOSENSITIVITY

As discussed previously, remediation is preferred to compensation/adaptation because this encourages use of the extremity; however, most strategies listed below are employed to allow greater safety until sensation returns. For clients with permanent sensory loss, these strategies may become maintenance techniques.

Changing the Task to Achieve Independence

- *Bathing example*: Clients should always check the temperature of water with the unaffected extremity to avoid any scalding.

- *Grooming/hygiene example*: Clients should look into any drawers prior to reaching in with the affected extremity. This will avoid cuts from sharp objects such as tweezers or razors. Client may also choose to reach in with the unaffected extremity, however cuts felt on this extremity will remain less safe than no cuts at all by looking first.

- *Feeding example*: When cutting food, the clients should always observe to avoid cutting the affected extremity.

- *Dressing example*: The client should check elastic sleeves to ensure they are not too tight on the affected extremity.

- *Toileting example*: If the affected extremity is the dominant side, the client may need to learn to clean him/herself with the nondominant hand. Women will also need to learn to apply feminine products with the nondominant hand.

Changing the Tools to Achieve Independence

- *Bathing example*: A thermostat can be installed on a single shower/bath or the hot water heater's thermostat can be adjusted to limit the temperature of water to avoid scalding.

- *Grooming/hygiene example*: If the hyposensitivity has occurred on the face as well as an extremity, electric razors are preferred to avoid any cuts.

- *Feeding example*: If holding food to cut it is unsafe, a one-handed cutting board can be utilized to avoid cutting the affected extremity.

- *Dressing example*: Clothing with elastic at the end of the sleeves should be avoided. This can cause pressure of which the client is unaware. This is true of outerwear and gloves as well.

- *Toileting example*: Generally, toileting is not impacted by hyposensitivity to the extent where introduction of tools is required.

Compensation/Adaptation Interventions of Self-Care for Clients With Decreased Performance Skills/Client Factors: Endurance/Energy

Energy is located in the AOTA *Framework* (2002a) under motor skills as well as process skills, but the definition is the same; therefore, it will be addressed as one area (Figure 3-16).

Decreased energy or endurance can be caused by a large number of pathologies. Most obvious is when a client has cardiac or pulmonary deficits that directly impact the ability to get oxygen to

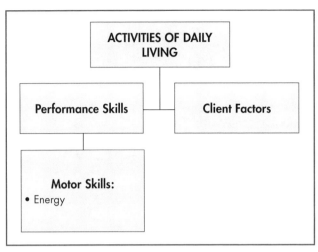

Figure 3-16. Relationship of energy/endurance to ADLs (adapted from American Occupational Therapy Association. [2002a]. *Occupational therapy practice framework: Domain and process.* Bethesda, MD: AOTA).

the muscles. Other clients will have decreased endurance due to immobility after a hospitalization or injury. Others have slowly limited activity over a longer period of time leading eventually to decreased endurance for activities.

The most common intervention methods used to increase endurance are two-fold. The first intervention is to build up the client's endurance by completing tasks. As stated earlier, this can be done using a bottom-up approach such as repetitive exercises with no or light weights. Examples of these include pulley exercises, or arm ergometers. These interventions are considered "remedial" and more information regarding these can be found in Chapter 2. A top-down approach will utilize graded functional activities to increase endurance.

The second aspect of increasing the client's functional skills is referred to as *energy conservation*. This is a compensatory/adaptive strategy because the education provided to the client is aimed at teaching the client to change behaviors, thus allowing the client to be less tired. Most of these principles have a similar theme: plan activities to limit exertion. Examples of these are listed below for each self-care activity.

Changing the Task to Achieve Independence

- *Bathing example*: Have all supplies required for bathing in one convenient location. Also, clients can complete showers or baths on a day where little else is planned and when energy is not typically drained (e.g., the end of the day is usually more tiring).

- *Grooming/hygiene example*: Have all supplies required for grooming/hygiene in one convenient location. Plan trips to nail salons for the midmorning and limit other plans that day.

- *Feeding example*: Eat meals in a relaxed environment with sufficient time allowed. Rushing through meals increases tension and can cause fatigue. If eating at a restaurant, limit plans for the remainder of that day. If eating a regular meal is too tiring, clients may choose to eat smaller meals throughout the day.

- *Dressing example*: Sit, rather than stand, while dressing. Put clothes away in outfits for ease of use each morning. Arrange clothes and drawers to allow easy access to clothes most often used. Rotate this with the seasons, if necessary.

- *Toileting example*: Straining while on the toilet can not only be dangerous for the heart, but can utilize a great deal of energy. Attempt to utilize the toilet for bowel movements when ample time is available. This will avoid significant straining in order to rush.

Changing the Tools to Achieve Independence

Many of the tools discussed previously will also assist the client with decreased endurance. It is important for the tools chosen to be lightweight so they are not contributing to fatigue. Larger equipment, such as seats, should be placed in a permanent location in order for the client to further conserve energy by not moving them.

- *Bathing example*: Use a shower seat to conserve energy when seated. Use a long-handled sponge to wash LEs, decreasing the need to bend/reach.

- *Grooming/hygiene example*: While standing at the sink, use a small footstool to rest on one leg while applying makeup or drying hair to limit fatigue. Lightweight blow-dryers or blow-dryer stands are available that can limit fatigue.

- *Feeding example*: Generally, no feeding tools are required.

- *Dressing example*: Adaptive equipment such as long handled shoehorns, elastic laces, sock aids, and reachers can decrease the need to bend/reach. As stated earlier, the weight of these tools should be considered. If too heavy, they may increase fatigue rather than decrease it.

- *Toileting example*: Utilization of laxatives, stool softeners, or fiber products, under the supervision of a physician, can reduce straining while on the toilet.

COMPENSATIONS/ADAPTATIONS OF SELF-CARE DEFICITS FOR CLIENTS WITH COGNITIVE, PERCEPTUAL, OR VISUAL LIMITATIONS: PERFORMANCE SKILLS/CLIENT FACTORS

This section will focus on the impact of cognitive, perceptual, and visual deficits upon ADL performance (Figure 3-17). Many conditions may lead to these deficits, primarily those of a neurological origin. As an example, Dodge, Kadowski, Hayakawa, & Yamakawa (2005) found cognitive impairment increases the risk of eventual decline in ADL/IADL skills with clients who have sustained a CVA. Depending on the amount of cognitive impairment, subjects who had baseline independence in ADL/IADL skills lost a significant portion of function within a short period of time, particularly in the older-adult group. Therefore, cognitive impairments and the effect on function should be carefully monitored in all client interventions, although more closely with older adults.

In general, cuing, as described in Chapter 1, is considered to be a useful tool for remediation as well as compensation/adaptation. For this reason, it will be addressed throughout the section. It is also important to note the below functions begin at the lowest skill level and are reliant upon the skill before. For example: A client must have good attention skills in order to have short-term memory, and must have short-term memory to have topographical orientation.

The AOTA *Framework* (2002a) presents perceptual and cognitive deficits within two sections of the document. The first section addresses basic cognitive skills in the general category of Performance Skills and the subsection of Process Skills. The AOTA *Framework* (2002a) defines these basic cognitive skills as necessary to complete, manage, and modify ADL tasks.

A second section of the AOTA *Framework* (2002a) also addresses cognitive as well as perceptual deficits. The deficits are discussed under the subsection of Client Factors, called Body Function Categories. These Body Function Categories are the affective, perceptual, and additional cognitive skills required to complete ADL tasks.

Body Function Categories are divided into *global mental functions* and specific mental functions:

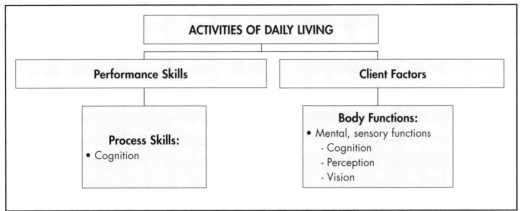

Figure 3-17. Components of performance skills/client factors related to ADLs (adapted from American Occupational Therapy Association. [2002a]. *Occupational therapy practice framework: Domain and process.* Bethesda, MD: AOTA).

- *Global mental functions.* These include consciousness functions (arousal level, level of consciousness) and orientation.
- *Specific mental functions*: Attention, memory, perception (visual-spatial), thought functions (recognition, categorization, generalization), higher-level cognitive functions (judgment, concept formation, time management, problem solving, decision making), and mental functioning (motor planning, specifically dressing apraxia) (AOTA, 2002a).

The format of this section of the text is a brief introduction to the topic and examples of compensation/adaptation interventions. Examples of appropriate activities will be listed. Some ADL examples will not be listed because these tasks may be inappropriate or not possible for a client with the deficits presented. For specific definitions, please refer to Chapter 2.

Compensation/Adaptation of Self-Care for Clients With Decreased Performance Skills/Client Factors: Cognitive Deficits

See Figure 3-18.

PROCESS SKILLS

Table 3-7 briefly presents the subcategories of Process Skills because these skills are typically addressed in a less formal manner within most ADL intervention plans.

Client Factors: Body Functions—Global Mental Functions

As stated earlier, *global mental functions* include consciousness and orientation. Consciousness is further divided to include arousal level and level of consciousness (AOTA, 2002a). Examples of appropriate activities will be listed below, although ADLs may not be possible to attempt with clients who have significantly decreased arousal levels.

AROUSAL LEVEL

Zoltan (2007) describes arousal level as "alerting" or a level of alertness that fluctuates depending upon the state of one's CNS and prepares for mobilization to attention.

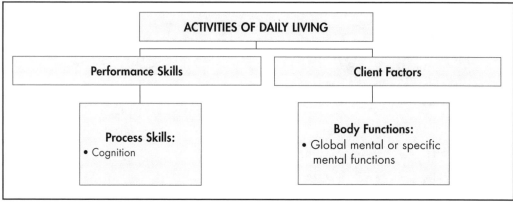

Figure 3-18. Relationship of cognition to ADLs (adapted from American Occupational Therapy Association. [2002a]. *Occupational therapy practice framework: Domain and process*. Bethesda, MD: AOTA).

The occupational therapy intervention at this level is very limited in terms of functional performance. Initially, the client's level of alertness may be very limited, not allowing for even the simplest of ADL training. Of particular concern with a low arousal level is the task of eating. This task will be addressed in the eating/dysphagia section later in this chapter.

Changing the Task to Achieve Independence

The client's *level of arousal* or ability to participate in the task will dictate the need or readiness to change the method. The therapist may need to see the client for several short sessions per day. Depending on the client's response, the physical context may need to be changed. For example, a less distractible environment may allow the client to better attend, or more than likely, a moderate amount of sensory stimulation such as noise/sound may improve the client's level of alertness (e.g., upbeat music).

The client may benefit from simple verbal instructions, and potentially, tactile cuing. Instructions and verbal communication may be upgraded as the client's level of alertness increases.

- *Bathing and hygiene example*: As levels of alertness increase and the client is able to sit upright in bed, the therapist may begin addressing simple ADL skills, which are continuously graded, as necessary. The basic intervention may involve asking the client to brush hair, brush teeth, or wash face and/or hands. In addition, as levels of alertness and attention improve, the therapist may begin to encourage the client to begin using ADL strategies to improve memory. (Refer to the memory section of this chapter for further details on memory.)

- *Feeding example*: Prior to feeding, arousal levels can be improved by providing a stimulating environment (bright and colorful), and positioning the client upright. (Refer to the positioning section of this chapter if adaptations are required to achieve an upright posture.) The texture and temperature of the food may also alert the client. For example, cold foods may increase alertness. Finger foods may also increase alertness.

- *Dressing example*: Dressing may not be appropriate until the level of alertness improves to the point where client can interact. The client may be able to participate in a simple task such as putting on a "johnny coat."

- *Toileting example*: Depending on the level of alertness, attempting to toilet out of the bed may keep the client more alert to complete the task. If toileting in bed, a task such as bridging may cause the client to become more alert. (Refer to the functional mobility section of this chapter for more information on bridging.)

Table 3-7

PROCESS SKILLS AND ADL EXAMPLES OF EACH

Process Skill Subcategories	*Examples of ADL Compensation/Adaptation Interventions*
Energy	
Paces	Provide client with a clock and chart with estimated amount of time required for each category of ADL tasks.
Attends	Refer to Specific Mental Functions category
Knowledge	
Chooses	Offer two or more options and play out scenario of choices with client. For example, allow client to choose the red shirt or the white shirt to match the purple pants.
Uses	Provide checklist of ADL items and brief description of what they are used for, such as a razor or step stool.
Handles	Demonstrate to client use of tools or materials. Observe for carryover upon next session. For example, demonstrate how to hang pants neatly in closet.
Heeds	Provide daily checklist to document each time ADL task is completed.
Inquires	Provide written directions for ADL tasks. Request client to ask one or more questions regarding safety in ADLs/session.
Temporal organization	
Initiation	Use external cues during intervention such as a bell or alarm clock to begin washing/dressing, for example. Address strategies to develop internal initiation cues.
Sequencing	Provide client with ADL board containing the written steps of bathing, dressing, etc.
Organizing space and objects	
Searches/Locates	Provide external cuing such as labels or signs to assist with locating ADL objects or tools.
Gathers	Provide checklist of items needed for bathing, dressing, or hygiene to assist client in gathering needed materials.
Organizes	Provide client with daily reminders, lists, or calendars. Assist client in organizing closet, drawers, and shelves, as needed.
Restores	Label shelves, drawers, closets to assist in putting items away.
Navigates	Use contrasting colors in physical contexts. Instruct client to use tactile cuing when navigating in bathroom and bedroom environments.
Adaptation	
Notices/Responds	Grade environmental, nonverbal, or perceptual cues in bathroom and bedroom, as appropriate.
Accommodates/Adjusts	Problem-solve alternative actions or scenarios with client. For example, client should attempt toileting skills in bathroom with different layouts.
Benefits	Assist client/family in problem solving various ADL issues that may occur upon discharge home and plan for adaptations.

Changing the Tools to Achieve Independence

Any tools used with clients who have a decreased level of alertness should be kept very simple with items added gradually, as the client tolerates. One tool should be introduced at a time, while ensuring safety.

- *Bathing example*: Begin with a familiar tool such as a washcloth that may be a very bright, alerting color and texture. Use the warm water and touch of the washcloth as an alerting tool.

- *Hygiene example*: Adapt oral care by assisting client to cleanse his/her mouth with a disposable oral swab. This adaptation is important because the client's level of alertness and/or oral motor status may not be ready for the amount of liquid created with using toothpaste. As levels of alertness improve, the activity may be graded to using a toothbrush and toothpaste.

- *Feeding example*: Brightly colored plates or placemats under the food may increase alertness. Providing foods of particular interest to a client, such as a favorite food, may also be alerting.

ORIENTATION

Orientation is an individual's awareness of time, person, and/or place. Deficits in orientation may typically present with memory loss and problems with new learning. Because the strategies for improving orientation must be reinforced with all skills throughout the day by the entire rehabilitation team and family, the interventions below are presented in general terms. In addition, much of orientation interventions are centered on visual/verbal cuing and consistency.

Changing the Task to Achieve Independence

- *General ADL examples*: The session may informally involve orientation training, as well. It is important to remember carryover with orientation is very much dependent upon memory skills. The client's daily patterns, such as routines, should be consistent and structured as much as possible, particularly as arousal levels improve. The client's physical context should be consistent, well organized, and if possible, simulate the client's natural environment for self-care tasks. For example, if feeding can occur in a small dining room rather than in the client's room, the client will be better oriented to mealtime.

The therapist may see the client either during or after breakfast, providing verbal orientation to the time of day as related to the ADL task. The method may be changed by asking the client basic orientation questions during the ADL task. This should occur throughout the day with the assistance of staff and family.

Changing the Tools to Achieve Independence

- *General ADL examples*: Basic orientation tools may begin with only a simple calendar or sign of the day and date. As the level of arousal improves, the method may be changed by introducing additional orientation boards. The boards may incorporate ADL information such as mealtimes, and bathing, dressing, and therapy schedules.

As the client's participation in therapy improves, familiar ADL items should be brought from home such as clothes, grooming items, and a watch.

Client Factors: Body Functions—Specific Mental Functions

Specific Mental Functions include attention, memory, perception (visual-spatial), thought functions (recognition, categorization, generalization), higher level cognitive functions (judgment, concept formation, time management, problem solving, decision making), and mental functioning (motor planning, specifically dressing apraxia) (AOTA, 2002a).

ATTENTION

Zoltan (2007) discusses the impact of attention deficits upon the client's ability to learn and focus on ADL skills. Attention is a building block for higher-level specific mental functions such as memory and problem solving and therefore, must be addressed first.

Changing the Task to Achieve Independence

Clients who have conditions that affect attention skills must begin ADL training with the simplest of tasks, in a short intervention time that is adapted with improvement. It is important for caregivers to speak simply and slowly, and allow for processing time (Zoltan, 2007). In addition, distraction should be kept at a minimum, although gradually introduced as the client is ready. The physical context should remain the same until the client demonstrates he/she is ready for generalization and/or gradation.

- *Bathing and hygiene example*: Intervention may begin at the bedside and progress to the bathroom sink by encouraging the client to brush hair, brush teeth, or wash face. ADL intervention may be adapted by asking the client to wash the upper half of the body and progressing next session to the entire body, as able. The task may be further adapted by progressing to the shower. The environment should be without distractions at first, with appropriate distractions added as the client improves.

- *Feeding example*: Prior to attempting feeding, the environmental distractions should be eliminated. Food items of particular interest to the client or with varied textures and colors can also increase attention to feeding. In order to decrease distractions, smaller meals should be presented to the client. Verbal or visual cuing to stay on task may be required, but should be graded.

- *Dressing example*: Provide only the required clothes with each step and gradually provide more clothing. The environment should be without distractions at first, with appropriate distractions added as the client improves. Backward chaining where the OT initiates the task and asks the client to complete it or forward chaining where the client is required to complete only a small portion of a task and then the OT finishes the task may be attempted. Chaining should be graded as improvement is noted.

- *Toileting example*: With a compensation/adaptive approach, Zoltan (2007) recommends that the client vocalize the task in a step-by-step manner. For toileting, the client should vocalize each step of what to do from the time he/she experiences the urge to void, to entering the bathroom, attending to perianal care, attending to clothing, and finally, washing hands at the sink.

Changing the Tools to Achieve Independence

In general, for all ADLs, the environment should be without distractions at first, with appropriate distractions added as the client improves. Tools utilized for the ADLs should be limited until the client has demonstrated improvement. Additional examples are provided for feeding and dressing regarding tools.

- *Feeding example*: To decrease distractions, limited utensils should be provided. Colorful plates may increase attention, but can also be distracting depending on the individual client.

- *Dressing example*: If a client is having difficulty donning pants, socks, and shoes, a step stool in front of the bedside chair may assist the client in reaching his/her feet with all three tasks. Additional tools may be added as appropriate and as the client's attention improves.

MEMORY

Although there are many types of memory and memory deficits, this section will focus specifically, on intervention strategies related to ADLs with an adaptive/compensation approach.

Changing the Task to Achieve Independence

Intervention strategies during ADLs, in general, may be adapted by providing the client with an ADL schedule. For individuals who have limited carryover, involve him/her in developing the schedule. The same strategy may be implemented for creating lists of items needed for bathing, dressing, hygiene, and toileting, as well as basic instructions for carrying out ADLs.

Chunking and grouping (Zoltan, 2007) is a method used to organize categories, objects, and function of items to be recalled. These methods can be utilized in general for all ADLs. The client is asked to group like items together (all items for brushing teeth), and repeat the steps verbally to increase retention of information. Additional specific examples are provided for feeding and dressing.

- *Feeding example*: Regularly scheduled meals with consistent routines will benefit memory skills.

- *Dressing example*: This "story method" (Zoltan, 2007. p. 223) is a strategy whereby a client is encouraged to create a story about what is to be recalled. The client will create a story regarding the steps involved, items needed, and physical context involved with getting dressed.

Changing the Tools to Achieve Independence

For all ADLs, cuing tools may be used as a strategy to increase memory through the use of alarm clocks/timers, memory notebooks, or labeling of ADL items and storage areas. The clocks and timers are utilized to remind the clients of a task or a portion of a task that requires completion. These are often used for IADLs such as cooking and medications, but can also be utilized for tasks such as toileting and bathing. A memory notebook will provide visual cues for completion of tasks. Another type of memory notebook suggested by Zoltan (2007) is the utilization of audio-tapes that provide step-by-step instructions for tasks. Visual cues can be used to label items as to their use or label storage for easy retrieval of items.

The *Specific Mental Functions*, which are addressed less formally and/or less frequently, within intervention plans, are presented in Table 3-8.

Compensation/Adaptation Interventions of Self-Care for Clients With Decreased Performance Skills/Client Factors: Perceptual Deficits

As depicted in Figure 3-19, the *Framework* (2002a) does address *Perceptual Functions* under Client Factors, however particular perceptual topics are not listed. The topics chosen for discussion below have been determined from the authors' clinical practice as well as current references that will be discussed throughout.

General compensatory/adaptive strategies that apply to clients diagnosed with perceptual deficits center around safety and environmental context. These general strategies include:

- Maximize safety in all situations by removing unsafe objects as necessary.

- Educate client and all caregivers regarding functional limitations.

- Practice in a variety of physical contexts.

Visual Fixation/Scanning

Visual fixation involves the voluntary ability to sustain gaze while visually attending to a task or an object in the environment. Scanning allows the eye to follow an object without simultaneous head movement. While saccadic eye movement is typically symmeticrital (e.g., reading), scanning during functional activities, however, involves less predictable patterns that are more complicated (Zoltan, 2007).

Table 3-8

SPECIFIC MENTAL FUNCTIONS AND EXAMPLES OF ADL COMPENSATION/ ADAPTATION STRATEGIES

Specific Mental Functions Subcategories	Compensation/Adaptation Intervention Strategies
Thought functions	
Recognition	During ADL session, ask client to identify typical ADL items, familiar individuals, or objects in the room. Label drawers an shelves.
Categorization	Educate client/family regarding organizing ADL items into categories such as shirts on one side of closet and pants on another or bathing items on one shelf of the bathroom and grooming on another.
Generalization	Address ADLs in a variety of possible situations, such as bathing at the sink and shower, and dressing in the bathroom and bedroom.
Higher-level cognitive functions	
Judgment	Teach client to ask for help when unsure of safety. Ask client open-ended questions in order to think out loud before acting.
Concept formation	Have client keep an ADL journal or log with daily schedule, progress, goals, and achievements.
Time management	Provide ADL schedule. Use clock or timer, as needed.
Problem solving	Alter environment to improve skills such as with external cues and written instructions. Explore possible strategies with client.
Decision making	Provide client with 2 or more options for safe and appropriate decision-making, before acting. Allow client to think-out loud.

Changing the Task to Achieve Independence

Provide cuing as needed. Cuing can be verbal or tactile when guiding the client to anchor the initiation of scanning (from left to right) and when controlling the speed of his/her scanning.

- *Bathing example*: The client should place his/her hands to the left/right of the labels on bottles to anchor reading. Bathing items should be routinely placed in certain locations to limit the scanning required to find needed items.

- *Grooming/hygiene example*: The client may experience difficulty in finding the toothbrush on the right side of the sink. The therapist may use or anchor the client to the middle of the visual field at the water spout. The therapist may then verbally cue the client to scan to the right of the spout. If verbal cuing is unsuccessful, the therapist may use tactile cuing by having the client touch the spout with the right hand and scan his/her eyes to the right, as the hand moves toward the toothbrush.

- *Feeding example*: Cuing may be required at first to find all items on the plate or table.

- *Dressing example*: When retrieving clothes from the closet, the client may be cued to anchor using touch as well as vision. Anchoring would begin on the left side of the closet with the

Figure 3-19. Relationship of perception to ADLs (adapted from American Occupational Therapy Association. [2002a]. *Occupational therapy practice framework: Domain and process.* Bethesda, MD: AOTA).

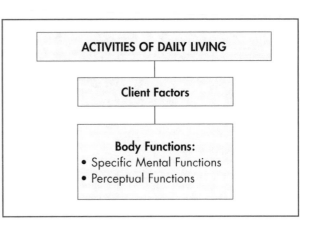

client gradually scanning to the right. With this method, the client would then retrieve all clothing needed, including cuing to scan toward the floor for his/her shoes.

- *Toileting example*: Cuing may be required at first in order to scan to find sanitary products or toilet paper.

Changing the Tools to Achieve Independence

- *Bathing example*: Brighten tools in shower/tub in order to increase ability to fixate on the object.

- *Grooming/hygiene example*: Brighten tools placed in a predictable pattern at the sink, tray table, or bureau.

- *Feeding example*: Brighten placemats or sides of tray table.

- *Toileting example*: A brightly-colored sticker may be placed to the left of the toilet tissue holder, in order for the client to anchor upon it and scan to the right in order to locate the paper.

VISUAL INATTENTION/NEGLECT

The impact of unilateral neglect on ADLs is significant. In reviewing various intervention approaches to unilateral neglect, Lin states, "unilateral neglect has been associated with poor recovery in everyday life functioning," and one conclusion of this research was that retraining to improve daily skills should include functional tasks (Lin, 1996). In addition, awareness of the inattention may play a role. Tham, Ginsburg, Fisher, and Tegner (2001) found clients who were educated regarding the disability and became more aware of the disability, demonstrated greater improvement in ADL skills even when specific ADL intervention was not provided.

For those clients who are unable to become aware of the inattention, the therapist will need to modify and simplify the physical context as much as possible. Gradual grading of activities will also be required. For example, begin by providing all objects within client's intact visual field and incorporate visual scanning through head as well as eye movements during functional activities.

Changing the Task to Achieve Independence

In general for all ADLs, placing the items required for the task within the available visual field will increase performance. As stated above, cuing the client to compensate by turning the head along with moving the eyes can also increase performance. Additional examples are provided below for hygiene and dressing.

- *Hygiene example*: While brushing hair, if client neglects affected side of the head, guide his/her hand to that side and verbally cue to attend.

- *Dressing example*: Use tactile and/or verbal cuing to encourage awareness of affected side. For example, as the client is donning a shirt, touch the client's affected UE while verbally cuing to attend to that side.

Changing the Tools to Achieve Independence

- *Bathing example*: Avoid a handheld shower to ensure the water washes over the entire body.

- *Grooming/hygiene and dressing example*: Utilize a mirror during tasks to encourage visualization of the entire body/face.

- *Feeding example*: Provide client with an adapted dish that has two to three dividers. Instruct client to turn dish clockwise into intact visual field each time a divider is emptied.

- *Toileting example*: Position toilet tissue within client's field of vision. After toileting, position client in front of bathroom mirror in order to fully hike pants and tuck in both sides of shirt.

BODY SCHEME

Body scheme is a foundation skill that uses sensory or internal awareness of the body and the spatial relationship of the body parts to one another (Jacobs & Jacobs, 2004; Zoltan, 2007). Because there are multiple forms of body scheme disorders, each one cannot be reviewed individually. For this reason, Table 3-9 identifies the most common forms of body scheme disorders as well as examples of compensatory/adaptive interventions for these.

VISUAL DISCRIMINATION

Visual discrimination involves the ability to distinguish between various objects or forms in relation to the environment (Zoltan, 2007). Because there are multiple forms of visual discrimination disorders, each one cannot be reviewed individually. For this reason, Table 3-10 identifies the most common forms of visual discrimination disorders as well as examples of compensatory/adaptive interventions for these.

MOTOR PLANNING

Motor planning involves the individual's ability to organize and perform movements in order to carry out purposeful activity (Jacobs & Jacobs, 2004). Apraxia is a category of motor planning deficits whereby impairments of purposeful movement or skills do not involve in coordination, sensory deficits, visual/perceptual issues, language deficits, or cognitive deficits alone (Crepeau, Cohn, & Schell, 2003).

Dressing apraxia is a specific motor planning deficit related to perceptual and cognitive skills. Zoltan (2007) describes dressing apraxia as a disorder in body scheme or spatial relations versus a motor or physical dysfunction. Clients demonstrate difficulty in proper orientation of clothing. For example, a client may put an arm in a pant leg, a sock on a hand, or a shirt on upside down. While dressing apraxia is a common motor planning deficit, other self-care examples are also provided below.

Changing the Task to Achieve Independence

- *Bathing, hygiene and toileting example*: Provide brief, one-step verbal cues or directions, such as "wash your face."

Table 3-9

BODY SCHEME DISORDERS AND EXAMPLES OF ADL COMPENSATION/ADAPTATION STRATEGIES

Body Scheme Disorder	Compensation/Adaptation Strategies: Task and/or Tools Changed
Autotopagnosia	During ADLs use verbal cues to increase awareness of body parts with a functional approach. For example: Ask client to pick up the part of the body that goes inside the shoe (Zoltan, 1996).
Finger agnosia	Adapt ADL environment to increase safety and finger dexterity.
Unilateral body neglect	Adapt ADLs by using reminders or daily activity list to complete entire task(s) to compensate for neglect.
Right–left discrimination	Provide adaptations to instructions during ADL instruction. For example, when dressing, provide tactile cuing to locate items, or state that the "shirt is next to the pants."

- *Feeding example*: Finger foods or foods easily placed on utensils (soup versus mashed potatoes) may decrease motor planning difficulties.

- *Dressing example*: The therapist should attempt the dressing task in several ways in order to assure success. First, various set-ups should be tried, such as dressing at the edge of the bed, in front of a mirror, or in a bedside chair. The therapist should consider presenting one piece of clothing to the client at a time or lay out all items at once.

Changing the Tools to Achieve Independence

In general for all ADLs, limit the use of tools because these may increase motor planning deficits. If tools are required, introduce them one at a time. For dressing, tools may include adaptation of clothing as described below.

- *Dressing example*: Adaptations may be made to the client's clothing such as labeling or color-coding the inside, top, right, or left. Buttoning a shirt may also be a very difficult task for a client with dressing apraxia. Strategies for success include having the client use tactile and visual input, as well as color-coding the button with the buttonhole. Instructions to button from the bottom-up or top-down may also work for a client with this deficit. Typically, the use of adaptive equipment may further confuse a client with dressing apraxia, particularly if ideational apraxia is also present, which affects the ability to use tools.

Compensation/Adaptation Interventions of Self-Care for Clients With Decreased Performance Skills/Client Factors: Vision

See Figure 3-20.

Table 3-10

VISUAL DISCRIMINATION AND EXAMPLES OF ADL COMPENSATION/ADAPTATION STRATEGIES

Visual Discrimination Disorder	Compensation/Adaptation Strategies: Task and/or Tools Changed
Form discrimination	Adapt environment by placing all hygiene items upright. Label item and store items in habitual pattern.
Depth perception	Teach client to compensate by using other sensory skills such as tactile. For example, client should use touch to locate the toothbrush when reaching for it.
Figure ground perception	Adapt ADL environment to increase cognitive awareness by carefully organizing items in a non-cluttered area. For example: put only a few items on shelf in bathroom.
Spatial relations	Label all ADL storage areas and replace items to consistent areas.
Topographical orientation	Adapt ADL environment through the use of simple pictures. For example, hang a picture of a dress on the clothes closet.

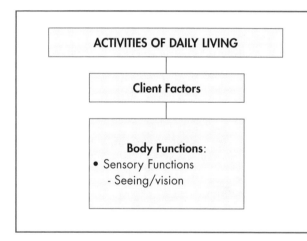

Figure 3-20. Relationship of vision to ADLs (adapted from American Occupational Therapy Association. [2002a]. *Occupational therapy practice framework: Domain and process*. Bethesda, MD: AOTA).

LOW VISION

When addressing low vision (visual acuity) with a compensation/adaptive approach, the focus is primarily on changing the task within the client's environment or physical contexts. Typically, individuals with low vision are able to independently perform basic ADL skills with or without simple task modifications. Higher-level ADL skills that involve safety issues (distinguishing hot from cold or identifying sharp objects) or require vision (such as reading directions) are usually a challenge.

There are many general issues to consider before providing ADL intervention with clients who have low vision. While specific examples will be described for each self-care task, the general strategies listed here should be utilized in conjunction with the specifics listed later in this section.

• Ensure client's glasses are available and fitted correctly.

- Provide any directions in simple, large print.
- Decrease clutter in environment.
- Use automatic, motion-controlled lighting.
- Control the amount of natural light in environment in order to decrease glare.
- Use Braille labels as appropriate.
- Use assistive technology, as described in Chapter 5, which provides auditory or tactile feed-back.
- Use contrast whenever possible.
- Organize belongings in a systematic, predictable routine in order to locate easily on a daily basis.
- To prevent slippage, remove bath mat when not in use.
- Install grab bars in tub/shower.

Changing the Task to Achieve Independence

- *Bathing example*: Organize items within reach, in a systematic location. For example: always place similar looking shampoo and conditioner in the same location to avoid confusion.
- *Grooming/hygiene example*: Organize items within reach, in a systematic location. For example: always place sharp razors in the same location to avoid cuts. Use fingers as a guide when applying makeup and purchase makeup that has been chosen in the past or have a friend evaluate a new color.
- *Feeding example*: Place food items in a consistent location, using a system such as the clock method. For example: place the juice at 12:00 and the coffee at 3:00.
- *Dressing example*: Do not place light clothes upon white bed sheets/blankets. When dressing, encourage client to use a systematic approach to organizing clothes by colors, styles, and appropriate weather (Cohen, 2001).
- *Toileting example*: If items are similar in shape or size, always place them in particular loca-tions so they do not get mixed up (tampons that are "plus size" versus "slim").

Changing the Tools to Achieve Independence

- *Bathing example*: When bathing, provide soap that is a different color than the sink and a bath mat, towel, slippers, and robe that are brightly colored.
- *Grooming/hygiene example*: Increase contrast using bright labels and large print. Braille can also be put on items if the client is taught how to use this. Another alternative is to place distinct textures on certain items that look similar, such as deodorant and hairspray. Use a magnifying mirror for makeup and shaving.
- *Feeding example*: Use brightly colored placemats, contrasting the color of the dining table and the tableware. If food items appear similar in color, place them on different color plates to distinguish.
- *Dressing example*: During dressing activities, encourage use of touch/texture to identify matching clothing (Cohen, 2001). Provide bright, solid-colored clothes, as able.
- *Toileting example*: Color-code baskets with bright colors to distinguish different feminine hygiene products (e.g., pantyshield versus maxi-pads) and other similar looking products.

VISUAL FIELDS

Visual fields are the areas of vision that are seen without movement of the eyes or head (Jacob & Jacob, 2004). Deficits may present on one side of the visual field in one or both eyes.

Changing the Task to Achieve Independence

- *Bathing example*: Provide client and caregivers with strategies for cuing into affected visual fields in order to locate all bathing supplies in the shower/tub. Place items in reach within intact visual field.

- *Grooming/hygiene example*: Provide client and caregivers with strategies for cuing into affected visual fields in order to locate all grooming and hygiene supplies. Place items in reach within intact visual field, particularly any items that can be sharp, such as a razor or tweezers.

- *Feeding example*: Provide client and caregivers with strategies for cuing into affected visual fields in order to locate all food and drink on the table. Seat client where items may be in reach of intact visual field.

- *Dressing example*: Provide client and caregivers with strategies for cuing into affected visual fields in order to locate all clothes in the closet or drawers. If clothes are picked out for a client, place items in reach within intact visual field.

Changing the Tools to Achieve Independence

For all self-care tasks, most adaptive equipment or tools will not provide assistance. Reminder cards can be placed within the client's visual field to remind the client to scan for other self-care items. Depending on the task, a large red strip can be placed to the affected side of the self-care tools and the client can be trained to scan until the strip is visualized. This will allow the client to view all items. In general, changing the task, as described above, will provide better compensation/adaptation by the client.

MAINTENANCE OF SELF-CARE SKILLS

For clients who are inappropriate for remediation and have plateaued with adaptation/compensation attempts—either due to prognosis, diagnosis, or their personal choices—maintenance will be the ultimate approach. For clients who are able to participate in remedial interventions, there will be a period of time when remediation is still being attempted and it is unclear when maintenance begins. It is difficult to determine when adaptation/compensation becomes maintenance; however, once it is determined a change in task or a change in tool is to be utilized long-term, maintenance has certainly begun. Maintenance is more likely to occur for clients with chronic illnesses, such as arthritis, or degenerative illnesses, such as Parkinson's disease. A particular symptom of any disease may become chronic, such as pain, causing maintenance to be appropriate.

It is important to note that the maintenance approach can still be a reimbursable service. While this is not the focus of this book, coverage is typically available for maintenance as long as skilled services are still required. Many clients, however, will not require skilled occupational therapy services once the above strategies are taught or the tools are mastered. If a diagnosis is progressive in nature, further evaluation of these strategies and tools may be required to maximize function throughout the progression of the disease.

FUNCTIONAL MOBILITY

INTRODUCTION

This section will focus on the impact of functional mobility upon ADLs. The *Occupational Therapy Framework* (AOTA, 2002a) categorizes functional mobility as a subsection of ADLs, which is an area of occupation. The *Occupational Therapy Framework* defines functional mobility as "moving from one position or place, to another (during the performance of everyday activities) such as in-bed mobility, wheelchair mobility, and transfers." Transfers include surfaces such as bed, bedside chair, wheelchair, toilet, tub/shower, floor, and car. In addition, functional mobility includes ambulation related to functional activities and transporting items. Pierson (1999) discusses trunk control, positioning, and bed mobility as components of functional mobility. These functional mobility categories must be addressed in a hierarchical nature (Trombly & Radomski, 2002). For example, adequate trunk stability and control must be achieved before trunk mobility. Furthermore, bed mobility should be addressed before chair transfers, and toilet transfers before tub transfers. More specifically, Pierson (1999) states that in order to achieve independence in functional mobility, important positioning/bed mobility activities are required, which include moving upward/downward, side-to-side, rolling, turning over, and from supine-to-sitting. These activities typically preclude attempts at actual transfers. In addition, functional mobility should be addressed in as many environmental contexts as possible in order to assure generalization and transfer of learning.

Necessary equipment for possible independence and safety in functional mobility will also be addressed. Functional mobility equipment generally includes devices for positioning, bed mobility, transfers, wheelchair mobility, ambulation, and overall safety.

Because mobility training is a top-down approach, it is discussed in this chapter. In addition, within the topic of mobility, it is important to note that the remedial and compensatory approaches to intervention often blend. Refer to Chapter 2 for discussion of mobility issues as related to ROM, strength, coordination, etc.

Remediation techniques for functional mobility include daily practice of skills through repetition, chaining (forward and backward), cuing, as well as incorporating preparatory methods into intervention sessions (refer to Chapter 1). There are several foundational skills necessary for progression to independent transfers and functional mobility. These skills include sufficient joint ROM and flexibility, adequate muscle strength, endurance to tolerate the activity, and adequate visual-perceptual and cognitive skills for safety. Specifically, sufficient UE strength is required for most transfers and functional mobility using an assistive device. A remediation example is as follows: Prior to transferring out of bed, the OT may supervise the client in an exercise program at bed level which includes ROM, Thera-Band (Hygenic Corporation, Akron, OH), and/or the use of handheld weights to increase UE strength. Next, the therapist may practice previously learned techniques such as rolling, supine-to-sit, and sit-to-stand at the edge of the bed using above remediation techniques, as applicable.

COMPENSATION/ADAPTATION OF FUNCTIONAL MOBILITY DEFICITS FOR CLIENTS WITH PHYSICAL LIMITATIONS

When addressing functional mobility issues during ADL tasks, several performance skills and client factors must be considered (see Figure 3-2). These have been previously defined in Chapters 1 and 2 and will follow the same format as discussed previously.

Performance Skills: Motor Skills

Motor Skills during functional activities involve moving and interacting with the environment, tasks, and objects (AOTA, 2002a). These skills include posture, mobility, coordination, strength and effort, and energy, which are defined below:

- *Posture* involves stabilization, alignment, and positioning of the body while moving and performing functional activities.

- *Mobility* involves moving the body, or its parts, in space and/or interacting with the environment during functional activities. Mobility includes walking, reaching, and bending.

- *Coordination* involves using body parts to interact with BADL objects in order to complete a functional performance activity. Coordination includes manipulation and the flow of movement to complete activity.

- *Strength and effort* involves skills that require adequate muscle force in order to complete a functional performance activity. Strength and effort include moving transporting, lifting, calibrating, and gripping task objects.

- *Energy* involves effort required to complete a performance skill activity and endurance for and pacing of a task.

Performance Patterns Related to Functional Mobility

When establishing an intervention plan, it is essential to determine the client's habits and routines regarding functional mobility. For example, a client may have habitually transferred out of bed on the same side for many years. After sustaining a cerebral vascular accident (CVA), the client may, because of hemiplegia, need to get out of bed on the opposite side, particularly for safety reasons. Therefore, while being sensitive to previous habits, the therapist must educate the client and family on the need to create a new habit.

A client's role(s) within the family may also be impacted by changes in functional mobility. A client who is now wheelchair-bound may not be able to partake in a habitual family hike, or take the family pet out every morning. It is the OT's job to work with the client and family to compensate or adapt the previous roles to the new disability.

Activity Demands of Functional Mobility

The activity demands of functional mobility include the required tools, space, time, foundational skills, and social skills to complete applicable tasks (AOTA, 2002a). Similar to performance patterns, aspects of activity demands are also related to the client's context. Table 3-11 provides examples of activity demands and functional mobility.

Client Factors: Body Function—Neuromusculoskeletal and Movement-Related Functions

- *Functions of joints and bones* include mobility and stability of joint and bone functions (PROM, postural alignment, and joint mobility).

- *Muscle functions* include muscle power (strength), tone, and endurance.

- *Movement functions* include motor reflexes, involuntary movement reactions/functions, motor control, and gait pattern functions.

There are many specific types of transfers that will be addressed in detail later in this section. Transfers are further designated by the level of assistance required. These levels are described in Table 3-12. Depending upon the physical abilities of the client, mental status, and safety abilities,

Table 3-11

ACTIVITY DEMANDS AND EXAMPLES OF IMPACT ON FUNCTIONAL MOBILITY

Activity Demands According to AOTA Framework (2002a)	Examples Related to Functional Mobility
Objects	Assistive devices such as a wheelchair, walker, or cane.
Space demands (relates to physical context)	Space available to maneuver assistive devices.
Social demands	Expectations of the individual to perform functional mobility independently.
Sequence and timing	Steps and proper sequencing required to complete functional mobility with or without an assistive device.
Required actions	Foundational skills required to complete functional mobility.
Body functions and structure	ROM and anatomical parts (hands/legs) required for functional mobility skills.

an additional therapist/health care professional may be needed during transfers, at least initially. The therapist should always ask for assistance before beginning the transfer if the need for a second individual is suspected.

It is very important to accurately assess the client according to these levels in order to accurately document baseline status and client progress. The accurate documentation of functional transfers/mobility is also vital for similar communication between health care professionals. Specific documentation includes the cross-discipline knowledge of transfer levels of assistance as depicted in Table 3-12. In addition, caregivers may also be provided with accurate training and education regarding the client's status.

Precautions and General Information for Functional Mobility

There are many precautions that must be considered and anticipated during all levels of assistance and types of transfers. General transfer precautions and safety techniques are listed in Table 3-13. The client's safety during transfers is a primary concern and the therapist is ultimately responsible for safe transfers. The therapist must have a baseline assessment of the client's mental and physical status in order to predetermine the type of transfer to attempt as well as potential level of assistance needed.

Prior to the transfer, the therapist must determine the best position for him/herself and the client in order to prevent injury. It is typically safest for the therapist to be in front of, and slightly to one side of the client (often the weaker side).

General Transfer Tools

Table 3-14 lists many tools that may be used for transfers from any surface, including bed level, standing, toileting, and showering during functional mobility. The tools will be referred to during the remainder of this section.

Table 3-12

LEVELS OF ASSISTANCE

Dependent Transfer	Client is unable to participate in transfer.
Maximum-Assist Transfer	Client performs 25% of transfer.
Moderate-Assist Transfer	Client performs 50% of transfer.
Minimum-Assist Transfer	Client performs 25% of transfer.
Contact Guard Transfer	Client requires hands-on for guidance or possible loss of balance.
Supervision Transfer	Client does not require physical assist, although may need verbal cues for safety/performance.
Distant Supervision Transfer	Client is approaching independence, although may need occasional reminders.
Independent Transfer (with or without an assistive device)	No assistance, cuing, or reminders needed for safety or performance.

Table 3-13

GENERAL TRANSFER PRECAUTIONS AND SAFETY TECHNIQUES

1. Client should wear proper shoes. If shoes are not available, then slipper socks should be worn.
2. Assess client's perceptual and cognitive status prior to performing transfers.
3. Assess client's physical capabilities prior to performing transfers.
4. Ensure all lines attached to client are protected.
5. Stabilize or lock all surfaces.
6. Adjust surfaces for safety and ease of transfer.
7. All unneeded equipment and furniture should not obstruct the transfer.
8. Preplan the steps and set-up of the transfer (selection and position of equipment).
9. Use a safety/transfer belt.
10. Anticipate possible safety issues that may occur.
11. Position the client properly before beginning the transfer.
12. Instruct client regarding safety issues and steps of the transfer, and demonstrate, as able.
13. Be knowledgeable of and use good body mechanics at all times. Instruct caregivers, as well.
14. Know your own limitations and ask for assistance, preferably before the transfer, if needed.
15. Instruct client not to hold onto the therapist when transferring. Do not grasp client's upper extremities during transfers.
16. Do not leave the client alone after transferring, particularly on an unfamiliar or less stable surface, such as a tub bench.
17. After the transfer is completed, ensure proper positioning and safety (lock wheelchair brakes, return side rails of bed).
18. Be aware of any special conditions which may be exacerbated during the transfer, such as a shoulder subluxation or total hip replacement.

Table 3-14	
FUNCTIONAL MOBILITY TOOLS	
Slide board	Made of wood or plastic, this device is placed under the client's buttocks to act as a bridge when transferring between one surface and another. This is typically used with clients who have paraplegia, amputation(s), severe LE weakness, or are unable to weight-bear.
Bed rails	May be permanently part of a hospital bed or portable to fit most typical bed mattresses.
Tub/toilet rails	Rails may be portable or installed permanently in the tub. Toilet rails are typically are permanent. Placement is important for accessibility.
Commode	A seat with a cut-out opening that holds a bucket. Used for toileting when necessary at the bedside or when the bathroom is inaccessible.
Walker basket	Typically a lightweight metal or plastic device which attaches to the front of the walker in order to transport small items safely.
Leg-lifter	A soft device with a large loop on one end in which the client places the foot or thigh of the affected LE. A loop on the opposite end is held in order for the UEs to move the limb in bed or to the edge of the bed.
Trapeze	A triangular metal device secured on a frame above the client's bed. The client uses the trapeze for leverage when performing bed mobility tasks such as supine to long-sitting and to the edge of the bed.
Rope ladder	An actual ladder device in which one end is attached to the foot of the bed and the others held by the client in order to pull to a sitting position in bed.
Transfer belt	A sturdy belt used during transfers, which gives the therapist something to hold onto (other than the client) while guiding/assisting the client. The belt serves as an additional safety method.
Draw sheet/pad	An additional sheet or thin pad placed directly under the client. It is used by health professionals/caregivers to hold onto while assisting the client with bed mobility.

COMPENSATION/ADAPTATION FOR TRUNK CONTROL

Trunk Control: Stability Before Mobility

Conditions that affect the client's central nervous system, such as stroke and spinal cord injuries, may impair trunk control. Individuals will not be able to engage in tasks that involve trunk mobility until adequate trunk control and strength have been achieved. Decreased trunk control will impact many areas of function including functional mobility, safe eating, independence in ADLs, interaction with the environment, and safety. Therefore, trunk or postural control must be a priority in order to achieve the simplest of functional outcomes.

Clients with decreased trunk control typically have the following postural weaknesses: Posterior pelvic tilt, unequal weight-bearing through ischial tuberosities, lumbar spine flexion, kyphosis, lateral flexion of the spine, and head/neck malalignments (Gillen & Burkhardt, 2004). Trunk control interventions should then begin with proper positioning of the client in order to address these postural issues.

Trunk Control: Mobility

Before beginning techniques to improve trunk mobility, the client must begin in a proper seated position. The therapist may use techniques throughout attempts at improving trunk mobility such as cuing, demonstration, hands-on techniques to "feel" the movement, or the use of a mirror. The overall goals are to improve trunk strength, balance, symmetry, and control during functional activities (Gillen & Burkhardt, 2004).

- *Examples of bed-level ADL tasks that may require trunk control movements*: Bathing and dressing, weight shifting while toileting, reaching at the sink for grooming items, and sitting at the kitchen table at mealtime.

CHANGING THE TASK TO ACHIEVE INDEPENDENCE

The therapist may provide handling techniques during ADL tasks. Handling includes providing external support to the trunk or allowing the client to feel the desired movement under the direction of the therapist. This handling may be graded according to the needs of the client (Gillen & Burkhardt, 2004). For example, the therapist may provide support to the client's lumbar area as he/she is leaning forward to don pants over feet. In addition, the therapist may encourage increased trunk motion during this task, through handling techniques, as the client is ready.

Reaching tasks may challenge and encourage improved trunk control by the placement of objects in various reaching distances from the client's position (Gillen & Burkhardt, 2004). For example, while seated in front of the sink for brushing teeth, the therapist may place the wheelchair slightly farther from the sink than typical, put the toothbrush on the counter, and the toothpaste in on a shelf slightly higher than the counter.

CHANGING THE TOOLS TO ACHIEVE INDEPENDENCE

As extremities are being incorporated into ADL tasks that involve weak trunk musculature, tasks will become increasingly more challenging. Therefore, trunk supports may be utilized to free the extremities for function. These aids include pillows, cushions, lap trays, and lumbar or lateral supports.

The client may not be ready to be challenged by increasing reach activities. In this case, the environment may be adapted by placing items at a closer distance. Adaptive equipment to enhance independence while improving trunk control/strength may be introduced such as a long handled sponge and shoe horn, reacher, and sock aid. The client may also need a commode or shower seat with a high back for increased trunk support when toileting and showering.

The client's home may require additional modifications as the trunk improves. Modifications may include: High back chairs with arms instead of sitting on a very soft, low couch or using a chair with arms at the kitchen table. If trunk mobility is significantly decreased, the client may benefit from a hospital bed with electronic controls and bed rails until strength improves.

Trunk control activities typically begin on a stable surface such as a chair or mat. As the client improves, an unstable or movable surface may be introduced (Gillen & Burkhardt, 2004). Unstable surfaces include the use of therapy balls, rocker boards, or bolsters. Basic trunk control exercises may be used as prepatory methods to ADLs, including reaching, catching, and throwing activities, for example, as the client is ready. Actual ADL activities may be encouraged on an unstable surface such as a bolster, beginning with a very simple task, such as buttoning a shirt. Activities must be graded very carefully in order to encourage success, safety, and security.

COMPENSATION/ADAPTATION FOR BED MOBILITY

Bed mobility activities include rolling from supine to side-lying, side-lying to supine, supine to prone, prone to supine, supine to sitting at edge of bed or long-sitting, bridging, moving upward/downward, and from side-to-side. Equipment for bed mobility may include bed rails, trapeze, draw sheet, leg-lifter, ladder rope, and special mattresses.

Bed mobility training is not only a precursor to transfer training and independence, but also vitally important for preventing decubiti and/or contractures, which result from lack of movement and position changing. In addition, rolling side to side and sitting upright in bed are tasks necessary for independence in ADLs (Trombly & Radomski, 2002). The client should be encouraged to assist the therapist as much as possible, whether it is with head movements, UE positioning, and/or LE movements. The amount of assistance given by the therapist should be graded and gradually decreased, as able (see Table 3-12). For example, rolling from supine to side-lying, the therapist may be initially offering moderate assistance at the knees and shoulder to complete the task. As the client improves, the movement may be graded by offering only minimal assistance at the knees and shoulder or grading may be completed by only offering moderate assistance at one body part versus two.

The first issue with bed mobility should be reducing the friction between the client and the surface of the bed or mat. For example, using a draw sheet under the client will help to decrease friction. Whenever possible, reduce the effects of gravity and/or use gravity to assist the activity. For example, by lowering the head of the hospital bed, the client may use gravity to assist when attempting to "scoot" back in bed. Proper body mechanics are also a priority for the safety of the client as well as the therapist and will be addressed later in this section as each movement and transfer is described.

Moving Side-to-Side

The client should be encouraged to assist with bed mobility as much as he/she is able. When moving side-to-side while in supine, the client should be instructed to flex at the hips and knees with feet flat on the mattress. One UE should be beside the trunk and the other abducted. The client is instructed to push both feet, elbows, and head into the mattress while lifting the pelvis upward. This technique is commonly referred to as *bridging* and is depicted in Figure 3-21. The pelvis should then move toward the abducted UE. Then, the client repositions the extremities in order to move again, if needed. The client should be instructed to move both to the right and left. Initially, the movement may be performed by the therapist offering assistance for bridging, and then the activity is graded by decreasing the amount of hands-on assistance offered.

Moving Upward/Downward

When moving upward while in supine, the client should be instructed to flex at the hips and knees with feet flat on the mattress with heels close to the buttocks. The elbows should be flexed and placed close to the trunk while the shoulders are pulled up towards the ears. The client is asked to bridge (as above) and move upward by pushing with the LEs and depressing the scapula. The client will reposition to move upward again, if necessary.

When moving downward while in supine, the client will partially flex the hips and knees with feet flat on the bed. The elbows are flexed next to the trunk and the shoulders depressed. The client is instructed to bridge while pushing into the bed with the elbows, head, and heels. The client moves downward by pulling the LEs, pushing upward with the shoulders, and downward with the elbows and forearms. The client is requested to reposition to repeat above, if needed.

Again, these movements may be graded by the therapist after initially offering hands-on assistance.

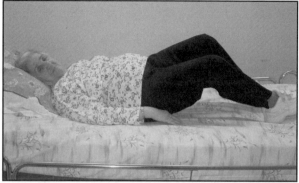

Figure 3-21. Client bridging in bed.

- *Examples of bed-level ADL tasks that may require these movements*: For a client on bed rest, the caregiver may rely on the client to perform/assist with these movements in order to make or change the bed. Clients tend to slip downward in the bed and not only are uncomfortable, but it is difficult to assist him/her to an upright position for safe eating. Therefore, the technique of moving upward is very important. Also, bridging is important when hiking pants in bed, placing a bed pan, and donning protective garments.

Changing the Task to Achieve Independence

The method may be changed by adjusting the levels of assistance. For example, the therapist may need to assist the client in flexing the hip and knees. The client may also need assistance in maintaining this position. The therapist may also assist with bridging, if needed. Instead of this strategy, the client may attempt the activity independently without flexing the hip/knees and only pushing down with the head and heels, with low extremities extended (Pierson, 1996).

Changing the Tools to Achieve Independence

The use of bed rails or trapeze may assist the client with bed mobility as needed. The therapist may assist the client with actually moving to the side by using a draw sheet, as needed.

Moving From Supine to Side-Lying

The client is initially requested to move to one side of the bed (see section on moving side-to-side). When rolling to the right, the client is instructed to reach across the midline with the left UE while lifting the flexed left LE over the right LE (Figure 3-22). The client flexes the neck and uses abdominal muscles in order to roll. Side-lying may be maintained by placing the right hand on the bed and flexing both LEs. The client may need to slightly lean the shoulders toward the left side to further maintain the position, but not too far as the client will fall into prone. The same technique may be used for the left side.

- *Examples of bed-level ADL tasks that may require these movements*: Moving to side-lying is important for placing a bed pan, cleansing the perianal area, hiking pants in bed, donning protective garments, and inspecting a client's back and buttocks for possible pressure areas/decubiti.

Changing the Task to Achieve Independence

As needed, the therapist may assist the client by facilitating movement at the hip, knee, shoulder, head, or UE. The therapist ascertains which areas may need the most assistance. As the client strengthens, less assistance is provided.

Figure 3-22. Client rolling to the right.

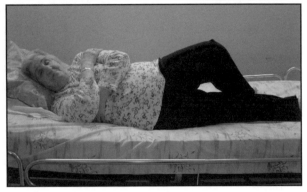

CHANGING THE TOOLS TO ACHIEVE INDEPENDENCE

The use of bed rails or trapeze may assist the client with bed mobility as needed. The therapist may assist the client with actually moving to the side by using a draw sheet, as needed.

Moving From Supine to Prone

The client is initially requested to move to one side of the bed. The client is then asked to roll as previously described, except the UE is placed under the side of the body or the shoulder is flexed close to the right ear. The client is then instructed to roll into prone (staying away from the edge of the bed).

CHANGING THE TASK AND TOOLS TO ACHIEVE INDEPENDENCE

These are described above under moving side-to-side and moving supine to side lying.

Moving From Prone to Supine

While in prone, the client is instructed to move to one side of the bed. In order to roll to the right side, the client should position the right UE under the right side of the body or flex the right shoulder and place it by the right ear. The left hand is placed flat on the bed near the left shoulder. The left hip and knee are either slightly flexed or extended. The client is instructed to push with the left UE, lift the LE over the right LE and roll to side-lying (staying away from the edge of the bed).

- *Examples of bed-level ADL tasks that may require these movements*: Most clients have difficulty moving out of a prone position or are not comfortable in it. If prone is comfortable, skin may be inspected in this position and pressure taken off the heels. Most ADLs do not require this position for completion of tasks. Therefore, lying or moving into prone is not typically a position of high priority.

CHANGING THE TASK TO ACHIEVE INDEPENDENCE

As needed, the therapist may assist the client by facilitating movement at the LE, head, or UE. The therapist ascertains which areas may need the most assistance. As the client strengthens, less assistance is provided.

CHANGING THE TOOLS TO ACHIEVE INDEPENDENCE

A draw sheet may be used to assist the client with this movement.

Moving From Supine to Long-Sitting

While in supine, instruct the client to prop on both elbows. The client must use abdominal muscles and gradually push up with alternating UEs in order to weight-bear on both hands.

- *Examples of bed-level ADL tasks that may require this position*: In a long-sitting position, the client may eat at bed-level, perform hygiene tasks, bathe UE, and/or don a bra, shirt, or hospital gown.

CHANGING THE TASK TO ACHIEVE INDEPENDENCE

As an alternative method, the client may roll into side-lying and gradually push with UEs into long-sitting.

CHANGING THE TOOLS TO ACHIEVE INDEPENDENCE

If the client is in a hospital bed and is unable to prop on elbows, he/she may use the electronic controls to elevate the head of the bed and position the client automatically into long-sitting. With the above alternative method, the client may use the bed rails for rolling into side-lying and pushing with UEs. A rope ladder or trapeze may assist with either method above.

Moving From Supine to Sitting at the Edge of the Bed

Instruct client to bridge slightly to the edge of the bed (see Figure 3-21), leaving enough room to roll into side-lying. Follow above procedures for rolling into side-lying. Position client with hips and knees flexed while maintaining side-lying (see Figure 3-22). Once in this position, the client pushes the lower extremity over the edge of the bed. Instruct the client to push with the UEs, head, and trunk following. The LEs gradually pivot in order to dangle over the edge of the bed.

- *Examples of ADL tasks at the edge of the bed*: As long as sitting balance is intact, the client may perform many ADL tasks at the edge of the bed such as feeding, hygiene, bathing and dressing the UEs, bathing the front of the LE, and donning socks and shoes. LE tasks may be more difficult as they require excellent sitting balance. Various mattresses such as those filled with air may not allow for safe sitting balance and activities at the edge of the bed.

CHANGING THE TASK TO ACHIEVE INDEPENDENCE

The therapist will offer assistance as necessary with each step of the task. The therapist may need to offer assistance with sitting balance at the edge of the bed.

CHANGING THE TOOLS TO ACHIEVE INDEPENDENCE

The client may use the bed rails, trapeze, or rope ladder for assistance with pivoting to a sitting position. The bed rail may assist in maintaining a sitting position. Long-handled adaptive equipment such a long-handled sponge may assist the client with ADLs at the edge of the bed.

Special Considerations for the Client With Neurological Symptoms

Typically, it is easier for a client with hemiparesis to roll toward the affected side as the unaffected side is able to actually perform the activity. Before rolling, the affected UE is positioned close to the body. Rolling towards the unaffected side requires more effort of the affected extremities, as able. The client reaches for and holds onto the wrist of the affected extremity while hooking the unaffected foot under the ankle of the affected LE. The client then uses the unaffected extremities to assist with rolling to the unaffected side. The therapist will provide levels of assistance as necessary (see Table 3-12).

Clients who have neurological weakness or paraplegia of the LEs will rely on UE function and strength for bed mobility. In particular, the client will use shoulder and scapula muscles for rolling and triceps, as well, for propping on elbows to long-sitting. The client will also use the UEs to move and position the LEs. Precautions must be taken to protect an unstable glenohumeral joint, which may be at risk for subluxation.

CHANGING THE TASK TO ACHIEVE INDEPENDENCE

The therapist or caregiver may assist with LEs and/or affected UE, as needed.

CHANGING THE TOOLS TO ACHIEVE INDEPENDENCE

Assistive devices such as a trapeze, rope ladder, leg-lifter, or bed rails may also assist with independence.

Special Considerations for the Client With Orthopedic Injuries

Clients who have had a total hip replacement will require specific precautions with bed mobility depending upon the surgical procedure. Clients who have had both an anterolateral approach and posterolateral approach are typically recommended to initially lie supine with a wedge between both LEs in order to ensure hip precautions. It is not typically recommended for a client to sleep on or roll to the affected side. Clients with hip replacements may benefit from a trapeze above the bed (Pierson, 1996).

Clients who have a LE amputation are instructed to use the unaffected side for eventual independent bed mobility. This is achieved through flexing the hip and knee while pushing the foot of the unaffected LE into the mattress (Pierson, 1996).

CHANGING THE TASK TO ACHIEVE INDEPENDENCE

The client should compensate by using the UEs for assistance with mobility whenever possible. The therapist or caregiver will offer assistance, as needed.

CHANGING THE TOOLS TO ACHIEVE INDEPENDENCE

Bed rails and/or a trapeze may assist with bed mobility.

ADAPTATION/COMPENSATION FOR TRANSFERS

The most important concept to remember with transfer training is that each client will be unique in his/her own assistance needs, limitations, safety issues, and frustration tolerance, to name a few (refer to Table 3-13). Adaptations must be made for each situation and physical context, as well, while keeping generalization of skills in mind. New therapists should never hesitate to ask for assistance when a transfer may be too difficult to perform alone, as safety is the priority. In addition, the therapist must be aware of the client's status at the time of the intervention session, as skill levels may change rapidly toward the positive or negative. The therapist not only needs to check the most recent documentation, but also inquire with nursing and/or other available team members prior to initiating the session. The proper steps of a transfer are listed below.

1. Always use a transfer belt during functional ambulation.

2. Maintain a wide stance closely behind or on the affected side of the client.

3. With one hand, hold the transfer belt and with the other, guide the client's anterior shoulder, across the chest or the trunk, as needed. Do not hold onto clothes or client's UE.

Table 3-15

WEIGHT-BEARING ABBREVIATIONS AND DEFINITIONS

- *Non-Weight-Bearing (NWB)*: The client is not to place any weight on the affected extremity.
- *Toe-Touch Weight-Bearing (TTWB)*: The client may rest the affected extremity on the floor, but no weight is to be applied to the foot.
- *Partial Weight-Bearing (PWB)*: The client can place some weight onto the affected extremity, but not full pressure.
- *Weight-Bearing as Tolerated (WBAT)*: This generally indicates that there are no medical restrictions, but pain may limit the client's ability to bear weight on the affected extremity.
- *Full Weight-Bearing (FWB)*: There are no medical restrictions, allowing the client to place all body weight on the affected extremity.

4. Position feet anterior-posterior: The outside foot should be in front of the other foot as well as between the client's foot and the assistive device. The inside foot should be positioned behind the outside foot as the client moves forward.

5. Move forward in the same direction as the client without crossing feet.

6. If the client loses balance backward, position behind the client in order for him/her to lean back, while assisting the client to re-gain balance.

7. If the client loses balance to the side towards the therapist, allow the client to lean into the therapist while using the transfer belt to assist in re-gaining balance.

8. Whenever it is too difficult to assist the client in re-gaining balance, the therapist or caregiver should quickly consider carefully assisting the client to the floor.

This section will cover all levels and types of transfers including sit-to-stand, stand-pivot, toilet, tub, car, and lift transfers. Performance of ADL skills will be incorporated where applicable.

Prior to asking a client to stand, the OT must be aware of the weight-bearing status of the client. The weight-bearing status is determined by the physician. The generally accepted abbreviations and definitions of weight-bearing are listed in Table 3-15.

Sit-to-Stand Activities

When performing sit-to-stand activities from any surface, it is important for the client to have supportive foot wear. The therapist will use a transfer belt and review procedures with the client. Before beginning, both transfer surfaces must be stable, which includes locking wheelchair and hospital bed brakes. The therapist positions him/herself in front of the client (and slightly to the weak side if necessary) offering LE stabilization, as needed with his/her own knee or foot (Figure 3-23). The client is requested to "scoot" to the edge of the surface (bed, wheelchair, chair, mat, etc) as much as safely possible, using one or both hands flat on the surface to push off. The client may also push off with the bedrail or armrest on one side, but not an assistive device such as a walker, as it will be unstable. Feet should be placed flat on the floor about 6 to 10 inches apart and slightly behind the knees (Pierson, 1996). The client is requested to lean forward with the shoulders above the knees. The therapist holds onto the transfer belt (and is using good body mechanics), while the client pushes off with the UEs and gradually straightens LEs into standing (Figure 3-24). At this time, the client may hold onto an assistive device such as a walker or quad cane in order to safely balance.

Figure 3-23. Start position for sit-to-stand.

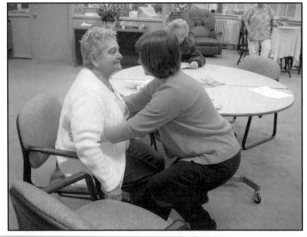

Figure 3-24. End position for sit to stand.

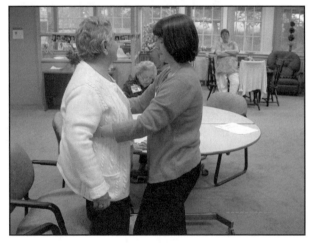

- *Examples of ADL tasks that use sit-to-stand activities*: Functional standing activities may be included in this area. Examples of functional sit-to-stand activities are toileting, bathing peri-anal area, hiking pants, and retrieving clothes from closet or bureau.

Changing the Task to Achieve Independence

If no rails or armrests are available, the client may push off of thighs or use both edges of the sitting surface.

Changing the Tools to Achieve Independence

Clients can use well installed grab bars to pull up into standing, rather than pushing off of the chair. Raised seat surfaces will generally allow greater ease of standing. For the bathroom, raised toilet seats are available. For other chairs, the legs can be made longer. There are rare instances when the therapist may allow the client to use one extremity held on the walker to stand with the other on the sitting surface. The therapist must supervise the client closely and provide instructions for safety.

Stand-Pivot Transfers

Stand-pivot transfers are used with clients who are unable to take at least a few steps to or from the transfer surface. This transfer is initiated in the same manner as a sit-to-stand activity, although the client will not have an assistive device ready for maintaining balance. As the client stands, the therapist stays close to assist with stability and balance. Once the client is in a full standing position, the client and therapist pivot simultaneously. The client is then gradually guided into sitting as he/she reaches back for the sitting surface (rail, armrest, cushion, etc).

- *Examples of ADL tasks that use stand-pivot activities*: See toilet transfers.

CHANGING THE TASK TO ACHIEVE INDEPENDENCE

It is advisable to perform this transfer to the affected side as well, in the event a nonpredictable environment is not set up for a transfer to the unaffected side. If a client requires assist of two individuals, a second may stand to the side or in back of the client, also using the transfer belt. The method may need to be changed completely if two or more professionals are unable to pivot the client. Alternative methods may include a manual "lift" by two or more professionals or a mechanical lift (refer to manual/mechanical lift information later in this section).

CHANGING THE TOOLS TO ACHIEVE INDEPENDENCE

Refer to the information regarding intervention with the client who has a neurological injury or illness below.

Issues for the Client With Neurologic Deficits

- Client typically will stand pivot to unaffected side and pivot on unaffected LE/foot.
- If one UE is hemiparetic, only one UE may be able to assist with the task.
- If client has a subluxation, a sling may be used for transfers and functional mobility only.

The use of the sling will help to protect the subluxation during the transfer. It should be removed when client is sitting/lying because extended use of the sling/shoulder immobility may encourage adhesive capsulitis.

Issues for the Client With Orthopedic Deficits

- Client typically will stand pivot to unaffected side and pivot on unaffected LE/foot.
- Total hip replacement (THR) precautions must be followed for clients who have sustained certain hip replacements (refer to section on THR precautions).

Transfers to Surfaces With an Assistive Device

Transfers using an assistive device are appropriate for a client able to take at least a few steps to or from the transfer surface. Again, ensure all surfaces are stable and locked. This transfer is initiated in the same way as a sit to stand activity with the device ready for maintaining balance upon standing (Figure 3-25). Once standing balance and stability have been achieved, the therapist may either assist or supervise the client to the transfer surface. When the client is ready to sit, if he/she is using a walker, the device should placed directly in front of him/her, but not be held while sitting. Instead, the client should reach back for the transferring surface with one or both UEs, as able (Figure 3-26). If the client is using a hemi-walker, quad cane, or cane, the device will remain on the side in which the client ambulates with it, but again, it is not held while sitting. Once sitting, the client should "scoot" fully back on the surface.

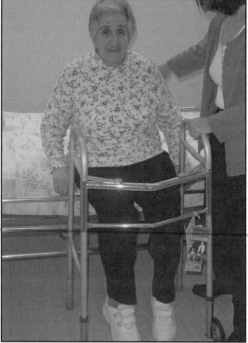 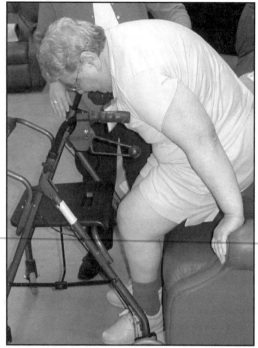

Figure 3-25. Sit-to-stand with adaptive ambulation device.

Figure 3-26. Client safely reaches back for chair prior to sitting.

- *Examples of ADL tasks that use transfers with an assistive device*: The client transferring with an assistive device may be carrying bath or clothing items from one surface to another in the bedroom or bathroom. Also, see toilet transfers.

CHANGING THE TASK TO ACHIEVE INDEPENDENCE

As the client progresses, the transfer surfaces may be placed farther away from each other.

CHANGING THE TOOLS TO ACHIEVE INDEPENDENCE

After consulting with the rehabilitation team, the client may be ready to progress to the next level of an assistive device or take a few steps to transfer without a device, if safe. The client who uses a walker may benefit from a walker basket.

Issues for the Client With Neurologic Deficits

- Possible need for a sling with UE subluxation, although a sling for the affected extremity should be used with extreme caution and only during transfers/functional mobility in order to protect the shoulder from subluxation (or further injury).
- Client with hemiparesis will most likely need a hemiwalker initially, as it provides a wider base of support for balance.

Issues for the Client With Orthopedic Deficits

- Client may need platform crutches or platform walker with UE injuries if weight-bearing is contraindicated on the wrist joints.

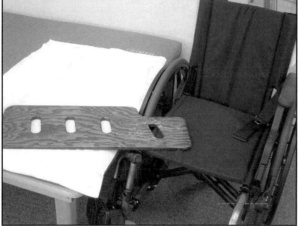

Figure 3-27. Slide board and wheelchair positioned.

Slide Board Transfers

Slide board transfers are appropriate for clients who have paraplegia of the LEs, bilateral amputations, severe LE weakness, or are unable to weight-bear on both LEs. The slide board is used as a bridge to transfer from one surface to another. The client must have adequate ROM and strength of both UEs, good sitting balance, and trunk mobility. The therapist applies the transfer belt. The transfer begins by equalizing the surfaces, as able. For example, with a hospital bed to wheelchair transfer, the bed should be positioned at a close level to the wheelchair. Both transferring surfaces must be stable and locked. Typically, a wheelchair is positioned at up to a 90-degree angle to the transferring surface (Figure 3-27). The client (with therapist's assistance as necessary) places the slide board under the buttocks by weight-bearing on the opposite extremity and elongating the trunk to the side. The client/therapist ensures the board is secured properly under the buttocks and on the transferring surface. The client leans forward slightly and weight-bears on both UEs, which should lift his/her body up slightly with each attempt. As this occurs, the client also moves across the board towards the transferring surface. The therapist positions in front of the client and may need to guide the LEs during the transfer.

- *Examples of ADL tasks that use slide board activities*: Slide board transfers are generally used to transfer to many surfaces during ADLs, including toilet and tub bench transfers.

CHANGING THE TASK TO ACHIEVE INDEPENDENCE

Typically, the therapist assists/supervises while positioned in front of the client. This positioning may vary depending on the set-up of the transferring environment. For example, in a small bathroom, the therapist may not fit in front of the client and may have to position behind or beside the toilet or tub bench during the transfer. Car transfers may also need an alternative method.

CHANGING THE TOOLS TO ACHIEVE INDEPENDENCE

A pillow case, towel, or powder may be put on the board to decrease friction and increase ease of transfer. If the client is unable to handle or place the slide board successfully, the transfer may be performed as a *bump-over* without the slide board. With this technique, there cannot be any armrests on chairs. Also, the transfer surfaces must be of equal height and as close together as possible. The therapist must first ensure client safety and cognitive skills.

Issues for the Client With Neurologic Deficits

- Client may need assistance secondary to poor sitting balance.
- Transfer toward strong side, if possible.
- Clients with paraplegia of both LEs may become independent with slide board transfers.
- Client with UE hemiparesis may not have sufficient UE strength/function to perform transfer.

Issues for the Client With Orthopedic Deficits

- Clients who have sustained bilateral amputations without prosthetic devices may require the use of slide board transfers.
- Clients who have a nonweight-bearing status of both LEs may require slide board transfers. This is typically a temporary situation.

Toilet Transfers

Toilet transfers may use any of the above transfer techniques depending upon the size and set-up of the bathroom(s) the client uses. The limitations of space within most bathrooms as well as safety procedures are the primary considerations when planning for eventual independence with transfer training. Often, a standard wheelchair will not fit into the client's bathroom, requiring alternative plans for toileting. For example, with a client who is unable to ambulate and the wheelchair does not fit in the bathroom, the best option would be to use a commode at the bedside. Aside from modifying techniques for limitations in space within most bathrooms, the above procedures for the many types of transfers remain the same.

- *Examples of ADL tasks that use toilet transfer activities*: Before the actual transfer, the therapist and client need to plan how LE clothing will be pulled down and hiked. Often, it is helpful to loosen belts and closures before transferring (being careful clothes do not fall to the floor during the transfer). Before toileting, the client will need to maintain standing balance to further loosen/pull down garments and then to cleanse and hike after toileting.

CHANGING THE TASK TO ACHIEVE INDEPENDENCE

The positioning of the wheelchair by the toilet may have to be modified due to the size and set-up of the bathroom. The position of the therapist may also need to be modified. The client may not be able to transfer to the unaffected or stronger side. An alternative method for slide board or bump-over methods may be a forward/backward toilet transfer. For example, the wheelchair is placed directly in front of the toilet and the client slides on and off the toilet in a forward/backward manner, facing the back of the toilet.

CHANGING THE TOOLS TO ACHIEVE INDEPENDENCE

The client may benefit from a raised toilet seat and rails. If there is a counter within reach, on one side of the toilet, it may be used to push off. A commode may be placed over the toilet with the bucket taken out, as an alternative tool. This commode may also be placed by the bedside at night.

Issues for the Client With Neurologic Deficits

- Whenever possible, client should transfer to/from the strong side.
- The client may benefit from a raised toilet seat or commode over the toilet.

Issues for the Client With Orthopedic Deficits

- Clients who have had back surgery, hip replacement, or knee replacement(s) may require a raised toilet seat for a successful transfer.
- Clients may also benefit from the use of rails.

Tub/Shower Transfers

Safety issues are of a higher concern with tub/shower transfers. It is recommended to have a skid-proof bath mat outside and inside of the tub/shower stall, rails, and handheld shower, and occasionally it is recommended to remove shower doors. Often tub benches cannot fit when shower doors are present. At least initially, clients are not recommended to transfer directly to the floor of the bathtub. Instead, a transfer tub bench or shower seat is recommended (Figure 3-28). Transferring to a transfer tub bench requires similar techniques to those presented above. The therapist may need to provide additional assistance with lifting LEs over the height of the tub. If no rails are present, the therapist may need to offer further assistance for safety, balance, and stability.

Transferring over the height of the tub or ledge of a shower stall will require additional explanation as well as strength, balance, and mobility on the client's part. The therapist applies the transfer belt and the client either ambulates to the tub/shower or stands from the wheelchair with procedures presented above. Example: The shower head is to the *right* when the client is facing the tub/shower. When standing beside the tub or shower, the client stands at an angle slightly facing, and to the side of, the tub or shower. If the client is able to hold the assistive device in the left hand, he/she may continue to do so. If it is held in the right, the client will need to let go of the device and grab onto a hand rail, which should be placed at the front of the tub/shower. If there is no rail, the client may hold the therapist's hand. The client will then step into the tub with the stronger LE while slightly facing the tub/shower and follow with the other extremity. The client may either grab onto a rail on the inner wall of the tub/shower with the left hand or reach for the shower seat. The client will then face the shower head, feel the seat behind his/her knees, continue to hold the rails, then reach back for the shower seat with one hand, and sit.

- *Examples of ADL tasks that use tub/shower activities*: While simulating the transfer and sitting on shower chair/bench, the client's trunk stability must be assessed. As applicable, one-handed shower techniques may be initiated, with or without use of handheld shower. Adaptive equipment may be used for one-handed bathing. The therapist must plan with the client how the peri-anal area will be bathed, particularly if there is no cut-out in the seat. If a sit-to-stand is required for this task, the client and therapist should simulate the skill prior to the actual shower.

Changing the Task to Achieve Independence

Instead of slightly facing the tub, the client may side-step into the tub. This method is preferable if the stronger LE is able to step in first. This method may be necessary due to lack of space. When the client is ready, transfers to sitting on the floor of the tub may be attempted with great caution, supervision, and good judgment.

Changing the Tools to Achieve Independence

The client may not be able to use a tub transfer bench due to lack of space or the expense of the tool. Often, a sturdy plastic lawn chair may fit in the tub as a shower seat and be much more affordable. Many prefabricated tub/showers have built-in shower seats, as well. The safety of these seats must be evaluated before use.

Figure 3-28. Transfer tub bench and shower seat.

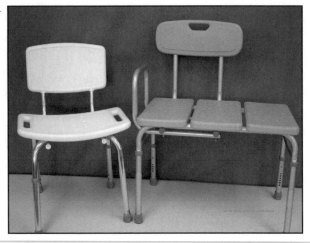

Issues for the Client With Neurologic Deficits

- Issues of concern surround safety, for example, the client who is impulsive, has neglect, or significantly decreased balance (to name a few) will have a greater risk of falling in a situation where the floor/bath is wet or slippery.

Issues for the Client With Orthopedic Deficits

- Secondary to possible THR precautions, casts, open wounds, staples, etc., the client may not be able to take a shower, and will need to sponge bathe.

Manual Lift Transfers

For clients who are fully dependent in transfers, two individuals may be needed to lift the client to a bed, mat, wheelchair, or commode. The techniques depend on the surface transferring to and from, as well as the size of the client. One technique is called the *cervical lift* or *through arm lift*. For example, if the client is beginning at wheelchair level, he/she will be positioned with the head and trunk flexed and UEs folded in front of the body (Pedretti, 1996). One therapist will position behind the client using a wide base of support. The therapist reaches under the client's axilla and around the chest to grasp the client's forearms. The second therapist faces side of the client's LEs and grasps them by holding one arm under the client's upper thighs and the other under the lower legs. (Alternative LE lift: the second therapist faces the client's LE in order to lift both LEs at the knees.) The therapists will count "one, two, three—lift". As the lift begins, they both must lift the client high enough to clear the height of the wheelchair while moving the client sideways toward the transferring surface. Proper body mechanics on the part of the therapists is vital.

- *Examples of ADL tasks that use manual lift activities*: Because this transfer is being dependent in nature, there are no ADL tasks directly related.

CHANGING THE TASK TO ACHIEVE INDEPENDENCE

See above. A third individual may either be needed to stand by or assist at the axilla or with the LEs. An alternative two-person method involves the therapists positioned on each side of the client distributing the client's weight more evenly. A negative aspect of the lift is that it often requires the client to be carried farther than the first method. Each therapist uses a forearm to cradle the client's thigh and the other crosses the client's posterior upper trunk to grasp the other therapists forearm. The client's UEs are placed over the therapist's shoulders (Pierson, 1996).

CHANGING THE TOOLS TO ACHIEVE INDEPENDENCE

If the client may be too heavy or his/her safety is an issue, a mechanical lift should be used.

Issues for the Client With Neurologic Deficits

- The client may be especially fearful of the transfer if visual/perceptual and/or cognitive issues are present.
- If a client is at Level IV of Ranchos Los Amigos Scale, for example, an agitated state may decrease the safety of the transfer.

Issues for the Client With Orthopedic Deficits

- Be aware of possible decubiti when rolling client and placing transfer pad. Client may be at risk for a decubiti secondary to friction from being manually transferred.

Mechanical Lift Transfers

Mechanical lift transfers are categorized as dependent in nature, as are manual lifts. A hydraulic lifting device, such as the Hoyer Patient Lifter (Pedretti, 2000) may be used for clients who are either too heavy and/or require extensive lifting and assistance (Figure 3-29). Caregivers need to be educated in the use of the mechanical lift, as with other transfers. Clients may be transferred to most surfaces, including the toilet and commode. Caution is necessary; however, if the client's mental status or sitting balance may necessitate supervision or assistance when arriving at the transfer surface.

The mechanical lift transfer also involves explaining the steps of the activity to the client before beginning. Steps are as follows:

1. While at bed level, the sling component of the lift must be positioned under the upper trunk, buttocks, and upper thigh of the client by rolling him/her from one side to the other. (see bed mobility techniques).
2. The lift should be positioned perpendicular to the bed and as close as possible with the spreader bar over the client's chest.
3. The chains or straps of the sling are attached to the spreader bar.
4. The control valve then is partially opened in order to gradually lower the spreader bar until the chains/straps can be attached to the sling.
5. Then the valve is closed to prevent the spreader valve from lowering further.
6. The chains or straps are attached to the sling, directing the "S" hooks away from the body.
7. Make adjustments and check all attachments as needed.
8. Ask the client to fold his/her UEs over the chest.
9. Elevate the client by pumping the handle until he/she is elevated off the bed.
10. Slowly move the lift from the bed with a second person guiding the client's LEs.
11. Guide the client to the transferring surface with his/her buttocks positioned directly over the seat/surface.
12. Gradually open the control valve, which will slowly lower the client to the surface.
13. Guide the client's body toward the surface and close the valve.
14. Remove the chains or straps from the sling, leaving the sling in place for the transfer back to bed or another surface.

Figure 3-29. Mechanical lift.

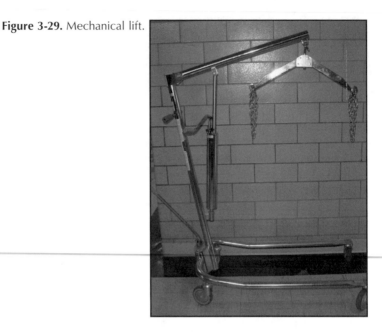

- *Examples of ADL tasks that use mechanical lift activities*: As stated, clients may be transferred via the mechanical lift to the toilet or commode. Adapted raised toilet seats, transfer pads with cut-outs, and rails are typically necessary for safety, hygiene, and sitting balance.

CHANGING THE TASK TO ACHIEVE INDEPENDENCE

As the client's ability to participate improves, the mechanical lift may not be needed.

CHANGING THE TOOLS TO ACHIEVE INDEPENDENCE

A sling with an opening at the peri-anal area may be used for clients who are lifted to a commode/toilet. A client may need to have multiple slings, with one at the upper body and one at the buttock area.

Getting Up From the Floor

Getting up from the floor is an important segment of rehabilitation for independence. If a client falls or needs to get up from the floor, the ideal position to begin with is in prone. The client will then push him/herself to a quadruped position and then to kneeling, half kneeling, and then standing.

- *Examples of ADL tasks that involve getting up from the floor*: This transfer may also be used when getting out of the floor of the tub.

CHANGING THE TASK TO ACHIEVE INDEPENDENCE

If the client is unable to position in prone, he/she may logroll to side-lying, push to side-sitting, and then move to quadruped position.

CHANGING THE TOOLS TO ACHIEVE INDEPENDENCE

The client may also hold onto a nearby stable object for assistance.

Car Transfers

Car transfers may be initiated with any of the various techniques above, as appropriate. For example, the therapist may perform a stand-pivot transfer with the client to the car seat. Slide board transfers or transfers using a walker or any other assistive device may also be attempted. The difference in a car transfer is with the approach to the car seat. With any of the types of transfers, the client will typically need to take a backward approach to the car seat. The client needs to back into the car seat and feel it behind the LEs before sitting. The client will need to reach back for the side of the car and/or dashboard when sitting. The open car door may be an obstacle for assistive devices as well as the therapist. Therefore, careful step-by-step planning of this transfer is necessary.

After the client sits, he/she may need assistance in pivoting in order to sit straight in the seat and lift both LEs over the edge of the car.

CHANGING THE TASK TO ACHIEVE INDEPENDENCE

The transfer approach may be easier for the client if he/she sits in the back seat of the car. Transferring into a van or SUV will be much more of a challenge. Clients will have difficulty because of the height of the vehicles and may either need to be lifted or use a ramp or step stool.

CHANGING THE TOOLS TO ACHIEVE INDEPENDENCE

As noted above, a ramp or step stool may be needed. Step stools may only be used with clients who have good mobility and strength. Because of the lack of stability with a step stool, the client must be closely assisted or supervised. Also, the client may not be able to access the car seat with his/her walker or wheelchair; therefore, for this transfer only, he/she may need to have handheld assist from the therapist, as appropriate.

Functional Ambulation for Clients With Physical Limitations

Basic foundation skills for functional ambulation include sufficient weight-bearing on the LEs, good LE ROM and strength, dynamic balance, and an adaptability to temporal and physical contexts.

Functional ambulation involves a repetition of movements called the *gait cycle*. The gait cycle involves two phases—the *stance phase* and the *swing phase*. The stance phase is when the heel contacts the ground and begins to bear weight until the foot is fully on the ground. Next, the heel lifts off the ground to make the mid-stance phase and then the push-off, which involves weight-shift forward onto the toes. Then, the foot is ready to leave the ground.

The swing phase involves the leg swinging forward with the foot clearing the ground. This is called *liftoff* or the early swing phase. The reach of late swing phase is when the leg decelerates and gets ready for heel contact.

It is important for OTs to have a basic understanding and working knowledge of the gait cycle in order to properly use observations, evaluate, plan, and execute interventions related to functional mobility, specific to the client's needs and related condition. Also, a good understanding of functional ambulation will allow for effective communication with physical therapy as well as other team members. For example, the OT may need to communicate with the physical therapist and/or other team members any changes in status or specific needs regarding of a client during functional mobility. Through this team process, making recommendations and decision making require basic knowledge of other health care practitioners' skills and roles.

CHANGING THE TASK TO ACHIEVE INDEPENDENCE

Compensation during functional mobility may require a change in the weight-bearing status of the client (see Table 3-15).

Table 3-16

FUNCTIONAL MOBILITY ASSISTIVE DEVICES

Wheelchair: manual, electric	Client with upper extremity function will typically use a manual chair.
Scooter	
Walker: standard, rolling, platform, 3-wheeled walker	Platform walker is used for clients who have sustained an UE injury and have weight-bearing restriction. Rolling walker is used with clients who do not have the strength to lift a standard walker. A three-wheeled walker offers more stability and has brakes.
Hemi-walker	One-handed walker with four legs to offer a wide base. It is held in the unaffected UE and is made for individuals with hemiparesis/hemiplegia.
Quad-cane: large and small-based (LBQC & SBQC)	A smaller base of support than a hemiwalker, but larger than a straight cane. Also has four legs. Base has two sizes.
Straight cane	Smallest base of support. May be used by client with neurological, orthopedic, or general balance conditions.
Crutches: axillary, platform, and Lofstrand	Platform crutches are also used for clients who have sustained an UE injury and have restrictions. Lofstrand crutches are used when less stability/support is needed than with axillary crutches (Pierson, 1996).

CHANGING THE TOOLS TO ACHIEVE INDEPENDENCE

Functional ambulation is an important aspect in achieving independence in ADLs. In order to achieve as much independence as possible, as well as ensure safety, stability, balance, and support, clients may require an assistive mobility device. Table 3-16 lists the many devices available, ranging from those offering the most assistance/stability (wheelchairs and walkers) to those offering the least (straight cane). See Figure 3-30 for sample assistive devices. The choice of assistive device also involves the client's ability to use one or both of the UEs.

Refer to the section on wheelchair mobility for descriptions of the power and manual wheelchairs. Clients who may only be able to ambulate short distances, such as from the bedroom to the bathroom, may need a manual wheelchair or a scooter for longer distances, such as community mobility. In addition, the use of a wheelchair/scooter during ADLs may allow the client to sit and rest, when needed, as well as free up the UEs, particularly where both hands are needed for a task.

In general, walkers offer maximal bilateral stability, balance, and support for individuals who have the use of both UEs. Types of walkers include standard, rolling, three-wheeled, and platform walkers. A *standard walker* must be slightly lifted off the ground with each step during ambulation. When negotiating corners, the standard walker must also be carried/lifted during the turn. The *rolling walker* is often helpful for individuals who cannot lift the walker or have an ataxic gait. For these individuals, it is usually easier to push the walker with each step, although turning corners may be more difficult. Also, clients who move too quickly or have difficulty stopping may not be safe with a rolling walker. These walkers may offer a folding option for fitting in a car, closet, or smaller space. A *walker basket* may fit in the front of most walkers in order to carry light items.

A *three-wheeled walker* that has larger, pneumatic wheels and hand brakes offers more stability and safety. Often, the three-wheeled walker will have a fold-down seat, offering rest periods for individuals with decreased endurance. This walker is capable of carrying heavier objects, although it is not indicated for clients who lean on the walker for support. The width and turning radius is larger and it is more difficult to store, particularly in a car.

Platform walkers may be the standard or rolling type and are fitted with either a single or double platform for the UE(s) to rest on. These are typically used for clients who require a walker for ambulation, but have either UE weight-bearing restrictions or significant deformities of wrists/hands that make grasping the walker too difficult. For example, a client with bilateral Colles fractures may need this type of walker not only because of weight-bearing restrictions, but also bilateral cast restrictions/immobility.

The *hemiwalker* is a one-handed walker typically used with individuals with hemiplegia who have limited to no use of the affected extremity. The hemiwalker offers a wide base of support and stability to be used on the unaffected side of the body.

Quad canes are four-pronged and provide less support and stability than the hemiwalker, although more than a straight cane. Quad canes are offered in two sizes: large-based (LBQC) and small-based (SBQC). Quad canes may be used for clients with neurological conditions who have progressed from a hemiwalker or for any individual who needs more support and stability than that offered by a straight cane, but does not need a walker.

Straight canes offer the smallest base of support and are used for individuals with mild balance and stability issues. Canes tend to be easier to use on stairs and narrow areas, and are more easily stored.

Axillary crutches are used for individuals needing less stability and support than a walker provides and allow increased speed of ambulation. Crutches require good standing balance and UE strength. They are easily used on stairs, stored, and transported. *Lofstrand crutches* allow the client to place the forearm in a cuff attached to the crutch versus positioning the device under the axillary area. Therefore, these crutches decrease injury to the axillary area and are easier to use on stairs. They are used when less stability/support is needed than with axillary crutches. *Platform crutches* use a similar attachment as the platform walker for individuals with weight-bearing or UE issues that limit gripping handles.

CHANGING THE TOOLS TO ACHIEVE INDEPENDENCE

The tools in Table 3-16 may be adapted depending upon the client's strength, ROM, balance, safety/cognition, and levels of assistance needed.

CHANGING THE TASK TO ACHIEVE INDEPENDENCE

The tasks of functional mobility may be adapted by changing the weight-bearing status of the client, as applicable.

- *Examples of ADL tasks that use functional mobility activities*: ADL tasks involving the above tools include: ambulating to the bathroom, toilet transfers, shower transfers, ambulating to the closet to retrieve clothes, etc.

COMPENSATION/ADAPTATION FOR WHEELCHAIR MOBILITY

A manual wheelchair is typically used by clients who have sufficient UE ROM and strength of one or both limbs for propulsion of the chair. One or both LEs may also assist with propulsion. A powered wheelchair or motorized scooter are appropriate for clients with limited or not

Figure 3-30. Sample ambulation devices.

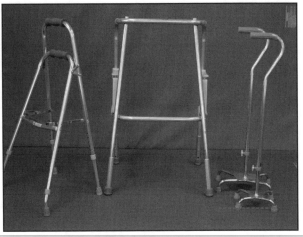

UE function or who have significantly decreased endurance. Typically, in order for a client to use a scooter, he or she will need to be independent with transfers and have good trunk control (Pedretti, 2000). When evaluating for the type of chair needed, the client's home, work, community, and transportation issues must be considered. The client must be instructed on mobility in all of the physical contexts of their lifestyle. Reid, Laliberte-Rudman, and Hebert (2002) suggest that occupational therapy intervention should focus more on wheelchair mobility in the appropriate clients. Through regularly practice, intervention has been shown to increase wheelchair speed, endurance, and handgrip strength, particularly when a functional approach is taken, such as with propelling to meals and social events. In addition, nursing home residents have reported wheelchair use increased feelings of independence, physical well-being, and emotional well-being (Simmons, Rahman, & Dietz, 1996). Increased wheelchair mobility will, furthermore, improve involvement in occupation, social participation, work, and roles, thereby, increasing quality of life and overall satisfaction.

Wheelchair mobility training typically begins in the rehabilitation clinic using a smooth surface in an uncluttered environment. The client must also be instructed in using the parts of the chair such as brakes and removable leg/armrests. Outside wheelchair mobility training must address propulsion on uneven surfaces/terrain, negotiating crowds and obstacles, narrow spaces, and accessibility in general.

- *Examples of ADL tasks that use wheelchair mobility activities*: Wheelchair mobility involves many functional activities such as transfers into and out of adapted shower stall, retrieving clothes from the closet/bureau, and general accessibility to the bathroom.

Basic Wheelchair Propulsion (Pierson, 1996)

- *Bilateral UE Propulsion*: The client grasps the top of the wheelchair handrims and pushes forward or pulls backward equally. When turning right or left, the client holds one handrim still, while pulling/pushing the other handrim in the desired direction.

- *Propulsion With One UE and One LE*: Typically, such as with hemiplegia, the functional UEs and LEs to be used are on the same side, although the technique may be adapted for contralateral sides. The client grasps the handrim on one side and pushes/pulls in the desired direction, while the LE works in the same direction. The foot may assist with turning as well.

- *Bilateral LE Propulsion*: The client uses the heels and soles of the feet to propel the chair in the desired direction, including turning the chair.

Changing the Task to Achieve Independence

The caregiver may offer assistance as needed with propulsion. The task may be broken down in small steps initially, such as with attempting turns or using both the UEs and LEs simultaneously.

Changing the Tools to Achieve Independence

The handrims may be adapted for ease of propulsion. The chair may also be lowered for clients using the LE(s) for propulsion. The client may need to wear leather gloves in order to increase grip on the handrims as well as for comfort.

Wheelchair Mobility on Ramps

Using a ramp for wheelchair mobility allows the client accessibility when stairs or the entrance to a van/bus or doorway are too high. The Americans with Disability Act ([ADA]28 CFR 36, §4) has specified regulations for the length, slope, and texture of a ramp. For every inch of rise, there must be 12 inches of ramp length and if the step is 4-inches high, the ramp must be 48 inches long.

Techniques for ascending (forward facing) a ramp involve leaning forward from the trunk, pushing on the handrims with a smooth forward motion. Moving the center of gravity forward is essential to avoid tipping backward. Descending (forward facing) a ramp involves positioning the hips to the back of the chair and sitting upright from the trunk (Pierson, 1996) or leaning backward slightly. The client should place the palms of the hands upon the handrims, keeping the fingers extended for safety. While applying even pressure on the handrims, the client controls or slows down the forward motion of the chair during the descent (Pierson, 1996). It is not recommended to use the handbrakes to slow the movement down the ramp.

Changing the Task to Achieve Independence

If a forward facing approach is not successful, the client may attempt a backward facing approach with ascending/descending. The client may require assistance for this task.

Changing the Tools to Achieve Independence

Wheelchairs may be adapted for specific needs, such as with a hemiplegic arm trough (Figure 3-31), antitip devices, high/low back rests, and desk arms, to name a few.

Wheelchair Wheelies

Wheelchair wheelies are an advanced skill that allows the client to elevate the caster wheels in order to manage curbs, sidewalks, or clear heights on the ground or floor. The therapist must first evaluate the client for safety, judgment, good UE strength, coordination, and balance while in the chair. While performing this technique, the therapist must also prepare for possible falls backward in the chair before the client fully acquires the skill (Trombly & Radomski, 2002).

Initiating the wheelie involves the client grasping onto the anterior handrim and quickly pulling back on the handrims with both hands. After this motion is completed, the hands are then moved posterior on the wheel rims. In this position, the chair frame is then rotated backward with a quick forward push on the wheel rims and a quick stop. This causes the caster wheels to elevate and the wheelchair balances only on the back wheels (Trombly & Radomski, 2002).

Wheelchair Mobility With Curbs and Steps

Although the need to negotiate curbs or steps in the community is becoming less and less frequent secondary to the ADA laws, there are still many circumstances where the client will need to know how to ascend/descend a curb or step. Clients who are deemed capable of performing a

Figure 3-31. Arm trough on a wheelchair.

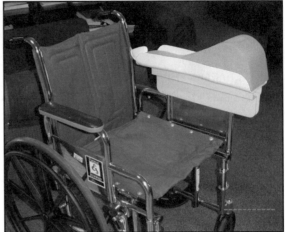

wheelie in a manual wheelchair may become independent with this skill. Ascending and descending a curb or steps using a powered chair or a scooter is not feasible, except for specialized chairs made for this purpose.

Ascending a curb or step is initiated by the client performing the wheelie with the casters positioned on the curb. Then, the client leans forward, gives a strong push on the handrims with the UEs, and propels the rear wheels onto the curb or step.

Descending uses a backward approach with the client leaning forward in the chair, pushing the handrims backward causing the back wheels to roll down the curb or step. The client may also use a forward-facing approach by using the wheelie position and pushing the back wheels off the curb/step.

In many instances, the client will need assistance with this task, particularly with decreased UE strength, decreased balance, and safety issues. For example, the client may be assisted with the wheelie component of the task or after the chair is in the wheelie position.

Descending more than one or two steps is a much more challenging and dangerous task, while ascending is not a feasible independent task. Two individuals should provide dependent mobility when ascending/descending several steps. When ascending, one individual stands behind the chair, which is positioned against the steps, while the second individual is in front. While tipping the chair backward, the individual in the back holds the handles and pulls the chair up each step. The individual in the front holds and balances the chair by the leg rests or frame. Descending involves the individual in the front guiding and holding onto the chair to control the speed, while the individual in the back assumes the same position, pushing the chair down each step. Proper body mechanics for both individuals providing the dependent mobility are essential (Trombly & Radomski, 2000).

Changing the Task to Achieve Independence

As above, the client may need the assistance of one or two individuals in order to complete the task. Forward facing and backward facing approaches may be attempted. In case of emergency, the appropriate client may be educated in ascending/descending stairs while sitting on the buttocks, using the UEs to bump up or down the stairs.

Changing the Tools to Achieve Independence

The wheelchair may be adapted with anti-tip devices. The weight of the wheelchair may also be a consideration.

Opening Doors While Propelling a Wheelchair

Propelling a wheelchair using a "self-closing" device to open/close doors involves client education in regards to safety techniques as well as working against resistance from the door (Pierson, 1996). When propelling through a door that opens away from the client, he/she must position the wheelchair at an angle facing the door latch. As this is done, the client reaches for the doorknob or latch with a quick, strong push. The client may need to stabilize the wheelchair by holding onto one handrim in order to prevent the chair from rolling backward. Then, the chair is quickly propelled through the doorway. The client may need to simultaneously hold the door open with one hand.

When propelling through a door that opens toward the client, the chair should be positioned at an angle facing the door hinges. The client reaches for the doorknob or latch with a quick, strong pull. Again, the client may need to hold the door open with one hand to prevent rolling backward. Several small pulls may be needed to open the door far enough.

CHANGING THE TASK TO ACHIEVE INDEPENDENCE

Moving through the door at an angle decreases the width needed to open the door and pass through, although if the chair does not fit at an angle, the approach should be facing the door. Because of the weight/resistance of a self-closing door, the client may require assistance

CHANGING THE TOOLS TO ACHIEVE INDEPENDENCE

Propelling the wheelchair without a self-closing device involves positioning the chair facing the door at an angle that is either facing the door latch or the hinges. The client will need to open the door only wide enough for the chair to fit through and follow the above procedures for opening the door, although less force is needed. The client will then turn the chair in order to close the door once through. When propelling the wheelchair through automatic doors, the client must first position him/herself far enough away for the doors to open safely without getting hit. The client may also benefit from an adapted doorknob turner or handle.

Getting On/Off an Elevator While Propelling a Wheelchair

The client may use a forward or backward approach when entering and exiting an elevator. Safety issues include: uneven surfaces between or a space between the floor of the elevator and the floor of the landing causing wheels to stop rolling or dropping into the space and/or the chair tipping forward; inability to reach the elevator buttons; or the doors attempting to close before the client is fully in or out of the elevator.

CHANGING THE TASK TO ACHIEVE INDEPENDENCE

The client may ask for assistance with either getting in/out of the elevator or using the control buttons. If the client has difficulty with one approach, such as entering forward-facing, he/she may attempt a backward approach.

CHANGING THE TOOLS TO ACHIEVE INDEPENDENCE

Again, the wheelchair may need anti-tip devices, one-arm drive, or adaptations to leg rests. The client who has had a THR may require a reclining wheelchair.

COMPENSATIONS/ADAPTATIONS OF FUNCTIONAL MOBILITY FOR CLIENTS WITH COGNITIVE, PERCEPTUAL, OR VISUAL LIMITATIONS: PERFORMANCE SKILLS/CLIENT FACTORS

As discussed previously, the AOTA *Framework* (2002a) presents perceptual and cognitive deficits within two sections of the document. The first section addresses basic cognitive skills in the general category of Performance Skills and the subsection of Process Skills. The AOTA *Framework* (2002) defines these basic cognitive skills as necessary to complete, manage, and modify ADL tasks.

Also a discussed previously, a second section of the AOTA *Framework* (2002) also addresses cognitive as well as perceptual deficits. The deficits are discussed under the sub-section of Client Factors, called Body Function Categories. These Body Function Categories are the affective, perceptual, and additional cognitive skills required to complete ADL tasks.

Specifically, this section will discuss cognitive and perceptual issues as they relate to functional mobility and ADL skills. The format is a brief reader introduction to the topic and examples of compensation/adaptation interventions. Examples of appropriate activities will be listed. For specific definitions, please refer to Chapter 2.

Compensation/Adaptation of Functional Mobility for Cognitive Deficits

See Figure 3-19.

PERFORMANCE SKILLS: PROCESS SKILLS

Table 3-17 briefly presents the subcategories of **Process Skills** as they are typically addressed less formally, within most mobility intervention plans.

Client Factors: Body Functions—Global Mental Functions

As stated earlier, *global mental functions* include consciousness and orientation. Consciousness is further divided to include arousal level and level of consciousness (AOTA, 2002).

AROUSAL LEVEL

Zoltan (2007) describes arousal level as "alerting," or a level of alertness that fluctuates (depending upon the state of one's CNS) and prepares for mobilization to attention.

Occupational therapy intervention at this level is very limited in terms of functional performance. Initially, the client's level of alertness may be very limited, not allowing for even the simplest of bed mobility training. The therapist may need to see the client for several brief sessions during the day, as able, focusing on sensory stimulation.

Changing the Task to Achieve Independence

The client's *level of arousal* or ability to participate in the task will dictate the need or readiness to change the method. As stated above, the therapist may need to see the client for several short sessions per day. Depending on the client's response, the physical context may need to be changed. For example, a less distractible environment may allow the client to better attend, or more than likely, a moderate amount of sensory stimulation such as noise/sound may improve the client's level of alertness (e.g., up-beat music).

Table 3-17

PROCESS SKILLS AND EXAMPLES OF COMPENSATION/ ADAPTATION STRATEGIES

Process Skill Subcategories (AOTA, 2002a)	Examples of Functional Mobility Compensation/ Adaptation Interventions
Energy	
Paces	Provide client with a clock and chart with estimated amount of time required to perform tasks such as transfers, functional ambulation, and transporting objects.
Attends	Refer to Specific Mental Functions category.
Knowledge	
Chooses	Before initiating a transfer, allow client to choose the appropriate assistive device that was used previously.
Uses	Ask client to describe the proper use of the above assistive device.
Handles	After verbally describing the use of the assistive device, ask client to physically demonstrate the use. Monitor for safety.
Heeds	Provide daily checklist to document each time a transfer is completed safely. For example, each time the client reaches back for the chair with both hands.
Inquires	Provide written directions for transfers/functional mobility. Request client to ask 1 or more question regarding safety with these tasks.
Temporal organization	
Initiation	Use external cues such as an audiotape with specific instructions to follow for each step of the transfer. Work with client to develop internal cues to initiate transfers.
Sequencing	Provide client with the written steps for safely completing transfers and functional mobility with/without assistive device, as appropriate.
Organizing space and objects	
Searches/locates	Provide external cuing such as labels or signs to assist with locating assistive device, bathroom, bedroom, etc.
Gathers	Provide checklist of items needed for transporting during functional mobility and transfers by using a walker basket or cart.
Organizes	Ask client to locate items in the environment that may hinder safe functional mobility, such as throw rugs, wet surfaces, or clutter.
Restores	Ask client to verbally instruct caregiver/therapist on how to safely return assistive device and/or transported objects to appropriate places.
Navigates	Teach client techniques for maneuvering in environment and/or around obstacles when using a wheelchair or assistive device.

continued

Table 3-17, continued

PROCESS SKILLS AND EXAMPLES OF COMPENSATION/ ADAPTATION STRATEGIES

Process Skill Subcategories (AOTA, 2002)	Examples of Functional Mobility Compensation/ Adaptation Interventions
Adaptation	
Notices/responds	Grade environmental, nonverbal, or perceptual cues as client notices/does not notice need to maneuver around obstacles.
Accommodates/adjusts	Problem-solve alternative actions or scenarios with client. For example, client should be able to modify functional mobility skills in order to safely maneuver in many different situations.
Benefits	Assist client/family in problem-solving various functional mobility situations that may occur upon discharge home and plan for adaptations.

The client may benefit from simple, very basic, verbal instructions, and potentially, tactile cuing. Instructions and verbal communication may be upgraded as the client's level of alertness increases.

In order to prepare the client for higher level skills and encourage sensory stimulation, basic bed mobility tasks may be attempted as the client's level of awareness improves. Refer to the section on bed mobility for more information. Depending on the client's level of alertness and attention span, functional mobility tasks may be graded, starting with simple bed mobility. Tasks such as those that require one- to two-step commands may be attempted such as bridging, rolling, reaching, and sitting upright. The client's level of alertness and attention span will also dictate the client's level of safety awareness and possible insight into his/her abilities.

As levels of alertness increase and the client is able to sit upright in bed, the therapist may begin addressing supine-to-sit transfers to the edge of the bed. While sitting at the edge, if the clients level of alertness allows, simple functional tasks may be attempted such as eating or brushing teeth.

In addition, as levels of alertness and attention improve, the therapist may begin to encourage the client to begin sit-to-stand activities.

Changing the Tools to Achieve Independence

At the most basic levels of bed and functional mobility, it is best to attempt tasks without tools, initially. As ability to attend improves, an assistive device may be introduced at the bedside for sit-to-stand activities, initially.

ORIENTATION

Orientation is an individual's awareness of time, person, and/or place. Deficits in orientation may typically present with memory loss and problems with new learning. Because the strategies for improving orientation must be reinforced with all functional mobility skills throughout the day by the entire rehabilitation team and family, the interventions below are presented in general terms. In addition, much of orientation interventions involve visual/verbal cuing and consistency.

Changing the Task to Achieve Independence

While performing bed mobility tasks, the therapist may informally involve orientation training as well. The session may include discussing the client's daily schedule for sitting up, sitting at the edge of the bed, and eventually getting out of bed for functional ambulation. These routines should be discussed and performed daily within the temporal context to encourage consistency and structure as much as possible, particularly as arousal levels improve. The client's physical context should also be well organized and neatly kept.

For example, the therapist may see the client either before or after breakfast, providing verbal orientation to the time of day as related to the functional mobility task. The method may be changed by asking the client basic orientation questions during the task. As another example, the therapist may progress the client to ambulate to the orientation board in order to read the schedule for the day. This should occur throughout the day with the assistance of staff and family.

Changing the Tools to Achieve Independence

As stated previously, basic orientation tools may begin with only a simple calendar or sign of the day and date. The method may be changed by introducing additional orientation boards as level of arousal improves. The boards may incorporate out-of-bed, functional mobility, and therapy schedules/information.

As the client's participation in therapy improves, additional tools may be added to assist with functional mobility such as a walker basket or a cart on wheels.

Client Factors: Body Functions—Specific Mental Functions

Specific Mental Functions include attention, memory, perception (visuospatial), thought functions (recognition, categorization, generalization), higher-level cognitive functions (judgment, concept formation, time management, problem solving, decision making), and mental functioning (motor planning, specifically dressing apraxia) (AOTA, 2002a).

ATTENTION

Attentional deficits may impact upon the client's ability to learn new functional mobility skills needed as a result of an illness or injury. For example, after sustaining a CVA, a client who needs to use a hemi-walker must have basic attention skills intact in order to be able to learn with higher-level specific mental functions such as memory and problem solving.

Clients who have conditions that affect attention skills must begin functional mobility training with simple tasks, in a short intervention time, which are adapted with progress. It is important for caregivers to speak simply, slowly, and allow for processing time (Zoltan, 2007). In addition, distraction should be kept to a minimum, although gradually introduced as the client is ready. The physical context should remain the same until the client demonstrates he/she is ready for generalization and/or gradation.

Changing the Task to Achieve Independence

Intervention may begin with bed mobility, progress to sitting at the bedside, and incorporate simple functional skills as attention skills improve. The client may then progress to standing activities and functional ambulation to the bathroom, closet, kitchen, etc. The client may be encouraged to "talk through" each step of the functional mobility activity. For example, the client may plan out the transfer from bed to chair with/without assistance from the therapist, before initiating the activity. Before each step of the activity is performed, the client may describe what he/she is going to do and what the safety issues are. The steps and difficulty of the functional mobility activities may be increased as the client is able to attend to task longer.

Changing the Tools to Achieve Independence

With clients being easily distracted, it is important to keep tools at a minimum and simplified. If needed, an assistive mobility device should be introduced first in order to safely initiate functional mobility. Additional tools such as a walker basket or push cart may be added as appropriate and the client's attention improves.

MEMORY

There are many types of memory and memory deficits, however, this section will focus specifically on intervention strategies related to functional mobility with an adaptive/compensation approach.

Changing the Task to Achieve Independence

Intervention strategies during functional mobility in general may be adapted by providing the client with a functional mobility schedule. For individuals who have limited carryover, involve him/her in developing the schedule.

The client may be assessed on a daily basis for carryover with the steps of functional mobility tasks, getting to and from specific areas, and safety precautions.

Changing the Tools to Achieve Independence

Cuing tools may be used as a strategy to increase memory through the use of signs to locate the bathroom, bedroom, memory notebooks, and labeling of storage areas.

An alarm clock may be set to remind the client of his/her out-of-bed, functional ambulation, and therapy schedule. The client may also be encouraged to wear a watch.

The Specific Mental Functions that are addressed less formally and/or less frequently within intervention plans are presented in Table 3-18. Those that require more detail and attention are discussed separately.

Compensation/Adaptation Interventions of Functional Mobility for Perceptual Deficits

As depicted in the table, the AOTA *Framework* document (2002a) does address "perceptual functions" under Client Factors, however particular perceptual topics are not listed. The topics chosen for discussion below have been determined from the authors' clinical practice as well as current references, which will be discussed throughout the information.

General compensatory/adaptive strategies that apply to clients diagnosed with perceptual deficits center around safety and environmental context. These general strategies include:

- Maximize safety in all situations. Remove unsafe objects as necessary.
- Educate client and all caregivers regarding functional limitations.
- Practice in a variety of physical contexts.

VISUAL FIXATION/SCANNING

Visual fixation involves the voluntary ability to sustain gaze while visually attending to a task or an object in the environment. Scanning allows the eye to follow an object without simultaneous head movement. While saccadic eye movement is typically symmetrical (e.g., reading), scanning during functional mobility activities, however, involves less predictable patterns that are more complicated (Zoltan, 2007). The client may have difficulty finding his/her way in the environment (topographical orientation), in particular with this deficit, while performing functional mobility tasks.

Table 3-18

SPECIFIC MENTAL FUNCTIONS AND EXAMPLES OF COMPENSATION/ ADAPTATION STRATEGIES

Specific Mental Functions Subcategories (AOTA, 2002a)	Examples of Compensation/Adaptation Interventions
Thought functions	
Recognition	During functional mobility session, items needed for bed to chair transfer include assistive device, slippers, and bedside chair. Ask client to locate bathroom during functional mobility.
Generalization	Address functional transfers in a variety of possible situations including chairs with/without arms, a couch, low/high surfaces, and a car. Functional mobility may include ambulating on ramps, stairs, grass, and in crowded/cluttered situations.
Higher level cognitive functions	
Judgment	Teach client to ask for help when unsure of safety. Ask client open-ended questions in order to think out loud before acting.
Concept formation	Keep a daily progress and achievement chart showing amount of assistance needed for transfers and amount of functional mobility achieved. Mark when goals have been achieved.
Time management	Provide out-of-bed and functional mobility daily schedule to encourage increased activity, particularly for discharge environment.
Problem solving	Ask client to assist with modifying environment for increased safety with functional mobility. Set up possible safety issues and ask client to identify them.
Decision-making	Provide client with two or more options for safe and appropriate decision making, before transferring. Allow client to think-out loud and verbally state the safe steps of the transfer.

Changing the Task to Achieve Independence

Provide cuing as needed. Cuing can be verbal or tactile when guiding the client to anchor the initiation of scanning (from left to right) and when controlling the speed of his/her scanning.

Scanning and anchoring tasks may be incorporated into bed mobility tasks when asking the client to roll and sit on one side of the bed, reach for the bed rail, and locate the assistive device and/or chair needed for the transfer.

During transfer activities, the client may be encouraged to scan a small area for the bedside chair and locate the arms of the chair for reaching back to sit. During functional ambulation, the client may scan the room for safety issues/obstacles, find the bathroom door, toilet/shower, and then head back to the bed or chair.

Changing the Tools to Achieve Independence

Brightly-colored stickers may be placed to the left of doorways in order for the client to anchor upon it and scan to the right without bumping into the side of the door when walking through. The same system may be used for the shower and toilet areas.

Table 3-19	
BODY SCHEME DISORDERS AND EXAMPLES OF COMPENSATION/ ADAPTATION STRATEGIES	
Body Scheme Disorders	*Examples of Compensation/Adaptation Interventions: Task and/or Tools Changed*
Somatognosia	During functional mobility activities, use verbal cues to increase awareness of body parts. For example: Ask client to pick up the part of the body that holds onto the hemi-walker.
Unilateral body neglect	Educate client on self-monitoring. For example, before standing, client should check to make sure both feet are in place on the floor and hands are pushing off to stand. A daily checklist may be used.
Right-left discrimination	Adapt instructions during functional ambulation training by using left/right directionality at request of client.

VISUAL INATTENTION/NEGLECT

Visual inattention/neglect is most concerning with functional mobility tasks as the client may be at a high risk for bumping into walls or furniture, falling, and/or injury. For those clients who are unable to become aware of the inattention, the therapist will need to modify and simplify the physical context as much as possible.

Changing the Task to Achieve Independence

During all functional mobility activities, encourage the client to increase visual attention by using his/her head and eyes to locate the bedrail, transfer surfaces, doorways, and assistive device. If needed, encourage the client to turn his/her body, as well. Use tactile and/or verbal cuing to encourage awareness of affected side. For example, as client is walking through a doorway, touch the client's affected UE while verbally cuing to attend to that side and prevent bumping into the doorway. If the client is unable to become aware of inattention, modify and simplify the physical context as much as possible. Gradually grade the tasks as appropriate (e.g., begin by providing all objects/items within client's intact visual field and grade).

Changing the Tools to Achieve Independence

Encourage client to wear a watch on the extremity of the affected side as a reminder to attend to that side and prevent bumping into doorways or walls. Attempt to use a mirror during sit-to-stand transfer activities to increase awareness of affected side.

BODY SCHEME

Because there are multiple forms of body scheme disorders, each one cannot be reviewed individually. For this reason, Table 3-19 identifies the most common forms of body scheme disorders as well as examples of compensatory/adaptive interventions for these.

VISUAL DISCRIMINATION

Visual discrimination involves the ability to distinguish between various objects or forms in relation to the environment (Zoltan, 2007). Because there are multiple forms of visual discrimi-

Table 3-20

Visual Discrimination and Examples of Compensation/ Adaptation Strategies

Visual Discrimination Disorder	Examples of Compensation/Adaptation Interventions: Task and/or Tools Changed
Depth perception	Adapt the environment by placing neon-colored tape at the edge of stairs and doorknobs.
Figure ground perception	Adapt functional mobility environment to increase cognitive awareness by carefully organizing items in a non-cluttered area. Adapt wheelchair brakes with neon stickers (Zoltan, 2007).
Spatial relations	Store assistive device and other needed items in a consistent manner.
Topographical orientation	Adapt functional mobility environment through the use of easy to read signs, pictures, and familiar landmarks.

nation disorders, each one cannot be reviewed individually. For this reason, Table 3-20 identifies the most common forms of visual discrimination disorders as well as examples of compensatory/ adaptive interventions for these.

Motor Planning

Motor planning issues may occur in relation to functional mobility with or without the use of assistive devices (tools). The client may have difficulty recognizing that assistive devices are used for functional mobility, even after instruction. In general, clients may also have difficulty negotiating each step involved with functional mobility. In addition, the client with motor planning deficits may present with difficulty following verbal directions when ambulating, which appears to be related to topographical orientation.

Changing the Task to Achieve Independence

- *General interventions with all types of functional mobility*: The therapist should attempt transfers in several ways. First, the client should be given simple verbal directions with minimal steps involved. If verbal cues are not successful, then tactile cuing may be attempted. The methods may be graded by increasing/decreasing the amount of cuing and steps of the directions involved.

  For deficits which resemble topographical disorientation, the environment may be adapted by simplifying cues for motor planning. For example, simple written cues posted for the client directing him/her towards the bathroom, stairs, chair, etc., may be provided. When supervised, the client may be given simple verbal commands or tactile cues in order to better negotiate the environment.

- *Example with transfers from bed to chair with walker*: The simplest method with apraxia may be a verbal command that briefly asks the client "please go to the chair." A more difficult two-step command may be to ask, "please get out of bed and sit in the chair." Because of physical limitations, the client may not be able to complete the task without the involvement of new learning. For example, if the client has a flaccid lower and UE, the command of "please go to the chair" will involve much more than it used to. Of course, the client will now need to learn how to negotiate right-sided flaccidity. The next method may be to attempt tactile cuing and physical assistance from the therapist, which is graded based on capabilities. (Refer to information on transfers in this chapter.)

- *Example with ambulation to the bathroom with walker*: The simplest method may be, again, to ask the client to walk to the bathroom. The therapist would place the walker in front of the client and wait to see if the client will be able to use it appropriately (see below). If the client does not initiate proper use of the walker, the therapist may attempt very simple verbal or tactile commands, as well as demonstration.

Changing the Tools to Achieve Independence

- *General interventions for all types of functional mobility*: Typically, the use of assistive devices may further confuse a client with apraxia, particularly if ideational apraxia is evident, which affects the ability to use tools. Usually, in terms of functional mobility, clients cannot safely perform tasks without the assistance of a walker, hemi-walker, cane, etc. This poses a significant challenge for the client who requires additional assistance secondary to balance and/or physical limitations, for example. Often, if two individuals are available, the client may do well with handheld assist. This offers the client tactile cuing as well as the guidance and support that may be needed with apraxia, as well as physical challenges.

COMPENSATION/ADAPTATION INTERVENTIONS OF FUNCTIONAL MOBILITY FOR VISION

GENERAL FUNCTIONAL MOBILITY STRATEGIES

- Maximize safety in all situations.
- Educate client and all caregivers regarding functional limitations.
- Practice strategies and adaptations in many possible environments and situations.
- Decrease clutter in environment.
- Use automatic, motion-controlled lighting.
- Control the amount of natural light in environment, as able, in order to decrease glare.
- Provide cuing, as needed.
- Use contrast whenever possible, for example:
  - ➤ Use markers on stairs.
  - ➤ Place neon-colored stickers on hand rail, water knobs (hot, in particular), light switches, and door handles.
  - ➤ Use colored toilet seat for contrast.
- Organize belongings in a systematic, predictable routine in order to locate them easily on a daily basis. For example: store bathroom items at a level within safe reach.
- Install carpeting in bathroom to prevent slippage and use bath mat.
- Install grab bars in tub/shower.

Low Vision

When addressing low vision (visual acuity) with a compensation/adaptive approach, the focus is primarily on changing the task within the clients' environment or physical contexts. Again, safety is the priority when considering the client's needs. The OT may need to refer to a low vision specialist in order to more specifically train the client on community functional mobility skills.

Changing the Task to Achieve Independence

Maximize contrast as able:

- *Functional mobility example*: When ambulating in bathroom and bedroom, encourage the client to use a systematic approach when moving in the environment. For example, the client should follow contrast on walls and flooring to maneuver in environment in the same manner upon each attempt.

- *Transfer example*: When transferring, use a systematic routine for organizing the environment and all transfer surfaces before moving.

Changing the Tools to Achieve Independence

- *Adapting walker*: Place bright green tennis balls or large neon stickers on the bottom of the walker legs in order for the client to easily identify where the walker ends and the floor begins.

- *Adapting wheelchair controls*: Paint wheelchair brakes and wheels with neon colors.

- *Adapting doorknobs*: Place neon-colored felt around doorknobs, or stickers in middle of doorknob.

Visual Field Deficits

Visual fields are the areas of vision that are seen without movement of the eyes or head. Deficits may present on one side of the visual field in one or both eyes (Jacobs & Jacobs, 2004). Functional mobility is especially challenging for these clients and all training must consider client safety.

Changing the Task to Achieve Independence

- *Functional mobility example*: Provide client and caregivers with strategies for cuing client into affected visual fields in order to prevent bumping into walls, furniture, or doors. Provide supervision during functional mobility whenever safety is not ensured.

- *Transferring example*: Teach client strategies for locating the transferring surface(s) safely. For example, remembering to reach back with both hands when sitting.

Changing the Tools to Achieve Independence

During functional mobility, provide all required tools/items with client's *intact* visual field as follows:

- *Transferring example*: For a client with a left field cut, transfer to the right side whenever possible.

- *Functional mobility example*: For a client with a left field cut, when turning around during ambulation, encourage client to turn to the right side.

- *Wheelchair mobility*: For a client with a left field cut, encourage client to stay on the right side of the hallway.

Maintenance for Functional Mobility

Positioning

Proper positioning is a continuous process that is necessary for the skin and joint integrity of all clients, as well as comfort. In addition, good positioning is vital for safe eating/feeding, most functional activities, eye contact, and effective communication. Although positioning is, of course, used with clients who are receiving rehabilitative occupational therapy services, it has been organized under maintenance as it often must or should be implemented long-term.

When considering positioning techniques and use of positioning tools (pillows, towel rolls, and bolsters), the individual needs of each client must be evaluated. Special attention must be given to clients with decreased/loss of sensation, paralysis, impaired skin integrity, poor nutrition, impaired circulation, and risk of contractures. For example, the therapist must observe areas were boney prominences may be experiencing pressure, causing redness, skin breakdown, eventual ischemia, and necrosis. Protective positioning restraints, such as wrist straps, should be used only on a short-term basis as their use may cause skin breakdown, as well (Pierson, 1996).

In general, positioning techniques should begin proximally as these techniques may influence the distal musculature (Crepeau, Cohn, Schell, & Boyt, 2003). For example, tone may be decreased in the distal extremity after positioning the UE properly. Caution should be taken when considering the placement of a pillow under the knee as the position may cause an eventual flexion contracture or deep vein thrombosis (Crepeau, Cohn, Schell, & Boyt, 2003).

Positioning schedules typically require the client's position to be changed approximately every 2 hours in order to prevent skin breakdown. Positions that provide weight-bearing into the involved extremity may assist with normalizing tone and enhance sensory awareness.

Purpose of Proper Positioning

According to Pierson, there are specific purposes of proper positioning. These are:

- Prevent contractures and soft tissue injury.
- Provide comfort.
- Support and stabilize the client.
- Allow for efficient function of organ systems.
- Provide relief of prolonged pressure through position changes (1996).

In addition, proper positioning allows for greater client interaction with the environment and greater participation in functional activities. Once a decubiti is formed, the client is often restricted in activity, which further emphasizes the importance of proper positioning, either in bed or in a chair. The typical boney prominences that are at risk for pressure ulcers are listed in Table 3-21. When positioning clients, certain precautions should be followed. According to Pierson (1996), these include:

- Observe the skin color.
- Protect the boney prominences listed in Table 3-21.
- Avoid excessive pressure to soft tissue, circulatory or neurological areas.
- Be aware of the special needs of clients with decreased mental status, decreased level of alertness, the frail elderly, individuals with paralysis, individuals with impaired circulation, and individuals with decreased sensation.

Table 3-21

BONEY PROMINENCES

Supine	Side-Lying	Sitting
Occipital tuberosity	Lateral ear	Ischial tuberosity
Spine of the scapula	Lateral ribs	Scapular/vertebral prominences
Inferior angle of the scapula	Lateral acromion process	Medial epicondyle of humerus
Spinous processes of vertebrae	Lateral head of humerus	
Posterior iliac crest	Medial/lateral epicondyle of humerus	
Sacrum	Greater trochanter of femur	
Medial epicondyle of humerus	Medial/lateral condyle of femur	
Posterior calcaneus	Malleolus	
Greater trochanter and head of fibula		

Adapted from Pierson, F. M. (1999). *Principles and techniques of patient care* (2nd ed.). Philadelphia, PA: W.B.Saunders.

Table 3-22

POSITIONING LYING ON THE INVOLVED SIDE

The Involved Side	*The Uninvolved Side*
• Scapular protraction • Shoulder flexion to 90° • Hip flexion • Shoulder external rotation • Full elbow extension • Neutral hip • Slight knee flexion	• Upper extremity positioned alongside the trunk and hip • Knee flexion • The hip and knee are supported with a pillow between them and the involved LE • An additional pillow is placed along the client's back in order to maintain the position

Adapted from Crepeau, E. B., Cohn, E. S., & Schell, B. A. B. (2003). *Willard and Spackman's occupational therapy for physical dysfunction* (10th ed.). Philadelphia, PA: Lippincott Williams & Wilkins.

Positioning in Bed

The typical *bed positions* include side-lying on the involved side, side-lying on the uninvolved side, and lying supine.

Ideal positioning for the client lying on the involved side is described in Table 3-22 and is pictured in Figure 3-32. These are general guidelines and may need to be adapted for particular clients.

Ideal positioning for the client lying on the uninvolved side is toward prone and described in Table 3-23 and pictured in Figure 3-33. These are general guidelines and may need to be adapted for particular clients.

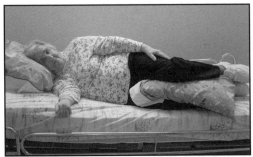

Figure 3-32. Client lying on the involved side.

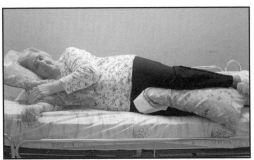

Figure 3-33. Client lying on the uninvolved side.

Figure 3-34. Client lying in supine.

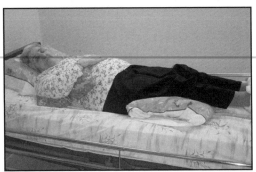

Table 3-23

POSITIONING LYING ON THE UNINVOLVED SIDE

Involved Side	*Uninvolved Side*
• Entire UE supported on a pillow supporting involved UE	• UE positioned under a pillow
• Scapular protraction	• LE in slight hip/knee flexion
• Shoulder flexion to 90 degrees	
• Elbow flexion up to 90 degrees	
• Full wrist and finger extension	
• The hip and knee flexed to 45 degrees	
• LE supported on a pillow	

Adapted from Crepeau, E. B., Cohn, E. S., & Schell, B. A. B. (2003). *Willard and Spackman's occupational therapy for physical dysfunction* (10th ed.). Philadelphia, PA: Lippincott Williams & Wilkins.

Ideal positioning for the client in supine is described below and pictured in Figure 3-34. These are general guidelines and may need to be adapted to particular clients (Crepeau, Cohn, Schell, & Boyt, 2003).

- A pillow positioned under client's involved scapula and hip.
- Involved scapula and hip are in slight protraction.
- Involved shoulder is slight abduction and external rotation.
- Involved elbow flexed, wrist, and fingers in extension.
- Involved hip and knee slightly flexed and positioned in midline

Sitting

Goal setting considerations for *sitting* should involve the client's medical/physiological status, the client's function and lifestyle, as well as the ultimate goals of the client. Medical considerations include potential for developing contractures, organ function, soft tissue integrity, and pain/discomfort levels. Functional considerations include the clients tolerance for activity, level of independence, motor control, and communication abilities. Personal and lifestyle considerations may include community involvement and mobility, client roles, environmental issues, and mobility in the home.

Considerations with sitting include promoting trunk stability in an upright midline position while allowing for mobility of the extremities and interaction with the environment. Further considerations include the type of chair chosen. The amount of support given by the chair includes the type of seating surface. For example, special seat cushions are available to prevent skin breakdown for clients with long-term needs. Firm cushions are typically used for prevention of internal hip rotation while in the chair, assisting with trunk stability and support by properly positioning the back and UEs, and providing support for sitting balance. Lumbar supports promote anterior pelvic tilt when needed. Proper positioning of the LE includes the hips, knees, and ankles in 90 degrees of flexion when sitting.

Foot stools, adjustable leg rests, wedge cushions, lapboards, adjustable arm rests, and straps may be used to enhance symmetrical and supported sitting positions.

Positioning for the Client With a Neurological Injury/Illness

Proper positioning of the client should begin immediately with all team members and caregivers educated and involved with this process. For example, a client with hemiplegia who initially presents with flaccidity of the involved extremities should be positioned preventing an eventual flexor synergy of hip, which includes external rotation, abduction, and knee flexion. Proper positioning is typically in the opposite pattern of the synergy, although each client must be considered individually. Therefore, positioning a client with a flexor synergy includes knee extension, lateral support of the LE with a pillow or rolled blanket to prevent hip abduction and external rotation.

Extensor synergy occurs when the later stages of hemiplegia cause spasticity of the extensor muscles, which are stronger than the flexors in the affected extremity (Pedretti, 2000). The extensor synergy includes extension and adduction at the hip, knee extension, and ankle plantarflexion. Recommended bed positioning for a client with extensor synergy includes lying supine with slight hip and knee flexion, which may be maintained with a towel roll or small pillow under the knee. In order to prevent adduction and internal rotation, a pillow or rolled blanket may be used to provide medial support between the LEs. While in the supine position, ankle plantarflexion must be prevented through the use of multipodus boots. Further ankle plantar flexion may be prevented by not allowing tight-fitted sheets/blankets to pull the feet into this position.

The affected UE should be positioned to prevent shoulder subluxation, soft tissue contractures, decreased ROM, and spasticity/flexor synergy resulting in general decreased function. The following positions should be avoided: prolonged shoulder adduction and internal rotation; elbow flexion, supination or pronation, wrist, finger, or thumb flexion; and finger/thumb adduction. Therefore, proper positioning of the affected extremity includes shoulder abduction, external rotation, elbow extension, neutral forearm rotation, slight wrist extension, thumb abduction and extension, finger extension, and slight abduction (all in varying amounts) (Pierson, 1996).

CHANGING THE TOOLS TO ACHIEVE INDEPENDENCE

Positioning may be provided with a pillow, small bolster, rolled towel/blanket, lap tray, or arm trough. The unaffected UE may also assist with positioning, particularly with maintaining the affected extremity in midline.

Caution should also be used with static positioning for long periods of time. Proper positioning *and* position changes should be alternated with regular ROM and self ROM exercises (refer to Chapter 2).

Positioning With for the Client With a Total Hip Replacement

PRECAUTIONS WITH THR (PIERSON, 1996)

Position the client in slight hip abduction from midline and neutral rotation. Hip adduction should not be beyond the midline of the body (e.g., do not cross legs). ADL activities with this motion may include crossing legs to don socks and shoes. The listing below describes proper positioning/precautions for clients with THR (Pierson, 1996).

1. The affected hip should not be *extended* beyond neutral.

2. While in side-lying, the affected hip should maintain *abduction and neutral rotation*. The client should be positioned with the affected LE on top of the non-affected extremity with pillows or a bolster supporting and maintaining the position.

3. *Anterior or anterior-lateral approaches* must not externally rotate the hip.

4. *Posterior or posterior-lateral approaches* must not internally rotate the hip.

5. Activities that involve rotation or twisting of the trunk with the LEs fixed must be avoided as these motions involve *hip rotation* (e.g., standing from the toilet and rotating the trunk around to one side in order to flush)

6. Do not *flex* the affected hip beyond 90 degrees with a posterior or posterior-lateral approach (e.g., when sitting on the toilet, a raised toilet seat is necessary to avoid 90 degrees of hip flexion).

ADDITIONAL PRECAUTIONS WITH POSITIONING AND FUNCTIONAL MOBILITY FOR THR

- *Lying*: Client should primarily lie supine while sleeping or resting with a pillow positioned between both UEs, above the knees, to prevent hip adduction. If the client needs to position in side-lying, a pillow should also be placed between the LEs, above the knees.

- *Transfers*: Scoot to the edge of the bed or chair before standing. Position the affected LE in front of the other when standing from bed or chair. Avoid low surfaces.

- *Sitting*: Chairs should be higher than knee height, have a firm sitting surface, a straight back, and arm rests. Avoid soft chairs, rocking chairs, sofas, or stools. Reclining wheelchairs will accommodate hip precautions by adjusting the backrest.

- *Ambulation*: Wear well-fitting, supportive, nonskid shoes. Avoid uneven surfaces as able. Follow weight-bearing status. Avoid pivoting on affected LE. Take small steps when turning.

- *Toileting*: Use a raised toilet seat or seat above knee height. Avoid twisting for personal hygiene.

- *Bathing*: Avoid bending or reaching for items, tub controls, etc. Avoid bending or squatting to bathe the LE. Use a long-handled sponge and reacher instead.

- *Dressing*: Avoid bending over, raising LEs, or crossing legs. Remain seated when donning clothes over feet. Use long-handled devices such as a reacher, dressing stick, and long-handled shoe horn. Use shoes that close with hook and loop fasteners, slip-ons, or elastic shoelaces.

- *Car transfers*: Avoid entering the car while standing on a curb or step. Avoid cars with deep or low seats. Use a pillow to raise seat heights.

Issues With Positioning Clients With Rheumatoid Arthritis (Pierson, 1996)

Because rheumatoid arthritis is a systemic disease that involves the musculoskeletal system—specifically the joints—prolonged immobilization or positioning should be avoided in order to prevent contractures. Gentle active and passive ROM of involved *and* uninvolved joints should be performed, as tolerated, on a regular basis. When rheumatoid arthritis is in an exacerbated stage of acute inflammation, extra caution should be taken. Refer to Tables 3-13 through 3-15 for general positioning techniques.

Issues With Positioning Clients With Burns (Pierson, 1996)

Positioning issues with burns include healing of skin, scar tissue development, contractures, and pain. Prolonged immobilization or positioning of affected joints should be avoided, particularly in the "position of comfort." Examples of the position of comfort are prolonged flexion or adduction positions involving the least amount of stress on the burn site or graft. Splinting is the primary positioning technique for burned extremities. Refer to Tables 3-13 through 3-15 for general positioning techniques.

Issues With Positioning Clients With Amputations (Pierson, 1996)

For clients with an above-the-knee amputations (AKA), the following positions should be limited or avoided due to risk of contracture of the hip flexor musculature: prolonged hip flexion, elevation of residual limb on a pillow while supine, sitting limited to 30 minutes at a time. Hip abduction of the residual limb should be avoided to prevent contracture of these muscles. The client should position the pelvis level in order to maintain trunk alignment while supine. This position will also help to prevent back pain and postural issues. When standing, the client should position the residual limb in extension. Occasional prone-lying is recommended to encourage hip and residual limb extension.

Clients with a below-the-knee amputation (BKA) should avoid the following positions in order to avoid the risk of contractures: prolonged hip and knee flexion, as well as elevation of the residual limb on a pillow while the client is supine. When the residual limb is elevated, the knee should be positioned in extension. The client should not sit longer than 30 minutes at a time in order to decrease the risk of hip flexor and knee contractures. Whenever the client is supine, sitting, or standing, the knee should be positioned in extension. Again, prone-lying is recommended to encourage extension of the residual limb.

The risk of contracture of the residual limb musculature will limit the client's ability to be fit with and use a prosthetic device; therefore, proper positioning is essential. Refer to Tables 3-13 through 3-15 for general positioning techniques.

ADL: EATING/DYSPHAGIA

INTRODUCTION

Before reading this section, it is important to note the information provided in this text regarding eating/dysphagia is considered entry-level. According to AOTA (2000), advanced skills are necessary for the OT to use various assessment or intervention tools safely, such as videofluoroscopic swallowing studies, videoendoscopy, fiberoptic endoscopic assessments, ultrasound, electromyography, and biofeedback. In addition, certain conditions typically require advanced skills, such as for clients with tracheotomies and laryngectomies. The advanced skill levels, which will not be addressed in this text, should build upon the entry-level skills as presented in depth throughout this section. For more information and training regarding advanced skills in eating/dysphagia interventions, refer to the resources provided in Appendix A.

DEFINITIONS

AOTA (2002a, p. 620) defines eating as "the ability to keep and manipulate food/fluid in the mouth and swallow it." Thus, eating is the ADL skill that is evaluated by the OT. The deficit that is addressed as a result of difficulty with eating is categorized as *dysphagia*. Dysphagia includes all the stages of swallowing which will be discussed in depth below. Feeding (as discussed earlier in this chapter) is a distinctly different activity of daily living skill and is defined by AOTA (2002a, p. 620) as "the process of bringing food from the plate or cup to the mouth." The specific difference is that dysphagia intervention addresses oral-motor deficits while feeding intervention addresses the actual skill of feeding oneself. It is common, however, to find deficits in eating and feeding at the same time (AOTA, 2002a).

ROLE OF THE OT AND COTA

Since eating is a basic human need, it is a primary focus of evaluation and intervention of ADLs. According to AOTA, "OTs and OTAs have the knowledge and skill, and are uniquely suited, to play a lead role in the evaluation and intervention of eating and feeding problems" (2002b, pg. 2). Academic institutions provide the basic, entry-level knowledge of eating and feeding issues. The entry-level practitioner may then choose to progress his/her skills to an advanced-level while working under supervision of a therapist experienced in dysphagia.

The role of the OT is as a dysphagia clinician—performing screenings, assessments, consulting, recommending, reporting, and carrying-out the intervention program (AOTA, 2000). The COTA, under the supervision of the OT, may contribute to, and implement the intervention plan (AOTA, 2002b). For specific details of entry-level and advanced-level knowledge and skills for eating and feeding, refer to AOTA's (2002b), *Specialized knowledge and skills in eating and feeding for occupational therapy practice*.

TYPICAL DIAGNOSES SEEN WITH DYSPHAGIA

- Cerebral vascular accidents
- Brain injuries

- Alzheimer's disease
- Huntington's disease
- Brain tumors
- Parkinson's disease
- Multiple sclerosis
- Myasthenia gravis
- Amyotrophic lateral sclerosis
- Developmental disorders
- Guillain-Barré syndrome
- Spinal cord injury
- Pneumonia
- HIV/AIDS
- Facial nerve paralysis
- Head, neck, and oral cancers, as well as the side effects of chemotherapy and/or radiation therapy
- Laryngectomy
- Respiratory issues
- Burns
- Chronic obstructive pulmonary disease
- Nasogastric tubes
- Tracheostomy
- Prolonged mechanical ventilation
- Psychiatric disorders (AOTA, 2002a)

SIGNS AND SYMPTOMS OF DYSPHAGIA

- Labored breathing/rales
- A wet, "gurgly" voice
- Aspiration
- Pocketing of food
- Coughing while eating/drinking
- Nasal regurgitation
- Rejection of food
- Sensory issues with food
- Open mouth posture
- Drooling
- Increased eating time (chewing and/or swallowing)
- Poor laryngeal elevation

- Poor tongue movement
- Complaints of food stuck in throat
- Painful swallow (Logemann, 1998)

DYSPHAGIA TEAM

The management of clients with dysphagia is often handled as a multidisciplinary team. Each member of the dysphagia team offers a specific expertise, whether it be in an acute care, subacute, skilled nursing, or home care environment. In addition to the OT, team members include:

- **Speech-language pathologist**: OTs and speech-language pathologists (SLP) often work together providing dysphagia evaluation and interventions. In addition, the SLP will offer interventions for voice, communication, and cognitive deficits, as appropriate.

- **Dietitian**: The dietitian's responsibilities include making sure the nutritional and fluid needs of the clients are met. The dietician also creates dysphagia diet levels.

- **Physician**: The physician determines the diagnosis and writes the referrals for dysphagia evaluations and interventions, specialty referrals, and medications.

- **Radiologist**: The radiologist conducts and analyzes assessments, which may include videofluoroscopy and ultrasound.

- **Nurse**: In addition to providing daily mealtime care for the client, the nurse observes for signs/symptoms of dysphagia, and reports information about the client's status to the team.

- **Respiratory therapist**: The respiratory therapist monitors the client's respiratory status in order to assure the client's airway and breathing is optimal for eating. This may include clients who are ventilator-dependent or those with tracheotomies.

- **Others**: Other disciplines who may consult with the dysphagia team include physical therapist, pharmacist, dentist, social worker, pulmonologist, or gerontologist.

PHASES OF THE SWALLOWING PROCESS AND RELATED DEFICITS

The phases of the swallowing process are the pre-oral phase, oral preparatory phase, oral phase, pharyngeal phase, and esophageal phase. Dysphagia may occur in one phase of the swallowing process, or in more than one phase. The first three phases are assessed through a dysphagia evaluation, while the pharyngeal and esophageal phases are assessed via a modified barium swallow (MBS) (Avery-Smith, 2003). A basic description of each phase and skills required are as follows:

- **Pre-oral phase**: The phase of eating when food/fluid is brought to the mouth. This process includes the skills of feeding as well as preparing for the next phases of the swallow (Logemann, 1998).

- **Oral preparatory phase**: The phase of eating when food is manipulated by the lips, cheeks, tongue, and jaw into a bolus that prepares the food for a safe swallow. Motor as well as sensory (taste, primarily) skills are required at this phase (Logemann, 1998).

- **Oral phase**: The phase of eating in which the bolus is propelled to the base of the tongue in order to swallow. Skills required include sensation, motor planning, sufficient tongue tone, movement, and coordination. The normal timing of this phase is between 1.0 to 1.5 seconds, after which the phase is considered to have a delay (Logemann, 1998).

- **Pharyngeal phase**: The phase of eating whereby the swallow is further triggered and initiated. Skills required include proper tongue base movement, closure of the soft palate, bilateral pharyngeal strength, sufficient laryngeal elevation, and sufficient airway closure during the swallow to prevent aspiration. This phase should last less than 1 second (Logemann, 1998).

- **Esophageal phase**: The phase of eating when the bolus moves from the esophagus into the stomach (Logemann, 1998). Skills required include sufficient esophageal function and motility.

REMEDIATION OF EATING/DYSPHAGIA

While the majority of this text discusses adaptation/compensation, remediation will be discussed in this section of eating/dysphagia because both approaches are closely tied to this skill.

AOTA (2003) categorizes remedial eating techniques as *indirect interventions* related to client factors which may not involve actual eating. These interventions are focused on facilitating and improving the swallow and include:

Decreased Range of Motion

Exercises include passive, active-assisted, active ROM, and self ROM of the tongue, lips, and cheek. Typically passive ROM may be performed with gloved fingers or the back of a spoon. In addition, laryngeal elevation may be completed by facilitating the Adam's apple into an upward/downward movement. Self-ROM may be performed as a passive or active-assisted form of exercise, as above. Active ROM may be performed in conjunction with passive ROM (as voluntary motion improves) or in isolation. Oral-motor ROM exercises include:

- Lip pursing
- Smiling (lip retraction)
- Tongue protrusion/retraction
- Tongue lateralization
- Jaw lateralization

Decreased Oral-Motor Strength

Oral-motor strengthening exercises may be an added intervention as active ROM increases. Decreased oral-motor strength involves resistance applied with fingers or tongue depressor to the movements as listed in *ROM*. In addition, lip, cheek, breath, and oral strength may be increased through sucking and blowing exercises using items such as:

- Blowing bubbles
- Sucking on a straw
- Holding a tongue depressor between the lips
- Blow pens, whistles
- Popsicles
- Lollipops
- Gum (Logemann, 1998)

Strengthening of pharyngeal and laryngeal movements may also include exercises that facilitate tongue retraction, such as yawning and gargling. In addition, asking the client to raise his/her voice when talking or throat clearing on a regular basis may also increase pharyngeal and laryngeal strength. *Note*: Contraindications for oral-motor strengthening/resistance may include conditions such as amyotrophic lateral sclerosis and myasthenia gravis because further weakness may be promoted. In addition, it is important to use care with the above tools to prevent aspiration (Avery-Smith, 2003).

- *Hypersensitivity*: The primary remedial intervention technique for facial and oral hypersensitivity is graded desensitization. Each client will be sensitive to his/her own individual textures, although typically, firm textures are most tolerable (AOTA, 2003). Therefore, desensitization techniques should begin with firm textures to the least sensitive areas of the face and/or mouth. Firm textures may include metal utensils, tongue depressor, or laryngeal mirror. Grading desensitization to lighter textures will include items such as a gloved finger, toothbrush, disposable oral swabs, and plastic utensils.

- *Hyposensitivity*: Sensory re-education and sensory stimulation programs are the primary remedial intervention techniques for hyposensitivity. Sensory re-education involves the use of familiar oral-motor objects such as utensils, a toothbrush, and hot/cold items that the client attempts to identify. Examples of sensory stimulation items include the use of a small vibrator, electric toothbrush, popsicles, or ice chips.

- *Low tone:* Increased tone may be facilitated using techniques such as a small vibrator, electric toothbrush, or a chilled laryngeal mirror applied to the cheeks, lip, and/or oral cavity. Quick stretch may also be used as a facilitation technique.

- *High tone*: The first remedial attempt at decreasing oral-motor tone should be proper positioning (refer to section on positioning). New techniques and materials should be gradually introduced in order to prevent anxiety that may further increase tone. In addition, slow passive stretch to the head, neck, and oral-motor area typically decrease tone.

- *Abnormal reflexes*: Once again, proper upright positioning should be the first remedial intervention performed to decrease abnormal reflexes. Items or strategies that promote these reflexes should be avoided. For example, to prevent tonic bite, a metal utensil should not touch the client's teeth (Avery-Smith, 2003).

- *Decreased initiation of the swallow*: A remedial technique intended to stimulate the swallow is performed with a chilled laryngeal mirror. The faucial pillars are stimulated by the mirror and then the client is asked to dry swallow, and when ready, attempt a specific texture of food or liquid (Avery-Smith, 2003).

COMPENSATION/ADAPTATION OF EATING DEFICITS/DYSPHAGIA FOR CLIENTS WITH PHYSICAL LIMITATIONS: PERFORMANCE SKILLS/CLIENT FACTORS

Avery-Smith (2003) categorizes the specific process of eating food as *direct intervention* for dysphagia. Therefore, the actual functional skills involved with eating/dysphagia will be addressed in this compensation/adaptation section. Motor skill deficits and body function limitations may cause choking, malnutrition, dehydration, and eventual aspiration. Prior to addressing dysphagia deficits, the OT should evaluate the client's ability to sit upright in order to increase safety during eating. See Figure 3-35 for an example of proper upright positioning while eating at bed level. Physical deficits, however, are not the only consideration with dysphagia.

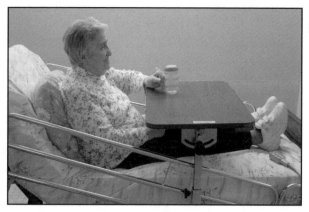

Figure 3-35. Example of proper upright posture at bed level for eating.

Eating, as a basic human need and satisfaction, involves performance patterns such as habits and routines. For example, we often set our clocks by when the next meal will be. The cultural context of eating is also an important consideration when working with clients who have eating dysfunction or dysphagia. For example, many cultures have family gatherings at the Sunday afternoon meal. A client diagnosed with dysphagia who is recommended to be NPO (nothing by mouth), and given a nasogastric or gastric tube, no longer can normally engage in these lifelong performance patterns.

In terms of activity demands, eating involves many social experiences. Most of our social activities involve eating, which may cause a client who is NPO to be isolated and embarrassed in these situations. Therefore, while the OT is facilitating safe and effective compensation/adaptations for the physical aspects of dysphagia, he/she should also consider the social, emotional, and cultural impacts of this condition.

Compensation/Adaptation Interventions of Eating Deficits/ Dysphagia for Range of Motion, Strength, and Coordination Deficits

ROM, strength, and coordination limitations will impact the client's ability to eat safely without aspiration. Typically, a client with dysphagia will be on an adapted diet, depending upon the motor skill or body function limitations. The dysphagia evaluation, modified barium swallow/videofluoroscopy , as appropriate, will help the OT when recommending a safe diet level for the client.

DIET LEVELS

The National Dysphagia Diet Task Force (NDDTF) (McCullough, Pelletier, & Steel, 2003) has developed national standards for food and fluid consistencies for dysphagia intervention. The four food consistency levels are described in Table 3-24, and fluid consistencies are described in Table 3-25. There are a number of foods that Groher (1997) states are best to avoid when working with clients who are experiencing dysphagia. These are listed below:

- Mashed potatoes
- Crackers
- Onions
- Carbonated beverages
- Plums

Table 3-24	
DIET LEVELS	
NPO: Nothing by mouth	Secondary to high aspiration risk and/or significant safety issues with eating, it is recommended for the client have an "alternative method of nutrition."
Level 1 Diet: Pureed Diet	The consistency of this diet is similar to pudding, requiring little to no chewing, and easy to swallow. Other examples include: mashed potatoes, cottage cheese, nectars, thick milkshakes, sherbet, yogurt, and custard (Jackson Siegelbaum Gastroenterology, 2002; Dorner, 2002).
Level 2 Diet: Mechanical Soft Diet	The consistency of this diet is ground, moist, and semisolid. Dry foods such as crackers and bread are avoided. Appropriate foods should form into a cohesive bolus. Other examples include: ground meats, potatoes, cooked vegetables, canned fruit, scrambled eggs, ripe bananas, and cooked cereals (Jackson Siegelbaum Gastroenterology, 2002; Dorner, 2002).
Level 3 Diet: Advanced Diet	The consistency of this diet is considered soft-solid requiring increased ability to chew. Food is chopped into bite-sized servings. Avoid foods which are dry, sticky, or crunchy. Examples of included foods are: chopped meats, potatoes, canned fruit, and cooked vegetables. Soft breads may be allowed (Jackson Siegelbaum Gastroenterology, 2002; Dorner, 2002).
Level 4: Regular Diet	All consistencies allowed.

- Prunes
- Any sticky boluses
- Any boluses that fall apart easily
- Dry boluses
- Mucus producers

With most dysphagia conditions, it is advised to crush medications (as able) in applesauce, jelly, custard, or gelatin.

The following are ROM, strengthening, and coordination adaptations/compensations for clients with dysphagia.

Changing the Task to Achieve Independence

- Attempt modified swallowing techniques to prevent aspiration, such as double swallows, supraglottic swallow (the client holds his/her breath while swallowing, and coughs before letting out the breath), and super-supraglottic swallow (the client holds his/her breath, bears down hard, swallows, and coughs after swallowing). Contraindications to the latter two techniques are cardiac or high blood pressure conditions (Logemann, 1998).

Table 3-25

DIET CONSISTENCIES FOR FLUIDS

Thick liquids (spoon-thick liquids)	Liquids are thickened to a puree or pudding consistency.* Refer to pureed diet level for examples (Jackson Siegelbaum Gastroenterology, 2002; Dorner, 2002).
Honey consistency liquids	Liquids are thickened to a honey consistency.* (Jackson Siegelbaum Gastroenterology, 2002; Dorner, 2002).
Nectar consistency liquids (medium consistency)	Liquids are thickened to a nectar consistency.* Examples of this consistency are: eggnog, nectars, tomato juice, and milk shakes. (Jackson Siegelbaum Gastroenterology, 2002; Dorner, 2002).
Thin liquids	Typical consistency of liquids with no modifications required.

*Commercial thickening agents include: Thick n Easy (manufactured by American International Products, Inc. [Los Angeles, Ca]) and Thick-it (manufactured by Milani Foods, Inc [Melrose Park, IL]).

- Ask the client to rotate the head and neck toward the affected side when swallowing in order to close off the weak side of the pharynx. This technique allows the unaffected side to propel the bolus and prevent pooling or aspiration (Avery-Smith, 2003).

- Ask the client to tuck his/her chin to the chest while swallowing in order to decrease the risk of aspiration with a weak swallow (Logemann, 1998).

- Ask the client to perform "effortful" swallows or swallow hard in order to decrease the risk of accumulating oral residue (Avery-Smith, 2003).

- The Mendelsohn Maneuver involves asking the client to hold the tongue into the hard palate while attempting to maintain elevation of the larynx during the swallow (Logemann, 1998).

- Clients with unilateral pharynx weakness may attempt eating in side-lying on the non-affected side if the above techniques fail, as appropriate (Avery-Smith, 2003).

- If a facial droop is present, ask the client to hold the affected side of the lips closed during the oral and swallowing stages to decrease risk of food loss (Logemann, 1998).

- Ask the client to concentrate chewing on the affected side (Avery-Smith, 2003).

- If pocketing of food is a problem, ask the client to sweep his/her cheek(s) with the tongue and/or massage the outside of the cheek in order to move food to the midline of the tongue. The therapist can also rub the outside of the cheek(s) in order to facilitate the clearance of food from the inside (Avery-Smith, 2003).

- Pocketing of food may be prevented by alternating bites of solids with sips of liquid.

- Ask the client to clear the throat and re-swallow if voice quality is wet or coughing occurs after drinking/eating.

- For clients who have difficulty with oral clearance, place the bolus at the middle of the tongue, and provide tactile cues to the cheek and jaw in order to facilitate tongue movement and initiation of the swallow (Avery-Smith, 2003).

- Present the utensil below the level of the bottom lip in order to prevent hyperextension of the neck, if needed (Avery-Smith, 2003).

- Attempt a swallow, clear throat, and re-swallow (double swallow) technique to clear food/liquids.

- Teach clients who have tongue thrust to position food on the posterior aspect of the tongue. Also, backward tilt of the head may help to prevent food from leaving the mouth.

- Sit upright for 30 minutes after meals.

Changing the Tools to Achieve Independence

- Introduce boluses with various characteristics to stimulate the swallow during meals (temperature, size, texture, and taste/flavor) (Avery-Smith, 2003).

- Thicken liquids, as needed, to increase control during the swallow.

- Avoid sticky boluses (Avery-Smith, 2003).

- As above, adapt the diet level per client needs.

- As above, adapt the placement of the utensils to the mouth, as needed.

- Alternate solids/liquids with ice-slush in order to stimulate the swallow (Avery-Smith, 2003).

Compensation/Adaptation Interventions of Eating Deficits/Dysphagia for Sensation Changes and Pain

Clients presenting with decreased sensation in the oral or facial areas must be educated regarding the limitations and safety issues involved (as able), in order to compensate. Examples of potential injuries include biting and hot foods. Adaptations during mealtime may be provided for the client who is unable to comprehend the safety issues involved (Groher, 1997).

CHANGING THE TASK TO ACHIEVE INDEPENDENCE

- Food should initially be placed in the areas of the mouth with the most intact sensation (Groher, 1997).

- Verbal cues should be given to clear areas where food may tend to pocket.

CHANGING THE TOOLS TO ACHIEVE INDEPENDENCE

- Alternate solids/liquids with ice-slush in order to increase sensation when eating and stimulate the swallow (Avery-Smith, 2003).

- Offer boluses with a variety of sizes, textures, tastes/flavors, smells, and temperatures (Avery-Smith, 2003).

- Offer diet levels that are easy to manage for the client who is experiencing pain, as appropriate.

- A laryngeal mirror may be used to check for pocketing of food (Groher, 1997).

- Clients with hypersensitivity may present with facial grimacing or refusals in reaction to an aversive food/texture.

For clients who are in any type of oral or facial pain, eating may be a negative and very exhausting experience. Groher (1997) recommends the consideration of requesting pain medication or topical antibiotics before or during mealtime. This approach may be contraindicated if oral sensation is further affected, decreasing the ability to safely swallow.

CHANGING THE TASK TO ACHIEVE INDEPENDENCE

- Create an environment of relaxation and a pleasurable experience at meal-time (provide relaxing music, decreased noise, and comfort) (Avery-Smith, 2003).
- The client may tolerate a desensitization program better if he/she controls the situation, such as feeding self various textures (Groher, 1997).

CHANGING THE TOOLS TO ACHIEVE INDEPENDENCE

- Provided graded textures of food, utensils, and plates/cups. Typically, desensitization begins with firm touch, such as eating with utensils. Softer objects or textures are introduced last (Groher, 1997).

Compensation/Adaptation Interventions of Eating Deficits/ Dysphagia for Endurance/Energy Deficits

Fatigue or decreased endurance, particularly in clients who have been on prolonged bed-rest or recently weaned from a ventilator, will most likely result in weakened oral-motor function. These clients, who typically have a very weak cough as well, are at significant risk of aspiration pneumonia. A weak, ineffective cough will not provide clearance of any aspirated food/liquid, allowing entrance into the airway. By observing the client in order to determine the times of day/conditions that cause decreased endurance, compensations may be implemented, as appropriate (Logemann, 1998).

CHANGING THE TASK TO ACHIEVE INDEPENDENCE

- Allow the client extended time to complete each meal.
- Adapt mealtime with pacing techniques such as rest periods in between courses or mouthfuls, and/or alternating solids/liquids.
- Begin eating with test trays of various textures/liquid consistencies. Progress to small snacks. Then, offer more frequent, smaller meals during the day.
- Provide positioning techniques that increase postural support for better endurance (Logemann, 1998).

CHANGING THE TOOLS TO ACHIEVE INDEPENDENCE

- Adapt diet levels by offering softer foods that take less time and energy to chew.
- Provide a smaller bolus (Avery-Smith, 2003).

Compensations/Adaptations of Eating Deficits/Dysphagia for Performance Skills/Client Factors

See Figure 3-18.

Compensation/Adaptation of Eating Deficits/Dysphagia for Cognitive Deficits

In general, when providing dysphagia intervention for a client who also presents with cognitive deficits, safety and decreasing risk of aspiration is of utmost concern. Examples of conditions that may present with concurrent cognitive deficits include dementia and traumatic or acquired brain injury. Clients who are deemed severely impaired, or unsafe to take nutrients by mouth (PO), may be recommended to have an *alternative method of nutrition*. The medical team would then consider the recommendations, collaborate with the family, and decide the best nutritional approach for the client, such as a nasogastric tube. This consideration has many medical, cultural, and ethical issues that must not be taken lightly and one always at the discretion of the family.

As will be discussed below, cognitive deficits related to dysphagia begin with the basic ability to sustain arousal and attention to task. If these cannot be maintained long enough for safe oral intake, alternative means must be recommended. As higher-level cognitive deficits present, clients may require supervision for safe eating with issues related to impulsivity, pacing, and handling of food, as examples. General intervention techniques may include cuing, hand-over-hand techniques, and visual reminders.

Table 3-26 briefly presents the subcategories of Process Skills as they are typically addressed less formally within most dysphagia intervention plans. Only the subcategories that apply to eating deficits/dysphagia have been included in this table.

Client Factors: Body Functions—Global Mental Functions

Global mental functions include consciousness and orientation. As stated earlier, a level of arousal or consciousness must be sufficient to allow for safe eating. Orientation is important when recognizing the time of day, as related to mealtimes. Also with eating, a consistent environment with routines should help to improve orientation, particularly in regards to mealtimes.

AROUSAL

Changing the Task to Achieve Independence

- Provide small, pureed snacks during heightened level of arousal times.
- Position client as upright as possible. Provide visual and verbal stimulation, such as natural lighting and verbal interactions.

Changing the Tools to Achieve Independence

- During safe levels of arousal, provide client with cold boluses.

ORIENTATION

Changing the Task to Achieve Independence

- During mealtimes, review with client the types of food being served as they relate to the time of day.

Changing the Tools to Achieve Independence

- Provide client with a daily mealtime schedule.
- Provide client with a daily menu in which appropriate foods may be chosen.

Client Factors: Body Functions—Specific Mental Functions

Specific Mental Functions include attention, memory, perception (visuospatial), thought functions (recognition, categorization, generalization), higher-level cognitive functions (judgment, concept formation, time management, problem solving, decision making), and mental functioning (motor planning) (AOTA, 2002a).

Table 3-26

PROCESS SKILLS AND EXAMPLES OF COMPENSATION/ ADAPTATION STRATEGIES

Process Skills Subcategories (AOTA, 2002a)	*Eating Deficit/Dysphagia Compensation/Adaptation Interventions*
Energy	
Paces	Introduce one food item at a time. Provide frequent small meals during the day and/or snacks.
Attends	Refer to Specific Mental Functions category
Knowledge	
Chooses	At the beginning of the meal, allow client to choose what he/she would like to eat or drink first, and so on.
Uses	Ask client to describe the proper use of the above assistive devices for safe eating.
Handles	Ask client to demonstrate safe and effective means of eating finger foods as well as handling of utensils. Monitor for safety.
Heeds	Provide daily checklist to document each time aspiration compensations are followed. For example, each time the client double swallows after drinking thickened liquids.
Inquires	Provide written directions for following aspiration precautions. Request client to ask one or more questions regarding safety with these tasks.
Temporal organization	
Initiation	Use external cues such as an audiotape with specific instructions to follow for each step of the transfer. Work with client to develop internal cues to initiate transfers.
Sequencing	Provide client with the written steps to be followed during mealtime to prevent aspiration and promote safe eating.
Organizing space and objects	
Searches/locates	Provide external cuing such as labels, signs, or color-coding of assistive devices in order to locate items before/during meals.
Gathers	Provide checklist of items needed during mealtime, such as thickener for liquids and adapted cup or straw.
Organizes	Ask client to locate items at mealtime that may hinder safety, such as food items that are contraindicated (e.g., unthickened liquids or crackers).
Adaptation	
Notices/responds	Provide cuing or environmental adaptations if observed that client does not notice safety issues at mealtime.

continued

Table 3-26, continued	
PROCESS SKILLS AND EXAMPLES OF COMPENSATION/ ADAPTATION STRATEGIES	
Process Skill Subcategories (AOTA, 2002a)	*Eating Deficit/Dysphagia Compensation/Adaptation Interventions*
Accommodates/adjusts	Problem-solve alternative compensations during mealtime if chosen interventions do not succeed, such as with swallowing techniques.
Benefits	Assist client/family in problem-solving various mealtime situations that may occur upon discharge home and plan for adaptations.

ATTENTION

Changing the Task to Achieve Independence

- For the client with attention deficits, massage cheeks to prevent pocketing. Attempt to feed client when he/she is hungry in order to maintain attention. Present one food item at a time with the most nutritious foods first. Assist client as attention decreases during the meal (Avery-Smith, 2003).

Changing the Tools to Achieve Independence

- For the client with attention deficits, provide flavorful foods that the client prefers. Cold foods may sustain attention.

MEMORY

Changing the Task to Achieve Independence

- During mealtimes, ask the client to recall dysphagia techniques taught previously.
- Ask client to recall what was eaten at the previous meal and use this as a means to improve orientation, as needed.

Changing the Tools to Achieve Independence

- Provide a daily planner for client to record menu, as above.
- Provide visual cues of dysphagia techniques, such as "swallow twice" after each mouthful.
- Provide supervision and verbal cues of dysphagia techniques during meals.
- The Specific Mental Functions that are addressed less formally and/or less frequently within intervention plans, are presented in Table 3-27.

In addition, safety issues include:

Changing the Task to Achieve Independence

- In the case of impulsivity issues, decreased safety, or judgment, provide the client with assistance, supervision, and cuing as needed during meals in order to prevent putting too much food in the mouth, controlling the bolus, and swallowing with each bite.

Table 3-27

SPECIFIC MENTAL FUNCTIONS AND EXAMPLES OF COMPENSATION/ ADAPTATION STRATEGIES

Specific Mental Functions Subcategories (AOTA, 2002a)	*Compensation/Adaptation Interventions*
Thought functions	
Recognition	During mealtime, ask client to locate items such as Thick-it, straws, and utensils.
Categorization	If client is alternating liquids and solids for ease of clearance, ask client to categorize which items are liquids and which are solids.
Generalization	When intervention is begun with only small snacks, for example, the compensations used should be generalized to all eventual mealtimes.
Higher-level cognitive functions	
Judgment	Teach client to ask for help when unsure of safety. For example, if client is thickening own liquids, he/she should check with the therapist initially as to whether the consistency is correct. Ask client open-ended questions in order to think out loud before acting.
Concept formation	Keep a daily progress and achievement chart showing amount of assistance needed for correct dysphagia techniques followed. Mark when goals have been achieved.
Time management	Educate client, before discharge, on allowing enough time for meals, particularly if client fatigues easily or eats too fast.
Problem solving	Set up possible safety issues and ask client to identify them, such as nonoptimal positioning for eating or unthickened liquids.
Decision making	Provide client with two or more options for safe and appropriate decision making, before eating. Allow client to think out loud, stating the compensations required for safe and effective swallowing, for example.

- Provide hand-over-hand guidance for the client who may eat too fast or demonstrate impulsivity. The client may need to be fed if he/she eats too fast and is at high risk for choking/aspiration.

Changing the Tools to Achieve Independence

- For the client who may eat too fast or demonstrate impulsivity, if a straw is used for liquids, pinch it in order to decrease the amount of fluid with each mouthful (AOTA, 2003).

Table 3-28

BODY SCHEME DISORDERS AND EXAMPLES OF COMPENSATION/ ADAPTATION STRATEGIES

Body Scheme Disorder	Compensation/Adaptation Interventions: Task and/or Tools Changed
Somatognosia	During mealtime, use verbal cues to increase awareness of body parts with a functional approach. For example: Ask client to point to the part of the body that chews food.
Unilateral body neglect	Adapt mealtime by using reminders to chew on the affected side of the body.
Right-left discrimination	During dysphagia intervention, use right-left terminology frequently.

Compensation/Adaptation Interventions of Eating Deficits/ Dysphagia for Perceptual Deficits

See Figure 3-20.

VISUAL FIXATION/SCANNING

Changing the Task to Achieve Independence

- Place instructions for dysphagia on a bulletin board (e.g., in the client's room). Ask client to scan the room in order to find instructions by anchoring to a certain spot on the wall to begin.

Changing the Tools to Achieve Independence

- Provide instructions on neon-colored paper, as above.

VISUAL INATTENTION/NEGLECT

Changing the Task to Achieve Independence

- Place reminders of dysphagia techniques or exercises within the client's visual field.

Changing the Tools to Achieve Independence

- Provide above reminders on colorful paper.

BODY SCHEME DISORDERS

Because there are multiple forms of body scheme disorders, each one cannot be reviewed individually. For this reason, Table 3-28 identifies the most common forms of body scheme disorders as well as examples of compensatory/adaptive interventions for these.

MOTOR PLANNING

Many individuals with dysphagia present with oral and limb apraxias. These clients with motor planning deficits are typically not able to perform verbal requests upon command, such as "please swallow your food" or "bring the cup to your lips." In general, the intervention plan should provide the client with a natural setting with food as the focus (Groher, 1997).

Changing the Task to Achieve Independence

- The therapist should demonstrate the desired movements. Verbal cues may also be used if proven effective (Groher, 1997).
- Tactile cuing or hand-over-hand guiding should be attempted to initiate eating and then, decreased as client follows-through.

Changing the Tools to Achieve Independence

- Initially, the client with apraxia may not be able to use previously familiar tools, such as utensils. Therefore, finger foods may be attempted.

Compensation/Adaptation Interventions of Eating Deficits/ Dysphagia for Visual Deficits

See Figure 3-21.

LOW VISION

Changing the Task to Achieve Independence

- Most of the examples for low vision and eating/dysphagia are similar to feeding, such as using brightly-colored set-ups for meals and setting up in a predictable manner.
- The therapist may use verbal and tactile cues.

Changing the Tools to Achieve Independence

An audiotape may be used to review dysphagia techniques and instructions, specific to the client.

VISUAL FIELD

Changing the Task to Achieve Independence

- Teach client compensation techniques for locating needed objects and instructions.

Changing the Tools to Achieve Independence

- Place instructions for dysphagia techniques and items needed within client's visual field.

MAINTENANCE PROGRAMS

Early in the dysphagia intervention process, it is important to consider whether or not the client will need a maintenance program. Clients who have long-term or chronic conditions such as dementia or cognitive disorders may need this type of program. Maintenance interventions typically involve compensation approaches such as swallowing techniques, positioning, and/or diet changes for chronic or long-term conditions (Logemann, 1998).

Re-evaluation of dysphagia should occur at least every 6 months to a year. For clients with progressively declining conditions, re-evaluation and/or follow-up may be required sooner (Logemann, 1998). In addition to evaluation/re-evaluation, the role of the OT in maintenance programs is to provide recommendations and caregiver teaching.

ACTIVITIES OF DAILY LIVING: SEXUAL ACTIVITY

Sexual activity is an ADL which is often over looked by OT. Cheng and Udry (2002) found fewer girls with disabilities were educated regarding sexual activity as compared to girls without disabilities. This lack of education can be due to erroneous assumptions on the part of the therapists, as well as society as a whole. Client with disabilities are not encouraged to engage in sexual activity by fearful parents and caregivers and others who believe these individuals are not interested (Glass & Soni, 1999). This is true particularly for women with disabilities. As Harilyn Rousso, Director of the New York Networking Project for Disabled Women and Girls, writes,

> *"So much of the traditional view of female sexuality is based on physical appearance, on meeting Madison Avenue standard of beauty and physical perfection. While disabled women are by no means unattractive, they often differ from these norms. In contrast, male sexuality, which is based less on physical appearance, includes other components, such as income level, status, and type of work; a disability in a man is thus less likely to detract from his sex appeal"* (1986, p. 4).

As for the elderly population, there is a societal myth that these individuals no longer participate in sexual activity. The increase in HIV/AIDs in the elderly population is evidence that these assumptions are incorrect (Henderson, Bernstein, St. George, Doyle, Paranjape and Corvie-Smith, 2004; Moore & Amburgey, 2000).

Another reason this topic is not addressed could be the apprehensions of individual therapists. Many therapists are not comfortable with the topic of sexual activity with clients because they are not comfortable with this topic in general. Occupational therapy education regarding sexual activity is limited (Friedman, 1997). In addition, many of today's elderly are not comfortable with the topic of sexuality; therefore therapists may be even more concerned about broaching this subject. As stereotypes of the elderly are changing, more elderly may ask questions of therapists, and the therapists need to be prepared to respond to these questions. In addition, there are many young adults and middle aged adults who require the services of OTs, including education regarding sexual activity.

According to the AOTA *Framework* document, sexual activity is defined as "engagement in activities which result in sexual satisfaction" (2002a, p. 620). It is important to point out this definition is not limited to sexual intercourse. Many clients will find sexual satisfaction from activities other than intercourse. The *Gale Encyclopedia of Nursing and Allied Health* defines sexuality to include, "body image, self image, gender identities, beliefs, and feelings about sex, capacities for love and friendship, and social behavior as well as overt physical expression of love or sexual desire. A person's sexuality is influenced by ethical, spiritual, cultural and moral concerns" (Gourley, 2002, p. 2203). Because sexual activity includes a variety of issues, the education for sexual activity is multidimensional. The physical issues related to a disability, the psychosocial issues related to social participation, as well as the issues of abuse must all be addressed.

This chapter will address the physical issues related to sexual activity, while Chapter 8 will address the social participation and sexual abuse issues.

Unlike other ADLs, sexual activity is not an occupation that can be practiced in the clinic. Because intervention is based on education, and success of the intervention is very subjective, based on each client, this chapter will focus on compensation/adaptation rather than remediation.

COMPENSATION/ADAPTATION OF SEXUAL ACTIVITY DEFICITS FOR CLIENTS WITH PHYSICAL LIMITATIONS: PERFORMANCE SKILLS/ CLIENT FACTORS: RANGE OF MOTION, STRENGTH, COORDINATION, SENSATION/PAIN, AND ENDURANCE/ENERGY

Sexual activity can be negatively impacted by motor skills deficits and body functions limitations. Limitations in motor functions may create clumsy or uncomfortable situations that clients choose to avoid by avoiding sexual activity as a whole. Body function changes following an injury or illness can result in a decreased desire for sexual activity. Korpelainen, Nieminen, & Myllyla found "Stroke caused a marked decrease in libido among both the patients and their spouses..." (1999, p. 716). This may be a result of the illness itself, or a result of secondary factors such as decreased body image or impaired sensation. In addition, fear of poor sexual function may limit libido.

Performance patterns, context, and activity demands need to be addressed as well. Performance patterns play a very large role in an individual client's sexual activity. As stated in Chapter 1, performance patterns include the client's habits, routines, and roles (AOTAa, 2002). Client habits and routines can range from an individual who rarely experiences sexual activity to a client who routinely experiences sexual activity. According to the AOTA *Framework* document, roles are defined as "a set of behaviors which have some socially agreed upon function and for which there is an acceptable code of norms" (2002a, p. 623). As stated above, the socially agreed upon standards and the acceptable code of norms may be based on stereotypes, not the actual code of a particular client. It is important for the OTs to determine the habits, routines, and roles of each client. When examining roles, the role of parent should not be overlooked. McAlonan (1996) completed satisfaction surveys with clients who had a spinal cord injury regarding their sexuality-related services and found "fertility issues were a major concern for both the female and male participants" (p. 832).

The areas of context that may impact sexual activity are the clients' cultural, spiritual, and social relationships. Culture and spirituality have a long tradition of having an impact on sexual activity. Within certain cultures, women's and men's sexual interests have different expectations. Some cultures do not allow sexuality to be discussed as openly as others. For example, according to the Muslim Women's League, an American Muslim organization, sexual education is acceptable and should be discussed within the community as it relates to pregnancy, as well as sexually transmitted diseases (www.mwlusa.org/publications/positionpapers/sexuality.html). While spirituality does not include religion alone, many religious beliefs will also impact sexual activity. For example, the Roman Catholic religion believes that sexual activity has a purpose of procreation over recreation. Clients who are widowed may feel guilty about sexual activity outside of a marriage relationship, even if beyond the age of procreation.

Social relationships can be strained because of injury or illness. Concerns over sexuality may put a further strain on these relationships. As stated above, fertility is a large concern for individuals after a spinal cord injury. Questions of fertility, as well as raising the children, need to be addressed with clients so they are well informed of the possibilities (McAlonan, 1996). If an adult has to move back in with parents following an injury or illness, this can further limit the individual's social and sexual activities due to family dynamics. All of these context factors offer opportunities for OT to open a dialogue with the client and assess the individual's needs.

Activity demands include social demands, required actions, and required body functions and structures. The required actions and required body functions and structures will be discussed. The social demands, as stated earlier, may be unrealistic for individuals with disabilities and for

Table 3-29

PLISSIT MODEL AND TRAINING

PLISSIT	Definitions (Adapted From Wallace, 2004	Training (Adapted From Friedman, 1997)
P	Permission from the client discuss sexual activity	Therapists are generally sufficiently trained to offer an opportunity for discussion regarding sexual activity
LI	Limited information provided to client	Adaptations/compensations listed below will provide this information.
SS	Specific Suggestions provided regarding sexual activity	Some advanced training may be required, depending on the specificity
IT	Intensive Therapy regarding issues of sexuality	Not generally provided by OTs unless advanced training completed.

the elderly. Poverty, substance abuse, race, sex, and educational levels can impact expectations. While expectations are important to know, it is more important to assess the particular roles to which an individual client wishes to return.

In general, OTs will be providing information and education to clients who have experienced a physical injury or illness. Some clients who have experienced cognitive or perceptual limitations will also require education. One tool that has been used by OTs and other health care practitioners to organize sexual activity education is PLISSIT. This tool was created in the 1970s, but the validity or reliability of this tool has not been established (Wallace, 2004). Despite this, it is a valuable guide to the level of specificity offered by an OT. Table 3-29 describes the PLISSIT model and training required for occupational therapy within this model.

Compensation/Adaptation Interventions of Sexual Activity Deficits for Range of Motion, Strength, and Coordination Deficits

ROM, strength and coordination limitations will impact positioning during sexual activity. Clients may have difficulty with sexual positions which were preferred in the past. OTs can discuss positioning without becoming sexually explicit. Examples of this include:

- Instruct clients with hemiparesis to lie on the affected side, thus allowing the unaffected side to be free for physical contact or additional support (TBI help.org).
- Instruct clients to discuss positions of comfort with partners in order to avoid being uncomfortable. Request the partner to take a more active role, allowing the client to assume a position that requires less movement (Friedman, 1997).
- Wedges or pillows may be required to support a particular position. General principles can be explained to the client, or if appropriate, specific positions can be reviewed with the client.

Compensation/Adaptation Interventions of Sexual Activity Deficits for Sensation Changes and Pain

As stated earlier, sensory changes can result in a decrease in sensation (hyposensitivity), such as after a CVA, or in increased sensation (hypersensitivity) and pain. For clients with decreased sensation, communication with the partner is vital. The partner can be asked by the client to caress the areas of intact sensation more often, allowing for greater pleasure for the client. If sensation is lacking to the point where pressure areas are a concern, such as after a spinal cord injury, the client should be educated to avoid prolonged positioning and to check the sitting/lying location for objects that can cause pressure or cuts prior to initiating any sexual activity (Friedman, 1997).

Decreased sensation can also result in bowel and bladder issues, which can embarrass clients during sexual activity. Clients who are not continent should be instructed to void prior to any sexual activity in order to avoid such situations. These clients should communicate the possibility of incontinence with their partner and be prepared with supplies for clean up if such an incident occurs (Friedman, 1997).

For clients experiencing hypersensitivity or pain, the education is centered on limiting pain so the clients can enjoy the sexual activity. If the pain is positional, such as back pain, clients can communicate with their partner regarding positions of comfort. These positions may be different than what couples are used to, such as sitting rather than lying down, therefore communication is vital. If the pain is due to contact, such as a burn or amputation of a limb, the clients again need to communicate with the partner regarding what contact causes this pain and how to avoid it.

Pain management techniques can also be incorporated. Massage or meditation prior to sexual activity can reduce pain due to stress or muscle tightness. Sexual activity can be planned when pain medication is most effective (Friedman, 1997). While this limits spontaneity, it will be beneficial for overall enjoyment if pain is absent during sexual activity (Friedman, 1997).

Compensation/Adaptation Interventions of Sexual Activity Deficits for Endurance/Energy Deficits

Decreased endurance can be a result of prolonged hospitalization or lack of activity as well as a particular illness. The elderly are particularly vulnerable to rapid declines in endurance with inactivity and are more likely to experience the most common forms of illness that result in decreased endurance: cardiovascular diseases.

For clients with cardiovascular disease, concerns regarding sexual activity are frequent. According to the American Heart Association, "many myths surround sex after heart disease or stroke. The most common one is resuming sex often causes a heart attack, stroke or sudden death. This just isn't true" (American Heart Association, 2005). While it is important for clients to discuss concerns with a physician, the OT can also offer suggestions. Most of these suggestions are general energy conservation principles, such as the following:

- Avoid stressful or rushed environments.
- Avoid sexual activity directly after meals or other physical activity.
- Be aware that fatigue may occur, and that this is normal.

For clients with other diagnoses resulting in decreased endurance, such as pulmonary diseases or progressive neurological diseases, these same principles will apply.

Compensation/Adaptation Interventions of Sexual Activity Deficits for Cognitive, Perceptual, or Visual Deficits

While there are some clients who will experience difficulty with sexual activity due to visual loss, this is rare and will not be discussed here. Individuals who experience perceptual deficits may have motor planning difficulties, body scheme disorders, inattention or certain agnosias that can, but do not necessarily have to, impact sexual activity. Intervention for these individuals would occur related to the specific deficit if the impact was of concern for the client; however, these deficits are often overcome by clients without intervention.

The appropriateness of education regarding sexual activity for clients with cognitive deficits depends largely on the severity of the deficits. If a client is unable to determine for him- or herself if a situation is voluntary or not, education regarding avoidance or reporting of abuse may be more appropriate. Rates of sexual abuse have been inconsistent, partially due to fear on the part of individuals to report sexual abuse. Another factor is that many individuals with disabilities are dependent on the caregivers/family members and these are often the abusers (Nosek & Howland, 1998). For clients with long-standing cognitive deficits, such as adults with developmental disabilities, education may be appropriate and this is addressed in Chapter 8. Clients with new cognitive disabilities, such as a client with a head injury, will need to be assessed individually to ascertain if education is appropriate. Education should not be avoided simply because a deficit exists or caregivers do not think it appropriate, but rather based on the safety and competence of each client.

MAINTENANCE OF SEXUAL ACTIVITY

Once the client has attained all information requested, these skills will become maintenance because they will remain beyond the time when intervention is being completed with the client. As this is a personal matter, it will be the choice of the client as to whether he/she utilizes the techniques provided or chooses to abstain from sexual activity once education has been completed.

CASE #1: JOSEPHINE

Josephine is a 75-year-old female who fell in the garage after tripping over her grandson's skateboard. She sustained a left hip fracture, was admitted to the hospital, and had surgery for a cemented bipolar hip arthroplasty. She was discharged to a short-term rehab facility 5 days after surgery in hopes to finally be discharged home.

Josephine lives in a mother-in-law apartment in her daughter and son-in-law's home. The apartment is above the garage and has 13 steps to enter. Once inside the apartment, there are no architectural barriers, except a traditional shower with glass doors. She also has a galley kitchen.

Josephine has a past medical history of Insulin-Dependent Diabetes Mellitus (IDDM), osteoarthritis, appendicitis, and had a hysterectomy 26 years ago. Prior to this fall, she was independent with all ADLs and IADLs. She did not use any assistive devices and drove short distances. Josephine attends the local senior center where she is active with bingo, line dancing, and senior water aerobics.

Josephine's goals are to "walk again and go to the senior center."

Current status is as follows: (R dominant).

ROM	WNL-BUE	
Strength	BUE grossly 4+/5 to 5/5	
Cognition	Occasionally forgetful as to the date, needs cuing for hand placement, hip precautions, and to use assistive device	
V/P	WNLs	
FM Skills	WFL-occ difficulty secondary to arthritis	
Functional Mobility and Transfers	Supine-to-sit with cuing and min (a), PWB'g, sit-to-stand with cuing and mod(a), Amb to w/c using RW and CTG	
ADL	(I) UE bathe/dress; requires adaptive equip for LE ADLs secondary to hip precautions and mod (a) with cuing	
Pain	4/5 at rest, 7/10 with mobility	

Case #2: Bill

Bill is 44-year-old male who sustained a CVA 1 week ago. He has an unremarkable past medical history. He lives in a two-story home with his wife and teenage daughter. As a result of the CVA, he will take a medical leave from his job as an accountant. Although Bill's job requires long hours, he is a devoted husband and father who makes breakfast for the family each morning. His wife works part-time as a social worker. Prior to his CVA, Bill enjoyed socializing with his wife and lifelong friends, bowling, and attending his daughter's soccer games.

After initial symptoms of left side numbness and weakness in his LLE, LUE, and left side of face, Bill's wife rushed him to the local ER. While in the ER, the symptoms progressed to full flaccidity in his LUE, difficulty swallowing, and blurred vision. After the ER, he was admitted to the medical ICU for 2 days, then transferred to a neuro step-down unit. His medical team is now evaluating Bill for the Intensive Rehab Unit within the hospital.

Bill's goals are to return to work, cook breakfast, and attend his daughter's soccer games upon d/c.

Current status is as follows: (R dominant)

ROM	Right: AROM-WNL	Left: PROM WNL, no active motion of LUE noted
Strength	Right: 5/5 grossly throughout	Left-flaccid
Endurance	c/o fatigue after 20 minute eval	
Sensation		
Proprioception	RUE-WNL	LUE-Impaired
Hot Cold	RUE-WNL	LUE-WNL
Localization	RUE-WNL	LUE-Impaired/L side of face, also
FM skills	RUE-WNL	LUE-Absent secondary to flaccidity
Visual/perceptual	Only complains of blurred vision	

Cognitive	A&O X 3 Tends to have difficulty sequencing simple ADL tasks	Safety: impulsive. Tries to get out of bed on own and out of w/c
Oral-motor	Choking with thin liquids, left side of mouth droops	Speech clear
ADL	Assist for meal set-up, cutting food and eating sandwiches	Mod (a) with grooming; Max (a) toileting; Mod (a) bathing
Transfers/functional mobility	Mod (a) supine-to-sit and sit-to-stand; Max (a) stand-pivot with walker.	Mod (a) to maintain sitting balance @ EOB
Affect	Flat, sad, difficult to motivate	
Other issues	Moderate subluxation, Left shoulder	Pain: 7/10 when shoulder is positioned or moved

SUMMARY QUESTIONS

1. Pick one ADL compensation/adaptation method and describe how it is related to one model/theory of occupational therapy.

2. Compare and contrast the remediation and compensation/adaptation approaches to ADL. Give specific examples.

3. Discuss safety issues as related to vision, perception, and cognition in ADLs.

4. Describe one general maintenance strategy in ADLs in relation to dressing techniques.

REFERENCES

American Heart Association. (June 3, 2005). Sexual activity and heart disease or stroke. Retrieved March 1, 2005 from www.americanheart.org/presenter.jhtml?identifier=4714.

American Occupational Therapy Association. (2000). Specialized knowledge and skills in eating and feeding for occupational therapy practice. *American Journal of Occupational Therapy, 54*, 629-640.

American Occupational Therapy Association. (2002a). *Occupational therapy practice framework: Domain and process.* Bethesda, MD: AOTA Press.

American Occupational Therapy Association. (2002b). Roles and responsibilities of the occupational therapist and occupational therapy assistant during the delivery of occupational therapy services. *Occupational Therapy Practice, 7*(15), 9-10.

American Occupational Therapy Association. (2004). *The reference manual of the official documents of the American occupational therapy association* (10th ed.). Bethesda, MD: AOTA.

Arnadottir, G. (1990). *The brain and behavior: Assessing critical dysfunction through activities of daily living (ADL).* St. Louis: Mosby.

Avery-Smith, W. (Ed.) (2003). *Dysphagia care for adults: A self-paced clinical course from AOTA.* Bethesda, MD: AOTA.

Avery-Smith, W. (1998). An occupational therapist-coordinated dysphagia program. *Occupational Therapy Practice, 3*(11), 20-23.

Cheng, M. M., & Udry, J. R. (2002). Sexual behaviors of physically disabled adolescents in the United States. *Journal of Adolescent Health, 31*(1), 48-48.

Cohen, J. R. (2001). Living with low vision. *Inside M.S., 19*(1), 46-54.

Cole, M. B. (1998). *Group dynamics in occupational therapy* (2nd ed.). Thorofare, NJ: SLACK Incorporated.

Crepeau, E. B., Cohn, E. S., & Schell, B. A. B. (2003). *Willard and Spackman's occupational therapy for physical dysfunction* (10th ed.). Philadelphia, PA: Lippincott Williams & Wilkins.

Dodge, H. H., Kadowski, T., Hayakawa, T., & Yamakawa, M. (2005). Cognitive impairment as a strong predictor of incident disability in specific ADL-IADL tasks among community-dwelling elders: The Azuchi study. *The Gerontologist, 45*(2), 222-231.

Dorner, B. (2002). Promoting an easier swallow. Focus on caregiving. *Provider, 28*(9), 69-70, 73-4.

Fasoli, S. E., Trombly, C. A., Tickle-Degnen, L., & Verfaellie, M. H. (2002). Context and goal-directed movement: the effect of material-based occupation. *Occupational Therapy Journal of Research, 22*(3), 119-128.

Fisher, A. G. (2001). *Assessment of motor and process skills* (4th ed). Retrieved June 12, 2005, from www.ampsintl.com.

Fisher, A.G. (2002, January). A model for planning and implementing top-down, client-centered, and occupation-based occupational therapy interventions. Short course presented at University of New Hampshire conference.

Friedman, J. D. (1997). Sexual expression: The forgotten component of ADL. *Occupational Therapy Practice, January*, 20-25.

Gibson, J. W., & Schkade, J. K. (1997). Occupational adaptation intervention with patients with cerebrovascular accident: a clinical study. *American Journal of Occupational Therapy, 51*(7), 523-529.

Gillen, G., & Burkhardt, A. (2004). *Stroke rehabilitation: A function-based approach* (2nd ed.). St. Louis: Elsevier/Mosby.

Glass, C., & Soni, B. (1999). ABC of sexual health sexual problems of disabled patients. *British Medical Journal, 318*, 518-521.

Gourley, M. M. (2002) Sexuality and disability. In K. Krapp (Ed.), *Gale encyclopedia of nursing and allied health*. (Vol. 4, p. 2203-2206). Farmington Hills, MI: Thomson Gale Group.

Groher, M. E. (Ed.) (1997). *Dysphagia: Diagnosis and management* (3rd ed.). Boston: Butterworth-Heinemann.

Henderson, S. J., Bernstein, L. B., St. George, D. M., Doyle, J. P., Paranjape, A. S., & Corbie-Smith, G. (2004). Older women and HIV: how much do they know and where are they getting their information? *J Am Geriatric Society, 52*, 1549-1553.

Jackson Siegelbaum Gastroenterology. (2002). Dysphagia diet: 5 levels difficulty in swallowing diet. Retrieved on March 20, 2005, from http://www.gicare.com/pated/edtgs07.htm.

Jacobs, K., & Jacobs, L. (2004). *Quick reference dictionary for occupational therapy* (4th ed.). Thorofare, NJ: SLACK Incorporated.

Korpelainen, J. T., Nieminen, P., & Myllyla, V. V. (1999). Sexual functioning among stroke patients and their spouses. *Stroke, 30*, 715-719.

Law, M., Baptiste, S., Carswell, A., McColl, M. A., Polatajko, H., & Pollock, N. (1998). *The Canadian occupational performance measure* (3rd ed.). Ottawa, Ontario: Canadian Occupational Therapy Association.

Lin, K. (1996). Right-hemispheric activation approaches to neglect rehabilitation post-stroke. *American Journal of Occupational Therapy, 50*(7), 504-515.

Logemann, J. A. (1998). *Evaluation and treatment of swallowing disorders* (2nd ed.). Austin, TX: PRO-ED.

McAlonan, S. (1996). Improving sexual rehabilitation services: The patient's perspective. *American Journal of Occupational Therapy, 50*(10), 826-834.

McCullough, G., Pelletier, C., & Steele, C. (2003). National dysphagia diet: What to swallow? *ASHA Leader, 27*, 16.

Moore, L. W. & Amburgey, L. B. (2000). Older adults and HIV. *Association of Perioperative Registered Nurses Journal, 71*, 873-875.

Muslim Women's League. (nd). An Islamic Perspective on Sexuality. Retrieved on May 10, 2005, from www.mwlusa.org/publications/positionpapers/sexuality.html

Nagel, M. J., & Rice, M. S. (2001). Cross transfer effects in the upper extremity during an occupationally embedded exercise. *American Journal of Occupational Therapy, 55*, 531-537.

Nelson, D.L., Konosky, K., Fleharty K., Webb, R., Newer, K., & Hazboun, V. P. (1996). The effects of an occupationally embedded exercise on bilateral assisted supination in persons with hemiplegia. *American Journal of Occupational Therapy, 50*, 639-646.

Nosek, M. A., & Howland, C. A. (1998). Abuse and women with disabilities. Retrieved May 31, 2005, from http://www.vaw.umn.edu.

O'Sullivan, N. (1995). *Dysphagia care: Team approach with acute and long-term care clients* (2nd ed.). Los Angeles: Cottage Square.

Pierson, F. M. (1999). *Principles and techniques of patient care* (2nd ed.). Philadelphia, PA: W.B. Saunders.

Rogers, J. C., & Holm, M. B. (1994). *Performance Assessment of Self-Care Skills (PASS – Home).* Version 3.1.

Tham, K., Ginsburg, E., Fisher A. G., & Tegner R. (2001). Awareness of disabilities in clients with unilateral neglect. *American Journal of Occupational Therapy, 55*(1), 46-54.

Trombly, C. A. & Radomski, M. V. (Eds.). (2002). *Occupational therapy for physical dysfunction.* (5th ed.). Philadelphia, PA: Lippincott Williams & Wilkins.

TBI help.org (nd). *Achieving sexual intimacy after a stroke.* Retrieved March 1, 2005 from www.tbihelp.org/sexual_intimacy_after_.htm.

Uniform Data System for Medical Rehabilitation. (1996). *Functional Independence Measure.* Amherst, New York retrieved from www.udsmr.org on June 12, 2005.

Wallace, M. (2004). Sexuality. *MedSurg Nursing, 13*(2), 122.

Zoltan, B. (2007). *Visual, perception, and cognition* (4th ed.). Thorofare, NJ: SLACK Incorporated.

4

Instrumental Activities of Daily Living

Mary Ellen Santucci, OTR/L

CHAPTER OBJECTIVES

By the end of this chapter, the student will be able to:

☑ Define **instrumental activities of daily living (IADL)** as it pertains to the *Occupational Therapy Practice Framework (Framework)*.

☑ Describe specific **models/frames of reference** as related to IADLs.

☑ Comprehend **safety issues** as related to IADLs.

☑ Delineate between the roles of the **occupational therapist** (OT) and the **occupational therapy assistant** (OTA) as they pertain to the occupation of IADLs.

☑ Comprehend and identify related **psychological implications** as related to decreased independence in IADLs.

☑ Describe the impact of **contextual factors** upon IADLs.

☑ Identify appropriate IADL intervention strategies based on various **performance skills and client factors**.

☑ Identify general IADL remediation strategies.

☑ Identify specific IADL compensation/adaptation strategies.

☑ Identify IADL compensation/adaptation intervention strategies related to vision, perception, and cognition.

☑ Identify general IADL **maintenance** strategies.

INTRODUCTION

According to the *Framework*, IADLs are defined as, "Activities that are oriented toward interacting with the environment and that are often complex (American Occupational Therapy Association [AOTA], 2002). IADL are generally optional in nature, that is, may be delegated to another (adapted from Rogers & Holm, 1994, pp. 181-202)." In general, included in IADL are the following areas of occupation: home establishment and management, meal preparation, shopping, financial management, community mobility, communication device use, care of others (including selecting and supervising caregivers), care of pets, child rearing, health management and maintenance, and safety procedures and emergency responses (AOTA, 2002). Intervention

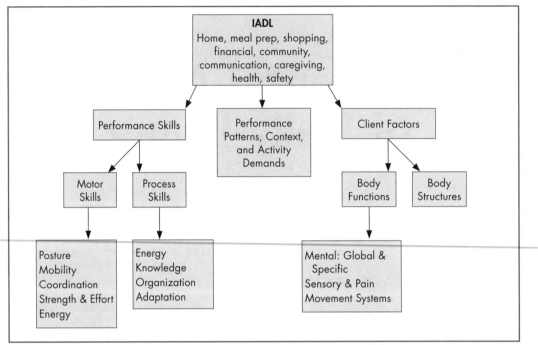

Figure 4-1. Components of IADLs (adapted from American Occupational Therapy Association. (2002). *Occupational therapy practice framework: Domain and process*. Bethesda, MD: AOTA).

in these areas of occupation will be discussed in greater detail throughout this chapter, with the primary focus being on remediation, compensation/adaptation and maintenance interventions. Frames of reference, safety concerns, implications for the psychological impact on IADLs, context, performance patterns, activity demands, and the role of the OTA will be addressed (Figure 4-1).

Throughout this chapter, the reader will be introduced to the management of clients with neurological, orthopedic, and cognitive/perceptual deficits to facilitate independence with IADLs in the above mentioned areas of occupation.

The role of the OT is to facilitate functional independence in all daily activities and participation in life roles to the greatest level of skill. The goal of this chapter is to introduce ways to assist the client in fulfilling both of these goals. As the client is going through the process of remediation of motor skills, process skills, and/or communication/interaction skills, the OT may offer recommendations for compensation or adaptation to increase the client's independence and safety. At the time that the client becomes appropriate for participation in IADLs, the OT must determine if continuing with the remediation process is appropriate. If so, the client may continue to practice normal movement patterns until mastery is achieved. If not, the therapist will begin instructing the client in compensation and adaptation strategies. For example, if the client is determined to return home alone, he/she will need to become independent with IADLs. If remediation of all skills has not yet been achieved, the client will need to implement compensation/adaptation techniques to facilitate this goal during the ongoing remediation process. If the client was to follow compensatory or adaptive methods from the onset of intervention, the OT will educate him/her in the most effective strategies to return to independent living. The goal of this chapter is to educate the OT in various means of facilitation of a client's functional independence and return to his/her life role.

The AOTA *Framework* document has defined various areas of IADLs. These definitions will be the basis for most of this chapter, with additions or clarifications added throughout. The definitions are as listed below.

- **Home establishment and maintenance** is defined as:

  "Obtaining and maintaining personal and household possessions and environment (e.g., home, yard, garden, appliances, vehicles), including maintaining and repairing personal possessions (clothing and household items) and knowing how to seek help and whom to contact." Meal preparation and clean-up refers to, "Planning, preparing, serving well-balanced, nutritional meals and cleaning up food and utensils after meals" (AOTA, 2002, p. 620).

  Specific tasks within this definition are not listed; however, the most common tasks have been chosen for review in this chapter. These tasks are: laundry, light cleaning, outdoor home maintenance, shopping, preparing a meal, setting a table, and wash/drying dishes and putting them away.

- **Financial management** is defined as, "Using fiscal resources, including alternate methods of financial transaction and planning and using finances with long-term and short-term goals" (2002, p. 620). In this section, financial management will include the following: check writing, payment by cash, and the use of credit cards.

- **Community mobility** is defined as, "Moving self in the community and using public or private transportation, such as driving, or accessing buses, taxi cabs, or other public transportation systems" (AOTA, 2002, p. 620). This section will focus on driving and public transportation.

- **Communication devices** is defined as, "Using equipment or systems such as writing equipment, telephones, typewriters, computers, communication boards, call lights, emergency systems, Braille writers, telecommunication devices for the deaf, and augmentative communication systems to send and receive information" (AOTA, 2002, p. 620). This section will focus on everyday use of communication devices, devices or systems for emergency alerting, and adapted devices for the visually impaired.

- **Care of others and pets** is defined as, "Arranging, supervising, or providing the care for" others and pets (AOTA, 2002, p. 620). This category of IADL addresses the care of others, including family members and pets.

- **Health management and maintenance** is defined as, "Developing, managing, and maintaining routines for health and wellness promotion, such as physical fitness, nutrition, decreasing health risk behaviors, and medication routines" (AOTA, 2002, p. 620).

Table 4-1 reviews the different aspects of each IADL category.

FRAME OF REFERENCE

Chapter 1 reviewed several frames of reference and models for occupational therapy. As stated in that chapter, occupational therapy has a humanistic philosophy as well as models that are client-centered and systems based. While a therapist's choice for a frame of reference depends on the setting of intervention, the therapist's preferences, and the needs of the individual client, for purposes of retraining clients in IADLs in this chapter, the Model of Human Occupation (MOHO) will be discussed. The OT will be assessing the client's level of volition, habituation, and performance. The client will be interviewed and the OT along with the client will determine the client's goals. Intervention programs will be established and intervention with the client revolves around facilitation of the client's desired role performance in IADL (Christiansen & Baum, 1991).

In addition to these, therapists using the top-down approach (as discussed in Chapters 1 and 2), may also use frames of reference based on the client's specific situation. For a client who is aging,

Table 4-1

COMPONENTS OF IADLs

Home establishment and maintenance, meal preparation and clean-up, shopping	• Laundry • Light cleaning • Outdoor home maintenance • Shopping • Preparing a meal • Setting a table • Wash/dry dishes and put them away
Financial management	• Check writing • Payment by cash • Use of credit cards
Community mobility	• Driving • Use of public transportation or community service transit systems • Mobilizing to bus stops
Communication device use	• Common communication devices (i.e., telephone, computer, pager systems) • Devices or systems for emergency alerting • Adaptive devices for those with visual impairment
Care of others	• Spouse • Children • Parents • Other family members • Friends
Care of pets	• Feeding • Exercise • Health maintenance
Health management and maintenance	• Exercise and fitness • Nutrition • Hygiene • Medication management and compliance

a developmental frame of reference, such as Jung's spiritual stages, Erickson's psychosocial stages, or Levinson's life transitions may be utilized (Cole, 1998).

For a client who has experienced a traumatic brain injury or a cerebral vascular accident and behavior changes are apparent, a behaviorist theory, such as behavior modification, may be employed. Behavior modification is based on environmental reinforcers in order to shape behavior (Cole, 1998). This same client may have cognitive deficits and require a cognitive frame of reference such as Toglia and Abreu's cognitive rehabilitation frame of reference. Originally based on learning theory, and now updated by Toglia to include metacognition (insight into own capabilities), this frame of reference emphasizes retraining cognition through hierarchical intervention and brain plasticity (Cole 1998).

Because behavior modification is based on environmental feedback, better carryover should be demonstrated again with the use of functional activities rather than rote exercise. This is also true of cognitive rehabilitation. According to Cole, "cognitive strategies are always taught in the context of an activity" (1998, p.149).

SAFETY DURING IADL INTERVENTION

According to the *Framework*, safety procedures and emergency responses include, "knowing and performing preventive procedures to maintain a safe environment as well as recognizing sudden, unexpected hazardous situations and initiating emergency action to reduce the threat to health and safety" (AOTA, 2002, p. 620).

The management of clients' performance demands focuses on safety with all aspects of IADLs. Many clients experience age-related physical and sensory changes that may be enhanced by an acute neurological, orthopedic, or cognitive/perceptual event. These acute events may precipitate client factor changes that may affect performance habits and/or performance skills. Driving, using public transportation, and managing medications for self or others are among examples of IADLs that need to be closely monitored with clients, and caregivers must be educated in all safety concerns. OTs must recognize implications for safety with respect to ADLs prior to facilitating a safe performance with IADLs. Safety concerns will be addressed throughout this chapter with respect to specific areas of IADL intervention.

IMPLICATIONS FOR PSYCHOLOGICAL IMPACT ON IADL

Psychological implications are important to consider with each client intervention. The OT must be sensitive to the mood and affect of the client and assess his/her level of motivation to increase function. A client who was functioning independently at home, but now requires supervision to shower and dress, may experience feelings of loss of dignity and self-worth. A client who is now unable to drive because of visual changes may experience feelings of sadness and confinement. An individual previously living alone may now need someone to stay with him/her all day or intermittently throughout the day. Changes in performance patterns can result, as the client may need to wait for assistance with self-care, whereas these tasks would have been completed at his/her own convenience prior to the onset of this illness. Home modifications may be required, along with the need to perform everyday occupations within a different context, in order to maintain safety. For example, a client may need to remain on one level of his/her home versus utilizing the upstairs and downstairs as in the past. Emotions such as sadness, depression, and despondence may be considered normal at first, but if they are prolonged, and are interfering with motivation towards independence, psychological intervention may be considered. The OT must be sensitive to these feelings to the same degree as being aware of the client's physical changes.

The impact of limited performance of a client may also affect family and other interpersonal relationships. The OT must be sensitive to the dynamics involved as well as offer support and guidance to the family or caregivers. This will facilitate ease and safety in the transition of the client to home in a dignified manner. At times, social work intervention may be indicated, recognized, and initiated even prior to the patient's discharge.

CONTEXT

Context or contexts "refers to a variety of interrelated conditions within and surrounding the client that influence performance. Contexts include cultural, physical, social, personal, spiritual, temporal, and virtual" (AOTA, 2002, p. 623).

Upon initial evaluation, OTs determine the role that context plays in occupational performance. For example, culture may play an important role in occupational performance. Some clients may be more receptive to the assistance of others for daily tasks and, therefore, may not be receptive to learning new techniques to advance their independence with IADLs. On the other hand, some clients may refuse the assistance of others or will not allow others in their home to provide them with care. These clients will need intensive rehabilitation to facilitate the return to home in a safe manner.

Physical environment will also have a large impact, particularly regarding safety concerns. Clients who have received home modification are more likely to function at a higher independence level (Stark, 2004). Particularly with the IADL of cooking, intervention should be provided regarding the safety of the kitchen environment, and adaptations should be made as necessary to ensure the safest possible context for the client. Adaptation of the actual home would be ideal; however, if this is not possible, some success has been found using the virtual component of context. While used during cooking only with clients who had a traumatic brain injury, the results of virtual reality for use with clients are promising (Zhang, Abreu, Seale, Masel, Christiansen, & Ottenbacher, 2003). For more information on physical context adaptations, see Chapter 3. Table 4-2 lists the areas of context and their impact on IADLs.

PERFORMANCE SKILLS

According to the AOTA, performance skills are defined as, "Features of what one does, not of what one has, related to observable elements of action that have implicit functional purposes" (2002, p. 621). Performance skills include motor skills, process skills, and communication/interaction skills. Table 4-3 lists the performance skill areas and their impact on IADLs.

An acute onset of deficits in the performance skills of motor, process, and communication skills will greatly influence functional levels and impact client safety. Clients manifesting deficits in any area of motor performance may be at risk for safety issues unless these areas are remediated or the client demonstrates use of compensation/adaptation strategies to increase independence and maintain safety. For example, the client who is able to ambulate safely with a rolling walker, but is unable to maintain balance with kitchen tasks that require carrying objects or reaching in low cabinets for items needed, may perform these tasks more safely at wheelchair level. A client who may be faced with a kitchen fire and is unable to process the methods of maintaining safety in an efficient and timely manner will not be able to live independently again. A client who comprehends the danger, but is unable to communicate via telephone or call out the need for help, may benefit from assistive devices for communication to assure safety. The OT will assess the client's level of safety based on these performance skills and their effect on function for the individual client.

PERFORMANCE PATTERNS

The *Framework* defines performance patterns as "patterns of behavior related to daily life activities that are habitual or routine" (AOTA, 2002, p. 623). Performance patterns include habits and routines. Table 4-4 lists performance patterns and their impact on IADLs.

Table 4-2

CONTEXTS AND IMPACT ON IADLs

Contexts (AOTA, 2002)	Impact of Contexts on IADLs and Intervention
Cultural	• Family teaching may be indicated. • Adaptive equipment/durable medical equipment may not be accepted. • ADL/IADLs may be limited to certain times of the day.
Physical	• Home environments may need modifications (i.e., ramps, durable medical equipment, living areas on first floor). • Limitations in mobility in familiar and unfamiliar environments.
Social	• Fear of participating in former social events. • Communication deficits limiting interaction. • Mobility deficits limiting social contexts.
Personal	• Impaired self image. • Impaired confidence. • Possible limitations with privacy.
Spiritual	• Inability to participate in spiritual services. • Possible loss of faith.
Temporal	• Modifications in daily routine times. • Increased time to complete tasks.
Virtual	• Inability to access the Internet can limit on-line shopping or communication capabilities.

Habits and routines play a strong role in daily function. An interruption in physical, sensory, or cognitive/perceptual skills may elicit a change in habit or routine to which it may be difficult for the client to adapt. OTs must remain sensitive to clients' former performance patterns and assist with facilitation and acceptance of new patterns to enhance function. For example, a client who generally awakens and walks outside for the morning paper independently and without an assistive device may need to wait for the assistance of a caregiver and may need to use a cane or walker for the task. It is often difficult for a client who has been accustomed to certain habits and routines to be receptive to an alternative lifestyle. Further discussion of the role of performance patterns in various areas of occupation will follow.

ACTIVITY DEMANDS

Activity demands refers to "the aspects of an activity, which include the objects, space, social demands, sequencing or timing, required actions, and required underlying body functions and body structures needed to carry out this activity" (AOTA, 2002, p. 624).

The activity demands of IADLs may require more effort and energy than they did previously. Often clients with an acute onset of neurological, orthopedic, and cognitive/perceptual impairments express feelings of fatigue and may be generally deconditioned secondary to a prolonged

Table 4-3

PERFORMANCE PATTERNS AND IMPACT ON IADLs

Category	AOTA Definition (2002, p. 621)	Impact on IADLs
Motor Skills • Posture • Mobility • Coordination • Strength and effort • Energy	Skills in moving and interacting with task, objects, and environment (Fisher, personal communication, July 9, 2001).	• Poor posture secondary to pain or prolonged use of an assistive device will limit endurance. • Use of walker, cane or crutches may limit ability to carry items. • Impaired fine motor coordination may limit safety with cooking tasks. • Impaired gross motor coordination may limit safety with community mobility. • Increased effort with performance due to muscle weakness may limit muscle energy and endurance for completion of tasks.
Process Skills • Energy • Knowledge • Temporal organization • Organizing space and objects • Adaptation	"Skills... used in managing and modifying actions en route to the completion of daily life tasks" (Fisher & Kielhofner, 1995, p. 120).	• Sustained effort with the motor components of IADL tasks will require pacing and may limit energy available for higher-level problem-solving skills and attention to task. • Impairments may be noted in choosing appropriate tasks, selecting appropriate tools, use of tools, or inability to ask for assistance. • Limitations may be evident in the client's ability to initiate, sequence, continue, and end an IADL task for success. • The client must be able to obtain needed items for a task and organize the environment for task performance as well as return objects to their designated space upon completion. • IADL tasks may often require modifications and adjustments for safe and effective completion.

continued

Table 4-3 continued

PERFORMANCE PATTERN AND IMPACT ON IADLs

Category	AOTA Definition (2002, p. 621)	Impact on IADLs
Communication/Interaction Skills • Physicality • Information exchange • Relations	Refer to conveying intentions and needs and coordinating social behavior to act together with people (Forsyth & Kielhofner, 1999; Forsyth, Salamy, Simon, & Kielhofner, 1997; Kielhofner, 2002).	• Limitations in range of motion (ROM) and strength may affect ability to communicate verbally or with gesture in the community. • The client may have difficulty requesting information by phone for financial matters. • Social interaction with family or friends may be limited.

Table 4-4

DOMAIN OF OCCUPATIONAL THERAPY

Category	AOTA Definition (2002, p. 623)	Impact on IADLs
Habits • Useful habits • Impoverished habits • Dominating habits	"'Automatic behavior that is integrated into more complex patterns that enable people to function on a day-to-day basis' (Neistadt & Crepeau, 1998, p. 869). Habits can either support or interfere with performance in areas of occupation."	• Selecting and placing clothing out for the next day when needing to be out early. • Forgetting to close kitchen cabinets and drawers. • Smoking.
Routines	"'Occupations with established sequences' (Christiansen & Baum, 1997, p. 6)."	Establishing a daily medication schedule.
Roles	"'A set of behaviors that have some socially agreed upon function and for which there is an accepted code of norms' (Christiansen & Baum, 1997, p. 603)."	Preparing the evening meal, role of caregiver.

hospital stay. Activities such as stair climbing on a daily basis or meeting social obligations can cause the client to experience fatigue. Meeting the demands of the day will require planning and organization in order to work efficiently and within an appropriate tolerance level. A client who is being introduced to new medications should also be monitored for changes in fatigue level as well as activity tolerance that may be a consequence of the change.

Table 4-5	
ACTIVITY DEMANDS AND IMPACT ON IADLS	
Space Demands	Home modifications may be indicated to accommodate assistive devices for gait.
Social Demands	Clients may need to entertain within their own home if accessibility to other environments is limited or if community mobility is an issue.
Sequencing and Timing	Both skills are needed for clients to be able to prepare a meal in an efficient manner.
Required Actions	The client must have the ability to complete all of the required actions necessary for driving to maintain safety.
Required Body Functions	A client may not participate in outdoor home maintenance activities if he/she demonstrates impaired balance on uneven surfaces.
Required Body Structures	A client with a nonfunctional UE will be unable to complete tasks requiring bilateral integration such as grasping and holding a laundry basket.

Continuous education in principles of energy conservation and work simplification may assist the client in participating in additional occupations more effectively. An introduction to adaptive equipment and durable medical equipment (DME) would also be indicated at this time. This area will also be addressed in greater detail throughout this section. Table 4-5 summarizes how activity demands can impact IADLs.

CLIENT FACTORS

Client factors are, "Those factors that reside within the client and that may affect performance in areas of occupation. Client factors include body functions and body structures" (AOTA, 2002, p. 624).

Any change a client may experience within his/her body may influence overall performance. Strength, mobility, ROM, muscle tone, postural stability, postural alignment, reflexes, control, and endurance should be assessed. Intervention in the form of remediation or compensation/adaptation will need to occur for the client to achieve independence in IADL. For more information on remediation of these skills, see Chapter 2.

ROLE OF THE OCCUPATIONAL THERAPY ASSISTANT

The role of the occupational therapy assistant (OTA) is to facilitate intervention in all aspects of IADL (AOTA, 2004). The OTA, under the supervision of an OTR, may implement an intervention plan utilizing remediation or compensation/adaptation techniques to facilitate independence in home management, financial management, community skills, communication devices, and care of others. For example, in an inpatient rehabilitation setting, the OTA may teach compensation/adaptation techniques to a client with a new CVA to facilitate independence with meal preparation. The

OTA may introduce adaptive devices such as a one-handed cutting board, a rocker knife, and/or a walker basket and educate the patient in hemi-techniques. For the client who has undergone a total hip replacement, the OTA may make recommendations for environmental changes within the home. These changes may include rearranging the refrigerator or cabinets to place the client's most frequently used items at waist level or above in order for the client to maintain total hip precautions. An adaptive device such as a reacher may be introduced to assist with certain tasks.

Prior to the intervention of IADL, it is understood that the OT has evaluated performance skills, performance patterns, and context. As a result of this assessment and interview with the client and/or the client's family, a method of intervention will be selected. A thorough understanding of the client's previous role within the family, the amount of support and assistance available, and quality of socialization outside of the home is important. This will assist the OT in determining intervention methods. The OTA will discuss with the OTR the findings of the evaluation and interview process in order to recommend intervention. Hence, the OTA will have a thorough understanding of the client's goals and the recommended method of intervention. The OTA may collaborate with the OTR with respect to the client's progress and together the two will determine new goals when indicated. The OTR will assist the client with recommendations for discharge planning in the inpatient setting and determine the safest plan and the services the client will require upon discharge to home. The OTA possesses the skills to observe the day to day progress that a client is making. In the event that the client has demonstrated a change in status, or if the client's set goals seem to be too high or too low, the OTA will need to bring this matter to the attention of the OTR for review.

EVALUATION OF INSTRUMENTAL ACTIVITIES OF DAILY LIVING

While the focus of this text is intervention, evaluations will be discussed briefly because they are an important component of the intervention plan. The first step of any evaluation is the completion of an interview or an occupational profile with the client. This allows the therapist to gather information regarding the client's motivating factors, goals, discharge needs, etc. One tool that can quickly and easily be administered to assist in this process is the Canadian Occupational Performance Measure (COPM). This tool allows the client to identify areas of occupation in which he/she would like to improve (Law, Baptiste, Carswell, McColl, Polatajko, & Pollock, 1998). Using a functional approach, the therapist would then begin to evaluate specific IADLs that the client desires to work on and that are required for discharge planning. While there are many evaluations available, a few examples of formal evaluations include the Performance Assessment of Self-Care Skills (PASS), the Kohlman Evaluation of Living Skills (KELS), the Arnadottir OT-ADL Neurobehavioral Assessment (A-ONE), and the Independent Living Scales (ILS). The PASS and A-ONE were discussed thoroughly in Chapter 3. The KELS, developed by Kohlman and Thomson, is an interview and activity-based evaluation. The evaluation includes five subsections with money management, transportation, and telephone use relating to IADLs (Thomson, 1992). This tool requires no training and the evaluation kit is inexpensive. The ILS addresses cognitive and perceptual skills while observing functional IADL tasks. This tool is standardized, therefore activities are completed in a set format rather than as the client may complete them at home. No training is required and the kit is relatively inexpensive (Psychological Corporation, 1996).

Informal evaluations include a kitchen evaluation and a home evaluation. Generally, these evaluations are created by individual facilities based on the needs of the client population. The kitchen evaluation includes the client's physical, cognitive, perceptual, visual, and endurance skills during a kitchen task. The home evaluation addresses the context, safety, and function of the client in whatever environment is planned postdischarge from occupational therapy. Refer to Appendix B for more evaluatuations.

INTERVENTION OF INSTRUMENTAL ACTIVITIES OF DAILY LIVING

Remediation of IADLs

In general, remediation of acute impairments involves relearning basic performance skills. Normal movement patterns are necessary for developing independence in all areas of IADL. For example, if a client who is right hand dominant has experienced a left CVA with resulting right hemiparesis, he/she may be unable to use the right UE functionally, as in writing a check. By utilizing the remediation approach, the client may develop functional ROM, strength, and coordination of the right UE to be able to complete a check-writing task. The client learns to use the affected UE for functional tasks versus learning compensation or adaptation techniques for use of the unaffected UE such as paying by cash or credit card. For more information regarding these foundational skills to IADLs, see Chapter 2.

By the time the client is advanced enough to participate in IADLs, utilizing the remediation approach will have involved practicing each task until mastery has been or is nearly achieved. For example, if the client wishes to manage his/her own checkbook, he/she will have had to practice writing skills to be able to legibly write a check. Basic mathematical skills will also need to be mastered if there is impairment in this area in order to manage money independently.

In conclusion, the remediation approach for clients who are ready to participate in IADLs involves practicing each task until mastery is achieved. The OT must give careful consideration to the client's allotted rehabilitation benefits as well as the client's disposition plan when working with the client and the rehabilitation team to determine whether or not the remediation approach is the best course for each individual client. Factors to consider are:

1. The client's overall readiness to learn.
2. The client's functional goals.
3. The client's prognosis and estimated rate and level of recovery.
4. The estimated length of occupational therapy intervention prior to discharge.
5. The amount of assistance the client will have upon discharge.

With careful consideration of these factors, the client and the rehabilitation team will determine the most appropriate approach for intervention. The selected approach may need to be reconsidered for efficacy if the client is not progressing as efficiently as expected or if recovery has been expedited. It may also be necessary to combine both approaches in order for the client to be discharged to home. Compensation/adaptation techniques may be utilized as the client continues with remediation of deficits. This will allow independence and safety with IADL while continuing to regain function.

Compensation/Adaptation of IADL Deficits for Clients With Physical Limitations: Performance Skills/Client Factors

Limitations a client experiences secondary to impairments in ROM, strength, coordination, sensation, pain, or endurance can greatly affect the client's ability to participate in IADL tasks in a safe and independent manner (Figure 4-2). These clients will have begun occupational therapy intervention once their physicians deemed them medically stable. Therefore, they may have recognized some of the limitations that they will encounter upon discharge to their home early after the onset of their illness.

Physical limitations will dictate the type of task chosen, the manner in which the client performs the task, the assistive devices he/she will need to use to facilitate independence, the level of

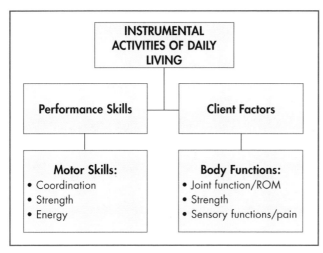

Figure 4-2. Components of performance skills/client factors related to IADLs (adapted from American Occupational Therapy Association. (2002). *Occupational therapy practice framework: Domain and process.* Bethesda, MD: AOTA).

activity tolerance, and the outcome. The client who is to participate in IADL tasks will need to have achieved a safe functional status through remediation of performance skills, or the client will need to have mastered adequate adaptation/compensation skills to facilitate the same. Whatever the approach, the client and his/her support system, along with the rehabilitation team, will need to determine what goals are feasible for this client.

Compensation/Adaptation Interventions of IADL for Clients With Decreased Performance Skills/Client Factors: ROM, Strength, and Coordination Deficits

HOME MANAGEMENT (HOME ESTABLISHMENT, MEAL PREP AND CLEAN-UP)

Laundry

Participating in the home management task of doing laundry involves collecting soiled clothing, carrying the load to the washer, separating clothing items, loading the washing machine, adding soap and bleach as indicated, and starting the cycle (Figure 4-3). It then involves removing clothing from the washer and placing it in the dryer, or hanging clothing on a clothes rack or clothesline. Once dry, the client will fold each piece of clothing and place it in a closet or drawer. For some clients, laundry management was a daily chore and for others a chore completed less frequently. Upon initial discharge to home, the client, along with his/her family and/or caregivers, will need to determine the amount of energy the client can allow for this task and still participate in other IADL tasks. It may be determined that the client should complete only one aspect of laundry management initially, and gradually work up to full management. Or it may be within the client's tolerance to complete all aspects of this task. Another consideration is the location of the washer and dryer and whether or not stairs are a factor. For the client with a neurological impairment, navigating stairs may be contraindicated upon initial discharge to home, and therefore completing the full task of laundry management may not be feasible. However, any aspect of the task such as collecting soiled clothing or folding clean laundry, may be completed.

Changing the Task to Achieve Independence

Clients with upper extremity (UE) physical impairments may experience many performance skill deficits. Some important points discussed are: safety, participation level, accessibility, and

Figure 4-3. Relationship of ROM, strength, and coordination to IADLs (adapted from American Occupational Therapy Association. (2002). *Occupational therapy practice framework: Domain and process.* Bethesda, MD: AOTA).

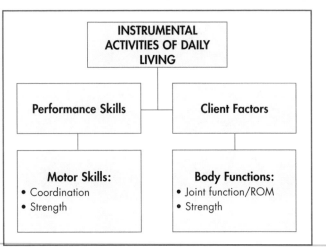

compensation/adaptation for balance and carrying items. Education in safety is of significant importance, and evaluation of a client's safety should be ongoing. The OT may need to perform home safety evaluations to assess the environment and make recommendations for modifications. In order to participate in the management of the laundry, the washer and dryer should be easily accessible to the client, especially with the use of an assistive device for gait. Laundry detergent and other laundry needs should be within reach. If hemiparesis is present, the client may need to use one-handed techniques to load the machines and to pour the detergent. Smaller, lighter detergent containers may be indicated for use. The receptacle for soiled clothing may need to be placed near the washer so the client will not need to carry the clothing. If that is not possible, a large duffle bag may be used so that the client can pull it along instead of carrying the clothing.

Placing newly washed laundry in the dryer should be less of a challenge to the client unless balance is an issue. If so, the client may need to remove clothing from the washer and place it on top of the dryer and sit to load clothes into the machine. Once the clothes are dry, the client will need to bring them to a table or other flat surface and fold them via one-handed technique. The client should then carry small bundles of clothing to the dressers and closets and put them away. If the client is unsteady with gait, the client may need to use a cart to complete this task in a safe and efficient manner. In extreme cases, a wheelchair may be required to maintain safety.

Clients with lower extremity (LE) or trunk limitations will experience different limitations. After joint replacement or back surgery, the client will have limited ROM and also may have to adhere to certain precautions. For example, the client who is recovering from a total hip replacement will not be able to bend at the waist beyond 90 degrees. The client who is status post back surgery will be limited in bending as well as twisting at the waist. These clients will need to stand for this activity. When sitting, the client may bend forward beyond 90 degrees to retrieve the clothing from its place of holding or to load the dryer. For purposes of maintaining precautions and balance, laundry baskets and all other working items should be placed on higher surfaces and not on the floor. Once the task is complete, the client will need to place his/her clothing in a drawer that is higher so as not to bend too far forward at the waist.

Changing the Tools to Achieve Independence

As previously noted, the client may use a duffle bag to carry laundry instead of a laundry basket, which would require the use of both hands. The client may then pull the duffle bag with one hand. If the client is using a walker, a lighter laundry bag may be attached to the front of the device and the client may need to make more trips to the laundry area. Also, smaller containers of laundry detergent may be indicated as noted above so that it will be easier for the client to grasp and pour with one hand.

For clients with limited ability to bend, a reacher may be required to assist with placing clothing in the dryer or removing the dry clothing. In addition, for the client with limited weight-bearing status, using a walker or crutches may limit his/her ability to carry clothing to and from the working area. A push cart may be required so that the client can push the clothes rather than carry them.

Light Cleaning

Light cleaning involves dusting, mopping floors, and organizing the home. Participating in the task of dusting involves bending and reaching to achieve thoroughness, grasping and lifting objects, and manipulation of dust cloths for the task. Mopping floors requires the ability to move furniture to reach all surfaces and to manipulate all required tools for the task. Organizing the home involves sorting out important items and placing them in their designated space and eliminating those items that are no longer wanted.

Changing the Task to Achieve Independence

For the client with physical deficits, one-handed techniques once again may be utilized to complete the above home management tasks. Utilization of energy conservation techniques may be necessary, as it will take the client a much longer time to complete these tasks. With dusting, the client will move more slowly from one area to the next, particularly if using an assistive device for gait. Removing items with one hand and then dusting and replacing items will take longer, especially if the client must use his/her nondominant hand. The client may be limited to dusting surfaces at waist level or slightly higher or lower if balance is an issue.

Mopping floors is a more challenging task for the client who manifests limited use of one UE and/or a deficit in balance. Light mops that may be pushed with one hand would be an appropriate choice. The client would benefit from mopping a small area at a time, moving slowly to change position.

Organizing the home is a general part of home management. Every client has a comfort level in terms of how his/her home looks. The client with a physical deficit will have to consider all aspects of his/her ability when determining the best way to organize the home. Modifications may be required in order to ensure safety. Regularly used kitchen items, for example, may need to be placed at more safe levels of reach. Items that are normally placed in cabinets or closets may need to be on countertops or on wall racks to assist the client with easier accessibility. Throw rugs may need to be removed, and pet care items will also need to be placed carefully to assure client safety. The client may need assistance at first to reorganize the home and subsequent organization should be easier. Of consideration to the client will be the level of ability to carry objects from one place to another, as well as maintaining use of the recommended ambulatory device while maintaining balance. It would be beneficial to clients if other members of the household organize their personal items and also maintain general organization to assist the client. If the client lives alone, it should be easier to maintain the home in the way the client desires.

For the postsurgical client who is limited in weight-bearing status on one LE, it may be best to delegate some of the tasks that involve challenging balance to a caregiver. Simple tasks may be accomplished if they do not jeopardize the client's safety. The client may require assistance to set up these tasks and sit while doing so. Once the client is as able to weight-bear as tolerated, he/she may be ready to attempt more involved tasks. The client must also maintain any movement precautions as indicated for total hip replacements, such as avoiding bending beyond 90 degrees either in sitting or in standing, or those precautions for clients who have had back surgery, such as avoiding forward bending or twisting at the waist. Therefore, performing certain tasks at wheelchair level may be contraindicated if they will involve bending forward or twisting at the waist.

Walker baskets may be indicated to assist with transport of items. A pushcart on wheels may also be an efficient method of transport. The client will need to make good use of adaptive equipment, such as a reacher, to retrieve items from high or low levels. Depending on the level of deficits and the availability, the client may utilize a wheelchair for these tasks or use outside services to assist with cleaning and organizing the home.

Outdoor Home Maintenance

This activity includes management of lawn, garden, landscaping, and patio. Outdoor home maintenance may be considered one of the more advanced IADL activities. Clients may view these tasks as work or leisure. Home therapy intervention by both physical and occupational therapists may be indicated in order to assure that clients maintain safety with each task. Clients must also be realistic in their expectations as these tasks may require a higher-level of endurance.

Changing the Task to Achieve Independence

Clients with limited physical skills may demonstrate impaired balance with gait on uneven surfaces such as grass or sand. It would be beneficial to the client to first practice ambulation on these surfaces and obtain a good level of balance prior to attempting any outdoor home maintenance tasks. Once ambulation is safe, the client may begin the challenge of maintaining the outside of his/her home. The client should be encouraged to choose tasks that are simple at first, yet provide enough of a challenge to feel a sense of accomplishment. Simple weeding tasks may be a good choice, for the client should be able to utilize one-handed techniques to complete this activity, if required. Watering the garden, flowers, or the lawn may also be a just right challenge for the client.

Another consideration is the area in which the client expects to work. A smaller working area would be indicated initially as the client begins to challenge him/herself with more advanced IADLs.

Lastly, outdoor home maintenance may be a difficult task for clients that are recovering from orthopedic surgery, especially if they maintain a limited weight-bearing status on the affected UE or LE. Of concern also would be limitations in forward bending of the trunk if seated, which would be the position of choice if a client were unable to bear full weight on one LE. Clients that are recovering from total hip replacement surgery or back surgery will be limited in their ability to bend at the waist, which would make gardening from a seated position contraindicated. While the client recovering from orthopedic surgery would need to wait until his/her restrictions are lifted before tackling many of the activities necessary to manage the outdoors, some tasks can be raised to higher surfaces to allow gardening. One example of this would be flowers or vegetables planted in pots on tables or in raised platforms.

Changing the Tools to Achieve Independence

The client may wish to participate in lawn care. Using a riding mower may be the easiest and most energy efficient method for the client. Assessment of the client's motor skills must first be obtained to assure that the client will have good control of the mower. The client must also be able to step on and off the machine safely. If a riding mower is not available, the client may benefit from pushing a lawn mower if he/she has enough UE strength and enough endurance to tolerate all aspects of the activity. Of consideration would be the client's ability to start the mower with one hand as indicated. If the client does not possess the strength to do so, he/she may require assistance or select a mower with an electric starter.

If the client has the motor skills sufficient to operate a power mower safely, he/she may consider a leaf blower as well to assist with management of leaves, and a snow blower to assist with snow removal.

Other tools may include a rolling garden chair with armrests to sit and complete planting or weeding, power equipment versus manual devices to compensate for deficits in motor skills, and garden tools with wider handles for easier grip. Work belts may be considered to carry necessary gardening supplies.

Shopping

The *Occupational Therapy Framework: Domain and Process* defines shopping as, "preparing shopping lists (grocery and other), selecting and purchasing items, selecting method of payment, and completing money transactions" (AOTA, 2002, p. 620). This includes the ability to organize and write or dictate a shopping list and the ability to mobilize in the community safely (discussed later in this chapter). Prior to visiting the store, the client must also determine the method to be used for payment and bring the appropriate money or credit/debit cards to be used. Upon arrival to the store, the client needs to determine what he/she needs to buy, select the necessary items from the shelves, place these items in a basket/cart, and pay for them in an appropriate manner. The client must keep in mind how much he/she is able to buy and carry. This is dependent upon the type of transportation being used to bring the client home and the limitations of the client's deficit. After shopping is completed, the client must bring the purchased items into the home and put them away.

Changing the Task to Achieve Independence

A client with physical impairment may demonstrate impaired motor skills. If the client's dominate UE is affected, and handwriting is impaired, the client may need to find an alternative method of recording a shopping list. While most of these alternatives include a new tool, the client can attempt to change the task by using the nondominant hand to write the shopping list. Shopping may be easier for some clients since most clients find that pushing the shopping cart helps with balance in the store. Endurance will still be an issue for consideration, and this will be addressed later in this section. Clients with LE impairment may have difficulty navigating the store. Also, the use of crutches may limit their ability to push a carriage.

Also of consideration may be the limited use of one UE. The client will have to reach for items with the unaffected UE. This may put the client at the risk of unsteadiness and possibly losing balance if he/she has no means of support. It may then be most beneficial for this client to have a companion when shopping.

If traditional shopping is not possible, the client may participate in home shopping and delivery services that are now available. This will generally be easier for younger adults because computer use is familiar to them. While not ideal, some clients may participate in a Meals on Wheels program to eliminate the need for extensive shopping.

Changing the Tools to Achieve Independence

If using the affected dominant UE, writing devices such as special grips for pens/pencils or other adaptive devices may assist. Figures 4-4 and 4-5 depict examples of adaptive writing devices. If using the unaffected nondominant UE, stabilization of the paper will be a factor to consider. Clipboards may be of assistance or the paper may be taped to the table. Whenever possible, the client using the unaffected UE should be encouraged to use the affected side for stabilization.

Should the activity of writing be deemed not feasible for the client at this time, use of a recording device may be indicated. The client may also be encouraged to use a computer if he/she is able to manipulate the keys and the mouse with one hand without experiencing frustration. If the client manifests a sufficient gross grasp, he/she may use a dowel to tap the computer keys for writing.

Those clients using a walker and who are not fully weight-bearing on the affected LE will not be able to use the grocery cart to assist with gait. Any of these clients may benefit from an electric riding device, or the assistance from friends or family for shopping.

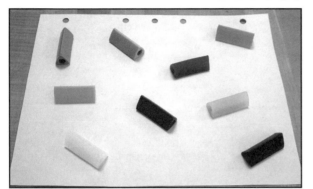

Figure 4-4. Adaptive pen/pencil grips.

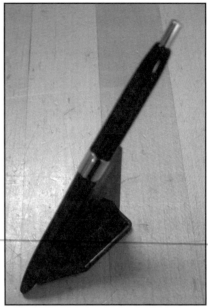

Figure 4-5. Adaptive writing device.

For clients with limited ability to reach items on shelves, a reacher may be utilized. Clients must be informed that items can fall from the reacher and cause injury to them, therefore the reacher should be used for lighter items. If there is a need to retrieve or carry heavier items, this client will need assistance from another. Often, grocery store clerks are willing to assist with such tasks, particularly in the smaller neighborhood stores. These clerks may also be available to bring the groceries to the car and load them as well.

Preparing a Meal

Preparation of a meal may have been an important occupation for the client before the onset of an injury or illness. Therefore, it may be very important for this client to be able to return to a level of function that will allow him/her to perform this task safely and as independently as possible once again. According to the *Framework*, meal preparation and clean-up includes, "Planning, preparing, serving well-balanced nutritional meals and cleaning up food and utensils after meals" (2002, p. 620). This author has included setting the table as well.

For preparation of a meal, the client must plan the meal menu, retrieve all ingredients, have the ability to measure them correctly, and follow directions for assembly of the selected recipe. The client will then assemble the ingredients and prepare the dish for cooking or baking. The client must then cook or bake the selected items and set the oven or stove correctly.

Changing the Task to Achieve Independence

The client with physical limitations may have limited use of one UE and may need a walker, cane, or crutches to navigate around the kitchen. One-handed techniques may be implemented to assist this client with meal preparation. The client who uses a cane may have the use of one UE to assist with this task, but may require increased time and effort to transport items one by one. Kitchen modifications may be indicated so that the client may be able to reach any items needed for meal preparation safely and without loss of balance. For example, frequently used cooking or baking pans normally placed in low cabinets should be placed in cabinets or on countertops at waist level or slightly higher. Refrigerated items should be placed on the higher shelves and towards

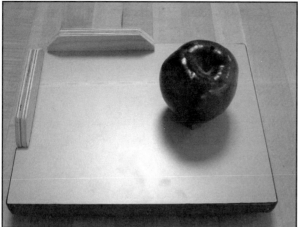

Figure 4-6. Adaptive cutting board.

the front for easier reach. This type of organization is also recommended for the client who is limited in LE or trunk movement.

The client with impaired balance may choose to sit for most of the task of meal preparation. If ambulating and carrying items puts the client at risk for falling, the client may seek help from family. If assistance is not available, the client may choose to use a rolling cart to transport items if he/she is deemed safe by the therapist to do so.

Changing the Tools to Achieve Independence

The use of adaptive devices will be of great assistance to the client with limited UE use. The use of a walker basket or walker tray, for example, may assist the client with transporting objects from one surface to another. Rocker knives, one-handed cutting boards, and dycem may also be devices of choice. Figure 4-6 depicts an adaptive cutting board. The OT working with the client in a rehab setting or in the home must educate the client in the use of these items to facilitate independence with meal preparation. The client with limited UE use will need assistance with placing and removing pans from the oven and the stove. Lighter weight pots and pans can increase independence, or the client will need to use the microwave or utilize stove-top cooking. If family is available to assist, the client may also ask for assistance with this task in order to maintain safety.

Although not ideal, if meal preparation is not safe, the client may utilize the services offered from others to prepare meals that the client will only need to reheat. Programs that provide hot meals delivered to the home may also be an option for the client to consider in order to eliminate the preparation of one hot meal for the day. Frozen dinners or prepackaged foods may also be used. However, attention must be paid to nutritional content.

Setting the Table

This task includes retrieving dishes and silverware from cabinets, carrying them to the table, and walking around the table to place the dinnerware at each setting. Napkins, condiments, and drinks must also be retrieved and placed on the table. In addition, the food must be served at the table.

Changing the Task to Achieve Independence

Participating in the task of setting the table is similar to the task of transporting items for meal preparation as outlined above. The client using a cane may be able to carry light items in one hand to the table if he/she demonstrates good balance and good strength of the affected UE since the client will be holding the cane with the unaffected side. This client may have to make

Figure 4-7. Cart utilized for transporting items in the kitchen.

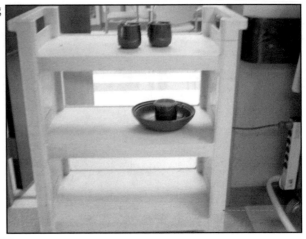

several trips to complete the task and avoid lifting heavy objects with just one hand. Once all the necessary items are carried to the table, the client will then need to ambulate around the table and set a place for each family member. The client may complete the task using a wheelchair, if necessary, or may sit to set the table if the table is small enough for the client to reach each setting area from one seat.

Changing the Tools to Achieve Independence

A walker basket, tray, or push cart may be used to transport some of the table settings (Figure 4-7). Lighter settings may be used, such as paper plates and cups, to increase ease and safety during transportation of the tableware.

Wash/Dry Dishes and Put Dishes Away

The last task within home management is cleaning and putting away the dishes. This task includes bringing all dishes, pans, and silverware that need to be cleaned to the sink, filling the washbasin, and then adding soap. The client must then wash and rinse all dishes, dry them and put them in their appropriate place. For those clients who use a dishwasher, they will load the dishes and silverware, add soap, and then set and start the device. When dry, the client will remove all items and place them in their appropriate place.

Changing the Task to Achieve Independence

Washing and drying dishes can be completed in standing or sitting. The client may require assistance to carry the items to be washed to the sink. If the client has limited or no functional use of one UE, he/she will have to attempt one-handed techniques for this task. Heavier pans or dishes may have to be left for someone else to wash and dry. If the client is able to use the affected UE, caution must be taken and the stronger arm should bear most of the work. Sensation should be assessed and if there is impairment, the client should be aware to test the water for dish washing with the unaffected hand prior to using the affected side.

In order to manage drying the dishes utilizing one-handed technique, the client may place a towel on the countertop and place the dish on the towel. With that towel or another, the client can wipe the dishes with one hand.

If the client has a dishwasher in the home, it may be easier to complete this task. The client will need to have good balance to load and unload the machine, especially if working towards the affected side. It may be safer for the client to stand with the machine to his/her unaffected side and load from that position instead of turning towards the affected side to load the dishwasher.

For example, if the client stands at the sink with the dishwasher to his/her right, and the right side is the affected side, the client should place dirty dishes to the right of the dishwasher, stand to the right of the machine, and load the dishwasher with his/her left hand. If possible, the client can use the affected UE to stabilize him/herself on the countertop while completing the task. To place the dishwasher soap in the machine, the client may use the same positioning technique.

To unload the dishwasher or to put hand-dried dishes away, the client should also work with the dishes to his/her unaffected side. The client may stack the dishes first on a counter near where they are to be placed, or place each piece in the drawer or cabinet as it is removed from the dishwasher. The client using a walker will place dishes on the countertop and move them along to the cabinet, taking a few steps with the walker after placing the dishes. The client using a cane may use the same technique, or may carry the dishes to their destination. As discussed previously, heavy pots, pans, or dishes will have to remain on the countertop until the client has assistance to put them away.

It may be difficult for this client to put dishes away from wheelchair level. If cabinets are high, the client will need to stand to put items away if he/she is able. If not, the client will need to find a new location within reach for these items or wait for assistance.

The clients who must adhere to total hip or spine precautions may not be able to complete the task of loading and unloading the dishwasher from a standing position because they may need to bend beyond 90 degrees at the hip to complete the task. Attempting this task from a seated position would also be contraindicated, as it would mean bending past 90 degrees. If this client has no assistance, he/she may need to resort to hand-washing and drying of dishes.

The task of putting dishes away may be accomplished if the client can complete the task and maintain the appropriate weight-bearing status/precautions. However, the client will only be able to place dishes in upper cabinets, as he/she will not be able to bend to place any items in the lower cabinets if maintenance of total hip or spine precautions is required.

Changing the Tools to Achieve Independence

If the client prefers to eliminate this task, paper dishes and plastic silverware may be used. A walker basket, tray, or push cart may also be utilized for transporting silverware or lighter dinnerware to and from the sink or dishwasher.

Financial Management

Finances are a very important aspect of IADL for all, but especially for those who have been hospitalized and have gone through rehabilitation, and for those with chronic illnesses. The cost incurred may be more than the client can put forth if he/she is not covered by insurance. Yet, even if a client is fortunate enough to have appropriate insurance coverage, other expenses may be accrued in an effort to help the client to live safely in his/her own home. For example, the client may need to pay out of pocket for additional help with ADL or IADL, for necessary durable medical equipment (DME) and adaptive devices, or for home modifications (Pynoos & Nishita, 2003).

Another consideration would be if the client was the main financial provider for the family or for him, or herself. If so, the client may now need assistance with financial planning and budgeting, especially if the client is unable to return to work or to the job he/she left. However, in addition to needing assistance for the long scope of care, the client will need financial assistance for normal day-to-day financial tasks such as paying for groceries and paying monthly bills.

Changing the Task to Achieve Independence

If a client has experienced an injury or illness that has resulted in motor deficits limiting use of the dominant UE, this will make the task of writing difficult. This could impact check writing or any financial matter requiring the client to sign his/her name. The client will need to continue to practice writing skills with the nondominant hand until the highest level of mastery is achieved.

The tasks of managing money and counting bills or change may also be difficult. The client may need to organize his/her bills in a wallet from largest to smallest or fold bills separately within the wallet to make them thicker to grasp from the wallet. In general, most clients can use the unaffected extremity to compensate with little difficulty.

Changing the Tools to Achieve Independence

If the client demonstrates some aspect of strength and coordination of the dominant UE, he/she may be able to relearn writing skills with the dominant hand and use of adaptive devices. Examples of these devices include built-up grips, a weighted pen to stabilize handwriting if tremulous, a weighted holder to slip onto pens for stabilization, or a gliding device that supports a pen or pencil to assist with limited strength or control of the arm. When writing, the client may need to position objects for use on his/her lap or on a tray versus using a table to maintain recommended positioning of the UE or for comfort.

If adaptive devices are not appropriate, the use of cash or debit/credit cards may be more manageable for the client. The client may also benefit from computerized bill paying, which is available through most banks.

For money management, a separate change purse may be utilized so that the client does not have to dig into a purse or pants pockets to locate change.

Community Mobility

Loss of independence in the area of community mobility for the client with a neurological deficit, the client who has experienced orthopedic surgery, or the client with cognitive/perceptual deficits can be devastating. Limitations in this area may mean a strong regression from socialization for a client. It may also mean difficulty keeping doctor's appointments, therapy appointments, and other important meetings. A client who is used to going out daily or being free to move about in the community on an as-needed basis may feel restricted with new limitations in this area. For example, in the past, if the client ran out of milk at home, he/she may have easily driven to the store to purchase it. Clients may now have to wait for a family member, caregiver, or friend to take them to the store or to bring the milk to the house. The OT needs to address the level of importance mobilizing in the community has with each client and determine the best approach towards this goal if it is significant to the individual. The therapist needs to discuss with clients where they will go in the community and how often there is a need to get around. Education regarding community transportation resources alone is insufficient according to Logan, Gladman, Avery, Walker, Dyas, & Groom (1994). This group found that intervention by occupational therapy, rather than education alone, resulted in increased community outings. More information regarding functional mobility intervention can be found in Chapter 3.

The client must determine if he/she wishes to return to driving again, and the therapist must determine if the client is safe enough and manifests the appropriate performance skills to carry out this task. For example, residual deficits in ROM, sensation, vision, endurance, hearing, and higher-level cognitive processing must be evaluated before the client can be referred for a driving exam. If the client manifests the appropriate motor and sensory skills, however, demonstrates impaired safety and judgment, the therapist should redirect the client's goals and avoid referring the client for a driving exam.

For the client who appears to be ready to begin driving soon after discharge, the therapist should make use of the clinical setting to begin retraining of the client in preparation for driving once again. There are some rehabilitation facilities that have an area designated for driving simulation. Often, there is a model car that the client may use to practice the motor components of driving such as placing and turning the key, shifting, steering, and transferring his/her foot from the gas pedal to the brake. It should be noted that driver retraining is not considered an entry-level skill for OTs and continued education is required prior to initiating this with clients. See Appendix A for further information regarding training.

If driving is unrealistic, the OT and other members of the rehabilitation team need to address other options with the client and offer suggestions and recommendations for alternative methods of transportation. The client may be fearful at first to use public transportation because the concept may be new to him/her. The elderly client may be concerned about being out alone or may have a fear of selecting the wrong transit system and becoming lost. They may have difficulty with transit fees. Also of concern to any client is the ability to mobilize independently on and off the transit vehicle in a safe manner, or walking safely to a bus stop. Weather conditions may also limit the client's ability to use public transport. The OT can work with a social worker to determine what means of transportation are available to the client. Some communities offer transport to and from the home for a minimal fee. If clients are fortunate enough to have family or friends to assist them, they may be sacrificing independence; however, the use of public transportation will be minimal.

Functional mobility within the community must also be addressed with all clients whether they return to driving or need to resort to an alternative means of transportation. The client must be able to step in and out of a car safely and be able to climb the stairs of a bus or other transportation vehicle independently. Clients recovering from any number of neurological or orthopedic injuries will need to be transported with their assistive device for gait such as a walker, cane, or wheelchair. If the client has limited or no functional use of one UE, he/she may not be able to use transportation that requires walking up steps secondary to the inability to then carry the walking device and hold on to a rail at the same time. See Functional Mobility in Chapter 2 for more information.

Changing the Task to Achieve Independence

While clients with a variety of diagnoses will experience difficulty with community mobility, the client with a neurological deficit is the client who needs special consideration for return to driving. After full interview, assessment, and intervention of the client, the OT will determine if the client demonstrates the ability to return to driving in a safe and appropriate manner. As previously discussed, the client will be referred for a driving exam if he/she demonstrates appropriate functional performance in all areas needed to perform the task. If the client does not manifest those performance skills necessary to drive safely, the OT will work with the client to determine the most effective means of transportation to replace driving. The client who is recovering from orthopedic surgery of the UE or LE may experience the same difficulties with public transportation as the client with a neurological insult. This client, however, should be able to return to driving if he/she wishes, with the consent of the doctor, once sufficiently healed. A driving test would not be indicated.

Changing the Tools to Achieve Independence

The client may rely on family, friends, public transportation, or taxicabs for rides as well as for trips to a shopping center. It is best if the client can select a method of transportation where he/she can be picked up and dropped off directly at his/her home until he/she achieves more independence with ambulation in the community. Many communities offer low cost transportation for the elderly as well. The client should use the device that he/she is most safe with for ambulation within the community, even if it is different from the device he/she uses within the home. The client may choose electric riding devices for tasks.

COMMUNICATION DEVICES

Communication is an extremely important aspect of living. All clients, in order to live at home, will need to be able to communicate their needs and wishes as well as respond appropriately in an emergency situation. For those clients who have experienced impairment in motor, sensory, or cognitive skills, effective communication may be limited without the assistance of an adapted device. The OT needs to confer with the speech and language pathologist to assess the effectiveness of the client's communication skills prior to making recommendations for discharge.

Changing the Task to Achieve Independence

For the client who has experienced a neurological deficit, communication skills may be strongly impaired. The client may be aphasic or dysarthric, making comprehension of the client's speech difficult. It may also be difficult for the client to express his/her needs. The client may manifest impaired motor skills that will limit efficiency. Any of the above will limit the client's ability to live home independently or remain at home alone for any period of time.

For the client with aphasia, assessment must be made as to whether or not the client can perform a task, although he/she may not be able to verbalize the steps of a task. For example, if a client is aphasic and is unable to state the emergency phone number 911, yet when given a telephone, the client is able to dial the number appropriately and efficiently, the client may be deemed cognitively appropriate to recognize the need for help. If, however, the client's aphasia limits the ability to express him- or herself once the call is made, the client will be unsafe. If the client's aphasia is manifested in his/her inability to dial the phone appropriately, this client may also be deemed unsafe to be alone. The client with dysarthria must be encouraged to speak slowly and clearly when communicating.

A client must be deemed appropriate for recognition of emergency situations prior to being discharged to home, particularly if 24-hour supervision is not available.

In summary, clients with aphasia and clients manifesting cognitive deficits need to be evaluated carefully in order for an appropriate discharge plan to be made. Clients who manifests aphasia and cognitive impairment may be most unsafe to be alone.

Changing the Tools to Achieve Independence

Impaired mobility may be addressed through the used of portable phones that the clients may have with them at all times. In-home intercoms or pager systems may also be used. If dexterity is impaired, use of one-touch dialing may be beneficial through the use of the unaffected UE if necessary. The client may also use a modified technique for computer use such as one-handed typing or use of a dowel in the affected hand for tapping the computer keys. Communication boards may also be effective in assisting the client with communication of his/her needs. The client may also benefit from an emergency call system where the touch of one button will alert personnel that he/she is in need of help.

CARE OF OTHERS AND CARE OF PETS

At times, the client who presents to the rehabilitation team to recover from a neurological insult or from orthopedic surgery has been the sole caregiver of a spouse or a part-time caregiver for grandchildren. It may be necessary to observe this client and recognize any feelings of depression and/or loss of self-worth secondary to limitations in assuming previous roles after rehabilitation. If the client admits to experiencing these feelings, a psychology or psychiatric consult may be indicated. The social worker assigned to the client must be available to assist the family with arrangements and to provide support to the client as he/she returns home to a new role. Rehabilitation team members (e.g., nurses, physical therapists, OTs, speech and language pathologists, care managers, and social workers) must educate the client's family prior to discharge as to what they can expect of the client when he/she goes home. If the client was the sole caregiver for a spouse prior to the onset of an injury or illness, and this role is no longer safe or appropriate, plans should begin immediately for changes in the client's role upon discharge.

In addition, Baun and McCabe (2003) discuss the impact of a client leaving a pet behind upon admittance to long-term care. The client must relinquish the role of caring for his/her pet, as well as the companionship and unconditional love. As a result, the caregiver must now assume the responsibility of pet care, if able. In turn, the authors also discuss the benefits of the companion animal for the caregiver and the role the pet now takes in terms of comforting the caregiver.

Changing the Task to Achieve Independence

Caring for others in the home may be as simple as supervising medication or as taxing as washing and dressing a spouse. The client and his/her family must discuss what expectations are realistic for the client upon returning home. Recommendations for intervention for the client with neurological deficits or for the client status post-orthopedic surgery should reflect the safest environment for all. Clients who have had surgical procedures will typically have lifting restrictions and clients with neurological diagnoses may have residual weakness that will limit their lifting abilities. A client with either neurological or orthopedic deficits may present with balance impairments that may require the use of a device, and therefore, may restrict the client's ability to care for another.

Child-rearing for a younger adult may be a particularly difficult task. Family and friends may need to be involved to assist the client and his/her family. Daycare centers and after-school programs may be considered to free the clients of some daily activities and supervision to allow them to focus on their own rehabilitation needs. Often, the older child may be involved in the rehabilitation process and in some of the household management tasks. This will allow the child to feel that he/she is contributing to his/her parent's rehabilitation as well as assist with fulfilling some of the needs of the family.

The client and his/her family must be educated in the importance of the client maintaining his/her own safety and health upon discharge. Often, the client's rehabilitation continues at home. Home physical and occupational therapists should evaluate the client's caregiver role if applicable and determine whether or not the client and family member are safe. It may be unsafe to discharge a client to home knowing that he/she will be caring for a spouse or other family member in addition to him- or herself. At this time, the client and his/her family may choose to acquire additional assistance for a family member in need.

The client who is to return to home as caregiver for a pet will need to be evaluated for safety as well. Those clients that have limited balance and are using a device to assist with gait will have to be especially careful of pets crossing their paths and also of any pet toys that may be left anywhere on the floor or carpet. The client that is used to bending forward to pick up a pet will have to maintain adherence to any weight-bearing or bending limitations. Placing food or water for the pet may be difficult for clients with an orthopedic diagnosis if they are unable to fully weight-bear on one LE, or, as in the case of clients who have had a total hip replacement or spinal surgery, they may not be able to bend to the floor. A client that manifests balance deficits may choose to sit to place food and water on the floor, or may choose to place the food on a raised surface. Cats generally will not have difficulty on a raised surface, but this may be problematic for dogs.

Upon the client's arrival home, pets may need to be introduced again when the client is sitting or lying down and not in a position to be pushed over by an excited pet. Often, the client's return home to his/her pet can be very therapeutic and enhance the healing process.

Changing the Tools to Achieve Independence

Pet bowls that are in a raised stand may be useful for clients who are unable to bend to the floor. A reacher may also be used to pick up or put down the bowl. Automatic feeders that need to be filled once per week and automatic litter box cleaners are a possibility to assist clients with limited mobility, strength, and endurance. Pet food may need to be purchased more frequently, in smaller bags, or it may be delivered via online or catalog shopping.

HEALTH MANAGEMENT AND MAINTENANCE

This aspect of IADL is of critical importance to the client and successful management will mean a greater chance for the client to maintain good health and quality of life. Upon initial discharge to home, the client may experience mixed emotions. He/she may be overwhelmed with transitioning from a more secure environment back to home and independent living. Routines must be established early on to assist the client with organization and planning.

The client must first understand the significance of medication compliance and of maintaining appropriate and recommended exercise programs as well as good nutrition and adequate hygiene. Home health care professionals will be available if assistance is needed in generalizing new learning from a rehabilitation setting to the home.

Changing the Task to Achieve Independence

With respect to physical fitness, the clients with neurological or orthopedic impairments will need guidance with developing an individualized exercise program that will promote strength, endurance, and overall good health. The clients should be encouraged to execute the home exercise program that was recommended by the rehabilitation team on a regular basis. Upon discharge from home care services, community exercise programs are also available for continuation of exercise. The client should get approval from the physician before beginning any community exercise program.

Good nutrition is also significant to the healing process. Education should be provided to the client as to what foods are important to consume to reduce any health risks, as well as what foods should be avoided because they are significant contributors to certain health problems. Clients who had been smoking prior to hospitalization should be encouraged to break this habit. We cannot expect all clients to recognize or admit the hazards that accompany smoking, but it is the health care provider's responsibility to provide education to the client concerning these risks.

Clients should also be sure to maintain good hygiene both inside and outside of the home. Improper hygiene is a known cause of spreading infections and of facilitating poor health.

Medication management and compliance is of utmost importance to a client's health and well-being. The client must understand the names and significance of all medications as well as the importance of taking these medications at the appropriate time and for as long as prescribed. Several studies have indicated that clients who begin self-medication prior to discharge from a facility have increased compliance. These clients do not necessarily have increased knowledge; therefore, it is vital that the client understands and is physically/cognitively able to call his/her physician with any questions as well as to reorder prescriptions when needed. (Kelly, 1994; Pereles, Romonko, Murzyn, Hogan, Silvius, Stokes, Long & Fung, 1996; Webb, Addison, Holman, Saklaki, & Wagner, 1990). In addition, collaboration with other rehabilitation team members regarding medications can improve compliance (Touchard & Berthelot, 1999).

Changing the Tools to Achieve Independence

A client may benefit from using a reacher to retrieve medications that are out of reach. Also to be considered are weekly and monthly medication organizers. The client with a neurological impairment limiting the functional use of one UE may need to have medications placed in uncovered containers or non-childproof containers to allow the client independence in retrieving medication. The client with orthopedic deficit may need to have medications placed within safe reach. A daily nutrition guide will also be helpful to assist the client in making the most effective food choices.

SENSATION CHANGES AND PAIN

Impairment in sensation may place a client at risk for injury when taking part in IADL tasks (Figure 4-8). Clients with impaired sensation must have intact cognition in order to be left unsupervised and be educated in the importance of thinking tasks through and concentrating on their performance with each activity. They must also visually focus on the task and guard the affected UE to avoid danger.

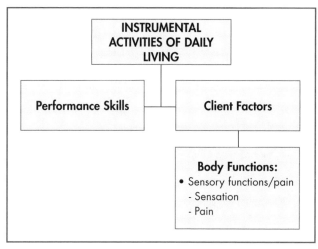

Figure 4-8. Relationship of sensation/pain to IADLs (adapted from American Occupational Therapy Association. (2002). *Occupational therapy practice framework: Domain and process.* Bethesda, MD: AOTA).

The IADL task of meal preparation needs careful attention, particularly when the client is using the stove or microwave and sharp utensils. Tasks involving use of electricity or power equipment also present a concern for the client with impaired sensation. Safety also becomes an issue if the client's impaired sensation affects his/her ability to carry objects such as dinnerware or laundry. The client must also be careful when using cleaning supplies that may include materials that are toxic to the skin.

Generally speaking, the client with either hyposensitivity or hypersensitivity of the UE must be extremely careful with tasks that place him/her at risk of injury. It is wise to use the unaffected UE whenever possible to safely complete a task. The client must also be careful when mobilizing in the home or in the community and use visual sense to avoid bumping into objects that may inflict any injury or pain. Table 4-6 summarizes the above IADL tasks as well as the compensatory/adaptive strategies.

Endurance/Energy

As discussed previously with ADLs, a lack of endurance will impact all areas of occupation (Figure 4-9). The inability to sustain activity for a period of time can impact even sedentary IADLs, such as balancing a checkbook. Principles of energy conservation and work simplification are provided to the clients in the form of education and practice in order to increase functional skills without excessive fatigue. These principles include the following:

- Organize work space.
- Organize the task to be completed.
- Select the most appropriate and effective time of day for each task.
- Limit activities to short periods of time on a daily basis.
- Work in areas that are waist level or slightly higher.
- Sit for completion of tasks when possible.
- Use adaptive equipment and DME when indicated.
- Select leisure activities that require less energy to complete.
- Make use of wheelchairs or driving shopping carts for community mobility and shopping tasks, or select stores that are smaller and more easily accessible.
- Use power equipment or tools when indicated.

Table 4-6

SUMMARY OF IADLS AND COMPENSATION/ADAPTATIONS FOR SENSORY DEFICITS

IADL Task	Compensatory/Adaptive Strategies for Sensation and Pain
Laundry	Use both hands to load/unload washer and dryer.
Light cleaning	Use a dust mitt instead of a cloth that may be frequently dropped.
Outdoor maintenance	Avoid use of sharp objects.
Shopping	Use both hands and/or vision to guide lifting and carrying grocery items.
Meal preparation	Wear an oven mitt to avoid a burn.
Table setting	Visually attend when reaching into drawers for sharp utensils and when carrying and placing them.
Dishes	Check water temperature with the intact hand to avoid a burn.
Financial management	If using a pen or pencil, place a hook and loop strip or other textured piece over grip area to enhance the sensation of grasp.
Community mobility	Visually attend to the environment to avoid bumping into objects.
Communication devices	Use the intact hand to control the device, especially in an emergency.
Care of others/pets	Avoid feeding pets by hand to avoid bites. Avoid grooming pet (use a groomer).
Health management	Keep pill bottles opened slightly and use the intact hand to grasp pills. Use wrist weights for UE exercise to avoid losing hold of hand weights.

Figure 4-9. Relationship of energy/endurance to IADLs (adapted from American Occupational Therapy Association. (2002). *Occupational therapy practice framework: Domain and process.* Bethesda, MD: AOTA).

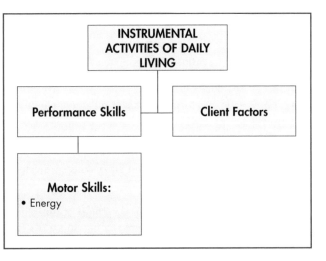

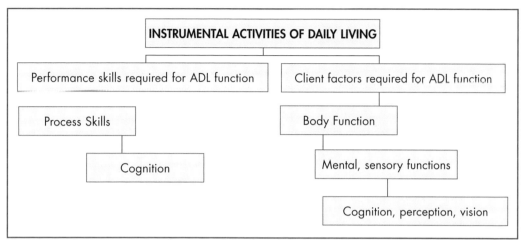

Figure 4-10. Components of performance skills/client factors related to IADLs (adapted from American Occupational Therapy Association. (2002). *Occupational therapy practice framework: Domain and process*. Bethesda, MD: AOTA).

The clients who incorporate these principles will find that they are more efficient and productive in all everyday tasks. They will have more time and more energy for leisure activities and social events.

PERFORMANCE SKILLS/CLIENT FACTORS

This section will focus on the impact of cognitive, perceptual, and visual deficits upon IADL performance (Figure 4-10). As stated in the ADL chapter, many conditions may lead to these deficits, primarily those of a neurological origin.

The use of cuing, as described in Chapter 1, will also be addressed throughout this chapter in terms of its use for remediation as well as compensation/adaptation. Again, the chapter is organized so that the lowest, foundational skill levels will build upon higher-level skills.

The *Framework* (AOTA, 2002) presents perceptual and cognitive deficits within two sections of the document. The first section addresses basic cognitive skills in the general category of Performance Skills and the subsection of Process Skills. The *Framework* defines these basic cognitive skills as necessary to complete, manage, and modify ADL tasks.

A second section of the *Framework* (2002) also addresses cognitive as well as perceptual deficits. The deficits are discussed under the subsection of Client Factors, called Body Function Categories. These Body Function Categories are the affective, perceptual, and additional cognitive skills required to complete ADL tasks. Body Function Categories are divided into Global Mental Functions and Specific Mental Functions (2002):

- *Global Mental Functions*: These include consciousness functions (arousal level, level of consciousness) and orientation.

- *Specific Mental Functions*: Attention, memory, perception (visuospatial), thought functions (recognition, categorization, generalization), higher-level cognitive functions (judgment, concept formation, time management, problem solving, decision making), and mental functioning (motor planning).

This section will also give examples of compensation/adaptation interventions for each topic. Examples of appropriate activities will be listed. Some IADL examples will not be listed because these tasks may be inappropriate or not possible for a client with these deficits For specific definitions, see Chapter 2.

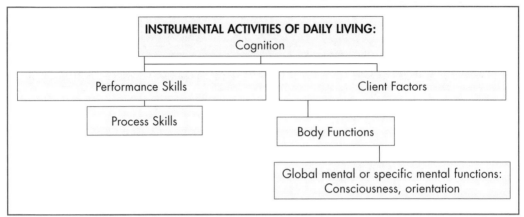

Figure 4-11. Relationship of cognition to IADLs (adapted from American Occupational Therapy Association. (2002). *Occupational therapy practice framework: Domain and process*. Bethesda, MD: AOTA).

A client who has experienced a neurological insult may present with deficits in the areas of cognition, perception and vision, which may limit the client's safety and ability to participate in IADL tasks. Verbal, visual, sensory and tactile cues may be needed in order for the client to function safely in his/her own home as well as in the community. The OT must determine the most effective method(s) to increase functional IADL performance. Education must then be provided to the client and his/her family or caregivers.

Cognitive Deficits

See Figure 4-11.

Process Skills

Table 4-7 briefly presents the subcategories of Process Skills because they are typically addressed in a less formal manner within most IADL intervention plans. Only the subcategories that apply to IADL have been included in this table.

Client Factors: Body Functions, Global Mental Functions

As stated earlier, *global mental functions* include consciousness and orientation. A client who is to participate in IADLs will need adequate global mental functions in order to complete these higher-level tasks safely and effectively. The client must choose times that he/she is most awake and alert and tasks that are goal-oriented and appropriate for his/her level of motor function. He/she must be sufficiently oriented to the specifics of the task, the demands involved, and the potential outcomes.

Client Factors: Body Functions, Specific Mental Functions

Specific Mental Functions includes attention, memory, perception (visuospatial), thought functions (recognition, categorization, generalization), higher-level cognitive functions (judgment, concept formation, time management, problem solving, decision making), and mental functioning (motor planning, specifically dressing apraxia) (AOTA, 2002).

Table 4-7

PROCESS SKILLS AND SAMPLE ADAPTATIONS/COMPENSATIONS

Process Skill Subcategories (AOTA, 2002)	*Examples of IADL Compensation/Adaptation Interventions*
Energy	
Paces	Assist the client in preparing a list of home management activities and develop a daily/weekly schedule for these tasks.
Attends	Refer to Specific Mental Functions category.
Knowledge	
Chooses	Ask the client to choose a dinner recipe for the week.
Uses	Have the client select from the recipe the items he/she needs to purchase at the store.
Handles	Observe the client in preparation of the meal.
Heeds	Create a list of safety measures the client must adhere to when preparing a meal and ask him/her to check off each item as completed.
Inquires	Encourage the client to ask questions regarding preparation of the meal when unsure.
Temporal organization	
Initiation	Give the client a time frame in which the meal preparation needs to be completed. Use a sounding device to signal time to begin the task.
Sequencing	Ask the client to read the recipe in the sequence that it needs to be completed and number each step.
Organizing space and objects	
Searches/locates	Select one cabinet for laundry supplies such as detergent, bleach, fabric softener, and dryer sheets.
Gathers	Have the client use two laundry receptacles that are appropriate for transporting, one for dark clothing and one for whites and gather and sort clothing appropriately.
Organizes	Devise a checklist with the client for all needed steps for laundry management in the recommended order and have him/her check off each step as completed.
Restores	Create a list of steps with the client to complete after the laundry is done in order to restore the machines and working area to the pre-working state (i.e., clean out dryer filter, return laundry receptacles to appropriate place, put away supplies).
Navigates	Educate the client in the safest carrying techniques for all needed supplies to complete the task.

continued

Table 4-7, continued

PROCESS SKILLS AND SAMPLE ADAPTATIONS/COMPENSATIONS

Process Skill Subcategories (AOTA, 2002)	Examples of IADL Compensation/Adaptation Interventions
Adaptation	
Notices/responds	Observe the client's performance with managing laundry and gradually substitute visual checklists with verbal cues as needed as the task becomes more automatic to the client.
Accommodates/adjusts	Problem-solve with the client how to determine whether a laundry load is small, medium, or large and adjust the amount of detergent, bleach, etc. needed.
Benefits	Discuss with the client the benefits of following the directions for loading the machine and for adding laundry detergent, bleach, and/or fabric softener and ask the client to discuss safety issues that may develop if instructions are not followed.

Attention

Decreased attention skills will affect the client's ability to learn and focus on IADL skills. Attention is a building block for higher-level specific mental functions such as memory and problem solving, and therefore must be addressed first (Zoltan, 2007).

Changing the Task to Achieve Independence

- *Light cleaning example*: A time schedule may be developed for each task to be completed with start time and approximate time of completion.

- *Outdoor maintenance example*: Choose activities that are goal-oriented to the patient to increase attention versus tasks that just need to be done.

- *Table setting example*: Select all items needed before setting the table to deter from distraction and elimination of some items.

- *Washing dishes example*: Have the client select some favorite music or listen to a favorite television show while completing this task.

- *Financial management example*: Select time of day when the client is most awake, use good lightening and have the client sit at a desk or table and maintain good posturing to enhance alertness.

Changing the Tools to Achieve Independence

- *Laundry example*: If the client does not have a machine that gives an auditory cue when it is done, a timer may be used to signify that the load is done or near completion.

- *Shopping example*: The client may prepare a list and adhere only to the purchase of those items listed.

- *Meal preparation example*: Use a timer for cooking and designate specific times for meals to increase attentiveness to task.

- *Community mobility example*: If using the city bus line, a written note of the client's destination can be provided to the bus driver in case the client loses his/her attention while traveling.

- *Communication device example*: Visual reminders such as flashing lights or auditory cues can remind the client to charge batteries. Daily calendar reminders would be helpful as well.

- *Care of others/pets example*: The client may benefit from a written schedule, an alarm, or a timer as reminders.

- *Health management example*: Daily nutrition guides and medication dividers will be helpful. Exercise videos/DVDs may also enhance attention.

Memory

Although there are many types of memory and memory deficits, this section will focus specifically on intervention strategies related to ADLs with an adaptive/compensation approach.

Changing the Task to Achieve Independence

Intervention strategies during IADLs, in general, may be adapted by providing the client with a schedule. For individuals who have limited carryover, involve him/her in developing the schedule. The same strategy may be implemented for creating lists of items needed for cooking, shopping, and cleaning, as well as basic instructions for carrying out IADLs.

- *Light cleaning example*: For each task, provide a list of instructions on how to complete, materials needed, and designate one day for each task and write on calendar.

- *Outdoor home maintenance*: Have the client review the instructions for all equipment, state safety precautions, and demonstrate use first.

- *Table setting example*: Draw a picture of a table setting for the client to follow and list all needed dinnerware.

- *Washing dishes example*: Provide verbal cues.

- *Financial management example*: Keep bills in one area, select a day of the month for payment, and write on calendar.

- *Community mobility example*: Have the client write down his/her destination, the name of the transit system he/she is taking, and the time of arrival and departure.

- *Communication devices example*: List all instructions for use of devices near the equipment and list all important phone numbers.

Changing the Tools to Achieve Independence

- *Laundry example*: Provide a checklist with all steps listed, designate 1 or 2 days a week as laundry days, and mark on a calendar.

- *Shopping example*: Have the client keep an ongoing list of items needed and use the list when at the store.

- *Meal preparation example*: Use written recipes and timers when cooking or baking, hang a sign over the stove to remind the client to turn it off.

- *Care of others/pets example*: Prepare a daily schedule of tasks and check off as they are completed.

- *Health management example*: Utilize daily nutrition guides, medication sorters, and written exercise programs. Write all appointments on calendars.

The Specific Mental Functions, which are addressed less formally and/or less frequently within intervention plans, are presented in Table 4-8.

Perceptual Deficits

See Figure 4-12.

Visual Fixation/Scanning

Clients who present with perceptual deficits involving visual fixation and limited ability to scan the environment will need continued practice and adaptation/compensation strategies in order to complete IADL tasks. The following compensatory/adaptive strategies may be implemented to assist the client. The client must first recognize that a deficit exists and be receptive to new strategies. Continued practice and repetition of purposeful activities should enhance the client's performance.

Changing the Task to Achieve Independence

- *Laundry example*: Have the client turn his/her head when reaching for and placing clothing. Place items far enough apart to encourage more head movement.

- *Light cleaning example*: When mopping or sweeping, give the client a point of visual focus to the left and right and tell him/her to stop once he/she has reached each point and move in the other direction.

- *Outdoor home maintenance example*: If the client is sweeping or raking, instruct him/her to visually attend to the broom or rake and follow the movements with his/her head and eyes; encourage wide and long strokes.

- *Shopping example*: The client will need to scan for all items he/she wishes to purchase; verbal cuing for a start and end point will be indicated.

- *Meal preparation example*: Ask the client to state the ingredient needed and ask him/her to locate the area in which it can be found, and then visually attend to that place.

- *Table setting example*: Instruct the client as to how many places need to be set.

- *Washing dishes example*: When loading or unloading the dishwasher, remind the client to turn his/her head when reaching and placing dishes.

- *Financial management example*: When balancing a checkbook, have the figures the client needs to add and subtract placed horizontally rather than vertically to encourage scanning from left to right with verbal cues if needed.

- *Community mobility example*: The client will need supervision for community mobility, with verbal cuing to turn his/her head in each direction to scan the environment. It would be helpful if the client remains with the most visual and auditory stimulation to his/her impaired side.

- *Care of others/pets example*: Have the client exercise the dog or play catch to trigger visual scanning and release fixation.

- *Health management example*: Have the client scan the calendar daily for any appointments or important matters for that day.

Changing the Tools to Achieve Independence

- *Communication devices example*: Raised surfaces for control buttons would be helpful so that the client can use his/her tactile sense while scanning to find the appropriate button.

Visual Inattention and Neglect

For clients who are unaware of inattention deficits, the therapist will need to modify and simplify the physical context of IADLs as much as possible. Gradual grading of activities will also be

Table 4-8

SPECIFIC MENTAL FUNCTIONS AND EXAMPLES OF COMPENSATION/ADAPTATION STRATEGIES

Specific Mental Functions Subcategories (AOTA, 2002)	Examples of Compensation/Adaptation Interventions
Thought functions	
Recognition	Given all adaptive devices, the client will select those appropriate for each IADL task to be performed. Choice selection can be graded beginning with a choice of two and increasing as appropriate.
Categorization	Given all cleaning supplies, the client will select those items needed for each specific task. Color coding may be useful using tape or marker with a general list (i.e., red for laundry supplies, blue for dishes, etc.).
Generalization	Discuss the principles of self-care that the client has learned and create a list of ways he/she can generalize this new learning to the care of others.
Higher-level cognitive functions	
Judgment	Discuss vignettes that may lead to unsafe conditions and ask the client to identify appropriate methods of handling them. Create a list of people the client may call with specific questions before acting if he/she is unsure of what to do.
Concept formation	Determine goals with respect to IADLs and chart progress weekly. Have the client state what accomplishments he/she has achieved.
Time management	Provide the client with a daily time schedule and ask him/her to plan the day incorporating daily routines as well as tasks or appointments that are specific to that day.
Problem solving	Ask the client to identify problems that he/she has encountered in the past and identify the solution that worked best. Have the client refer to this learning when encountering a new challenge.
Decision-making	Have the client discuss the pros and cons of each choice he/she is to make and then select the best choice and determine the reasoning behind this choice for future decision making.

required. For example, begin by providing all objects/items within the client's intact visual field; incorporate visual scanning through head as well as eye movements during functional activities, etc.

Changing the Task to Achieve Independence

- *Laundry example*: Have the client with left inattention/neglect stand to the right of the washer and dryer if possible and turn to the left to load the machines.

Figure 4-12. Relationship of perception to IADLs (adapted from American Occupational Therapy Association. (2002). *Occupational therapy practice framework: Domain and process.* Bethesda, MD: AOTA).

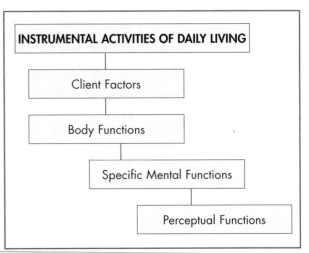

- *Light cleaning example*: Cue the client to reach all four corners of the counter or table when cleaning and count as he/she reaches them.

- *Outdoor home maintenance example*: Place marker points at each side of the garden as points of reference when the client is weeding.

- *Shopping example*: Identify one item in the aisle that the client needs and ask him/her to look towards the impaired side of vision to locate it.

- *Meal preparation example*: Place all adaptive cooking devices to the impaired visual side of the client's working area, and place commonly used spices in cabinets to the client's impaired visual side.

- *Table setting example*: Have the client set the table clockwise or counter-clockwise depending on which visual field is impaired (e.g., clockwise for right inattention/neglect and counter-clockwise for inattention/neglect to the left).

- *Washing dishes example*: Stack soiled dishes to impaired side, and have the client stand with the dishwasher on his/her impaired visual side.

- *Financial management example*: Place a border on each check on the side of the client's visual impairment.

- *Community mobility example*: The client will need to rely on family or community transportation.

- *Care of others/pets example*: Have feeding dishes and food placed on the client's impaired visual side.

- *Health management example*: Place all medications or health supplies in cabinets to the client's impaired visual side.

Changing the Tools to Achieve Independence

- *Communication devices example*: Raised surfaces to enhance tactile sensation will assist the client in finding control buttons.

Body Scheme

Body scheme is a foundation skill that uses sensory or internal awareness of the body and the spatial relationship of the body parts to one another (Jacobs & Jacobs, 2004; Zoltan, 2007). Because

Table 4-9	
BODY SCHEME DISORDERS AND SAMPLE COMPENSATION/ADAPTATION STRATEGIES	
Body Scheme Disorder	*Compensation/Adaptation Interventions Strategies: Task and/or Tools Changed*
Unilateral body neglect	Use verbal cuing as well as visual demonstration to encourage bilateral integration with meal preparation.
Right-left discrimination	Have the client wear a ring or bracelet on the dominant hand and use this as a point of reference when performing IADL activities.

there are multiple forms of body scheme disorders, each one cannot be reviewed individually. For this reason, Table 4-9 identifies the most common forms of body scheme disorders as well as examples of IADL compensatory/adaptive interventions for these.

Visual Discrimination

Visual discrimination refers to the ability to detect differences and similarities between objects, thereby determining whether they are alike or different (Okkema, 1993). The client who wishes to return to the tasks of IADLs will need to learn compensation/adaptation strategies in order to participate in an independent and safe manner. Caregivers will need to be educated in the specifics of the client's deficit and how it will relate to the client's ability to function. Education will need to be provided as to what can be expected of the client and what strategies he/she will need to perform in order to complete the tasks. The client will need to possess intact cognitive skills such as deduction and reasoning in order to learn to compensate and adapt to functional activities (Okkema, 1993). Table 4-10 describes sample compensation/adaptation strategies for visual discrimination disorders.

Motor Planning

Motor planning involves the individual's ability to organize and perform movements in order to carry out purposeful activity (Jacobs & Jacobs, 2004). Apraxia is a category of motor planning deficits whereby impairments of purposeful movement or skills do not involve in-coordination, sensory deficits, visual/perceptual issues, language deficits, or cognitive deficits alone (Crepeau, Cohn, & Schell, 2003).

Zoltan (1996) states that a client with apraxia will present with errors in performance skills such as perseveration, inability to perform upon command, and limitations in tool usage. In general, apraxia may be addressed through adapting the environment, limiting tool usage, hand-over-hand activities, chaining, using familiar activities for interventions, presenting activities in small steps, and limiting verbal commands.

Changing the Task to Achieve Independence

- *Laundry example*: If laundry is a familiar task for the client, begin with backward chaining and offer hand-over-hand assistance versus verbal cuing.

- *Shopping example*: Reintroduce shopping in a familiar but small store, such as a neighborhood market or drug store. Begin with only a short list of familiar items. Offer hand-over-hand assistance when necessary.

Table 4-10

VISUAL DISCRIMINATION AND SAMPLE COMPENSATION/ ADAPTATION STRATEGIES

Visual Discrimination Disorder	Compensation/Adaptation Interventions: Task and/or Tools Changed
Form discrimination	Have client sort laundry by similar items and by color (i.e., white t-shirts, black socks, etc.).
Depth perception	Instruct the client to utilize the sense of touch and feel for surfaces and boundaries when attempting tasks such as pouring liquids or batters or placing items in containers.
Figure ground perception	Adapt containers holding most commonly used spices and other meal preparation items with colors to distinguish them from other items in cabinets.
Spatial relations	Color code cleaning supplies and cabinets in which they belong and ask client to return all supplies as used.
Topographical orientation	Label cabinets or use picture representations of items to be found inside. Identify place settings by placemats.

- *Washing dishes example*: Provide hand-over-hand assistance and backward or forward chaining activity as needed. Eliminate glass items and sharp objects as necessary.

Changing the Tools to Achieve Independence

- *Light cleaning example*: If this task is familiar to the client, begin with using cleaning supplies that may be familiar to the client, such as a sponge or feather duster. Add more tools as client improves.

- *Meal preparation example*: Begin activity with having the client prepare a simple sandwich or snack that does not require the use of kitchen tools. As the client improves, gradually implement the use of a simple, safe utensil, such as a spoon or butter knife.

- *Table setting example*: Begin activity by setting the table for one person with only a few items such as a plate and spoon or plastic fork. Add more place settings or utensils as able. Use backward chaining to set the table, as needed (adaptation of task).

VISION

See Figure 4-13.

Low Vision and Visual Field Deficits

Because these deficits tend to have similar issues in relation to IADLs, they are presented below in a general compensation/adaptation approach.

A client who has experienced a neurological deficit may also manifest changes in vision. These changes may include double vision, otherwise known as diplopia, a visual field cut, and/or deficits in depth perception. Any change in vision will impact IADL in some way. The client will need to learn to compensate or adapt to these changes in order to regain functional independence. Recommendation should be made for the client to see an ophthalmologist or an optometrist spe-

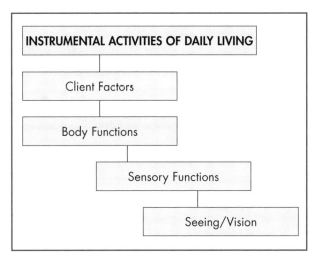

Figure 4-13. Relationship of vision to IADLs (adapted from American Occupational Therapy Association. (2002). *Occupational therapy practice framework: Domain and process.* Bethesda, MD: AOTA).

cializing in neurological deficits, especially if he/she wishes to participate in IADLs. Deficits may be more evident in these activities than were noted in basic ADLs (Okkema, 1993). Upon evaluation, it may be determined that the client may benefit from specially made glasses containing prism to assist with facilitation of normal vision. Visual training may also be indicated. The OT should instruct the client in visual compensation techniques until the client is able to visualize in a normal manner. These include the following:

- Position materials in the unaffected visual field to assist with reading or identifying objects.
- Use magnifiers or magnifying lamps to enhance reading (Figure 4-14).
- Memorize the phone dial, use one-touch or speed dialing, purchase a telephone with larger, easier to read numbers.
- Utilize audible rather than visual devices such as talking clocks/watches, temperature scales and calculators (Figure 4-15).
- Use tactile aids that raise surfaces of appliance controls.
- Maintain proper lighting with all mobility and avoid sun glare by using eye shades and shades or curtains in the home.
- Reposition the head to scan the environment of the affected side.
- Use bright tape to mark each step of a flight of stairs.
- Listen to books on tape or invest in large print magazines.
- Visit a low vision store for various cooking and leisure activity items specifically made for clients with low vision.
- Avoid working with hot surfaces, sharp objects, or toxic materials.
- Use tactile sense whenever possible to enhance vision.
- Modify the home to eliminate clutter and try to keep furniture and other items in the same place.

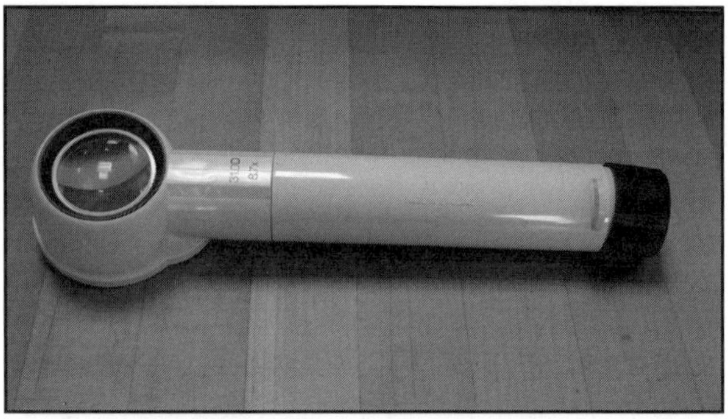

Figure 4-14. Magnification lamp for reading.

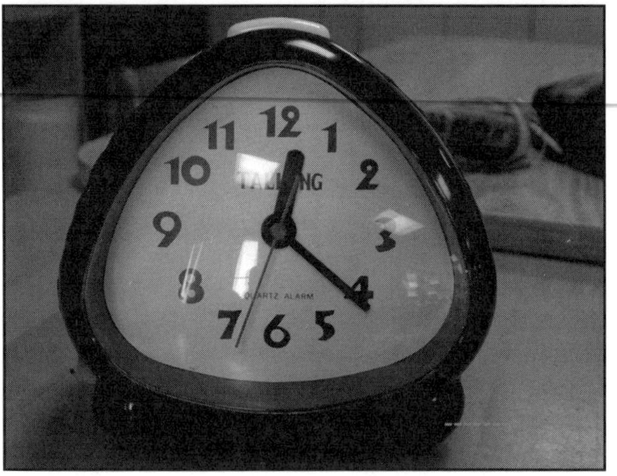

Figure 4-15. Talking clock.

MAINTENANCE OF IADL

One of the basic precursors for IADL maintenance is a good understanding of all teaching and the necessities of compensation or adaptation techniques to maintain safety along with independence for all areas of IADLs. The client must be educated regularly throughout rehabilitation, both in a facility and subsequently in the home. Generalization of new learning to the home setting may at times be challenging. It is important, therefore, that the client have continued rehabilitation to assure that new techniques are being generalized. Practice is also important in order for new techniques to become automatic to the client. With a good basis for relearning of performance skills, new performance patterns and habits should become inherent in the client's behavior. The client will then have the opportunity to generalize this new behavior to many contexts.

CASE STUDY 1: JIM C., CVA

Jim C. is a 57-year-old single male who lives alone. A very close group of friends noted significant changes in his mental status one day as they were visiting. These friends subsequently reported that Jim was having trouble expressing himself for 2 or 3 days prior to this, although he refused to seek medical evaluation. Emergency medical service was called on this particular day and Jim was found to have an elevated blood pressure of 240/120. He was brought to the emergency department of the local hospital and was diagnosed by head CT (cat scan) as having a left parietal lobe infarct, with no bleeding. Jim had recently been discharged from the hospital for treatment of bilateral LE cellulites, which was also noted to be present at the time of this admission. He was noted to be aphasic. After evaluation, Jim was admitted to the hospital for treatment of the cellulites and control of his high blood pressure, along with monitoring and intervention of his acute left CVA.

Jim's past medical history is significant for hypertension, and chronic LE edema and cellulites. He lives alone in a one level home with one step to enter. He was independent with all ADLs and IADLs prior to admission, including dressing changes of his LEs. He was driving and working part-time at a local restaurant. His family was limited to one distant relative who lived out of the area.

Jim was evaluated by physical, occupational, and speech therapy after his admission to the hospital. His overall strength of the UEs and LEs was graded at 4 of 5, however, the question was raised as to whether or not the client was stronger as he was noted to have difficulty following commands. He demonstrated no deficits with coordination or sensation of the UEs or LEs. He ambulated without a device with contact guard assistance initially. He was alert; however, orientation was difficult to assess as the patient manifested severe receptive and expressive aphasia of the Wernicke type. He was able to follow simple one-step commands intermittently with visual and tactile cues as needed.

The speech therapist's evaluation results found Jim to be severely aphasic. He demonstrated deficits in auditory comprehension, conversational speech, and the ability for new learning. Jim often used sound substitutions in naming objects. For example, he would say "bable" instead of "table." He would often substitute words saying "shoe" for "sock" or "chair" for "table." Often, Jim fabricated words in conversation and he was found to have perseverative speech as well. The OT's evaluation found Jim to be pleasant and cooperative, requiring max verbal, visual, and tactile cuing for testing and subsequently for treatment. He was noted to be at supervision level to shower and dress, with contact guard assist for functional transfers using grabber assistance when available.

As previously noted, Jim manifested overall functional strength. He demonstrated good balance and physical therapy intervention focused on higher-level balance skills and community mobility. He was able to navigate stairs without difficulty and he required no assistive devices for gait. Physical therapy intervention also focused on management of Jim's LE wounds and subsequent infection.

Interdisciplinary intervention was based on cognitive retraining, auditory comprehension, following commands, identifying objects appropriately, wound care, strengthening, and facilitating independence with BADLs and IADLs in a safe manner. Jim was evaluated shortly after his hospital admission for transfer to the hospital's intensive rehabilitation unit, as he was deemed unsafe to be discharged home alone.

Jim was admitted to the intensive rehabilitation unit 5 days after initial admission. Upon evaluation by physical, occupational, and speech therapy, he demonstrated approximately the same status as was noted upon acute care evaluation. He received daily physical and occupational therapy, and speech therapy was administered approximately three to four times per week. Occupational therapy's main focus in the rehabilitation setting was on safety and cognitive retraining for IADLs because the client was soon independent in BADLs. Physical therapy's focus was on strengthening, gait, and mobility within the hospital community, higher-level balance skills, and wound care for the LE cellulites. Speech therapy focused also on cognitive retraining, but their main focus was the client's aphasia. Simple object identification tasks and following simple one-step commands was the intervention of choice initially.

Although Jim was progressing well with the motor and functional aspects of therapy, safety remained a primary concern. Jim was not functioning in an unsafe manner within the rehabilitation unit; however, concern was that he would be unsafe if discharged home to an uncontrolled, unsupervised environment. Jim's safety deficits revolved around his aphasia. He was unable to dial 911 correctly on a consistent basis, and even when he did, he was unable to state appropriately his problem or his address. He was independently managing his finances prior to his CVA, yet he was now unable to perform simple money management tasks accurately.

Occupational therapy intervention initially focused on remediation of cognitive skills. It appeared it would be a long process to complete, and in the interim, Jim needed to be able to function at home. Intervention was re-evaluated and focus was placed on compensation/adaptation techniques. These will be further addressed. Although improvement was seen, it was still evident that Jim was going to require some assistance throughout the day for some IADL tasks.

The OT focused on the performance areas of safety and financial management during the course of Jim's rehabilitation stay. To assess safety with meal preparation, Jim was given the cooking task of baking corn muffins. He prepared the muffins with supervision and no verbal cuing except to direct him to where the needed items could be found in the occupational therapy kitchen, as this setting provided a new context for him to perform in. Although Jim verbalized the instructions incorrectly when reading them from the box, he prepared the mixture with 100% accuracy and no cuing. He safely placed the muffins in the oven, needing assist only to set the oven timer. When they were ready to come out, he removed the pan safely and remembered to turn the oven off. Jim completed the task of clean-up appropriately, utilizing good safety. Throughout this meal preparation task, Jim executed appropriate performance skills requiring mobility and processing; however, he was noted to have continued impairment in communication/interaction skills. The demands of the activity were appropriate for his level of performance, and all client factors were noted to be within functional limits. The OT deemed him safe for performance in the kitchen.

Throughout his rehabilitation stay, Jim was independent in making his bed and doing his own laundry. He functioned safely and appropriately, but his aphasia persisted and certain cognitive deficits still needed to be addressed.

Financial management was a greater challenge for Jim. He had difficulty naming coins and identifying their value. The OT created a guide for Jim, with the individual coins taped to a sheet of paper and their names and money denominations written next to them. Continued drills in naming the money types as well as problem solving the tasks of making change and giving the correct amount needed for a purchase were performed. Ultimately, Jim improved and was able to provide the correct coin or bill upon request 90% of the time. He was also able to select the appropriate monies needed upon request. For example, if the OT asked Jim to give her $2.54, Jim was able to do so. When Jim was told that he made a purchase of $8.64 and gave the clerk $10, he was able to make the correct change with minimal cuing 100% of the time. Check writing was not a normal habit for Jim, nor was the use of credit cards. He paid only by cash. Therefore, it was essential that money management intervention focused on cash management skills.

The OT also worked on creating a grocery shopping list with Jim, to identify items by name and to calculate the cost. He was able to write the list appropriately, copying the names of items from a store flyer. Jim required maximum assistance with the problem-solving aspects of this task. For example, he was asked how much it would cost if he wanted to purchase 2 pounds of bananas at 69 cents a pound. He was unable to add or multiply to obtain the correct answer.

The OT took Jim to the hospital cafeteria to assess generalization of the newly relearned money management skills. They went at a time when the cafeteria was quiet to minimize the stress of the task. Jim selected an item of purchase, and upon arriving at the cashier he was able to provide the correct amount of money for payment. Both Jim and the OT were pleased at his ability to perform this task in a new context where activity demands were different and slightly greater for him.

Intervention of home safety and client safety revealed that Jim was unable to state the 911 emergency phone number consistently and upon demand. The OT provided Jim with a telephone and asked him what he would do in the case of an emergency such as a fire. Jim responded that he would run out of the house, but was unable to state the emergency number consistently. The OT worked with Jim on dialing the number and he quickly was able to do so; however, difficulty was noted in verbalizing his needs, his name, or his address secondary to his aphasia. The OT designed a written dialogue for Jim to recite stating that he had aphasia, what his name was, where he lives and that he needed help. Jim practiced continually with this dialogue, but was still inconsistent with his verbalizations. The OT challenged Jim with various emergency vignettes and was pleased that Jim was able to at least recognize danger even though his verbal response to it was limited. She felt confident that he would be able to remove himself from any danger if needed. Yet she was concerned that he would have difficulty stating his needs if medical attention was indicated. It was recommended that Jim purchase an emergency call system to assure his safety in a time of emergency. He said he would consider it.

Jim's discharge plan was an issue secondary to his limited insurance and subsequent inability to receive home health care or home therapy. He remained on the rehabilitation unit for an extended period of 8 weeks. The care manager/discharge planner in charge of Jim's case was in touch with his distant relative on a regular basis, and he was insistent that Jim would need further rehabilitation until arrangements were made for him to be eligible for home services. Jim was in the process of applying for Medicaid. He was not happy with the recommendation that he could not go home as he felt that he would be fine. He stated that friends would be there to assist with cooking and transportation as needed. This was confirmed by the OT and the care manager after discussion with these friends. Jim stated he would not drive. He had concerns about his home as the weather was changing from early to late fall during his admission. He was expecting his last paycheck and wondering if it had come and if so, where it was. His social work representative had been contacted and was in the process of assisting Jim with his financial concerns and his family was notified about his concerns regarding his home.

Despite the above interventions, Jim decided that he was unwilling to transfer to a short-term rehabilitation facility and he signed himself out of the intensive rehabilitation unit one evening against medical advice. Contact was made with Jim the next day to be sure that he would visit his primary physician for continued monitoring of his blood pressure and his chronic cellulites. Subsequent contact with the client found him to be functioning fairly well at home alone with improvement noted in certain aspects of his speech. The rehabilitation team hoped that Jim followed through with all recommendations and that he was educated sufficiently to maintain his safety at home.

Case Study 2: Annie D., Parkinson's Disease and Fractured Humerus

Annie D. is a 75-year-old married white female with known history of Parkinson's disease. She lives with her husband on the second floor of a three-level home. Annie was independent with all ADLs and most IADLs prior to her recent fall and subsequent fractured rib and fractured left humerus. She ambulated with a straight cane, but also owned a walker. Annie and her husband have one married daughter and one granddaughter who live out of state. Annie's daughter and son-in-law come into town often and assist Annie and her husband with grocery shopping and with transportation to appointments since neither Annie nor her husband drive. Annie's husband is not well and requires assistance from a home health aide for ADL, although he does participate in cooking tasks with Annie. He has been in and out of the hospital frequently and on one particular evening he fell at home. Annie rushed from her bed to assist him and consequently fell herself. Annie had an emergency call system and was able to call for help. She was taken to the hospital where she was diagnosed with a fractured rib and a left humerus fracture.

Annie had been discharged from the hospital a few months earlier after treatment for dehydration and frequent falls. She was admitted for rehabilitation and discharged home at her current level of function. Annie's husband remained at home during Annie's hospital stays with home health aide assistance as well as assistance from his daughter and son-in-law.

Annie's past medical history is significant for Parkinson's disease, coronary artery disease (CAD), hypertension, coronary stent placement, myocardial infarction (MI), noninsulin dependent diabetes mellitus (NIDDM), osteoarthritis, bilateral LE cellulites, and pneumonia. Outward symptoms of her Parkinson's were noted to be slight hand tremors and gait imbalance.

Annie was admitted to surgery for an open reduction internal fixation (ORIF) of the left humerus. Her postoperative orders indicated that Annie was nonweight-bearing on her left UE. When medically stable, she was evaluated by physical and occupational therapy. Annie was noted to be alert and oriented to self, time, place, and situation and followed all commands appropriately. She was able to make her needs known. She complained of pain in her rib area and in the left UE for which she was receiving medication.

Annie was right hand dominant. Right UE strength was assessed to be 4-/5 throughout. Passive ROM and strength of the left UE was unable to be assessed secondary to pain. She was noted to have edema of the left hand and was given a compression glove for edema control. Annie was instructed in the purpose of the glove and she was educated in further edema control techniques including positioning of the left UE in elevation and active fisting exercises. Annie was receptive and compliant with all teaching. Coordination and sensation of the right UE was intact. Left UE coordination was unable to be assessed and Annie complained of numbness and tingling of the third through fifth digits of the left hand. Functional evaluation involved assessment of Annie's ability to don her hospital booties. She was noted to require maximal assistance for this task.

Physical therapy evaluation noted that Annie's LE strength was assessed at 4 of 5 bilaterally with intact coordination and sensation. Neither the physical therapist nor the OT was able to assess mobility upon initial evaluation secondary to Annie's complaints of pain. Upon treatment of Annie, it was noted that she required maximal assistance of two for bed mobility and moderate assistance of one for sit-to-stand transfers.

It was determined that Annie would once again need intensive rehabilitation prior to returning home secondary to her impaired motor skills and new and challenging activity demands. Annie needed to relearn independence with ADL and IADL with training within the context of the intensive rehabilitation unit and consequent generalization to living in her own home again.

Upon admission to the rehabilitation unit, Annie was re-evaluated by physical and occupational therapy. Her functional status was approximately the same as it was upon initial hospital assessment. Annie was able to tolerate assessment now of her left UE. She was able to complete active shoulder flexion against gravity to approximately 90 degrees and was assessed at 3-/5 strength. Elbow and forearm strength were unable to be assessed secondary to the fracture. Left wrist flexion/extension and left grip were also assessed at 3-/5.

Since Annie had received therapy services at the rehabilitation unit in the past, she was familiar with rehabilitation and the benefits of physical and occupational therapy. Initial occupational therapy goals for Annie were:

1. Increase Annie's ability to perform bathing and dressing with minimal assistance and adaptive equipment as needed.

2. Complete toilet transfers with minimal assistance and grabber as needed.

3. Increase right UE strength to 4+-5/5 and left shoulder and wrist strength to 3/5.

4. Decrease left hand edema to none.

5. Increase left hand grip to 4/5.

Annie's orthopedic MD recommended active ROM activities of the left UE to facilitate increased extension of the elbow. He also recommended passive stretching of the left elbow into extension. Annie did not tolerate the stretching too well because of the pain it elicited, despite receiving pain medication prior to stretching. Therefore, she was encouraged to actively use the left UE for functional tasks. She remained non-weight-bearing on that arm.

Upon first weekly assessment by occupational therapy, Annie had achieved minimal assistance level for grooming and bathing; however, she continued to require maximal assistance for dressing. She had been provided with a reacher but required continued practice. She was not receptive to a sock aid, although she had one at home, because she was unable to manipulate it well enough secondary to the motor limitations of her left arm. Toilet transfers were now with contact guard assistance with right grabber. Right UE strength was increased to 5/5 throughout; however, left UE shoulder, wrist and grip strength remained at 3-/5. She no longer manifested any edema of the left hand but was encouraged to maintain elevated positioning when sitting or sleeping. Annie was ambulating 75 feet with a straight cane and minimal assistance.

Occupational therapy intervention continued to focus on increasing Annie's independence with bathing, dressing, and grooming, as well as with functional mobility. At week 2, introduction was also made to intervention of simple home management tasks, and increasing ROM of the left elbow. Annie was fitted for a progressive extension splint as recommended by her MD. The OT educated Annie and the nursing staff in donning and doffing techniques and in the method of adjusting the splint. Prior to discharge, Annie's daughter was also instructed verbally in these techniques and written instructions were provided. Although Annie made good attempts at donning the splint, she was unable to do so. Her husband would be unable to help her upon discharge to home. It was then determined that Annie would wear the splint only when her daughter was there, unless the home health aide provided for her upon discharge could be instructed in placing the splint. The tension was preset with Annie, only able to tolerate the lowest level of tension. She and her daughter were instructed to allow the home therapist to adjust the tension and gradually increase it if Annie was able to tolerate more.

By the end of week 2, Annie had shown further progress. She was now able to shower because the staples in her left arm had been removed. She completed a tub transfer with right grabber with contact guard assistance. She showered with minimal assistance for thoroughness secondary to limitations in motor performance of the left arm. Annie was now able to complete upper body dressing with minimal assistance, including both button down and pullover tops, and completed donning of her underwear and skirt with supervision. She remained dependent for her socks, but was able to don her shoes with hook and loop fasteners with supervision. Toilet transfers were now completed independently and Annie was ambulating 125 feet with the straight cane and supervision. Left shoulder flexion remained at 3-/5 strength; however, left wrist and grip strength increased to 3/5. Left elbow ROM was assessed at -40 degrees extension to 105 degrees of flexion, a minimal change from her original status.

Home management tasks were an excellent choice of intervention for Annie because she enjoyed them and they were part of her habits and routine patterns prior her admission. Also, Annie used her left UE volitionally with light baking tasks, kitchen cleaning and organization, folding her laundry, and also in decorating the rehabilitation unit's Christmas tree. The OT noted greater use and extension of the left UE with all home management tasks.

Annie was considered to be safe with all aspects of ADL and IADL evaluated within the rehabilitation setting. Of concern was her discharge to home and her role in caring for her husband. These concerns were discussed with her family, who assured the rehabilitation team that Annie would not be responsible for her husband's care, but only for herself.

Annie was discharged to home approximately 3 weeks after admission to the intensive rehabilitation unit. As previously stated, her daughter was invited in for teaching in the use of the extension splint. The care manager/discharge planner in charge of organizing Annie's home services was looking into the possibility of Annie receiving home health aide services in the evening to assist with donning the splint prior to Annie retiring to bed. Annie's daughter was willing to educate the home health aide in donning the splint. If it were not feasible, Annie would resort to wearing the splint only when her daughter was there to help and she was instructed to inform her orthopedic surgeon of this upon discharge.

Annie was ambulating within her room and to and from the bathroom with the straight cane at an independent level. Toilet transfers, hygiene, and clothing management were all performed independently upon discharge. Tub transfer remained at contact guard assistance and it was recommended to Annie that she wait for her daughter or the home health aide before showering. Annie verbalized understanding of this recommendation. Bathing abilities were advanced to supervision level and dressing abilities remained at minimal assistance, except Annie was still dependent for donning her socks. Grooming abilities were assessed at independent level. Annie required assistance with meal preparation with the lifting and transporting of heavier items. She was able to perform clean up tasks using the right UE for grasping most items and assisting with the left.

Right UE strength remained 5/5 throughout. Left UE shoulder and wrist flexion/extension was assessed at 3/5, and Annie was now able to complete pronation and supination of the left forearm with 2+-3-/5 strength. Left elbow PROM was assessed at -40 degrees of extension to +95 degrees of flexion demonstrating slight improvement.

Annie demonstrated good advancement towards her IADL goals of independent living once again. However, she was unable to care for her husband without assistance.

Summary Questions

1. Discuss how contextual factors affect IADLs and give at least two specific examples.

2. Discuss how psychological implications may impact IADL performance.

3. Describe the role of the OTA in IADL intervention.

4. Discuss how three Body Function Categories, if impaired, may affect IADL.

References

American Occupational Therapy Association. (2002). *Occupational therapy practice framework: Domain and process.* Bethesda, MD: AOTA.

American Occupational Therapy Association. (2004). *The reference manual of the official documents of the American Occupational Therapy Association* (10th ed.). Bethesda: MD: AOTA.

Baun, M., & McCabe, B. (2003). Companion animals and persons with dementia of the Alzheimer's type. *American Behavioral Scientist, 47*(1), 42-51.

Cole, M. B., (1998). *Group dynamics in occupational therapy* (2nd ed.). Thorofare, NJ: SLACK Incorporated.

Christiansen, C., & Baum, C. (Eds.) (1991). *Occupational therapy: Overcoming human performance deficits.* Thorofare, NJ: SLACK Incorporated.

Crepeau, E. B., Cohn, E. S., & Schell, B. A. B. (2003). *Willard and Spackman's occupational therapy for physical dysfunction* (10th ed.). Philadelphia, PA: Lippincott Williams & Wilkins.

Jacobs, K., & Jacobs, L. (2004). *Quick reference dictionary for occupational therapy* (4th ed.). Thorofare, NJ: SLACK Incorporated.

Kelly, J. M. (1994). Implementing a patient self-medication program. *Rehabilitation Nursing, 19*(2), 87-90.

Law, M., Baptiste, S., Carswell, A., McColl, M. A., Polatajko, H., & Pollock, N. (1998). *The Canadian Occupational Performance Measure* (3rd ed). Ottawa, ON: Canadian Occupational Therapy Association.

Logan, P. A., Gladman, J. R. F., Avery, A., Walker, M. F., Dyas, J., & Groom, L. (1994). Randomised controlled trial of an occupational therapy intervention to increase outdoor mobility after stroke. *British Medical Journal, 329*, 1372-1374.

Okkema, K. (1993). *Cognition and perception in the stroke patient: A guide to functional outcomes in occupational therapy.* Gaithersburg, MD: Aspen.

Pereles, L., Romonko, L., Murzyn, T., Hogan, D., Silvius, J., Stokes, E., Long, S., & Fung, T. (1996). Evaluation of a self-medication program. *J Am Geriatric Soc, 44*(2), 161-165.

Psychological Corporation. *Independent living scales.* (1996). San Antonio: Author.

Pynoos, J., & Nishita, C. M. (2003). The cost and financing of home modifications in the United States. *Journal of Disability Policy Studies, 14*(2), 68-73.

Stark, S. (2004). Removing environmental barriers in the homes of older adults with disabilities improves occupational performance. *Occupational Therapy Journal of Research, 24*(1), 32.

Thomson, L. K. (1992). *The Kohlman evaluation of living skills* (3rd ed.). Bethesda, MD: AOTA.

Touchard, B. M., & Berthelot, K. (1999). Collaborative home practice: nursing and occupational therapy ensure appropriate medication administration. *Home Health Nurse, 17*(1), 45-51.

Webb, C., Addison, C., Holman, H., Saklaki, B., & Wagner A. (1990). Self-medication for elderly patients. *Nursing Times, 86*(16), 46-49.

Zhang, L., Abreu, B. C., Seale, M. S., Masel, B., Christiansen, C. H., & Ottenbacher, K. J. (2003). A virtual reality environment for evaluation of a daily living skill in brain injury rehabilitation: reliability and validity. *Archives of Physical Medicine and Rehabilitation, 84*(8), 1118-1124.

Zoltan, B. (2007). *Vision, perception, and cognition* (4th ed.). Thorofare, NJ: SLACK Incorporated.

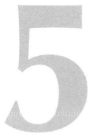

Education

Jennifer Ruisi Cosgrove, EdD, OTR/L
Rebecca L. Simon, MS, OTR/L
Amy Darragh, PhD, OTR/L
Guest Editor: Kimberly Hartmann, PhD, OTR/L, FAOTA

CHAPTER OBJECTIVES

By the end of this chapter, the student will be able to:

- ☑ Define **education** as it pertains to the *Occupational Therapy Practice Framework (Framework)*.
- ☑ Comprehend the **legal rights** of adult learners with disabilities.
- ☑ Describe specific **models/frames of reference** as related to adult education.
- ☑ Delineate between the role of the **occupational therapist** (OT) and the **occupational therapy assistant** (OTA) as they pertain to the occupation of adult education.
- ☑ Identify issues related to **access to support services** in adult education.
- ☑ Identify issues related to **access to classroom information**.
- ☑ Describe the impact of **contextual factors** upon education.
- ☑ Identify appropriate educational intervention strategies based on various **performance skills and client factors**.
- ☑ Identify specific education **compensation/adaptation** strategies.
- ☑ Identify general education **remediation** strategies.
- ☑ Identify education compensation/adaptation intervention strategies related to **vision, perception, and cognition**.
- ☑ Identify general education **maintenance** strategies.

INTRODUCTION

Education plays an important role in North American culture. Postsecondary education in particular represents social status, improved job prospects, and higher socioeconomic status (Unger, 1994). As such, the *Framework* (American Occupational Therapy Association [AOTA], 2002) identifies education as an area of occupation for occupational therapy practitioners to consider in their evaluation and intervention plans for the clients with whom they work. Figure 9-1 contains the components of education according to the *Framework*. These components will be addressed throughout the chapter.

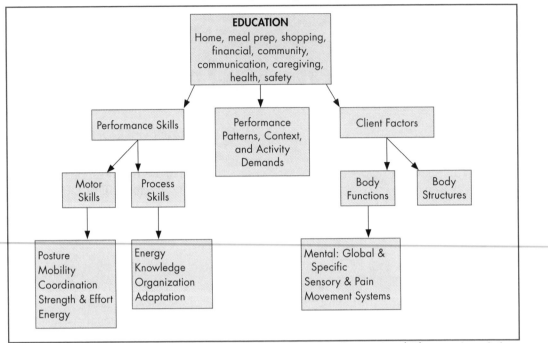

Figure 5-1. Components of education (adapted from American Occupational Therapy Association. (2002). Occupational therapy practice framework. *American Journal of Occupational Therapy, 56*(6), 609-639).

The *Framework* defines education as "activities needed for being a student and participating in a learning environment" including participation in formal education, informal personal educational needs or interests exploration (beyond formal education), and informal personal education participation (AOTA, 2002, p. 620). AOTA offers these definitions of terms:

- *Formal education participation*: Including the categories of academic (e.g., math, reading, working on a degree), nonacademic (e.g., recess, lunchroom, hallway), extracurricular (e.g., sports, band, cheerleading, dances), and vocational (prevocational and vocational) participation.

- *Exploration of informal personal educational needs or interests (beyond formal education)*: Identifying topics and methods for obtaining topic-related information or skills.

- *Informal personal education participation*: Participating in classes, programs, and activities that provide instruction/training in identifying areas of interest (2002, p. 620).

The purpose of this chapter is to discuss the roles of occupational therapy practitioners in facilitating and supporting adult clients as they pursue postsecondary education, providing a framework for evaluating their functional needs, and selecting appropriate remediation and accommodation interventions to promote success with educational goals, and to provide resources that may prevent future barriers to successful performance in the academic environment. For the purposes of this chapter, education as an area of occupation will be examined in the context of adults age 21 and over. Components of the above described AOTA definitions of the education domain particularly applicable to children (e.g., nonacademic and extracurricular participation) are not included. Although these components can be an integral part of postsecondary education, they are related primarily to leisure and social participation and are not discussed in this chapter (see Chapters 7 and 8).

This chapter will begin with the background and significance of adult education, including the applicable laws and legal responsibilities of postsecondary institutions and the students, learning theories, and learning styles. Next, occupational therapy roles in postsecondary education including evaluation and intervention information for adults with a variety of disabilities, both from a direct service provision model and a case management model, are presented. Finally, resources including funding, services, and Web sites available for individuals with disabilities are discussed. The occupational therapy client will be referred to as the "student" or "client" throughout this chapter as appropriate.

Postsecondary Education

DEFINITIONS AND STATISTICS

While more difficult to quantify, postsecondary education, which occurs after high school at a public, independent, technical, community, or junior college or university, has an essential role and many benefits in our society. Providing financial gains to individuals brings more financial resources to the society as a whole. In addition, many postsecondary programs require students to complete courses in a variety of subjects, such as sociology, anthropology, and psychology, along with the student's major of choice. Over the last 10 years, the proportion of individuals graduating from high schools and graduating with a bachelor's degree has increased steadily to 85% and 27%, respectively (Stoops, 2004). The proportion of students who enrolled in college immediately following high school graduation increased from 49% in 1972 to 62% in 2001 (National Center for Education Statistics, 2003). Between 1992/93 and 2002/03 the number of people earning associate degrees is increased 29%, bachelor's degrees 13%, and master's degrees 33% (National Center for Education Statistics, 2003a). Postsecondary education increasingly is a prerequisite to employment for many occupations and is associated with higher pay and better benefits when compared to high school education (Megivern, Pellerito, & Mowbray, 2003; Unger, 1994). For example, in 2000, full-time male workers over the age of 25 with a bachelor's degree earned a median annual salary of $56,334 as compared to $34,303 among male workers with a high school diploma. Full-time female workers received a median annual salary of $40,415 with a bachelor's degree as compared to women with a high school diploma who received a median annual salary of $24,970 (National Center for Educational Statistics, 2003).

In addition to better pay, postsecondary education benefits may also include increased work stability, job satisfaction, and upward mobility (Kasworm, 2003, Unger, 1994). In 2002, approximately 79% of adults (25 and older) with a bachelor's degree or higher were employed, while only 64% of adults with a high school diploma were employed, and 44% who were not high school completers were not in the labor force (National Center for Education Statistics, 2004). Unemployment rates follow the same trends. The 2002 unemployment rate was as 8.4% for adults (age 25 and over) who had not completed high school, compared with 5.3% for those with a high school diploma, and 2.9% for those with a bachelor's degree or higher (National Center for Education Statistics, 2004). Interestingly, 87.4% of individuals receiving a bachelor's degree were employed within 1 year after graduating from college in 1999-2000 (National Center for Education Statistics, 2004).

Learning, however, is not just an economic issue; it is important for social and cultural growth also. Education provides important information about societal norms and helps to expose individuals to information that may have not been obtained simply by going about one's daily life. Some students are able to study abroad or meet students studying in the United States from other cultures and further broaden their knowledge base. Some adults will seek educational opportunities for leisure purposes, such as a cooking or art class. Others may seek education, such as attending college, because of the leisure opportunities educational environments can provide such as sports, clubs, and organizations. Recognizing the importance of adult education or postsecondary education in a client's life, for either the continued pursuit of knowledge or for the leisure aspects it may satisfy, is important for occupational therapy practitioners to recognize and take into consideration during intervention planning.

The number of adults with disabilities entering postsecondary institutions continues to rise. The proportion of college students reporting disabilities has increased from 3% in 1978 to 9% in 1998 (National Center for Education Statistics, 2002). According to the recent statistics, roughly 9% of all undergraduate students in the 1999 to 2000 academic year reported having some type of disability or disabilities (National Center for Education Statistics, 2002). These disabilities are classified as orthopedic or mobility impairments (29%), mental illness or depression (17%), health problems (15%), hearing (6.7%), attention deficit disorder (6.4%), vision (5.2%), specific learning disability/dyslexia (5%), speech (.2%), and others (16.4%) (National Center for Education Statistics, 2002). In addition, students with disabilities enrolled in postsecondary institutions were older, with an average age of 31, as compared to students without disabilities whose average age was 26. Interestingly, students with disabilities enroll in a variety of educational institutions: 2-year public institutions (49%) and 4-year public institutions (25%), 4-year private not for profit (14%), and "other" public institutions, which includes for-profit vocational institutions (11%) (National Center for Education Statistics, 1999). It is important to note that students with disabilities experience the same financial and employment benefits from postsecondary education as their nondisabled counterparts. This is evidenced by the fact that students with disabilities and an earned bachelor's degree have jobs in areas closely related to their degree and have similar full-time starting salaries when compared to students without disabilities (National Center for Educational Statistics, 1999).

Legal Rights of Adult Learners With Disabilities

Adults with disabilities have certain civil rights that enable them to attend postsecondary institutions. These rights are a result of primarily two acts: Section 504 of the Rehabilitation Act of 1973 (PL 93-112) and the Americans with Disability Act of 1990 (ADA, 1990, PL 101-336). Because of these acts, postsecondary institutions cannot discriminate on the basis of disability and must allow equal access for individuals with disabilities, otherwise qualified, to attend classes as long as they meet the academic and technical standards for admission/participation (Madaus, 2005). Students accepted into the institution have the right to reasonable accommodations, program accessibility, and auxiliary aids/services (Brinckerhoff, McGuire, & Shaw, 2002).

Section 504 of the Rehabilitation Act of 1973 prohibits discrimination on the basis of disability in programs and activities that receive federal financial assistance. This applies to all colleges and universities because they receive federal funds. At these institutions, individuals with disabilities have the right to have access and/or the opportunity to participate in the same programs and activities as other students with the use of supplementary aids and services as needed (www.section508.gov).

The ADA created new and comprehensive civil right protections for individuals with disabilities. It prohibits discrimination on the basis of disability in private employment (Title I), all state and local government agencies (Title II), places of public accommodation such as museums, restaurants, and theaters (Title III), and mandates accessibility to communication services for people who are deaf, hard of hearing, or speech impaired (Title IV) (Americans with Disabilities Act, 1990). While public colleges/universities are covered under Title II, most private colleges/universities have activities for the general public and are covered under Title III.

ACCOMMODATIONS AND ESSENTIAL FUNCTIONS

Two important concepts associated with these rights are accommodations and essential functions. "Accommodation means any change to a classroom environment or task that permits a qualified student with a disability to participate in the classroom process, to perform the essential tasks of the class, or to enjoy benefits and privileges of classroom participation equal to those enjoyed by adult learners without disabilities" (University of Kansas Institute for Adult Studies, 1998, p. 54). Under Section 504 and the ADA, institutions may require adequate documentation/verification of a disability and the need for accommodations before such accommodations are made. Verification is usually required in the form of a medical or psychological evaluation or statement. However, evaluations from vocational rehabilitation agencies, or formal/informal evaluations from the institution's disability support services officer or coordinator may be accepted as verification of a disability (1998, p. 108).

For college or adult education students with disabilities, academic accommodations may include adaptations in the way specific courses are conducted, the use of equipment and support staff, and modifications in environments and academic requirements. Accommodations, if basic enough, can be achieved by the adult learner individually without assistance from the educational program. Examples of this include the use of adaptive writing devices such as pencil grips or universal cuffs or using a tape player to record lectures.

Before an accommodation will be provided by the academic institution, several steps must be accomplished:

1. Students must apply to the academic institution (which includes meeting the essential functions if applicable).

2. Students must disclose their disability.

3. Students must provide documentation of disability.

4. If above criteria are met, students will be eligible for accommodations and will begin to work with the disabilities coordinator at the academic institution to establish an accommodation plan.

Specific examples of accommodations that may be requested of the educational program include extended time for test taking/completion of assignments, note-takers, sign language interpreters, modifications to desk/chair height, assistive technology, and written instructions/lecture notes. Cost and effects of the accommodation on the requirements of a course are factors that educational programs can take into consideration when determining the ability to fulfill the accommodation request. If a requested accommodation is a fundamental alteration of a program or would impose an undue hardship, the institution is not required to provide it (42 U.S.C. §12111). In these cases, other alternatives must be explored.

Another resource for students is the coordinator of these programs. Educational programs with 15 or more employees must designate a Section 504 Coordinator and 50 or more employees must designate a responsible employee as the ADA coordinator (28CFR35.107, 34CFR104.7). One person may serve both functions. Occupational therapy practitioners should collaborate with the 504/ADA coordinator, often referred to as the disabilities coordinator, when working with clients on educational goals.

A new movement in postsecondary education, Universal Design for Instruction, is a proactive approach to teaching that uses inclusive instructional strategies that benefit a broad range of learners, including students with disabilities (Scott, McGuire, & Embry, 2002):

> *"The nine Principles of UDI provide a framework for college faculty to use when designing or revising instruction to be responsive to diverse student learners and to minimize the need for 'special' accommodations and retrofitted changes to the learning environment. UDI operates on the premise that the planning and delivery of instruction as well as the evaluation of learning can incorporate inclusive attributes that embrace diversity in learners without compromising academic standards"* (Scott, McGuire, & Embry, 2002, p.1).

The nine principles of Universal Design for Instruction are based on the principles of universal design (which originated in the field of architecture) and effective instruction and were developed as part of a 3-year federal grant from the U.S. Department of Education at the University of Connecticut's Center on Postsecondary Education and Disability. The principles are undergoing rigorous construct validation through a series of procedures and continue to be refined (Scott, McGuire, & Embry, 2002). Presently they are defined as:

1. Equitable use: Instruction is designed to be useful to and accessible by people with diverse abilities. Provide the same means of use for all students—identical whenever possible, equivalent when not.

2. Flexibility in use: Instruction is designed to accommodate a wide range of individual abilities. Provide choice in methods of use.

3. Simple and intuitive: Instruction is designed in a straightforward and predictable manner, regardless of the student's experience, knowledge, language skills, or current concentration level. Eliminate unnecessary complexity.

4. Perceptible information: Instruction is designed so that necessary information is communicated effectively to the student, regardless of ambient conditions or the student's sensory abilities.

5. Tolerance for error: Instruction anticipates variation in individual student learning pace and prerequisite skills.

6. Low physical effort: Instruction is designed to minimize nonessential physical effort in order to allow maximum attention to learning. Note: This principle does not apply when physical effort is integral to essential requirements of a course.

7. Size and space for approach and use: Instruction is designed with consideration for appropriate size and space for approach, reach, manipulations, and use regardless of a student's body size, posture, mobility, and communication needs.

8. A community of learners: The instructional environment promotes interaction and communication among students and between students and faculty.

9. Instructional climate: Instruction is designed to be welcoming and inclusive. High expectations are espoused for all students (Scott, McGuire, & Shaw, 2003).

In addition to meeting entry requirements, students with disabilities must be sure they meet any *essential functions* associated with their courses or programs of study. Essential functions, as distinguished from academic standards, refer to the cognitive, physical, and behavioral abilities that are necessary for satisfactory completion of a course or program curriculum, with or without accommodation (Association of the American Medical Colleges, 1993, 29CFR1630.2). Colleges and universities that establish essential functions can ensure they will not have to lower their academic standards to accommodate individuals with disabilities. Individuals with disabilities may request accommodations in order to meet the established essential functions. Essential functions are typically associated with academic programs of a professional nature and are rarely a prerequisite for adult education programs. Essential functions are usually described within several categories including, but not limited to, sensory and observational skills, cognitive skills, motor skills, behavioral and social skills, communication skills, and intellectual/conceptual abilities. Occasionally, and depending on the type of educational program, endurance, coordination, and emotional health may also be included. When assisting clients with the return to or the integration into a structured educational environment, occupational therapy practitioners should be aware whether essential functions exist at a particular institution in order to plan intervention appropriately. Figure 5-1 provides an example of essential functions established at the University of South Dakota for the Master of Science Degree in Occupational Therapy. Students wishing to attend the program must meet the essential functions established for the program, which include criteria outlined in the following sections: sensory processing demands, cognitive demands, physical demands, psychosocial demands, communication demands, environmental demands, and professional behaviors.

OCCUPATIONAL THERAPY ROLES IN POSTSECONDARY EDUCATION

Although there is minimal discussion in the literature regarding occupational therapy practitioners working to attain adult educational goals, practitioners can use their unique skills in a variety of ways. Examples of these include assisting clients with determining accommodations that will be necessary at the postsecondary level, training of clients in the use of assistive technology devices, assessing and adapting environments, and case management. These roles fall into one of three types: consultant, direct care provider, and educator (AOTA, 2002).

The occupational therapy practitioner's role as case manager is debated (Lamb, 2003; Daykin, 2001). Social workers and nurses are most often placed in the role of case manager. Social workers receive training in social policy, community organization, and community resources to help them most effectively provide resources for their clients (Case-Smith, 1991). Nurses too have played an important role in case management, particularly in acute care settings (Lohman, 1999). Occupational therapy practitioners, however, also receive education on health care, social, educational, governmental, and community systems as they relate to the practice of occupational therapy (ACOTE, 1998). Despite the community debate, the AOTA's Scope of Practice (2004) includes case management as an appropriate occupational therapy intervention.

In some settings, it is a natural extension of the occupational therapy practitioner's roles and responsibilities. For example, early intervention services recognize occupational and physical therapists as potential case managers (Case-Smith, 1991). As students approach graduation, occupational therapy practitioners have participated in the transition planning phase of high school. Transition services are included as part of the Individuals With Disabilities Education Act (IDEA) Amendments of 1997 (IDEA: Public Law, 105-17). These services are designed to facilitate the move from high school to postsecondary activities, including postsecondary education. The participation of the occupational therapy practitioner in transition planning is critical for the success of the student (Asher, 2003; Davidson & Fitzgerald, 2001; O'Reilly, 2000). Occupational therapy practitioners are able to identify what many of the postgraduation needs may be and are able to identify resources that are available.

Occupational therapy practitioners working with adult clients also serve as case managers. Occupational therapy practitioners in geriatric, outpatient, mental health, and acute care settings all may find themselves taking on the role of case manager (Lamb, 2003; Jacobs, 2002; Lohman, 1999). Mental health centers use occupational therapy practitioners as case managers, either as part of their role as OT or with the job title of case manager (Lamb, 2003; Jacobs, 2002). In other settings, case management responsibilities may require more specialized training. For example, in an acute care setting, the OT may have to participate in advanced training classes on medical processes and medical economics in order to effectively perform the duties of a case manager (Lohman, 1999).

The following sections will discuss these roles in the context of evaluation and intervention.

The first step in any role is evaluation. With education, the evaluation includes interest exploration with the client, knowledge of appropriate frames of reference, and knowledge of learning theories/learning styles.

For interest exploration, occupational therapy practitioners may choose to use an interest inventory to determine the client's goals and interests. Often, with onset of injury, clients may feel

ESSENTIAL FUNCTIONS OF THE UNIVERSITY OF SOUTH DAKOTA OCCUPATIONAL THERAPY STUDENT

A Master of Science degree in Occupational Therapy signifies that the holder is eligible to sit for the National Board for Certification in Occupational Therapy Examination, and the holder is prepared for entry into the profession of occupational therapy. Therefore, it follows that graduates must have knowledge and skills to function in a broad variety of clinical, community, or school environments and to render a wide spectrum of occupational therapy services. All students admitted to the Occupational Therapy Program at The University of South Dakota must meet the abilities and expectations outlined below.

Regarding those students with verifiable disabilities, the University will not discriminate against such individuals who are otherwise qualified, but will expect applicants and students to meet certain minimal technical standards (essential functions) as set forth herein with or without reasonable accommodation. In adopting these standards, the University believes it must keep in mind the ultimate safety of the clients whom its students and graduates serve. The standards reflect what the Occupational Therapy Program believes are reasonable expectations required of students and practitioners in performing essential functions of the profession.

I. **Sensory Processing Demands**: Participating as a student requires functional use of vision, hearing, and touch along with awareness of body position and movement. Specific visual skills required include near and far vision, peripheral vision, color vision, and depth perception. Students must be able to perceive and interpret sensory information accurately to provide quality client care.

II. **Cognitive Demands**: The successful occupational therapy student maintains a high level of alertness and responsiveness during classroom and fieldwork situations. The student must possess the ability to focus on a task for a prolonged period of time to allow for successful learning to take place. In addition, the occupational therapist must be able to recall information and organize information in an efficient and useful manner. This includes the ability to acquire, retain, and prioritize informational data, conceptualize and integrate abstract information, apply theoretical knowledge to specific client populations and justify a rationale for therapeutic interventions, and problem-solve to create innovative and practical solutions.

III. **Physical Demands**: The successful occupational therapy student must possess sufficient motor abilities to allow for treatment intervention with a variety of clients. This includes functional use of all four extremities, which would allow the student to carry out assessments and to provide therapeutic interventions. Quick reactions are necessary not only for safety, but for one to respond therapeutically in most clinical situations. The student also needs to demonstrate good mobility skills including the ability to walk, climb, stoop, kneel, crouch, and crawl to allow one to complete therapeutic interventions on all types of surfaces. The student is regularly required to maintain positions for extended periods of time such as sitting, standing, and writing. The student frequently is required to demonstrate good arm placement to allow for reaching and positioning of hands to successfully manipulate large and small objects. The student must be able to lift and carry up to 50 pounds, and push or pull up to 100 pounds.

IV. **Psychosocial Demands**: The student must display the emotional maturity to interact with a variety of individuals with diverse ages, diagnoses, cultures, and socioeconomic backgrounds. The student frequently needs to address multiple, demanding tasks simultaneously and therefore needs to have established strategies for stress management

V. **Communication Demands**: *Written*: The student must be able to effectively communicate in written English. The format can range from a brief note with appropriate use of abbreviations to a descriptive narrative. *Verbal and Nonverbal*: The student must be able to produce the spoken word and to interpret factual information along with nonverbal cues of mood, temperament, and social responses from clients, supervisors, and peers. Response to emergencies/crisis situations, as well as more routine communication, must be appropriate to the situation. Communication must be accurate, sensitive, and effective. *Reading*: The student must be able to read and comprehend information in English from a variety of written sources (e.g., textbooks, professional journals, medical/school records, and government regulations).

VI. **Environmental Demands**: The occupational therapy student must be able to negotiate and successfully achieve access to multiple environmental situations. These environmental situations may be physical, social, or cultural. The physical environment would consist of nonhuman aspects. The student is occasionally exposed to

continued

wet or humid conditions (nonweather); and must sometimes work near moving mechanical parts, fumes or airborne particles, hazardous materials, blood borne pathogens, outdoor weather conditions, risk of electrical shock, risk of radiation, and vibration. The noise level in the work environment will range from a classroom situation in which the noise level is low to an industrial or clinical environment where the noise level may be high. The social environment would consist of norms, expectations, and routines of different environments. The occupational therapy student will be exposed to multiple treatment environments, which have implicit and explicit rules for behavior.

The occupational therapy student must demonstrate multicultural competency to interact with multiple client populations. Multicultural competency as outlined by the American Occupational Therapy Association includes awareness of one's culture, willingness to explore and become knowledgeable about another culture, being respectful to individual diversities, and being able to select culturally sensitive therapeutic interventions.

VII. **Professional Behaviors**: The student is expected to demonstrate professional behaviors and attitudes during his/her participation in the classroom and clinical settings. This includes, but is not limited to: commitment to learning, dependability, written and verbal communication, interpersonal skills, professionalism, cooperation, clinical reasoning, and intrapersonal coping skills. Faculty will assess and mentor the development of each student's professional behavior. Students must be able to give and receive constructive criticism. Responsiveness to constructive criticism from faculty, clinical instructors, and peers is essential for success.

Comments: The description above is intended to reflect the essential functions in a general manner. It is not all-inclusive, and is not a contract, expressed or implied. The description also attempts to describe functions in multiple contexts from the didactic experience to the fieldwork experience. Keeping this in mind, some essential functions may increase or decrease depending on the context.

The Department will not discriminate on the basis of race, color, creed, national origin, ancestry, citizenship, gender, sexual orientation, religion, age, or disability. Students having concern regarding their ability to meet these essential functions must contact the Office of Disability Services at the University of South Dakota. Accommodations may be arranged through this office.

Figure 5-2. Essential Functions for University of South Dakota Occupational Therapy Student (reprinted with permission from The University of South Dakota Occupational Therapy Program).

their chance for continued education is lost and goals to continue to pursue postsecondary education or other form of adult education may not be reflected in an individual's stated goals. With proper education on options for assistive technology and other methods of accessing education, clients may feel empowered to return to their pursuit of education and therefore a better quality of life.

Based on the previously stated statistical information, occupational therapy practitioners working with clients in postsecondary education will likely see adults with newly diagnosed or existing disabilities including mobility or orthopedic impairments, neurological impairments, sensory disorders, and/or cognitive impairments. As this text focuses on clients with physical disability impairments, information related to mental illness and learning disabilities is limited, although these are recognized as possible issues that occupational therapy practitioners may encounter when working with adults on goals related to postsecondary education. In addition, there are other individuals who could benefit from occupational therapy services who do not have a disability such as immigrants considering formal education for the first time, single parents, and women who are incarcerated. For example, OTs can serve in social service agencies or work for social welfare projects providing transitional living services to women at risk (Jacobs, 2002). OTs are able to serve those people transitioning to a postsecondary institution from the special education system in high school, entering the institution following a newly diagnosed physical disability, or re-entering the academic environment following a life-changing illness or injury. In all of these varied situations, the goals of the client to begin or re-enter education must be established first.

FRAMES OF REFERENCE

Occupational therapy practitioners can use the information from Chapter 1 on occupational therapy theories in conjunction with the theoretical knowledge presented in this chapter, as well as their own professional experiences, to form an approach for working with adults wishing to pursue postsecondary education. Theories related to adult learning will be discussed under the following categories: behaviorist, cognitive, humanist, and social learning.

The basic assumptions of the *behaviorist* theory include the belief that learning is manifested by a change in behavior and learning is determined by the environment rather than the learner (Merriam & Caffarella, 1991). Early theorists included J. B. Watson, E. L. Thorndike, Pavlov, Guthrie, and B. F. Skinner. In the behaviorist theory, the purpose of education is to promote a desirable behavioral change, the teacher has ultimate authority, and the learner is a passive listener. Incentives, feedback, and emphasis on mastery and competence describe the basic approaches and methods of learning (Merriam & Caffarella, 1991; Cole, 1998). Learning activities may include hints, cues, or consequences which guide students to desired behavior(s).

In contrast, the *cognitive* theory views learning as a process occurring inside the learner in an attempt to make sense of the world and give meaning to experiences. Some of the major theorists include Piaget, Bruner, and Ausubel. Gestalt learning theorists include Wertheimer, Kohler, Koffka, and Lewin. In the cognitive theory, the purpose of adult learning is knowledge acquisition. Instructors create the proper conditions for learning and the learner is actively involved in the learning process (Merriam & Caffarella, 1991; Cole, 1998). Learning will include challenging learners beyond their current ability but within their potential level of development, thus allowing the material to be internalized.

While the cognitive theories examine the mental processing of information and the behaviorist theories focus on the environment shaping observable behavior, the *humanist* theories examine the potential for growth as a motivation for learning (Merriam & Caffarella, 1991). Key theorists include Maslow, Rogers, and Knowles. In the humanistic perspective, experience separates adults from youth when learning. The purpose of education is to enhance personal growth, development, and self-actualization. In the humanist perspective, students learn how to learn and there is a relationship between the facilitator of learning and the learner. Learning activities may include group discussion, self-directed learning, and experiential learning (Merriam & Cafarella, 1991; Cole, 1998).

Finally, the *social learning* theories suggest that people learn by observing other people. Key theorists include Bandura and Rotter. The purpose of learning in the social theories is to promote desirable changes in knowledge, attitudes, and behavior. The role of the learner is one of an observer, decision-maker, and processor of information, while the instructor serves as a model or provider of models as well as a facilitator. Approaches to learning may include demonstration, modeling, apprenticeships and mentoring, tutorials, peer partnerships, and on the job training (Merriam & Cafarrella, 1991).

Each of the theory groupings discussed have very different assumptions about the way adults learn. Occupational therapy practitioners should identify the most appropriate theory of learning based on each client and the context of intervention in order to develop strategies that will enhance their client's learning in therapy.

Adult Learning Theories and Learning Styles

Occupational therapy practitioners working with adults in an education setting must be familiar with the key theories of learning for adults. They also must be able to identify the learning styles of their clients to better assist them in attaining their educational goals. Understanding how adult students learn will be important when working with other professionals assisting the client, such as the disabilities coordinator at the school or university, professors, and any other professional assisting with client's goal of attending postsecondary education classes. Understanding this information will assist the occupational therapy practitioner in problem solving and offering suggestions to both professionals and the client as it relates to the client's physical disability. Merriam and Caffarella (1991) suggest "learning as a process (rather than an end product) focuses on what happens when learning takes place. Explanations of what happens are called learning theories" (p. 124). Learning theories are discussed at length in Chapter 9.

Lastly, the occupational therapy practitioner should determine the client's primary method of learning. Everyone has a particular way in which he/she prefers. This will be especially important for clients whose physical limitations include cognitive impairments. A learning style does not suggest how intelligent a person is, but does define how a person's brain works best and most efficiently when attempting to learn new information (Halsne, 2002). Understanding personal learning styles can assist with success during any type of educational activity. Occasionally, depending upon the reason a client is being seen in occupational therapy, a preferred learning style may not be possible any longer and assisting the client with adapting to a new learning style may be necessary. Learning styles have traditionally been classified as auditory, visual, and tactile/kinesthetic (Halsne, 2002). This classification is one of the simplest forms and it is suggested for those interested in further study on learning styles to review the literature for the many theories and classifications that exist.

As the name would suggest, *auditory* learners prefer learning by hearing such as listening to a live lecture or audiotape. *Visual* learners, on the other hand, prefer to learn new information by reading or viewing a demonstration. Learners who prefer to manipulate materials when first being introduced to them are often classified as *tactile/kinesthetic* learners. Tactile/kinesthetic learners prefer to learn by doing, with hands-on practice being the best way for this type of learner to master a concept (Halsne, 2002). Refer to the list of strategies for visual, auditory, and tactile/kinesthetic learners. Depending on the client's disability, some of the strategies listed may need to be modified or accommodations may need to be requested in order for them to be achieved. For example, if color coding materials is recommended to assist learning and the client has an upper extremity (UE) physical disability which will prevent him/her from being able to do this, the occupational therapy practitioner may teach the client how to highlight text using a computer equipped with assistive technology, eliminating the need for use of the UEs.

STRATEGIES FOR VISUAL, AUDITORY, AND TACTILE/KINESTHETIC LEARNERS

Visual learners may benefit from the following strategies:

- Color coding material into categories (highlighter pens may be one way of accomplishing this).
- Flash cards with key concepts.
- Translating illustrations and diagrams into written summaries or vice versa.
- Using computers to translate notes and important learning material into well-organized printouts.

Auditory learners may benefit from the following strategies:

- Joining study groups.
- Talking out loud while reading or studying new concepts.
- Tape recording lectures.
- Using textbook tapes/CDs (textbooks often have additional study aids available for purchase that include tapes and CDs of material discussed in the text).

Tactile/kinesthetic learners may benefit from the following strategies:

- Spending time in the field to gain first-hand knowledge of the subject matter.
- Writing out notes on the computer or by hand.
- Ambulating or moving about while studying.
- Acting out learning concepts if possible.

Occupational therapy practitioners working in this area need to include an assessment of the client's learning style in their overall assessment. To do this, the occupational therapy practitioner may request that the client take a learning styles inventory. The Learning Type Measure (LTM) published by About Learning is one example of an assessment tool that profiles individual approaches to learning. The LTM provides personal strengths and weaknesses as a learner. It is designed to assist with improving individual potential, motivate learners with strategies crafted to their unique learning style, and identify situations in which different people function most effectively. The LTM is a 26-point self-report questionnaire that measures individual preferences for selecting, organizing, prioritizing, and representing knowledge, information, and experience. The LTM can be taken online and the test taker is provided with immediate scoring and feedback. Examples of questions asked include:

- Part A (15 questions) asks you to place yourself in a learning situation as you respond to the questions and then rank the answers given between 4 and 1, with 4 = most like and 1= least like. One question asks, "I learn best by": a) testing how things work, b) working in groups, c) self-discovery and thinking, d) reflecting (The Learning Type Measure [About Learning, Inc., Wauconda, IL]).
- Part B (11 questions) examines your watching and doing behaviors. Each question gives you two choices, for example: "When learning, I prefer to" a) reflect before I act, and b) act and then reflect (The Learning Type Measure, About Learning, Inc.).
- Part C (8 questions) asks you to rate each question on a scale of 1 to 5, with 5 being very true or important and 1 being not true at all. One question asks: "Generally I enjoyed my schooling" (The Learning Type Measure, About Learning, Inc.).

Once the exam is taken, the scores are submitted for scoring and a learning profile is created with both strengths and weaknesses. The LTM can be taken online for a small fee at www.about-learning.com and more information can be obtained by contacting About Learning, Inc.

INTERVENTIONS FOR ACCESSIBILITY

Once the evaluation is complete, and depending on the role of the therapist as discussed earlier, the OT will be concerned with three types of accessibility: (1) access to support services, (2) access to educational facilities, and (3) access to classroom information.

Access to support services, similar to case management, has been used in transition planning, discharge planning, and service coordination. Case management interventions aimed at facilitating transitions to community supports or coordinating community and university services to assist the student with attaining his/her educational goals are both remedial and compensatory in nature. Remediation and compensation associated with case management is discussed below.

Access to facilities and to classroom information is a more direct service, and this type of service is provided both off- and on-campus, either privately or through the university. Interventions based on a direct service model include assessing existing and recommending structural accommodations and assessing and providing assistive technology, as well as including or providing remedial and compensatory approaches. More details regarding direct service provision will be discussed later in the chapter.

Access to Support Services—Case Management

The services available to students seeking postsecondary education are both university- and community-based. For a student with a disability, understanding and making sense of these services can be difficult and overwhelming. As case managers, occupational therapy practitioners can assist by facilitating connections with these supports and/or coordinating communication between these services.

The authors of this chapter use the term *facilitation* to describe a remedial approach, by which the occupational therapy practitioners gradually shift responsibility for accessing and using support services to the client, based on gradual improvements in the individual's ability to assume the role of self advocate. Occupational therapy practitioners have specialized training in the grading of activity and occupation and in the use of this strategy to promote independence (for more information regarding grading, see Chapter 1). The authors use the term *coordination* to describe a more adaptive or compensatory approach, in which the occupational therapy practitioner serves as the strategy for maintaining support access and usage, and coordinating the communication between services to assist the client with meeting educational goals. Again, this strategy is one in which occupational therapy practitioners receive specialized training. They are able to determine the need for compensation, as opposed to remediation, and are skilled in the therapeutic use of self in practice. These strategies can be used both with students with developmental/physical disabilities who have transitioned from high school to postsecondary education, and with individuals who have experienced a new diagnosis or impairment and are attempting to return to college or university.

STUDENTS TRANSITIONING FROM HIGH SCHOOL

As stated earlier, the transition from high school to postsecondary education is included as part of the IDEA Amendments of 1997 (IDEA: Public Law, 105-17). As a member of the transition team, the occupational therapy practitioner makes recommendations based on the students' needs and abilities, and makes predictions regarding possible areas of challenge in the postsecondary environment. However, once discharged from the school-based services, the student no longer has access to these school-based professionals.

The occupational therapy practitioner who takes on the student's care, through a variety of traditional and nontraditional sources, can use either case management approach of facilitation and/or coordination to promote academic success. Using the facilitation approach, the occupational therapy practitioner examines the supports that are available on campus and in the community to assist the individual with postsecondary participation. As the individual becomes more comfortable with the transition and the service providers, the occupational therapy practitioner gradually shifts the responsibility for campus support to representatives from the various involved agencies and to the individual client.

Occupational therapy practitioners can take a more active role in the coordination of services. In this role, the occupational therapy practitioner serves as the adaptation. For the client who cannot negotiate the service agencies independently, the occupational therapy practitioner can coordinate on- and off-campus services, the communication between agencies and service providers, and periodic team meetings to discuss the student's progress. Under this model, the client does not assume responsibility for his/her own care coordination and the OT either will continue throughout the postsecondary experience or will have to transfer care to another involved professional.

The community agencies that may be involved with this population include:

- Group home service providers.
- Independent living centers.
- Departments of vocational rehabilitation.

- Community mental health centers, if applicable.
- Campus-based services for students with disabilities.
- Campus-based counseling centers.
- Community supported employment agencies.

The value of such services can be inferred from studies of adults with mental illness. For example, one study reported 16.3% of their participants with mental illness who dropped out of college reported that a case manager who could coordinate and facilitate both educational and mental health goals would have helped them remain in school (Megivern, Pellerito, & Mowbray, 2003).

STUDENTS RETURNING TO COLLEGE OR UNIVERSITY

Occupational therapy practitioners also may support individuals with a new diagnosis or physical disability, such as a traumatic brain injury, spinal cord injury, or multiple sclerosis. The case management approach remains the same, though the community agencies may differ. The occupational therapy practitioner will need to consider many agencies and services including:

- Division of vocational rehabilitation.
- Local independent living centers.
- Campus office of resources for students with disabilities.
- Campus counseling centers.
- Community mental health centers.
- Community physicians, nurses, and other medical personnel.
- Community psychologists, neuropsychologists, and counselors.
- Local social security offices.
- Local social service agencies.

The occupational therapy practitioner must determine whether each client has the ability to assume the role of case manager. Many factors enter into such a decision. Cognitive status, important among individuals with brain injuries, for example, may require the OT to assume the role of coordinator. The complexity of service coordination may add too much cognitive stress to the individual's academic life, impeding academic performance. Individuals with physical impairments may present with different challenges. Students with spinal cord injuries may require initial coordination of services, but once campus supports have been established, they are able to coordinate on their own. Other physical impairments such as fatigue, for example, become more complex. Fatigue itself can impair cognitive acuity and the OT must carefully assess and interview individuals with fatigue to determine which approach will best promote academic success.

The OT as case manager must have a thorough knowledge of community resources and agencies in order to provide effective service provision. These resources include the agencies above, but also local grant supported projects, state funding initiatives, and campus systems. These resources can be critical to the success of the individual returning to school, whether by allowing assistive technology to be purchased or by providing on-campus support.

Access to Educational Facilities

Accessibility is one of the barriers that students with physical disabilities may face once deciding to return/continue with postsecondary education or adult education programs. Structural accessibility includes the accessibility of physical facilities including ramps, automatic doors, elevators, accessible restrooms, pay phones, classrooms, libraries, computer centers, and cafeterias. In addition, the presence of the following will impact many students with disabilities: curb cuts, handicapped parking, and adaptive on-campus transportation or shuttle services in all buildings and on all campuses. Additionally, structural accessibility includes nontraditional methods of accessing campus services such as the various options available through distance learning.

One important role that occupational therapy practitioners play when working with clients is the role of educator. Educating our clients about acceptable methods of program accessibility in educational institutions is an important foundation to provide. Both Title II of the ADA and Section 504 of the Rehabilitation Act require educational programs that are accessible and usable by individuals with disabilities (Scott, 1994). Structures built after January 26, 1992, must follow the ADA Standards for Accessible Design. These newer buildings, therefore, usually do not pose a problem to individuals with physical disabilities. However, many educational institutions operate in older buildings, which make structural modifications difficult. In these cases, schools can meet accessibility accommodations through nonstructural methods. Although these methods are not considered ideal and must not result in any type of segregation of individuals with disabilities, they can be effective in achieving a student's access. Some examples of remedial and adaptation/compensation accommodations are listed below. In addition, occupational therapy practitioners need to consider the possible barriers clients with physical disabilities may face when attending events in specialty classrooms such as labs, theaters, and gymnasiums. Although most of these types of classrooms will be in compliance with the ADA Standards for Accessible Design, there will be cases when they are not and the occupational therapy practitioner should problem-solve with the client on the preferred method for accessibility.

ACCESSIBILITY ACCOMMODATIONS THROUGH NONSTRUCTURAL METHODS (UNIVERSITY OF KANSAS INSTITUTE FOR ADULT STUDIES, 1998)

Remedial

- Reassignment of services or classrooms to an accessible location such as the ground floor of a building or relocation to completely different building.
- Moving computers in libraries and computer labs to an accessible location.

Adaptation/Compensation

- Assignment of aides to assist in nonaccessible areas such as retrieving a book from a shelf or library that is inaccessible.
- Providing accessible workstations.
- Modifying hardware on doors to allow for access.

As stated earlier, the ADA does provide certain rights to students regarding structural access. Occupational therapy practitioners should educate their clients about their accessibility rights. Although the following points are only a small sample of what the ADA Standards for Accessible Design stipulate, they are a good place to start. Those interested in the detailed version of the ADA Standards can access them on the ADA Homepage: http://www.usdoj.gov/crt/ada/adahom1.htm.

- Parking: Students should have access to accessible parking spaces that are closest to the accessible building entrance.
- Stairs: Students should have alternate ways to access buildings and classrooms if stairs are present, such as ramps, elevators, lifts, curb cuts, etc.
- Doors: All doors should have at least 32 inches of clear opening, meaning any person using a wheelchair or other type of mobility device should be able to fit through the door opening. Door handles should be operational by individuals with limited strength and/or coordination.

- Elevators: All elevators should have the following in place to accommodate a variety of disabilities: call buttons that are no higher than 42 inches, visible and audible door opening/closing and floor indicators, and raised and Braille lettering on the control buttons and floor indicator signs.

- Seats and tables: Accessible tables/seating should be available in all classrooms and other areas within buildings. The tops of tables and counters should be between 28 and 34 inches high.

- Restrooms: Students should have access to lavatories with faucets that can be operated with one closed fist. Soap and towel dispensers should be 48 inches or lower from a front approach and 54 inches or lower from a side approach. Stalls should be wheelchair accessible with grab bars mounted to the side and behind the toilet, and toilets should be 17 to 19 inches in height.

- Telephones: If pay phones are provided, students should have access to phones that are no more than 48 inches to the highest operable part, are hearing aid compatible, and/or have volume control.

Access to Classroom Information

Academic accessibility, or access to classroom information, includes the institution's ability to satisfy necessary accommodations, such as extended time for examinations and assignments, note takers, and doing work in a different way or in a different place. Accessibility issues will be discussed using the following categories: orthopedic/neuromuscular mobility, cognitive, visual, and hearing. However, let us first discuss some important points about assistive technology, as technology allows access to postsecondary education for most disability impairments in a way little can mimic.

ASSISTIVE TECHNOLOGY

This section will attempt to clarify the role of the occupational therapy practitioner in evaluation and provision of assistive technology as a tool to provide equal opportunity for the student to achieve the best results possible in postsecondary education. Assistive technology is considered to be a compensatory approach, modifying or adapting the student's environment for increased function and maximum independence.

While there are many ways to define assistive technology, the definition that has been most widely accepted by professionals is from the Assistive Technology Act of 1998. It states that an *assistive technology device* is: "Any item, piece of equipment or product system whether acquired commercially off the shelf, modified, or customized which is used to increase or improve functional capabilities of individuals with disabilities." The act further states *assistive technology service* means: "Any service which directly assists individuals with a disability in the selection, acquisition, or use of an assistive technology device" (Assistive Technology Act, 105-394, S. 2432, 1998).

This term also includes:

- The evaluation of the needs of individuals with a disability.

- The purchasing, leasing, or provision of the device.

- The selection, designing, fitting, customizing, adapting, applying, maintaining, repairing, or replacing of the device.

- Coordinating and using other therapies, interventions, or services such as those associated with education and rehabilitation plans and programs.

- Training and technical assistance for the person with a disability, or if appropriate, the family of the person.

- Training or technical assistance for professionals, including individuals providing education or rehabilitation service, employers, or other individuals who are substantially involved in the major life functions of individuals with disabilities (Assistive Technology Act, 105-394, S. 2432, 1998).

As described previously, Section 504 is accessed by the student and accommodations are primarily student driven. The role of the occupational therapy practitioner in addressing assistive technology issues would likely be to provide information on, and access to, the most beneficial assistive technology for the student and the setting. In a study completed in 1993 by the Board for Rights of Virginians with Disabilities, a satisfaction survey indicated 86% of the adult students in postsecondary education had encountered barriers to their education because of their disability. Many students indicated they were "unaware of the services to which they were entitled or which were available" (West, Kregel, Getzel, Ming, Ipsen, & Martin, 1993, p. 461). The study also found that the accommodations they received were too little or too late and the students did not receive the support of the classroom teachers, school personnel, and other students in accessing and utilizing accommodations and modifications. A large number of students noted social isolation was also common (West, et al., 1993). It is the role of the occupational therapy practitioner to educate the students on their options and rights within the constraints of Section 504, so adult learners do not feel they can no longer participate in educational activities because there are no options for them or it would be too difficult to continue.

An assumption can also be made that the students who do choose to continue or begin an educational experience as adults with a disability may make minimal requests for accommodations when uneducated about the options. This may be especially true if they feel the support is not there or the use of a piece of assistive technology may negatively impact instructors' perception of them or even further isolate them from classmates.

A role change or goal change based on a disability can have a negative impact on psychosocial functioning and decrease clients' social participation, sense of self-efficacy, and overall quality of life. As mastery generally leads to self-esteem, teaching students how to access the most appropriate assistive technology in the classroom environment may considerably impact their ability to flourish socially, culturally, and economically.

It is the occupational therapy practitioner's role to work in a collaborative model with the student to determine the best fit for assistive technology. It may also be the role of the OT to work directly in collaboration with the disability services coordinator on site at the educational institution to advocate for the most appropriate device. It is also possible that a school, required only to provide equipment within reasonable accommodation guidelines (according to Section 104.44 part D of The Rehabilitation Act of 1973, Section 504), will provide a more complex and perhaps more appropriate piece of equipment if it is recommended by a qualified professional such as an occupational therapy practitioner.

Whether or not occupational therapy practitioners are "qualified professionals" has been argued by some universities. One example is the following case. In the case of Guckenberger v. Trustees of Boston University (Mass. 1997), a class action suit was filed by 10 students with disabilities against Boston University and its administration. The students maintained the policy changes implemented by the president of the University regarding the documentation of their learning disabilities, the provision of accommodations, and the possibility of course substitutions resulted in discrimination by denying equal access to the educational opportunities available to students without learning disabilities at the University. Boston University contended that only those individuals who are physicians, clinical psychologists, or licensed psychologists could provide acceptable documentation of a learning disability. Moreover, the University maintained that only those individuals who hold a doctoral degree or higher could have the training and expertise necessary to diagnose a learning disability or appropriately prescribe accommodations in response to available diagnostic information.

While the judge acknowledged the appropriateness of establishing the credentials and expertise of the diagnosticians providing information in support of a student's request for accommodation, she found Boston University had not demonstrated any practical or educational necessity for its exclusive reliance on information provided by its restricted listing of professionals. In a decision released on August 15, 1997, Judge Patty Saris found that some of the actions taken and some of the procedures did result in discrimination against students with disabilities. Jane Jarrow, PhD wrote in her article, Students with Disabilities in Higher Education: Confirmations and Cautions from the Boston University Lawsuit, that the Boston University case highlighted the following principles regarding treatment of students with disabilities in higher education:

> *Institutions have the right to demand documentation of disability and requests for accom-modation be current and complete and such documentation clearly demonstrate the need for requested accommodations in order to assure equal access. However, the standards established for accepting such documentation may not be applied so narrowly or be so restrictive as to become overly burdensome for the student attempting to access appropri-ate accommodations under the law, thus screening out eligible individuals from enjoying their full right to equal access. Institutions also may expect documentation of disability and the need for accommodation be provided by qualified professionals on the basis of testing and assessment, in keeping with established professional guidelines. However, the institution may not discount the documentation submitted from appropriate professionals on the basis of its arbitrary decision to rely solely on the opinions or input of individuals with training and credentials within a more narrowly confined range than those generally accepted within the field. (Jarrow, 2000)*

In accordance with the Assistive Technology Act definition, the OT's role with an adult learner is to evaluate the needs of the person: thinking in terms of how a piece of equipment may best match the individual strengths and weaknesses of the student as well as looking at the environment in which the student will be functioning. One must continually be aware of the context (the insti-tution itself and the student's role in the setting), the activity demands (the course requirements), client factors (the individual's disability status), and how a piece of assistive technology would inter-face with all of these. For example, if an occupational therapy practitioner is working with a client with cerebral palsy who will be living on the campus of a 4-year institution majoring in computer programming, the assistive technology needs will be vastly different from a client with cerebral palsy who is commuting to a 2-year program and earning a degree in nursing.

While David Edyburn (2002) describes 12 models of assistive technology assessments, and there are more beyond, the authors have chosen one model, the HAAT (human, activity, context and assistive technology) model (Figure 5-3) described by Cook and Hussey (2002), for inclusion here. This model flows nicely with the *Framework* (AOTA, 2002) model of evaluation and assessment. In this assessment process, information regarding the consumer is gathered and analyzed so that the most appropriate assistive technology can be recommended and a plan can be developed. The skills and abilities of individuals are measured and the ability of the client to actually use the device is considered. This requires collaboration with other professionals including speech thera-pists, physical therapists, educational counselors, professors, caregivers, and the student. It also requires an understanding of how to gather and interpret relevant data.

A needs assessment is completed including performance areas; in this case it would be edu-cation. The activity demands are listed, tasks that are difficult for the client are described, and contexts in which the activity occurs are included. Previous experience with assistive technology is also viewed as valuable information to assist in that assessment process. This would be most

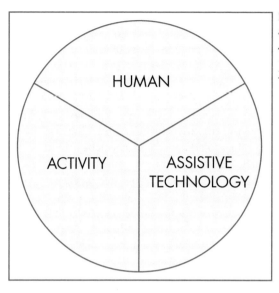

Figure 5-3. The HAAT (Human, Activity, Context and Assistive Technology) Model (adapted from *Assistive Technologies: Principles and Practice (2nd ed.),* Cook and Hussey, p. 41, Copyright 2002, with permission from Elsevier).

pertinent in the case of a student who does not have a new injury or disability status and has been functioning in the classroom setting prior to postsecondary level given certain devices. The occupational therapy practitioner would strive to avoid duplication of items already in the client's possession or those that have been tried without success.

An occupational therapy practitioner or facility can also purchase comprehensive evaluation tools to determine the most appropriate and effective assistive technology for their clients. One such tool, *The Functional Evaluation of Assistive Technology* (FEAT) created by Marshall H. Raskind and Brian R. Bryant is available through PRO-ED Catalogs for a relatively low price. This tool is a systematic, comprehensive, ecologically-based assessment protocol that can be used with students from elementary school though postsecondary education. The scale assists with determination of the most effective assistive technology that will help individuals with learning problems compensate for their difficulties and meet the demands of the school environment. The five scales of the FEAT are:

- *Contextual Matching Inventory*: Provides information about setting-specific demands.

- *Checklist of Strengths and Limitations*: Used to gather data regarding the person-specific characteristics.

- *Checklist of Technological Experiences*: Offers information about the person's past/current use of technology.

- *Technology Characteristics Inventory*: Examines device-specific characteristics such as dependability and product support.

- *Individual-Technology Evaluation Scale*: Used to determine whether the proposed assistive technology application offers legitimate potential for compensatory effectiveness.

There is also a summary and recommendations booklet that is used to summarize the assessment information and plan subsequent progress monitoring. The scales can be completed by various members of an evaluation team or by the occupational therapy practitioner independently. While this tool is primarily for those with learning disabilities, it can be helpful to the occupational therapy practitioner working with a client with multiple physical needs as well.

Once the needs are identified, the student's skills need to be closely evaluated to determine the type of device that is most appropriate. In the case of the adult learner, the assistive technology recommended by the occupational therapy practitioner will be *hard technology*. Hard technologies are readily available components that can be purchased and assembled into assistive technology systems (Cook & Hussey, 2002, p. 6). Hard technologies can include computers, software systems, mouth sticks, adapted switches, and other types of traditional devices.

According to the U.S. Department of Education, National Center for Educational Statistics, 1999-2000 National Postsecondary Student Aid Study (NPSAS: 2000), disability categories for students enrolled in higher education that would be impacted by assistive technology are hearing loss, visual impairment, mobility/orthopedic issues, and cognitive disorders (learning disabilities, dyslexia). Most institutions provide at least one support to students with needs based on Section 504 guidelines. These include alternate exam formats, tutors, readers, note takers, and scribes.

Assistive technology devices are typically listed as textbooks on tape, assisted listening devices, and talking computer programs (Brinckerhoff, Shaw, & McGuire, 1992). The occupational therapy practitioner is qualified to venture beyond these typical devices and guide the student, as well as the disabilities service coordinator, into looking at other devices which will be more appropriate and individualized for the student, and perhaps more economical based on the longevity and variability of usage.

While there are many options, occupational therapy practitioners need to utilize assessment findings to realistically match the device characteristics to the needs of the student and the setting in which it will be used. While voice activated software may seem like the perfect recommendation for a student who cannot use his/her hands to type or write due to an orthopedic or neurological impairment, many factors need to be considered. For example, if the student will be using the program within a classroom, other students may be extremely distracted by the sound. This would not be a good match and most likely will not be accepted or provided by the disability coordinator. Similarly, if the student needs a seating and positioning device, the context plays a large role in decision making. If the student needs to change classrooms frequently, the device must be mobile; however, if access is only required in a lab setting or other particular classroom environment, something more static can be installed. It is also important to remember the institution is not required under Section 504 of the Rehabilitation Act to provide anything that will be used in the client's home, therefore the practicality of the item and the necessity in the educational environment must be at the forefront at all times (Rehabilitation Act Section 504, PL 93-112, 1973, 1977). Figure 5-X presents various assistive technology options in combination with the impairment area it will best address. Most of the examples will be discussed throughout the chapter.

It is also important to understand that there are options for accessibility in computers which generally come installed with basic options for accessibility. Located in the Control Panel window of most computers (Figure 5-4), there are a variety of options that may assist students with independence without having to purchase additional technology. In the Accessibility Option (Figure 5-5), there are choices for applying "sticky keys," which would mean the student does not have to hold down the shift key and a letter simultaneously if he or she can only use one hand, or one digit, for typing. Other options include a visual marker when the computer makes a sound and the ability to control the contrast of the screen as well as the blink rate and width of the cursor. The keyboard can also be set to not repeat a letter even if it is held down for a long period of time. This feature may be beneficial for those with motor control issues and can prevent many typing errors. Another icon, Keyboard Options, also allows the user to change the properties of the keyboard to allow for delays and can assist with incoordination difficulties. In addition, the icon Mouse Properties allows users to vary the speed of the mouse or touch pad as well as vary the pointer size and speed. Many other options are available within this window and settings can be varied easily depending on the student's preferences. For more information on the accessibility options available, visit: http://www.microsoft.com/windowsxp/using/accessibility/default.mspx.

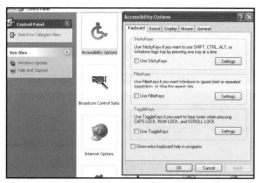

Figure 5-4. Microsoft Control Panel window.

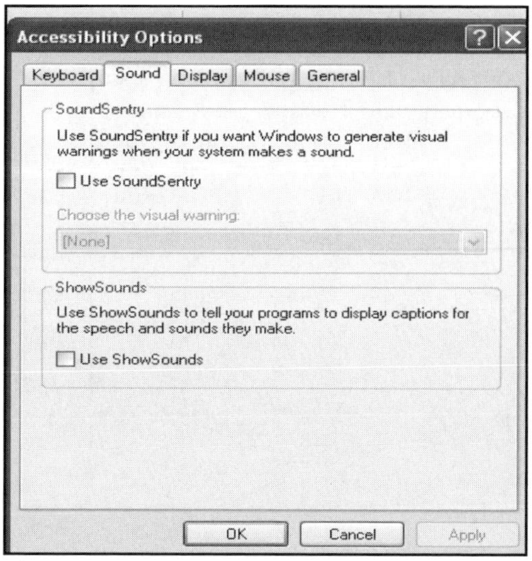

Figure 5-5. Accessibility options window on the Microsoft Control Panel.

Lastly, many computers have a text-to-speech option built into their systems. Once the software is loaded (Windows Office XP has it as an available download), the computer will take users through a 15-minute training that will allow them to choose a computer voice to "read" the text aloud. A set of earphones can be plugged into the computer to avoid distraction in the classroom. This option will work well with CD versions of textbooks that can be ordered, if available, by contacting publishers of required texts. Students can then have access to reading assignments for homework and other reading assignments without having to purchase special equipment.

As each computer model and brand varies in the options available, it is important to review the available programs on each student's individual system. At times, separate software packages may need to be ordered through an assistive technology catalog (see Appendix A) or through the Microsoft Web site, which supports those with disabilities: http://www.microsoft.com/enable.

INTERVENTION FOR ORTHOPEDIC/NEUROMUSCULAR MOBILITY-RELATED FUNCTIONS THAT IMPACT EDUCATION

Clients may be seen in occupational therapy for a variety of movement-related issues (Figure 5-6). Certainly, clients with movement issues wishing to participate in postsecondary education or adult education programs may face barriers depending on their specific issues. Orthopedic, neuromuscular, and movement-related functions are a body function client factor that includes functions of joints and bones, muscle functions, and movement functions (AOTA, 2002). Strategies related to UE and LE orthopedic and neuromuscular issues will be discussed from an adaptation/compensation perspective including environmental modification, adaptive techniques, and adaptive equipment/assistive technology. See Chapter 2 for remediation and maintenance strategies. Impairments commonly seen with clients who have these types of physical disabilities include limited mobility and joint range of motion (ROM), limited strength, decreased coordination, and decreased or fluctuating endurance.

Figure 5-6. Components of performance skills/client factors related to education (adapted from American Occupational Therapy Association. [2002]. Occupational therapy practice framework. *American Journal of Occupational Therapy*, 56(6), 609-639).

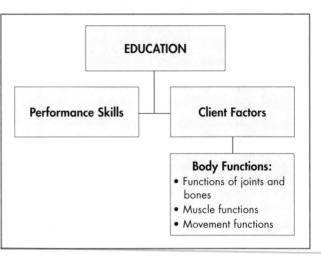

Modes of injury for these types of limitations include:

- Trauma: Fractures, soft tissue damage, spinal cord injury, etc.

- Acquired Brain Injury (ABI): Neurological insult affecting tone and/or strength, traumatic brain injury (TBI), cerebrovascular accident (CVA), tumors, intracranial bleed, arteriovenous malformation, etc.

- Pathology: Degenerative diseases such as multiple sclerosis, Guillain-Barré Syndrome, amyotrophic lateral sclerosis, etc.

- Prolonged illness with debility: Multitrauma, transplantations, chronic obstructive pulmonary disease, respiratory arrest, etc.

Environmental modifications for individuals with physical disabilities pursuing postsecondary education will most likely be achieved through the school's compliance with the ADA *Guidelines for Accessible Design*. However, in the classroom it may be necessary to request several accommodations depending on the physical disability, such as:

- A personal assistant or aide to get settled in the classroom, take notes, assist with mobility within the classroom as required by the class, etc.

- Classroom furniture may need to be modified for different heights or easier access.

- Temperature may cause fatigue and may need to be addressed if the environment is too cold or hot.

- Assistive technology devices may be required.

In conjunction with environmental modifications, occupational therapy practitioners should include adaptive techniques during intervention such as energy conservation techniques. Energy conservation techniques, which involve educating clients regarding ways to preserve energy throughout their day, will be especially important for individuals with physical disabilities because of the extra demands placed on the body. Although each case will need to be addressed individually depending on the physical disability and the type of educational activity the client has chosen to participate in, the following recommendations may be adapted as appropriate and provided to the client:

- Schedule classes during a time that is best for your energy level. If possible, avoid times of day that will require extra travel time because of traffic.

- If necessary, use a wheelchair to ensure that you will be able to make it through a class or classes. A personal assistant or aide may be requested to assist with propelling the wheelchair to and from parking lots and classes if a manual chair is not available.

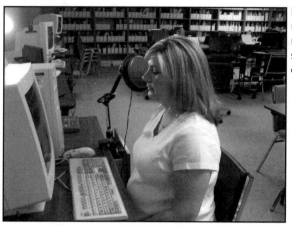

Figure 5-7. The client's inability to use her upper extremities for keyboarding is corrected through the use of a head activated switch that controls the commands on the computer.

- Schedule classes with a break in between to allow a rest period, which may include eating or drinking to help restore your energy level. Discuss the possibility for short breaks with teachers/professors to enhance your functional performance throughout the length of the class.

- Take the elevator whenever possible.

- If possible, remain seated during all class activities.

- Limit the amount of books and other items you carry with you. Whenever possible, attach backpacks to wheelchairs or use backpacks on wheels. Requesting an assistant or aide to assist with transporting necessary materials from the car or to and from class is an accommodation that can be discussed with the office for students with disabilities.

- Instead of writing notes in class, use a tape recorder. Notes can be translated into written copies during a less energy-consuming time after class.

- Plan ahead. Use date books and calendars in conjunction with course syllabi and outlines to plan for assignments, tests, and other activities that will add to the amount of work in a given day/week/month.

Different types of adaptive equipment may be helpful for individuals with physical disabilities. For example, an individual with decreased strength, limited ROM, or abnormal tone may require assistance with holding a textbook and turning the pages of the book. Several types of book holders are available through adaptive equipment catalogs. In addition, modifications for turning pages in the book may be accomplished through adaptive equipment such as a mouthstick with friction tip end, electric page turner, and a stick placed in a universal cuff. Writing may also be an issue for individuals with UE physical disabilities. Some examples of adaptive equipment that can be used include a slip-on writing aid; an easy glide writer, which requires the arm rather than finger to operate; and one-handed writing boards, which secures paper for individuals who are only able to use one of their UEs.

The technology for those with limited UE movement use, either from a limited joint ROM, strength, or endurance, is expanding rapidly. Voice recognition technology, a variety of different mice, and switch accesses are the most readily available of the options for the student who cannot access a computer through traditional methods. Voice recognition software is sold in almost every catalog and is made for a variety of different programs and applications. Computer mice come in a variety of shapes and sizes and can be purchased in most retail stores, as well as in catalogs specifically designed for those with disabilities. Switch options range from a simple head activated button (Figure 5-7) to a switch that can detect even the slightest of muscle movements in any part of the body. These switches can be used to highlight letters and words to type and are often used

Figure 5-8. Relation of cognition to education (adapted from American Occupational Therapy Association. [2002]. Occupational therapy practice framework. *American Journal of Occupational Therapy,* 56(6), 609-639).

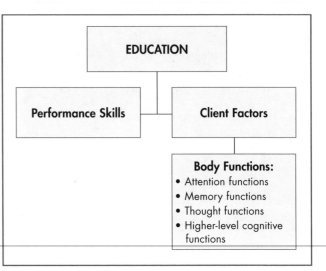

in conjunction with software that will begin to recognize common words and complete them for the student with limited key strokes or switch clicks. As technology continues to advance, so do the tools of the trade for those with movement impairments. Access is sometimes only limited by one's imagination and ability to create.

INTERVENTIONS FOR COGNITIVE IMPAIRMENTS THAT IMPACT EDUCATION

Clients who are being seen by occupational therapy and have identified areas of concern in cognition may have accessibility issues in the classroom related to the actual task of learning (Figure 5-8). Cognitive impairments may be the result of an ABI or a degenerative disease such as:

- CVA
- TBI
- Tumors
- Intracranial bleeds
- Seizure disorders
- Developmental delays
- Brain chemistry imbalances
- Multiple sclerosis
- Parkinson's disease
- Alzheimer's disease

Typically, occupational therapy practitioners working with adults who need assistance with returning to or beginning a postsecondary education program because of cognitive impairments will have had some life-changing event such as one of the acquired or progressive diseases listed. According to the *Framework* (AOTA, 2002), cognitive function is a body function client factor and is listed under the category of mental functions. Specific mental functions related to cognitive impairments include:

- Attention functions: Sustained attention and divided attention.

- Memory functions: Retrospective memory and prospective memory.

- Thought functions: Recognition, categorization, generalization, awareness of reality, logical/coherent thought, and appropriate thought content.

- Higher-level cognitive functions: Judgment, concept formation, time management, problem solving, and decision making.

If a client has a deficit in one or more of the areas listed above, intervention will be determined based on the client's goals and rehabilitation potential. Pursuit of postsecondary education with a documented deficit in mental function will require various intervention approaches including remediation, adaptation/compensation, and maintenance techniques. While cognitive remediation is discussed here as it relates to education, further information regarding cognitive remediation in general can be found in Chapter 2.

Attention Functions

Attention functions include both sustained attention and divided attention. Sustained attention is necessary to complete cognitively planned activities (Duchek & Abreu, 1997). One example is reading a chapter in a textbook. In order to complete the task, individuals must focus on the activity of reading. Inability to ignore distractions can interfere with a client's ability to sustain his/her attention on a task. Divided attention is the ability to focus on more than one activity or task at one time (Yakil & Hoffman, 2004). An example is the ability to listen to a lecture and take notes at the same time. Intervention for attention may include one or more of the following methods: remediation, adaptation/compensation, and maintenance.

When attempting to remediate either sustained or divided attention, the initial goal of intervention will focus on the development of process skills. Process skills will include the establishment of an environment that will allow clients to attend to activities for the longest amount of time without distraction. Graded intervention for complexity, length of time, and amount of environmental distractions is necessary. As clients demonstrate improvement, process skills will progress to the establishment of attending to more complicated tasks in more distracting environments, and for greater lengths of time. The occupational therapy practitioner should provide feedback and rewards for improved performance. The goal is to progress the client's performance in attention so he/she can fully attend to classroom activities and homework assignments as required by the educational environment.

If attention does not improve through remediation activities, the occupational therapy practitioner may need to adapt the task or educate the client in compensatory techniques. Many of the adaptations will be viewed as accommodations, which must be discussed with the disabilities coordinator at the school. Modifications may be made to the context, activity demands, or performance patterns of the task. Adaptations and compensatory techniques may include, but are not limited to:

1. Use of a tape recorder to record lectures, which can be listened to in a less distracting environment once the class is over.

2. Instruct the student to sit in the front of classrooms, thus eliminating as many distractions as possible.

3. Allow the student to use a note taker in the classroom.

4. Ask the instructor to:
   a. Provide notes or information regarding activities that will be required during the class ahead of time to allow the student time to prepare.
   b. Accept alternative forms of information sharing, such as taped instead of oral reports.

    c. Allow the student to submit in-class assignments a day or two after the class.

    d. Break work into smaller amounts or smaller work intervals.

    e. Have the student work with a partner who will instruct him/her to stay on task.

    f. Provide instructions or explanations in small steps.

Maintaining attention performance will be different for all individuals. In order for individuals with attention deficits to have continued success in postsecondary school environments, they will need to work with the disabilities coordinator at the school and each instructor for each and every class they choose to enroll in. As accommodations will be different in each class and as each instructor will have a different level of understanding as to how to support an individual's requested accommodations, ongoing dialogue will be necessary for success and maintenance.

Memory Functions

Memory functions include both retrospective memory and prospective memory. Retrospective memory is memory for the content of the intended action, or remembering what to remember (Duchek & Abreu, 1997). A prospective memory is the ability to remember to do things at appropriate times, or simply stated, the ability to remember to remember (Duchek & Abreu, 1997). An example of retrospective memory is remembering instructions given in class for a particular assignment. Prospective memory would be remembering to record the due date of the assignment in an assignment date book so you don't forget to complete and submit the assignment when it is due.

Studies examining memory remediation interventions have been inconsistent (Thornton, 2000; Carney, Chestnut, Maynard, Mann, Patterson, & Helfand, 1999). In addition, the level of memory impairment will determine how likely it is that the specific strategies will work (Strangman, O'Neil-Pirozzi, Burke, et al., 2005) with some clients the interventions strategies suggested may prove successful (2005). Remediation and compensation/adaptation strategies are discussed together as separation of the two types of interventions proves to be difficult with this type of impairment. In general, intervention does not focus on restoring memory, but providing functional and useful strategies to reduce the impact of the memory impairment on functioning and independence. However, many of the adaptation/compensation techniques employ strategies that may eventually lead to remediation.

Internal and external memory strategies focus on improving the client's ability to encode, store, and retrieve information. Internal memory aids require individuals to use mnemonic strategies such as visual imagery, verbalization, association, categorization, rhyming, and storytelling, to name a few. The difficulty most clients encounter when using mnemonic strategies is remembering to remember them. These strategies require clients to plan ahead in order to use them. External memory strategies may include aids used by clients to assist with memory or cuing by another individual. Some clients will require an external cue to remember to use an external aid, which may include calendars, journals, planners, timelines, alarm clocks or other types of alarms, labels throughout the environment, memory wallets, and memory books. Instructions for memory books and wallets are listed below. In addition, assistive technology now exists that can be used as external memory aids. See Table 5-1 for a list of memory strategies for intervention.

- Memory Wallets and Books (Burgeouis, 1992)
  - Memory Wallet
    - Materials: Index cards, contact paper, O-Ring
    - Content: Pictures, text, and phrases to aid memory
    - Headings may include: Daily schedule, directions to class, my classes, my teachers, etc.
  - Memory Books
    - Materials: Three-ring binder, heavy duty paper, page protectors or contact paper, dividers

Table 5-1

MEMORY STRATEGIES

Strategy	Purpose
Watch alarms	Can be set to alarm at specified time. Models also available with talking feature, which allows a command to be spoken at a specific time. Example: "it is time to leave for school now."
Electronic planners	Acts as a portable calendar with the ability to alarm at set times to aid memory.
Mini recorders (Figure 5-9)	Records audible feedback. Many can be worn around the neck to aid in remembering to use device. Students can immediately record important information they need to remember.
Cassette recorders	Can record instructions given in class to assist in retrieval of information at a later time.
Memory wallets and books	External cue which contains pictures, text, and phrases to aid memory such as daily schedules, directions and other important information.
Labeling	Labels can be placed throughout the environment to serve as an external cue for important information. Example: Note on door to exterior of house that states "Remember your book for class."
Mnemonic strategies (visual imagery, verbalization, association, categorization, rhyming, storytelling)	Mnemonic strategies are intended to be used to enhance recall. Example: Student's biology science class is on the fifth floor; teach the student to think science starts with s, and s looks like the number 5.
Calendars/journals	Calendars and journals are used to record all important information and must be used constantly throughout the day as an external cue for remembering important information.

○ Content: Pictures, text, phrases to aid memory

○ Divided sections may include: Home, school, special events

As memory demands fluctuate, intervention approaches may need to be modified to allow individuals to preserve performance. This will be true with individuals attending postsecondary education activities. Classes, teachers, demands, schedules, and content will change often. Maintenance of memory will primarily include revision of environmental conditions to meet the client's specific and current needs. They may include reorganizing the client's environment, including removing and reorganizing clutter, identification of specific areas for needed items, and labeling. In addition, external cues such as visible calendars and environmental signs will need constant maintenance. In order to ensure the greatest success, clients, in conjunction with the occupational therapy practitioner or disabilities coordinator, must re-examine strategies used and determine changes that will encourage ongoing successful memory performance.

Figure 5-9. The client uses a mini recorder to help with remembering assignments and other important information throughout the day.

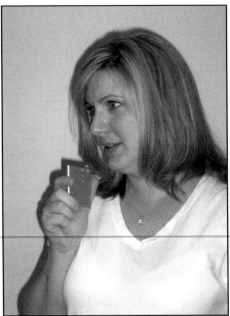

Thought Functions

Thought functions include recognition, categorization, generalization, awareness of reality, logical/coherent thought, and appropriate thought content (AOTA, 2002). Deficits in thought functions are often seen immediately following an accident or traumatic health event. As the mental state clears, individuals will often display spontaneous improvements in these basic cognitive functions. Individuals who continue to display limitations in thought functions beyond the time frame in which these deficits are commonly seen will rarely have the cognitive ability to identify individual goals. Cognitive deficits in thought functions will limit participation in postsecondary education and therefore will not be discussed in this chapter.

Higher-Level Cognitive Functions

Higher-level cognitive functions include judgment, concept formation, time management, problem solving, and decision making (AOTA, 2002). Please see Chapter 2 for intervention related to judgment, concept formation, problem solving, and decision making. Higher-level cognitive functions are essential skills for anyone participating in a learning environment. Strategies related to the functions of time management will be discussed from an adaptation/compensation perspective in this chapter. See Chapter 2 for remediation and maintenance intervention strategies.

Strategies related to time management can be discussed in occupational therapy intervention. However, it will be necessary to discuss many of the proposed strategies with the disabilities coordinator for the school as well as the specific instructor for the class or course.

The most common way to compensate for time management issues is through the use of schedules. Individuals may need to develop different types of schedules including daily, weekly, and monthly. Depending on the severity of the impairment, daily schedules can be broken down into 15-minute increments to ensure success. Planners are available in several formats and are easy to incorporate into a daily routine. In addition, the following strategies may also prove successful for individuals with time management impairments:

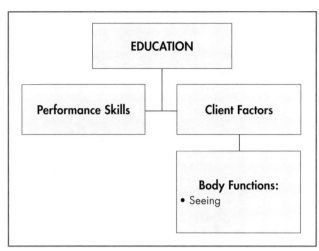

Figure 5-10. Relationship of vision to education (adapted from American Occupational Therapy Association. [2002]. Occupational therapy practice framework. *American Journal of Occupational Therapy*, 56(6), 609-639).

- Ask the student to work with a class partner who will cue him/her to stay on task.
- Ask the instructor to assist student in the following ways:
  - ➤ Setting time goals for each task.
  - ➤ Knowing what to expect in class by providing a daily class outline.
  - ➤ Providing checklists with timeframes for assignments.
  - ➤ Using a timer in class to cue student regarding remaining time for a task or assignment.

Clients can improve time management by setting a schedule ahead of time and then evaluating the effectiveness of the schedule at the end of the day or week. Evaluative methods will include determining tasks that were not accounted for in the schedule, tasks that took more or less time than scheduled, and how well the individuals followed the schedule or the ability of the schedule to assist with overall time management.

INTERVENTION FOR VISUAL IMPAIRMENTS THAT IMPACT EDUCATION

Clients who are being seen by occupational therapy and have identified areas of concern with their vision may have accessibility issues in the classroom (Figure 5-10). According to the *Framework*, seeing functions as a body function client factor and is listed under the category of sensory functions and pain (AOTA, 2002). Seeing functions include visual acuity and visual field functions. *Visual acuity* is the ability of the eyes to see objects clearly and distinctly. Acuity is typically measured on the Snellen eye chart where normal vision is said to be 20/20. The visual field is the area one sees when looking at the environment. There are two types of visual fields: central and peripheral. The central field of vision is used for clear and focused vision including such activities as reading, while the peripheral field of vision is not as clear but aids with motion detection and spatial orientation. Anyone with vision worse than 20/200 that cannot be improved with corrective lenses is considered legally blind (American Foundation for the Blind, 2005). In addition, people with a visual field of less than 20 degrees diameter (10 degrees radius) are also considered legally blind (2005). Approximately 10 percent of those deemed legally blind, by any measure, are actually sightless (2005). The remainder have some vision, from light perception alone to relatively good acuity. Those who are not legally blind, but nonetheless have serious visual impairments, possess low vision. Low vision is a general term used to describe lowered visual acuity, and a specific legal term in Canada and the U.S. used to designate someone with vision of 20/70 or less in the better eye with correction (Watson, 2001).

Figure 5-11. The client uses a video magnifier to increase the size of the text in a book she is reading for an assignment.

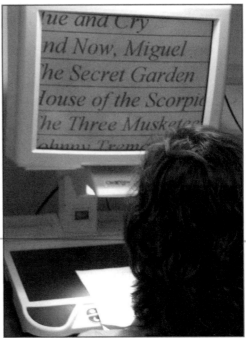

Occupational therapy intervention for individuals with visual acuity and visual field deficits will not retrain the eye to see better. Therefore, intervention strategies will focus on adaptation and compensation. Through adaptation and compensatory strategies, clients may improve their ability to see and for clients with total blindness, strategies are available to aid in functional performance. Numerous assistive technology devices are available to individuals with low vision. Many catalogs are specifically devoted to visually impaired individuals and options for students range in price and accessibility depending on the needs of the consumer. Refer to Appendix A for sample catalogs.

Software to enlarge electronic information, as well as to read information found online aloud, can be extremely helpful to the student who does most work either on line or simply on the computer. In addition, this type of software may also aid students in completing home assignments. One example of a magnification software program is ZoomText (Ai Squared, Manchester Center, VT), a computer software package that can increase text on the computer screen from 2x to 16x magnification. In addition, students may benefit from color coded keyboards, calculators, etc., and computer software that has speech recognition capabilities.

For accessing printed material, one of the most common tools is a video magnifier (Figure 5-11). This piece of equipment lacks portability and is quite expensive but can be extremely beneficial to individuals who need it. Most are large computer screens (14 inches or larger) with a magnification component that scans books and other items and enlarges them on the screen. Some can be focused on a variety of different surfaces, including a white board or other vertical writing surfaces utilized by a teacher in the classroom. A more portable and less expensive option is a handheld camera, which can be purchased directly from a catalog and connected to any television screen for viewing. For those who have less vision or who cannot access information by sight at all, there are hardware and software products that are capable of scanning written work and read the material aloud to the student. Many of these can be connected to headphones to avoid distraction in a classroom. Braille options are numerous as well and can be found in almost every assistive technology catalog.

For note-taking or other written work, a simple voice dictation system can be utilized as well as other speech recognition systems that will actually type words as the student speaks. For those requiring Braille, printers, note-takers, and refreshable Braille display boards are available and easily purchased through a variety of catalogs. In combination with the assistive technology examples listed, students with low vision may benefit from the following accommodations (as previously discussed, many accommodations will need to be discussed with the disabilities coordinator for the school and/or with the specific course instructor):

- Request an assistant in the classroom to read and explain items presented in visual format.
- Use an adjustable lamp for increased lighting.
- Wear a brimmed cap to reduce visual glare.
- Use magnification devices.
- Use a typoscope (a sheet of black cardboard or plastic with a cut-out the size of a line of print).
- Use large type text when available or large print books.
- Use the book on tape version of the class text (audio books).
- Use yellow acetate overlays and yellow filters on documents to provide enhanced contrast and decreased glare.
- Ask the instructor to:
  - Allow for extra time when vision is required for a classroom activity.
  - Allow student to sit close to materials that must be viewed.
  - Allow student to seek out the best position in the classroom with regards to the light source.

In combination with the assistive technology discussed, students with no vision or total blindness who will benefit from only a few of the accommodations listed for students with low vision may use the following adaptations to aid in functional performance in the educational environment:

- Use of Braille texts.
- Provide an assistant in the classroom to read and explain items presented in visual format.
- Use of a brailler or slate and stylus to take notes in class.
- Use of a tape recorder to take notes in class.
- Use of voice recognition computer software.
- Use of Braille keyboard labels.
- Use of text-to-speech programs.

Currently, new legislation exists that will allow primary and secondary students who are blind, or who have print disabilities, to access printed instructional materials in a streamlined fashion. This will be achieved through the Instructional Materials Accessibility Act (H.R. 1350). This act creates a system for acquiring and distributing publishers' electronic files of textbooks and other instructional materials, so these materials can be made available in Braille, synthesized speech, digital text, digital audio, or large print.

Each state educational agency receiving federal financial assistance under the IDEA will be required to develop and implement a written statewide plan to ensure printed instructional materials required for classroom use in elementary and secondary schools are made available in specialized formats to individuals who are blind or have other print disabilities at the same time that such materials are provided to individuals without such disabilities (Sollenberger, 2005).

Figure 5-12. Relationship of hearing to education (adapted from American Occupational Therapy Association. [2002]. Occupational therapy practice framework. *American Journal of Occupational Therapy, 56*(6), 609-639).

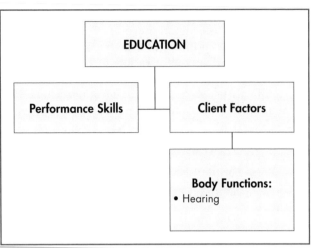

There is no such provision at this time for postsecondary students, but options do exist. For Braille and electronic texts, The American Printing House for the Blind (APH) offers accessible instructional materials and supplies can be purchased. The Louis Database of Accessible Formats for people who are blind or visually impaired, housed at the APH, acts as a centralized clearinghouse of over 145,000 titles in accessible formats produced by over 200 agencies.

Finally, Recording for the Blind and Dyslexic (RFB&D) is a useful resource for taped books. RFB&D's library contains more than 98,000 titles in a broad variety of subjects including literature, history, math, and the sciences. They serve all academic levels, including postsecondary, postgraduate, and professional. For more information, visit www.rfbd.org.

INTERVENTION FOR HEARING IMPAIRMENTS THAT IMPACT EDUCATION

Occupational therapy practitioners will most likely work with individuals who have age-related hearing loss, also known as *presbycusis* (Figure 5-12). According to the *Framework*, hearing function is a body function client factor and is listed under the category of sensory functions and pain (AOTA, 2002). Hearing function is defined as the response to sound and this function is assessed in terms of its presence or absence and its effect on engaging in occupations and in daily life activities. Many older adults choose to participate in various types of postsecondary educational activities including attending classes at a college, university, or an adult education program. If hearing loss is a functional barrier, occupational therapy practitioners can assist by suggesting accommodations for improved performance (AOTA, 2002). However, audiologists and other qualified professionals should be consulted to assist with fitting clients with hearing aid devices that will provide the most hearing possible.

Once clients have been evaluated for and properly fit with a hearing device, the occupational therapy practitioner can focus on intervention, which will improve function within the limitation of the client's ability to hear in the educational setting. As with previous disabilities discussed, occupational therapy intervention will not retrain the ear to hear better; therefore, intervention strategies will focus on adaptation and compensation.

For those students who present with a hearing loss, amplified hearing and captioning devices are available in addition to the traditional methods of hiring notetakers and providing lectures

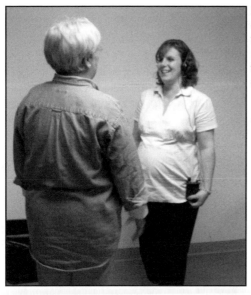

Figure 5-13. Pocket Talker amplification system. This client is able to converse with her professor through the use of the amplification system she wears. The microphone located on the unit is attached to her trousers and amplifies the professor's voice, which the client hears through the headphones she is wearing.

in written format. Amplification systems are extremely beneficial to individuals who have had a mild to moderate hearing loss and can be ordered directly out of a catalog. They vary in price and complexity depending on the needs of the client and the environment in which they will be utilized. Most types of systems are worn individually (generally as headphones) and have a microphone that amplifies the speaker and diminishes the background noise; they are easily portable from one location to another and are often referred to as a Pocket Talker (Williams Sound, Eden Prairie, MN) (Figure 5-13). A personal FM educational system is also an option. With this piece of wireless equipment, the teacher wears the transmitter and microphone and students use a portable receiver. This system allows numerous students to utilize the technology and is significantly more expensive. Table 5-2 presents additional information and pricing.

If the client has lost all hearing, captioning, Communication Access Realtime Translation or (CART), can also be utilized. This is the instantaneous translation of the spoken word into English text using a stenotype machine, notebook computer, and real-time software, and it displays the text on a laptop computer for individuals or on a larger monitor for larger groups. Personal CART service is often provided in classroom settings for students who are hearing impaired. The text displayed includes identification of the speaker (when known), the dialogue, and (where possible) a description of sounds. In some cases, schools have resisted provision of CART services due to expense, but precedents have been set using ADA legislation and most higher education institutions have been required to provide this service to a student in need regardless of the cost.

In combination with the assistive technology options available for individuals with hearing loss, the following compensatory strategies may assist in the functional performance of students with hearing impairments in the educational environment:

- Use of a sign language interpreter.
- Holding classes in rooms that are acoustically engineered to decrease background noise or rooms with carpeting and/or drapes that will reduce the amount of echoing.
- Asking the instructor to:
  - Use a microphone or amplifier.
  - Provide a written copy of lectures and oral directions presented in class.
  - Provide visual cues whenever possible (flashing lights or visible timers).

Table 5-2

ADAPTIVE TECHNOLOGIES

The following devices are all available as standard order catalog items. Pricing is based on EnableMart (Vancouver, WA), which is just one option for purchasing equipment. See Appendix A for more information on ordering through EnableMart and for other catalog options.

Deficit Area	Possible Assistive Technology	Description	Cost*
Orthopedic/ neuromuscular impairments	Ribbon Switch	Activated by bending the soft handle in any direction with head, arm, or hand	$
	OnScreen	Places keyboard on screen for mouse access for those who cannot look down at keyboard and back up to screen (also addresses diminished focus/saccade issues)	$
	Soothsayer Word Prediction	Software that helps type faster and more accurately based on word prediction technology	$
	Big button switches	Alternate input device to computer for those who are unable to operate a mouse	$
	Programmable Foot Switch	Three button keyboard/mouse accessed by one foot or both feet	$
	Touch Window	Eliminates the use of a mouse and allows user touch access to select and move objects on screen	$$
	SCATIR Switch	Self-Calibrating Auditory Tone Infrared Switch works directly or indirectly with eye-blink, eyebrow movement, or facial movement and has auditory feedback component	$$$
	Tracker One	Head pointing device operating from USB port in computer	$$$$
	Quick Glance System	Users place mouse pointer anywhere on screen by looking at desired location; clicking done with eye blink	$$$$
Hearing Loss	Pocket Talker Pro	Personal Amplification System with headphones	$
	Personal FM Educational System	Portable wireless listening system where the teacher wears transmitter and microphone and each student wears earphones	$$$
	Closed Captioning System	Captioning system that requires a stenographer or other word detection software and a screen for user to read what is being stated	$$$$

*$: less than $200.00 $$: $200.00-$400.00 $$$: $450.00-$650.00 $$$$: >$700.00

continued

Table 5-2, continued

ADAPTIVE TECHNOLOGIES

Deficit Area	Possible Assistive Technology	Description	Cost*
Visual Deficit	Scan & Read (Lite & Pro)	Reads text in up to 12 languages and magnifies text up to 400%	$
	Gh Player™ 2.0	Speaks written words in both Talking Book and TXT format	$
	4-Track Players	Handheld cassette player for recording voice	$
	ZoomText software	Enlarges text and has capability to read it aloud	$$
	Max Portable Video Magnifier	Mobile, connects to television, up to 30X in black and white	$$
	Duxbury Braille Translator	Converts regular print to Braille in an automated format	$$$
	Reliant Video Magnifier	Static magnification system with monitor	$$$$

*$: less than $200.00 $$: $200.00-$400.00 $$$: $450.00-$650.00 $$$$: >$700.00

> ➤ Arrange class discussions in a circle or semi-circle set up so the individual can view each person who is talking.
> ➤ Stand directly in front of the individual when lecturing or provide instructions to allow for lip reading.
> ➤ Eliminate background noise by keeping classroom doors and windows shut.

DISTANCE LEARNING ACCESSIBILITY

Distance learning is an option for participating in educational programs off-campus via cable television, Internet, satellite classes, videotapes, correspondence courses, or other means. Between 1995 and 1997, the percentage of 2- and 4-year degree-granting institutions offering distance education courses rose from 33% to 44% and the number of courses offered just about doubled (National Center for Education Statistics, 2003b). Distance learning may be a viable alternative to traditional classroom methods of learning for individuals who are homebound or who, because of physical or other limitations, choose not to attend on-site classes. Although distance learning may be a wonderful alternative for many because it provides increased access related to distance and time, it may not be completely accessible for students with disabilities. In 1996, the United States Department of Justice clarified the ADA Act on access to the Internet for individuals with disabilities: "Covered entities which use the Internet for communications regarding their programs, goods, or services must be prepared to offer those communications through accessible means as well" (ADA Accessibility, 1996). Assistive technology can be applied to the distance learning model to aid access for students with physical disabilities.

Students with visual disabilities may need a computer with screen reader software and a speech synthesizer which will read the text which appears in the distance learning course. Printed materials and other educational aids provided by the instructor to aid in the online class may pose a barrier to these students. Accommodations may include audiotapes, Braille printouts, and tactile drawings (Burgstahler, 2000). For students with hearing impairments, necessary accommodations may include text captioning or transcription for audio output. Distance learning programs also often use real-time chat communications to aid class discussion. This type of communication will be difficult for students whose physical limitations prevent the rapid response time often required in these types of "discussions." Other forms of discussion, such as e-mail or discussion boards, will be a better alternative and will accommodate most accessibility issues.

For students with UE physical limitations, it will most likely be necessary for the computer to be adapted with assistive technology devices such as the ones discussed earlier. Keyboard access and cursor control access may be common computer barriers for individuals with UE physical disabilities and are often rectified with the use of text-to-speech software programs. When distance learning courses are designed to meet the needs of all types of learners, they can serve as wonderful opportunities for individuals with disabilities (Burgstahler, 2001).

FUNDING

Funding for the recommended device will vary based on a variety of factors, including the Section 504 disability coordinator's discretion at the individual institution but, as stated above, the recommendation of a qualified professional is highly regarded and can impact the receipt of equipment for clients. Funding sources beyond the institution include, but are not limited to, the following (Table 5-3 provides a listing of more funding options):

- **Personal funds**, especially in cases where the device will be utilized in the home more than in the school.
- **Health insurance**, which will, in most cases, cover the occupational therapy assessment and possibly the training involved in utilizing the equipment.
- **Programs for the developmentally disabled**, which will vary from state to state.
- **Vocational rehabilitation**, which is funded through the federal government and includes assistive technology to allow individuals to attain maximum potential in the workplace.
- **The Plan for Achieving Self-Sufficiency (PASS)**, which is funded through the Social Security Administration and allows individuals to put aside income to find equipment or services that will assist them in achieving vocational objectives (Cook & Hussey, 2002).

It is the responsibility of each occupational therapy practitioner to become familiar with the resources in the community in which they work as well as to develop relationships with the personnel in each agency. Connecting clients to resources is an important aspect of the OT's role with the adult student. There are many methods of identifying resources for clients. Asking team members, supervisors, and other individuals in the field of education and training of adults with disabilities, are all appropriate methods of acquiring information on funding for assistive technology. Identifying local independent living centers in the area through www.ilru.org can provide the practitioner with a wealth of resources. Another method of finding funding is to perform a web search for your area in relationship to assistive technology. In Rhode Island, for example, Central Information and Resource Center is the lead agency for the Assistive Technology Access Partnership (ATAP), which is designed as a "statewide partnership of organizations and agencies, each with a targeted assistive technology focus, working together providing information and improving access to assistive technology for individuals with disabilities" (http://www.atap.ri.gov). Such a resource can be extremely beneficial to clients and practitioners as well.

Table 5-3

FUNDING OPTIONS FOR ASSISTIVE TECHNOLOGY

Public Programs

Medicare

Medicaid

Required and optional services

Intermediate care facilities for persons who are mentally retarded (ICFs/MR)

Early and periodic screening, diagnosis, and treatment (EPSDT)

Home and community-based (HCB) waivers

Community-supported living arrangements

Maternal and Child Health

Maternal and child health block grant to states

Children with special health care needs

Special projects of regional and national significance (SPRANS)

Education

Individuals with Disabilities Education Act (IDEA) state grants (Part B)

IDEA programs for infants and toddlers with disabilities and their families (Part H)

State-operated programs

Vocational education

Head Start

Vocational Rehabilitation

State grants

Supported employment

Independent living, Parts A, B, & C

Social Security Benefits

Title II: Social Security Disability Insurance (SSDI)

Title XVI: Supplemental Security Income (SSI)

Work incentive programs

Developmental Disability Programs

Department of Veterans Affairs Programs

Older Americans Act Programs

Alternative Financing

Revolving Loan Funds

Lending library

Discount program

Low-interest loans

Private foundations

Service clubs

Special state appropriations

State bond issues

Employee Accommodations Program

Equipment Loan Program

Corporate-sponsored loans

Charitable organizations

US Tax Code

Medical care expense deduction

Business deductions

Employee business deductions

Americans with Disabilities Act (ADA) credit for small business loans

Credit for architectural and transportation barrier removal

Targeted jobs tax credit

Charitable contributions deduction

Private Health Insurance

Health insurance

Worker's compensation

Casualty insurance

Disability insurance

Civil Rights

ADA

Rehabilitation Act, Section 504

Universal Access

Rehabilitation Act, Section 508

Decoder Circuitry Act

Telecommunications

Telecommunications for the Disabled Act of 1982

Telecommunications Accessibility Enhancement Act of 1988

The Alliance for Technology Access (ATA) is a network of community-based resource centers, developers, vendors, and associates dedicated to providing information and support services to children and adults with disabilities, and increasing their use of standard, assistive, and information technologies. ATA members are nationwide and can be found at www.ataccess.org.

In addition, for information specifically related to postsecondary education and those with disabilities, the Association for Higher Education and Disability (AHEAD) can be found at http://www.ahead.org and contains links regarding assistive technology as well as many other adult student options. Disabled Student Service Organizations can also be a valuable source of information on assistive technology options and funding.

CASE EXAMPLE OF ON-CAMPUS SUPPORT

As a model of emerging practice, an OT working at Edinboro University in Pennsylvania is part of a team of professionals that evaluates and coordinates services for students with disabilities directly on campus. According to Michaels (2004), Edinboro University's disability service program began in 1974 and has expanded considerably since that time. Initially, the role of the OT was established to teach students the life skills they needed to succeed in the educational setting. The Office of Students with Disabilities (OSD) wanted students to graduate and function independently in society. It was felt that an occupational therapy practitioner was best suited for providing life skills training in the college setting, and therefore, a therapist was hired to work with students directly on campus. The salary of the therapist is paid from the OSD's budget with no direct billing submitted, as all services are free of charge to the students.

In the past 12 years, the role of occupational therapy at Edinboro University has expanded considerably. The OT meets the needs of students by providing assistive technology for enhanced learning, environmental modifications, and a variety of other forms of therapy such as wellness education, consumer advocacy, and transition options from campus to community living. In addition, major service components of the OSD include personal care, van transportation, wheelchair maintenance, learning disability support services, Living Skills Center, academic aide system, tactile laboratory, assistive technology center, and recreation/multipurpose room. Table 5-4 provides a description of the major service components.

The role has also expanded through collaboration with other divisions of the University such as the Health and Physical Education Department. For example, every student at Edinboro, regardless of his/her disability, must complete a three-credit Physical Education requirement. The OT works with the Health and Physical Education Department to adapt the physical activity component for students with disabilities in order to allow for successful completion of the program.

In addition to other accomplishments, the OT expanded the role of the assistive technology team to perform evaluations for students as well as vocational rehabilitation clients in Pennsylvania who do not attend the school. The OT is also developing a student fieldwork program with neighboring universities to train and expose occupational therapy students to this unique occupational therapy practice area in a university environment.

Other educational programs include a disability awareness "wheelathon." This program is held each spring for disability awareness week through the OSD. With occupational therapy in the lead role, the OSD sponsors this program to increase campus and community awareness. Participants push a 1-mile route around campus to educate the campus community about some of the environmental issues students with disabilities face on a regular basis. The event also raises funds for an organization on campus or in the community that benefits students with disabilities

Most of the students with disabilities who come to Edinboro receive funding through their home state vocational rehabilitation office. This funding pays for other support services such as

Table 5-4

MAJOR SERVICE COMPONENTS—OFFICE FOR STUDENTS WITH DISABILITIES AT EDINBORO UNIVERSITY

Personal Care	The Office for Students with Disabilities (OSD) trains attendants who assist students with grooming, bowel and bladder routines, showering, dressing, room cleaning, and other activities of daily living. These services are coordinated by a full-time registered nurse.*
Van Transportation	The University owns and maintains a fleet of seven vans. These vans are used to transport students from their residence halls to their classrooms on a daily basis. Also, van service may be requested for medical appointments, internships, and other transportation needs.*
Wheelchair Maintenance	The OSD maintains a wheelchair repair room that employs personnel trained in repairing electric and manual wheelchairs. An inventory of wheelchair parts and supplies are in stock to minimize "downtime" of the students' wheelchairs.*
Learning Disability Support Services	Support services are offered at three levels for students with learning disabilities. Services for the two higher levels include supervised study sessions with a trained peer mentor and writing specialist assistance.* The lowest level provides the basic services of assistance in arranging academic accommodations, including alternate test arrangements, priority scheduling for classes, consultation with staff, and tape-recorded textbooks. These basic services are also included in the higher levels.
Living Skills Center	The Living Skills Center is an intermediate step designed to "bridge the gap" between home, residence life, and off-campus apartment life. This center encourages a self-directed approach for students to gain the information, skills, confidence, and responsibility to make the transition to independent, self-directed living.
Academic Aide System	The academic aide system is designed to help students with the mechanics of school work. The academic aide is a reader or writer for students who cannot complete these activities independently. An academic aide can also provide library assistance.
Tactile Laboratory	The Tactile Laboratory was designed to meet the needs of students who are blind or have visual impairments. It develops educational materials in tactile, audible, and enlarged form for both students and faculty.
Assistive Technology Center (ATC)	The ATC staff work with any device or technique that can be used by a person with a disability to minimize the cognitive, sensory, motor, or linguistic limitations that the disability might otherwise impose. A broad range of services is provided to enable individuals with severe disabilities to function in school, home, and the workplace. These services include wheelchair evaluations and adaptations, physical mobility and life skills training, alternative access and computer evaluations, home and work-site evaluations, and school-to-work transition support.*

continued

Table 5-4, continued

MAJOR SERVICE COMPONENTS—OFFICE FOR STUDENTS WITH DISABILITIES AT EDINBORO UNIVERSITY

Recreation/Multipurpose Room	This facility, designed for use by students with and without disabilities, has a variety of recreational components including video games, TV, billiards, table tennis, air hockey, and various pieces of adapted physical fitness equipment. This room is also a meeting place for student-run adapted recreational and sport opportunities for students wishing to use off-campus facilities.

*Additional fees are associated with these services.

Reprinted from *OT Practice* (2004, August 9), Michaels, E., Campus Inclusion. Pages 10-13, Copyright 2004, with permission from The American Occupational Therapy Association.

personal care, van transportation, and wheelchair repair. While there are students who arrive on campus with adaptive equipment and assistive technology, the OSD assistive technology program provides students with equipment recommendations and training upon arrival on campus. The ATC team then works with the vocational rehabilitation offices to fund assistive technology equipment needed for school, work, or internships.

Students meet with the OT upon entering the program or prior to discussing services. This allows the students to become acquainted with the facility as well as how occupational therapy may be a part of their educational experience. The students decide whether or not they want to be involved with the OSD services and then can begin their journey.

As described, the role of occupational therapy may be expanded to assist students in achieving their full potential as adults. The Edinboro program should be used as a model to educate administrators as to how the needs of adult learners can be met when utilizing occupational therapy practitioners as well as other therapy service providers in their setting. Occupational therapy practitioners should be encouraged to apply for positions in colleges, universities, and other educational facilities in order to use their unique skills and talents in this area.

The knowledge an occupational therapy practitioner possesses in the areas of physical disabilities, psychosocial issues, environmental access, and the holistic approach to intervention can be valuable in any educational setting. Although occupational therapy practitioners have found a home in primary and secondary school environments, this model proves our services should not stop there. Although an adult education facility may not be recruiting occupational therapy practitioners specifically, advocacy for our profession within these settings is a must. More information on this model can be found by accessing Edinboro University on the web at: http://www.edinboro.edu/cwis/tac/dis_serv/dseup.htm or http://www.edinboro.edu/cwis/tac/dis_serv/osd.htm#OT_services.

RESOURCES

For other resources, please refer to Appendix A.

General Community Resources

- Offices for students with disabilities: Required by Section 504 of the Rehabilitation Act of 1073 to provide mandated services such as disclosure letters, extended time, separate environment testing, in-class note takers, interpreters on technical services for hard of hearing, alternative forms of testing, books on tape, course substitutions.

- Campus-based counseling centers: Provide no or low-cost counseling services for students.

- Campus-based assistive technology centers: Provide assistive technology services and information to students and community members.

- Campus-based support groups

- Department of Vocational Rehabilitation: Will sometimes provide funding for post-secondary education and related supports as part of clients' rehabilitation plan.

- Independent Living Centers: Local resource for community funding and available services. May have equipment loan closet.

- Community programs: For example, supported education and/or employment programs

- Community mental health centers

- Community-based support groups

- Medicaid Waiver and other federal, state, or local funding programs

CASE EXAMPLE #1: LEANN, TRAUMATIC BRAIN INJURY

Leann is a 19-year-old female who sustained a traumatic brain injury at the age of 16. She was a passenger in a car that slid on black ice and ran into a ditch. After 3 weeks in a coma, Leann began the long process of rehabilitation. She missed her junior year of high school, though she returned the following year. She was eligible for special education services and completed high school successfully with the support of the education team and the individualized education program (IEP). She decided to attend the local community college and her school-based team helped design a transition plan to help support her.

Following graduation, Leann underwent two surgeries, one to increase her speech volume and one to address a severe contracture in her left elbow. She was referred to outpatient occupational therapy following the surgeries. The OT evaluated her and determined she has limited functional use of both UEs due to bilateral UE paresis, decreased mobility due to limited ambulation, poor balance, and poor endurance, and almost inaudible speech, even following the surgery. She has intact cognition and perceptual skills, though reports sometimes she needs to hear information more than once to "get it all." She uses a power wheelchair independently and can walk for limited distances. She is independent in toileting and feeding light finger foods, but requires help lifting a heavy beverage.

She reported to her OT that she is committed to beginning classes at the community college, and supplied the transition plan drafted by her team in high school. Based on the plan from the team and the results of her evaluation, the OT has the following primary concerns:

- Leann is easily fatigued, especially when using her arms excessively. She needs assistance with writing, page turning, carrying and manipulating textbooks, opening doors, and drinking beverages. She also will need alternative test-taking methods, and perhaps extra time for test taking.

- Leann must travel with her wheelchair between classes, get to class on time, and access bathroom and other campus facilities independently. She needs adequate time between classes to travel and accessible buildings and bathrooms (ramps, automatic doors, accessible classrooms).

- Leann must coordinate both support services and her schedule to meet her needs and so she needs to contact people in the DSO and the registrar's office.

The OT takes the following steps.

Case Management Services

1. The OT takes a facilatory role, believing Leann can take over her own case management once she has connected with necessary services. She contacts the DSO and arranges for an intake meeting with Leann and a counselor in that office.

2. She reviews the course list with Leann and they contact the registrar to determine where the classes are held, the distance between classes, and the amount of time between classes. She and the registrar identify a contact person in the registrar's office to provide this information each semester so Leann can do this independently.

ACCESSIBILITY

The OT and Leann go to the campus together and assess her mobility, including access to buildings, the student center, and bathrooms. They discover the bathroom doors are too heavy for her to open independently and refer this to the DSO, which agrees to have the in-class note taker assist with bathroom access in between classes. All other campus facilities are accessible.

ASSISTIVE TECHNOLOGY

The OT recommends:

1. A laptop computer for the in-class note taker to use.

2. Software to read text out loud so Leann can listen to lecture notes if she becomes fatigued.

3. Voice-activated software for paper writing and computer control.

4. Environmental control unit (ECU) at home to assist with lights, computer, music, television, VCR/DVD. Leann has a small room that is very difficult for her to access. The ECU gives her more control over her studying environment, allows her to view videos for class, turn her lights on and off, and control other general elements of her environment.

5. Recommendations for other assistance include extended and alternative test-taking strategies, texts on CD which her computer can read aloud, and student readers if necessary for texts which are not available on CD.

CASE STUDY #2: RAYMOND E., MULTIPLE SCLEROSIS

Raymond E. is a 21-year-old male who recently completed his junior year at an Ivy League college. Raymond is pre-Law and has been on the dean's list since his freshman year. He is a popular student who has served in various student leadership roles on campus. He was named captain of the football team for his upcoming senior year and has been a star player since high school.

He has lived on campus for 3 years and has rented an apartment near campus with two friends for his senior year. Raymond's family lives an hour away but he sees them frequently. He returns home at least once a month to visit for the weekend or have Sunday dinner with his extended family.

Over the summer, he was brought into the emergency room by his football teammates when he could not participate in a practice session due to extreme numbness and tingling in his UEs and double vision. Once a complete battery of tests was completed, Raymond was diagnosed with multiple sclerosis. When a complete history was taken, it was discovered that Raymond had been having symptoms for the past 6 months. He had been ignoring the symptoms, which included frequent numbness and tingling in his extremities as well as fatigue and other visual disturbances, because he believed they were due to his academic lifestyle and the demands football had placed on his body.

This diagnosis was shocking to Raymond as well as to his family, friends, and others in his life. Raymond moved home for the remainder of the summer, subletting his apartment for 3 months to a friend, and began outpatient rehabilitation approximately 1 month before school began. His symptoms were exacerbated by the heat of the summer and his hopes for a quick recovery were diminished.

His most recent occupational therapy evaluation revealed significant visual deficits, diminished short-term memory, and noticeable spasticity in both UEs. He is having difficulty initiating movement and cannot use his hands and fingers in a coordinated manner. These are all impacting his daily life: the low vision is limiting his ability to use a computer and read books, magazines, and newspapers; his short-term memory loss is affecting his ability to remember to take his medication effectively, and his UE weakness and spasticity is limiting his ability to perform self-care tasks (dressing, bathing, hygiene) and writing and computer-related tasks (he can no longer write or type effectively due to weak grasp and finger incoordination). During the occupational therapy evaluation, it was also noted that Raymond is becoming increasingly depressed about his status.

During intervention sessions, the OT notes, once engaged in conversation about his former roles, he becomes most animated when discussing his academic and athletic accomplishments and appears to have a desire to return to school. At other times, however, when the subject of school is brought up directly he states he can, "never go back" because, "what good would it do." He feels his ability to participate in college as he once did is gone and he is embarrassed to be in class and not be able to participate.

Case Study Questions

- What is the role of the outpatient OT as related to Raymond's educational status?
- If Raymond decides he would like to attempt to return to school, what resources would need to be recruited and why?
- What evaluation/assessment procedures would need to be completed if the occupational therapy practitioner wants to assist him in returning to his former educational role?
- What assistive technology would be most appropriate for him and how might the occupational therapy practitioner assist him in attaining it?
- What are the boundaries and limitations of which the occupational therapy practitioner must be aware if Raymond returns to school while still being treated in the outpatient setting?

SUMMARY QUESTIONS

1. What laws related to education protect individuals with a disability? Discuss these laws in relation to contextual factors.
2. Discuss two important issues related to access in adult education for individuals with a disability.

3. Name three adaptation/compensation strategies using assistive technology in adult education.

4. Discuss the role of the OT in adult education interventions.

ACKNOWLEDGMENTS

We thank Eileen Michaels, MEd, OTR/L from Edinboro University for her information regarding the role of OT at the University. We would also like to thank Judith Hammerlind Carlson and the staff at TechACCESS of RI for their assistance with information related to assistive technology and for the use of their lab for picture taking.

REFERENCES

ACOTE. (1998).

ADA accessibility requirements apply to Internet Web pages. 1996. *The Law Reporter,* 10(6), 1053-1084.

American Foundation for the Blind. (2005). Key definitions of statistical terms. Retrieved March 29, 2005, from http://www.afb.org/Section.asp?SectionID=15&DocumentID=1280

American Occupational Therapy Association. (1998). Standards for an accredited educational program for the occupational therapist. Retrieved April 29, 2005, from www.aota.org.

American Occupational Therapy Association. (2002). Occupational therapy practice framework. *American Journal of Occupational Therapy,* 56(6), 609-639.

American Occupational Therapy Association. (2004). Occupational therapy scope of practice. *American Journal of Occupational Therapy,* 58.

Americans with Disabilities Act. 42 U.S.C. §12101 (1990).

Americans with Disabilities Act. 42 U.S.C. §12111 (1990).

Americans with Disability Act, 34 C.F.R. §104 (1999).

Asher, A. (2003). From student to employee: helping students with disabilities make the transition. *Developmental Disabilities: Special Interest Section Quarterly,* 26(4), 1-4.

Assistive Technology Act. (1998). *Public Law,* 105-394, S. 2432.

Association of American Medical Colleges. (1993). Americans with Disabilities Act (ADA) and the disabled student in medical school: Guidelines for medical schools. Association of American Medical Colleges, Washington, DC. (ERIC Document Reproduction Service No. ED370491).

Bourgeois, M. (1992). Evaluating memory wallets in conversations with persons with dementia. *Journal of Speech and Hearing Research,* 35(6), 1344-1357.

Brinkerhoff, L. C., McGuire, J. M., & Shaw, S. F. (2002). *Postsecondary education and transition for students with learning disabilities* (2nd ed.). Austin, TX: PRO-ED.

Brinckerhoff, L. C., Shaw, S. F., & McGuire, J. M. (1992). Promoting access, accommodations, and independence for college students with learning disabilities. *Journal of Learning Disabilities,* 25(7), 417-429.

Burgstahler, S. (2001). *Real connections: Making distance learning accessible to everyone.* University of Washington, Seattle.

Carney, N., Chestnut, R. M., Maynard, H., Mann, N. C., Patterson, P., & Helfand, M. (1999). Effect of cognitive rehabilitation on outcomes for persons with traumatic brain injury: A systematic review. *Journal of Head Trauma Rehabilitation,* 14(3), 277-307.

Case-Smith, J. (1991). Occupational and physical therapists as case managers in early intervention. *Physical and Occupational Therapy in Practice,* 11(1), 53-70.

Cole. (1998).

Cook, A. & Hussey, S. (2002). *Assistive technologies: Principles and practice* (2nd ed.). Sacramento, CA: Mosby.

Davidson, D. A. & Fitzgerald, L. (2001). Transition planning for students. *OT Practice,* 6(17), 17-20.

Daykin, W. (2001). Yet another role: the community occupational therapist as care manager. *British Journal of Occupational Therapy,* 54(1), 46.

Department of Justice. (1994). ADA Standards for Accessible Design. Title III Regulations, 28 CFR Part 36.

Dote-Kwan, J. (1995). Information accessibility in alternative formats in postsecondary education. *Journal of Visual Impairments & Blindness, 89*(2), 120-129.

Duchek, J. M. & Abreu, B. C. (1997). Meeting the challenges of cognitive disabilities. In C. Christiansen & C. Baum (Eds.), *Occupational therapy: Enabling function and well-being* (2nd ed.). Thorofare, NJ: SLACK Incorporated.

Edyburn, D. L. (2002). Models, theories and frameworks: contributions to understanding special education technology. *Special Education Technology Practice, 4*(2), 16-24.

Fuller, W. E., & Wehman, P. (2003). College entrance exams for students with disabilities: Accommodations and testing guidelines. *Journal of Vocational Rehabilitation, 18*, 191-197.

Guckenberger v. Trustees of Boston University, 974 F. Supp. 106, 10 NDLR 277 (D. Mass. 1997) (Guckenberger II).

Halsne, A. (2002). *Online versus traditionally-delivered instruction: A descriptive study of learner characteristics in a community college setting.* (ERIC document Reproduction Services No. ED465534). Retrieved March 30, 2005, from EDRS Online.

Individuals with Disabilities Education Act Amendments of 1990 (Public Law 101-476). 20 U.S.C., 400 et seq.

Individuals with Disabilities Education Act Amendments of 1997 (Public Law 105-17). 20 U.S.C., 1400 et seq.

Intons-Peterson, M. J., & Fourrier, J. (1986). External and internal memory aids: when and how often do we use them? *Journal of Experimental Psychology: General, 115*, 267-280.

Intons-Peterson, M. J., & Newsome, G.L. III. (1992). External memory aids: effects and effectiveness. In D. Herrmann, H. Weingartner, A. Searleman & C. McEvoy (eds.), *Memory improvement: Implications for memory theory*. New York: Springer-Verlag.

Jacobs, K. (2002). Navigating the road ahead. *OT Practice*, June, 24-30.

Jarrow, J. (2000, October). *Students with disabilities in higher education: Confirmations and cautions from the Boston University lawsuit*. Retrieved April 9, 2005, from http://www.janejarrow.com/tv_station/bu/maintext.html

Kasworm, C. E. (2003). Setting the stage: Adults in higher education. *New Directions for Student Services, 102*, 3-10.

Lamb, M. (2003). Case management for a geriatric outreach program in British Columbia. *Occupational Therapy Now*, Sept/Oct, 30.

Lohman, H. (1999). What will it take for more occupational therapists to become case managers? Implications for education, practice, and policy. *American Journal of Occupational Therapy, 53*(1), 111-13.

Madaus, J. W. (2005). Navigating the college transition maze: a guide for students with learning disabilities. *Teaching Exceptional Children, 37*(3), 32-37.

Mass. (1997).

McCarthy, B., & St. Germain, C. (1993). *The Learning Type Measure*. Wauconda, IL: About Learning Inc.

Megivern, D, Pellerito, S, & Mowbray, C. (2003). Barriers to higher education for individuals with psychiatric disabilities. *Psychiatric Rehabilitation Journal, 26*(3), 217-231.

Merriam, S. B., & Caffarella, R. S. (1991). *Learning in adulthood*. San Francisco, CA: Jossey-Bass.

Michaels, E. (2004, August 9). Campus Inclusion. *OT Practice*, 10-13.

Mull, C., Sitlington, P. L., & Alper, S. (2001). Postsecondary education for students with learning disabilities: A synthesis of the literature. *Exceptional Children, 68*(1), 97-118.

National Center for Education Statistics. (1997). *National postsecondary student aid study, 1995-96 (NPSAS:96), Methodology Report, NCES 98-073*. Washington, DC: Office of Educational Research and Improvements, U.S. Department of Education.

National Center for Education Statistics. (1999). *Students with disabilities in postsecondary education: A profile of preparation, participation, and outcomes, NCES 1999–187*. Washington DC: Office of Educational Research and Improvements.

National Center for Education Statistics. (2002). *Profile of Undergraduates in U.S. Postsecondary Institutions: 1999-2000, NCES 2002-168*. Washington DC: Office of Educational Research and Improvements.

National Center for Education Statistics. (2003). *The Condition of Education, 2003, NCES 2003-067*. Washington DC: Institute of Education Sciences.

National Center for Education Statistics. (2003a). *A profile of participation in distance education: 1999-2000, NCES 2003-154*. Washington DC: Institute of Education Sciences.

National Center for Education Statistics. (2003b). *Mini-Digest of education statistics 2003, NCES 2005-017.* Washington DC: Institute of Education Sciences.

National Center for Education Statistics. (2004). *Digest of education statistics 2003, NCES 2005-025.* Washington DC: Institute of Education Sciences.

O'Reilly, A. (2000). Transition services planning and the school-based services. *OT Practice, 5*(20), 16-17.

Rehabilitation Act of 1973. Section 504, 29 U.S.C. §794 (1977).

Rehabilitation Act of 1973, Section 504, 28 C.F.R. §35

Ross-Gordon, J. M. (2003). Adult learners in the classroom. *New Directions for Student Services, 102,* 43-52.

Scott, S.S. (1994). Determining reasonable academic adjustments for college students with learning disabilities. *Journal of Learning Disabilities, 27*(7), 403-412.

Scott, S., McGuire, J. M., & Embry, P. (2002). *Universal design for instruction fact sheet.* Storrs: University of Connecticut, Center on Postsecondary Education and Disability.

Scott, S., McGuire, J., & Shaw, S. (2003). Universal Design for Instruction: A new paradigm for teaching adults in postsecondary education. *Remedial and Special Education, 24*(6), 369-379.

Section 504 of the rehabilitation act.(nd). Retrieved from www.section508.gov on June 8, 2005.

Singh, D. K. (2003). Students with disabilities and higher education. *College Student Journal, 37*(3), 367-378.

Sollenberger, K. (2005). Victory for textbooks on time. *Future Reflections, The National Federation of the Blind Magazine for Parentsand Teachers, 23*(4), 40-45.

Strangman, G., O'Neil-Pirozzi, T., Burke, D., Cristina, D., Goldstein, R., Rauch, S., et al. (2005). Functional neuroimaging and cognitive rehabilitation for people with traumatic brain injury. *American Journal of Physical Medicine and Rehabilitation, 84*(1), 62-75.

Stoops, N. (2004). Current population reports. United Stated Census Bureau, June. Retrieved May 2, 2005 from http://www.census.gov/prod/2004pubs/p20-550.pdf.

Thornton, K. (2000). Rehabilitation of memory functioning in brain injured subjects with EEG biofeedback. *J Head Trauma Rehabil, 15*(6), 1285-1296.

Unger, K. (1994). Access to educational programs and its effect on employability. *Psychosocial Rehabilitation Journal, 17*(3), 117-126.

University of Kansas Institute for Adult Studies. (1998). *Accommodating adults with disabilities in adult education programs.* Lawrence, KS: University of Kansas for Research on Learning.

U.S. Census Bureau. (2005). PEOPLE:Education. United States Census Bureau, January. Retrieved June 6, 2005 from http://www.factfinder.census.gov/jsp/saff/SAFFInfo.jsp-pageID=tp5_education

U.S. Department of Education. National Center for Education Statistics. Profile of Undergraduates in U.S. Postsecondary Institutions: 1999–2000, NCES 2002–168.

Watson. (2001).

Wattenberg, T. (2004). Beyond legal compliance: Communities of advocacy that support accessible online learning. *The Internet and Higher Education, 7,* 123-139.

West, M., Kregel, J., Getzel, E.E., Ming, Z., Ipsen, S.M., & Martin, E.D. (1993). Beyond Section 504: satisfaction and empowerment of students with disabilities. *Exceptional Children, 59*(5), 456-467.

Westby, C. (2000). Who are adults with learning disabilities and what do we do about them? *Topics in Language Disorders, 21*(1), 1-14.

Yakil, E. & Hoffman, Y. (2004). Dissociation between two types of skill learning tasks: the differential effect of divided attention. *Journal of Clinical and Experimental Neuropsychology, 26*(5), 653-666.

6a Work

Martha Sanders, MA, MSOSH, OTR/L, CAPS
Robert Wright, OTR/L

CHAPTER OBJECTIVES

By the end of this chapter, the student will be able to:

- ☑ Define **work** as it pertains to the *Occupational Therapy Practice Framework (Framework)*.
- ☑ Describe specific **models/frames of reference** as related to work.
- ☑ Comprehend **safety issues** as related to work.
- ☑ Delineate between the roles of the **occupational therapist** (OT) and the **occupational therapy assistant** (OTA) as they pertain to the occupation of work.
- ☑ Comprehend and identify related **psychological implications** as related to decreased independence in work.
- ☑ Comprehend issues related to **ergonomics, industrial rehabilitation, work hardening, and work conditioning**.
- ☑ Describe the impact of **contextual factors** upon work.
- ☑ Identify appropriate activity of daily living (ADL) intervention strategies based on various **performance skills** and **client factors**.
- ☑ Identify specific work **compensation/adaptation** strategies.
- ☑ Identify general work **remediation** strategies.
- ☑ Identify work compensation/adaptation intervention strategies related to **vision, perception, and cognition**.
- ☑ Identify general work **maintenance** strategies.

INTRODUCTION TO WORK

Definition of Work

Work is central to human existence as a means of providing sustenance, self-worth, and self-identity (Bing, 1989). Although the meaning attributed to work may vary according to the individual worker, occupational therapy has acknowledged the health-promoting purpose of work since its inception (Harvey-Krefting, 1985). The profession of occupational therapy has been instrumental in using work both as a *method* to enable physical and psychiatric rehabilitation

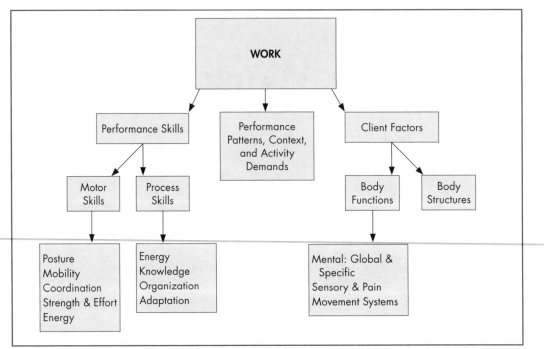

Figure 6a-1. Components of work (adapted from American Occupational Therapy Association [2002]. Occupational therapy practice: Domain and process. *American Journal of Occupational Therapy, 56,* 609-639).

as well as a *goal* for industrial rehabilitation following work-related injuries (Harvey-Krefting, 1985; Jacobs, 1991; Stein & Cutler, 1998). Work continues to be an important performance area of occupation as identified in the *Framework* (American Occupational Therapy Association [AOTA], 2002) (Figure 6a-1).

According to the *Framework* (AOTA, 2002), work "includes activities needed for engaging in remunerative employment or volunteer activities (Mosey, 1996, p. 340)." Work therefore includes all activities required to perform the role of a worker or volunteer both inside and outside of the home. The specific content areas included in the work performance domain are employment interests and pursuits, employment seeking and acquisition, job performance, retirement, and volunteering (AOTA, 2002).

Employment interests and pursuits include identifying work interests based on an individual's skills, abilities, interests, and the opportunities available. The process of identifying employment interests actually begins with the imitative play of young children who simulate the actions of adult role models and heroes. Young children learn about the world of work through school and home responsibilities that provide rewards for productivity, goal achievement, and leadership. Career choices become gradually crystallized throughout adolescence and young adulthood as individuals identify their strengths, specific skills, and the job opportunities available to them (Erikson, 1997).

Prevocational planning may utilize standardized and nonstandardized skills assessments, vocational interest tests, and career inventories to promote the process of self-discovery (Jacobs, 1991). Vocational interest tests provide potential career options for individuals based on the similarity of their responses to those who have demonstrated success in a particular field (Murphy & Davidshofer, 2001).

Employment seeking and acquisition, an important aspect of vocational planning, refers to the process of identifying employment opportunities, developing a resumé, completing a job application, preparing for the interview, completing the interview, and negotiating terms of employment (AOTA, 2002). This process is undertaken and practiced as adolescents seek various part-time or temporary jobs. These skills become further honed as individuals search for jobs in which their personal subsistence and future career are related to job performance.

Job performance, the focus of this chapter, includes developing work habits, learning and performing job tasks, as well as complying with the norms or culture of the work setting (AOTA, 2002). Part-time work in adolescence often serves as a means to learn about, and establish, such fundamental work habits as punctuality, attendance, learning a task, and relating to supervisors and peers (Atwood, 1992). Although adolescents readily become competent in the physical job tasks, the interactional aspects of the job, such as coping with angry customers (in the food service industry) and communicating with supervisors, are not well-developed at this age (1992). This chapter will focus on work hardening and ergonomic modification because these areas are typical practice areas for work programming. Retirement and volunteering aspects of work programming will be addressed in Chapter 6b.

Components of Work According to the Framework

Effective intervention for work involves a thorough examination of **client factors** that impact the client's ability to meet the demands of the workplace. Client factors will include body functions (such as mental functions, sensory functions, neuromuscular, and cardiovascular functions) and body structures that support these functions. Clients who have been injured on the job will commonly have limitations in neuromusculoskeletal functions that make some aspect of the job difficult or unsafe to perform. For example, a client with low back pain may be unable to perform a manual material handling job that requires frequent lifting from the floor due to pain and decreased trunk motion, strength, and flexibility. Another client with carpel tunnel syndrome may have difficulty performing fine motor assembly tasks due to a weak pincer grasp, deficits in finger coordination, or sensory discrimination deficits caused by changes in the sensory cortex over a long period of time (Prosser & Conolly, 2003). Client factors will need to be evaluated for most work interventions.

Performance skills refer to the functional components of performing the job. Performance skills are composed of motor, process, and communication/interaction skills that interact to enable successful job performance. **Motor skills** include one's posture during work and use of proper body mechanics while performing the task (AOTA, 2002). The concept of "neutral posture" is fundamental to preventing work-related injuries associated with awkward postures. *Mobility* refers to the myriad of motions that workers assume while performing job tasks, such as reaching for an object, squatting to change a tire, walking to shelve items, or standing at a cash register. *Coordination* relates to manipulative activities integral to most assembly, computer, and fine motor tasks. *Strength* is the force necessary to lift, push, pull or move objects or loads. *Energy* refers to workers' abilities to moderate their pace of work so the required amount of work can be accomplished during the work day (Alexander, 2004).

Process skills enable workers to organize their workplaces, sequence jobs, modify the job as necessary, and effectively apply knowledge to the tasks at hand (AOTA, 2002). Process skills become automatic for highly skilled, experienced workers. However, workers who are returning to an adapted job, learning a new job, or learning a new technique that requires them to modify a pre-existing process may need retraining or practice to resume their preinjury level of productivity. For example, a plumber who has returned to work from experiencing wrist tendonitis may decide to use ergonomic tools to improve his/her wrist position while working. However, the individual may need to adapt his/her usual hand position on the tool to accommodate the extended handle. Workers with psychiatric disabilities may also need assistance in organizational aspects of the job (Stein & Cutler, 1998).

Communication and interaction skills may be well-established in seasoned workers. However, as stated, younger workers (Atwood, 1992), workers with psychiatric disabilities (Stein & Cutler, 1998) and young adults with learning disabilities (Stacey, 2001) may not have developed strong interactional skills in responding to authority figures, taking feedback (particularly criticism), making "small talk," and following the formal and informal rules of the workplace.

The **activity demands** in the workplace refer to the environmental, physical, and social demands of the workplace that would commonly be included in a job analysis (Ellexson, 2004). OTs who work with clients returning to a job need to clearly understand the job demands in order to develop goals that will enable clients to safely perform their jobs. The activity demands will include the objects or equipment workers use, the environmental conditions (such as the size of the workspace, the illumination levels, noise levels, temperature, and flooring, among others), the required actions, sequence, and productivity demands (AOTA, 2002). A task analysis will provide the required performance skills, body structures, and body functions for the job.

The **social demands** of a job may refer to the informal means of working together as a team, the attitudes toward injured workers on disability, the type of dress code for "dress down days," or the informal rules common to a group or culture of workers. The social demands of the workplace are considered to be critical to an individual's success in a particular job (Stein & Cutler, 1998). Social skills become critically important for workplaces dependent upon the input and collaboration of many workers.

Performance patterns refer to the habits, routines, and roles that support one's job (AOTA, 2002). Habits may include clearing one's desk before leaving for the day or writing a "to do" list for the following day (Alexander, 2004). Habits are considered to be integral to time management skills (Stein & Cutler, 1998) and become particularly important in prevocational skills development. Routines involve completing a sequence of tasks. Examples of routines may be checking e-mails in the morning while drinking a morning coffee, donning personal protective equipment for certain types of work, completing end-of-shift procedures for "cashing out," or other established sequences performed on a regular basis.

The **context** refers to the overall conditions in which the job is embedded. Cultural aspects of the job may include the ethnic background of workers or the work group cultures formed by individuals who perform a particular job skill, trade, or occupation. The ethnic backgrounds of the workers may impact their means of relating to authority, their educational level, and career goals. The culture of a work group impacts their choice of tools, definition of quality of work, ways of organizing their day, and the informal "ways of doing things" that are critical to mastery over one's job (Baker & Sanders, 2004).

Frames of Reference

Frames of reference that are commonly applied to work programming are the biomechanical frame of reference and the rehabilitative/acquisitional frame of reference. The *biomechanical frame of reference* focuses on maximizing human movement in order to facilitate occupational performance (Green & Roberts, 1999; Trombly & Radomski, 2002). Impairments in body structures due to injury, disease, or pain may cause dysfunction in the movement system. According to the biomechanical frame of reference, human movement is enabled through adaptations or modifications which increase an individual's strength, endurance, and range of motion (ROM) (Cole, 1998).

The fundamental concepts of kinetics (study of forces) and kinematics (the study of human movement) are applied to workplace interventions to maximize the workers' capacities. For example, work heights may be adjusted to enable proper positioning for hand motion or use; workloads may be decreased to minimize the forces necessary to accomplish the job. As discussed in

Chapter 2, interventions under the biomechanical frame of reference commonly include exercises or techniques that gradually increase an individuals' strength and ROM such as pulleys, aquatics, use of weights or exercise equipment, or aerobic activities (Leveau, 1992). In work hardening, job simulations are used to increase individuals' endurance or tolerance to job tasks (refer to section on Industrial Rehabilitation).

The biomechanical frame of reference is not a client-centered approach, and therefore needs to be used in conjunction with an approach that integrates individuals' needs and goals into the intervention plan. The **rehabilitative approach**, also called **acquisitional**, focuses on enabling an individual to function as independently as possible. (Trombly & Radomski, 2002; Cole, 1998). Within this approach, environmental modifications and adaptive equipment are used to compensate for deficits that limit effective functioning. The rehabilitative approach supports the individual's need to work in order to support him- or herself. Interventions therefore focus on means by which to restore work-related skills and prevent further dysfunction through education, purposeful activity, and active problem-solving.

Role of the Occupational Therapy Assistant

The role of the OTA in the performance area of work parallels other intervention areas. OTAs may work alongside the OT to carry out work hardening interventions, education, and ergonomic modifications, provided they have demonstrated competency in that skill. OTAs may also contribute to work evaluations by completing standardized aspects of a functional capacity evaluation (FCE) or a job analysis for which they have demonstrated competence. However, the OT is responsible for interpreting results of the FCE and job analysis and developing a plan with the client to meet his/her vocational goals.

Safety Issues

WORKER SAFETY

Concerns for client safety are paramount in work programming. The Occupational Safety and Health Administration Act (OSHA) of 1970 was promulgated in order to provide a safe workplace for all workers (OSHA, nd). To that end, employers identify the safety regulations relevant to that work environment and develop safety procedures to which workers are expected to comply.

Safe practices for the workplace begin with using the proper technique to perform one's job. The proper technique refers to using **process skills** such as choosing the proper tools for the job, sequencing aspects of the job, positioning one's body correctly, using personal protective equipment, such as hardhats and steel-toed shoes, and implementing the proper work methods. *Personal protective equipment* refers to garments that act as a barrier to protect the body from potential harm (Kjellen, 2000; Krause, 1997).

Organizational and individual worker variables also impact workplace safety. Individual behaviors may include worker knowledge, training, level of fatigue, and risk-taking behaviors. Over a period of time, workers may often develop "shortcuts," or quicker ways of performing a task that circumvent safety practices and increase the risk of developing further injuries (Kjellen, 2000; Krause, 1997). Workers must acknowledge the impact of physical or psychological deficits on the ability to safely perform one's job. At the worksite, ergonomic modifications or treatment-related interventions, such as splints, must not interfere with job performance.

THERAPIST SAFETY

Although most therapists focus on the safety of their clients, therapists need to acknowledge their own safety when working at a job site or in the clinic. In the clinic, therapists need to acknowledge electrical safety when working with frying pans filled with water or multiple appliances plugged into one fuse or circuit (Bracciano, 2000). Ground fault circuits (GFCs) should always be installed to prevent short-circuiting of faulty equipment.

Thermal electrical equipment may cause burns if precautions are not taken to protect oneself from heat guns, hot packs, or hot water from splinting pans or hydroculators. Similar to industrial workers, therapists should develop safe practices when using potentially hazardous equipment, such as using tongs (not fingers) to remove hot packs, turning off a heat gun when not in use, and positioning oneself correctly when using a razor blade knife (to prevent the knife from injuring the thigh on a follow-through swipe). Proper maintenance of equipment helps to prevent unnecessary mechanical malfunctions. The importance of using proper body mechanics for assisting clients in using job simulation equipment cannot be underestimated. Therapists will need to learn the proper body mechanics for using a hand truck, assisting a client with transfers, and using tools correctly.

Implications for Psychosocial Issues

The majority of clients enter industrial rehabilitation with a physical injury resulting in pain, functional deficits, and inability to work. Social and psychological consequences further disrupt the family and impact quality of life for many workers (Kirsh & McKee, 2003). Much of the problem arises from a tone of distrust that sometimes develops among the health care providers, work supervisors, human resource personnel, compensation systems, and workers. Each player has a different perspective when interacting with the injured worker. Supervisors want a quick return to work to maintain productivity, human resource personnel are concerned with insurance costs, health care providers want to avoid reinjury, and the workers wants a full paycheck and a sense of self-worth. Since chronic pain is not a visible injury, workers feel they must legitimize the pain. Research studies report that injured workers feel misunderstood and not respected by employers, society, their community, and coworkers (Kirsh & McKee, 2003).

ERGONOMIC MODIFICATIONS

Introduction

Ergonomics addresses the interface between the work and the worker so that jobs can be performed in the safest, most productive, and most comfortable manner possible (Kroemer & Grandjean, 2001). While the broad field of ergonomics includes many specialty areas, such as designing rehabilitation equipment, industrial tools, computer systems, and controls and displays (e.g., pilot cockpits and car dashboards), most OTs work in the area of musculoskeletal ergonomics (Rice, 1998). This area of ergonomics focuses on the prevention of work-related musculoskeletal disorders (MSDs) in business and industry. More recently, ergonomics has been applied to non-work activities such as leisure, housework, and caring for children (Sanders, 2004).

The simplest definition of ergonomics, fitting the work to the worker, implies the client-centered nature of ergonomics and the focus on designing work tasks and equipment to be most easily used by the worker or "end user"(Rice, 1998; Sanders & McCormick, 1993). In a proactive manner, ergonomic design is a health-promoting intervention that improves the efficiency for all workers performing a certain job task. Tasks that are ergonomically designed attempt to minimize, if not eliminate, hazardous exposures for workers performing that task. More often, however, ergonomic interventions are modifications or adaptations that are applied retroactively to work tasks or work processes that have contributed to a diagnosed MSD in individuals or groups of clients. In this regard, ergonomic interventions focus on modifying the work tasks, the work environments, and the organization of work in order to minimize risks that may contribute to musculoskeletal pain.

In ergonomics, the terms *adaptation* and *modification* are similar and therefore will be addressed together.

This chapter will focus on intervention strategies for the workplace involving ergonomic adaptations (such as the use of specialized ergonomic tools) and ergonomic compensations (such as lifting assists to minimize heavy forces to the low back) notwithstanding the importance of accurate evaluations in determining the intervention required.

Goals and History

As stated, the goals of ergonomics are to decrease musculoskeletal discomfort and increase work productivity, efficiency, and comfort. Although these goals may seem distinct, in actuality, a worker who is more comfortable is also more productive. Studies show that comprehensive ergonomic intervention programs can increase worker productivity while decreasing health care costs and the risk for developing an MSD (Noack, 2005; Oxenburgh, 1997). Ergonomic intervention benefits both the employee and the employer.

History of Ergonomics

The science of ergonomics dates back to 1717 when Ramazzini, the father of occupational medicine, speculated on factors within the work environment that contributed to his patients' illnesses. Ramazzini described the "violent and irregular motions," "bent posture," and "tonic strain on the muscles" as factors that contributed to musculoskeletal pain in his patients (Ramazzini in Wright, 1940). He documented the fundamental physical and psychological risk factors found to contribute to MSDs today (Sanders & McCormick, 1993).

As the Industrial Revolution took hold, Frederick Taylor and Frank and Lillian Gilbreth revolutionized the organization of work by applying scientific methods to modern factory management. Taylor used scientific management to reduce entire jobs to a series of repetitive tasks efficiently performed by individual workers. He thus promoted assembly-line pacing, motion and time measurements for each job, paying workers according to production standards and incentives (Sanders & McCormick, 1993).

The era following World War II was a time of considerable growth in ergonomics as technology was applied to military procedures and equipment. An appreciation for the "human element" as the weak link in a mechanical operation was recognized. The Human Factors and Ergonomics Society was formed in 1957 that advanced the science of ergonomics among civilian companies producing pharmaceuticals, automobiles, and consumer products. In the 1980s and 1990s burgeoning computer use became the focus of many ergonomic studies. However, the disasters at Three Mile Island nuclear plant in Pennsylvania and the Union Carbide pesticide plan in Bhopal, India underscored the critical importance of human factors in worker safety today (Sanders & McCormick, 1993).

Legislation Affecting Ergonomics

Presently, no federal ergonomic standard exists, although an ergonomic standard has been in the making for over 15 years. The recent history of ergonomic regulations began in the early 1980s when the OSHA began to issue voluntary guidelines designed to assist industry with controlling the increasing number of MSDs in the workplace. In 1981, the National Institute of Occupational Safety and Health (NIOSH), the agency performing research on occupational safety and health, developed the *Work Practices Guide for Manual Lifting,* which provided industry with analytical procedures used to determine the amount of weight employees could safety lift in a given situation. In 1991, these lifting calculations were revised and widely distributed for use in industry (NIOSH, 1994a). In 1991, OSHA also introduced *The Ergonomics Program Management Guidelines for Meatpacking Plants* in response to skyrocketing rates of MSDs (OSHA, 1991). This manual outlined a comprehensive ergonomics program designed to prevent upper extremity (UE) injuries in the meatpacking industry. In 1997, the *Elements of Ergonomics Programs* was developed and distributed by NIOSH to enable managers to perform ergonomic workplace evaluations and devise ergonomic programming to decrease MSDs in all industries (NIOSH, 1997).

In 2001, a Federal Ergonomic Standard was passed and subsequently rescinded in 2002 with a change of governmental offices. Although the standard survived only a few months, the act sensitized employers to the importance of ergonomic interventions in managing employee's injuries and provided a comprehensive written ergonomics program for industry to emulate.

At present, industries can be cited for obvious and willful ergonomics violations under the "General Duty Clause" of the OSH Act (5a)(1) of 1970. This clause states employers must "furnish to each of its employees employment and a place of employment which is free from recognized hazards which are causing or likely to cause death or serious physical harm." Therefore, companies who repeatedly ignore obvious ergonomic hazards can be cited and fined for not providing a safe workplace for its workers (OSHA, nd).

A Model of Ergonomics and the Development of MSDs

Although ergonomics has traditionally focused on the physical or biomechanical aspects of performing a job, such as the tools, the postures, and forces, researchers find that injuries still occur even when the most well-designed equipment is utilized.

Consider the following scenario:

Joe is a 37-year-old male who works as an instructional technologies programmer at a local college. Joe works 6 to 7 hours per day on the computer and plays video games at lunch. Joe has monthly deadlines necessitating that he work overtime toward the end of the month in order to meet these deadlines. Joe moved into a new work area that was equipped with an ergonomic keyboard, adjustable chair, adjustable keyboard tray, and an ergonomic mouse. Joe's workstation was adjusted to his height of 5'6" and to his body dimensions. Joe was given stretches to perform every hour and a free pass to the gym at lunch. However, after 1 month of working in the new workstation, he began to complain of numbness, tingling, and paresthesias in his right hand, and elbow pain in his left arm. An OT observed him at his workstation and found he had moved his computer to the right corner of the desk (to give him more room), and he was sitting on the edge of his chair with one foot tucked under his body. He had brought his personal laptop computer to work, and was working on two computers simultaneously. He therefore spent much of his day twisting his body and keying in a manner that placed pressure on his wrists. Further inquiries about his hobbies revealed that he played the drums 2 nights per week.

This case reveals that the design of the tools and equipment are not the sole components of an ergonomics plan. Joe was given the proper ingredients for an ergonomically correct workstation. However, he was not educated in proper use of the equipment and therefore personalized his workstation in a manner that negated the intent of the original set-up of the equipment. Nor did Joe understand the impact of all activities on the development of MSDs, including playing video games on his computer at lunch and playing the drums at home.

The National Research Council (1998), in its extensive review of the scientific research relevant to MSDs, outlined a broad conceptual framework to examine all the factors that contribute to MSDs in the workplace (Figure 6a-2). MSD refers to injuries that develop gradually over time due to repeated stressors to a particular part of the body (NIOSH, 1997). MSDs include lateral epicondylitis, deQuervain's disease, rotator cuff tendonitis, and wrist tendonitis. MSDs may also include nerve entrapments such as carpal tunnel syndrome and Guyon's canal syndrome (NIOSH, 1997; Prosser & Conolly, 2003). The model suggests that the primary factors in the initial development of an MSD are physiologic loads that are placed on body tissues throughout the day. Body tissues

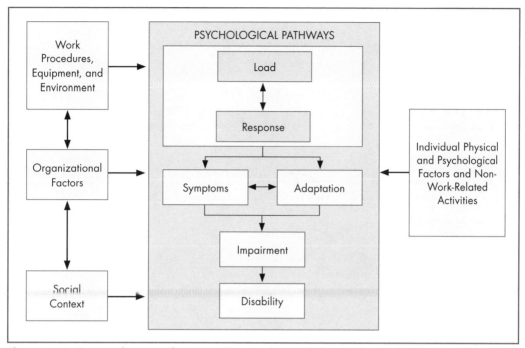

Figure 6a-2. Factors that contribute to MSDs in the workplace (adapted from National Research Council. [1998]. *Work-related musculoskeletal disorders: A review of the evidence.* Washington, DC: National Academy Press).

respond to these loads by gradually strengthening and becoming conditioned, or by fatiguing and becoming injured, depending on the condition of the tissue, extent of the loads, and opportunity for rest. Signs and symptoms of MSDs, such as pain or inflammation, may progress to a disabling condition if intervention is not provided.

As the model indicates, factors in the home and work environments may contribute in varying degrees to the development of MSDs. In the workplace, the type of tools used, height of the equipment, and forces used on the job all impact tissue loads. *Organizational* factors such as the pace of the job, the necessity for overtime, and workers' abilities to exert control over their job tasks also influence the development of MSDs. In fact, strong causal relationships exist between the development of cardiovascular disease and high job strains (high job demands with low control over the job) (Karasek & Theorell, 1990). Further, psychosocial issues such as the degree of social support, relationships with authority and peers, and organizational culture may influence the development or perception of illness. For example, piece rate incentives may motivate employees to work faster and longer hours, thus contributing to overuse of muscle groups.

In the model, the individual worker's physical and psychological factors that influence the development of MSDs refer to client factors such as the worker's health history, level of physical conditioning, stress, attitude, personal work style, and the performance of hobbies or nonwork-related activities. Table 6a-1 delineates the areas that are addressed by ergonomics.

In short, ergonomics addresses not only the activity demands of the workplace (work tasks and procedures), but also the psychosocial components of the job including work organization and individual characteristics such as size, work style, home and work stressors, hobbies, and other responsibilities. Research indicates a greater prevalence of MSDs when both biomechanical and psychosocial factors are present in a job situation (NIOSH, 1997).

Table 6a-1

AREAS ADDRESSED BY ERGONOMICS

Work Tasks (Physical)

- Work procedures
- Work tasks
- Tools
- Work environment

Workplace Organization (Psychosocial)

- Job content
- Organizational factors
- Worker support
- Work culture

Worker Contributions (Individual)

- Personal stress level
- Homework responsibilities
- Personal size
- Worker style
- Hobbies

OTs are in a unique position to address all these factors because they are trained to analyze tasks, systems, and individual characteristics as related to overall health. The following section will discuss biomechanical factors, as they tend to be the initial focus of risk factor reduction.

Biomechanical Risk Factors

The biomechanical risks inherent in work tasks have been the primary focus of research in the industrial arena. This discussion will address the primary biomechanical risk factors: repetition, force, awkward postures, static postures, contact stresses, and vibration.

- *Repetition*: Repetition refers to performing the same motions over and over within a given time period. Jobs are typically classified according to the percentage of similar motions performed within a certain cycle time. Jobs are characterized as *low repetitive* if similar movements are repeated less than 50% of the time. Jobs are considered to be *highly repetitive* if similar movements are performed more than 50% of the time (Silverstein, Fine & Armstrong, 1987).

- *Force*: Force is commonly expressed as the amount of effort required by a worker to overcome external loads by pushing, pulling, grasping, or handling objects. In reality, two types of force exist: *external forces* are the loads exerted on the body during work-related activities; *internal forces* are the amount of muscle tension developed to overcome external loads. In industry, external forces are usually the reference point. A high force job is considered to be one in which workers use >10% to 15% of their maximal strength during a job task (Kroemer & Grandjean, 2001).

- *Awkward Postures*: Awkward postures are those that deviate from a *neutral* posture. A neutral posture is one in which muscle forces are approximately balanced throughout the body so the head is upright, shoulders are at one's side, elbows flexed to 90 degrees, back straight, and knees slightly flexed. The ears, neck, shoulders, hips, knees, and ankles should be approximately aligned from a lateral view (Leveau, 1992). Awkward postures that are associated with the gradual development of MSDs are neck flexion, shoulder protraction, shoulder flexion and abduction greater than 45 degrees, elbow flexion greater than 90 degrees, trunk flexion, and wrist flexion, extension and deviation greater than 30 degrees (NIOSH, 1997). Therapists should understand that muscles and tendons must generate increased internal forces to accomplish a task when working in an awkward position versus when working in a neutral posture (Leveau, 1992).

- *Static Postures*: Static postures are those maintained in the same position for greater than 20 minutes. Static postures stabilize the body proximally, resist the force of gravity, and allow for distal mobility.

- *Contact Stresses*: Contact stress is pressure placed on the skin and underlying **soft tissue structures.** Contact stresses may contribute to tendon, nerve and other soft-tissue injuries over a period of time (Tichauer & Gage, 1977; Chaffin & Anderson, 1984). Compression can occur from the edges of desks, work surfaces, tool edges, tool handles, or other workstation components.

- *Vibration*: Prolonged exposure to vibration from vibrating hand tools or surfaces has been known to affect workers' overall health and to contribute to hand arm vibration syndrome (HAVS) in an average of 50% of all workers who use vibrating tools (NIOSH, 1989).

Ergonomic Evaluations

Ergonomic evaluations identify the risk factors involved in performing the job tasks. Ergonomic evaluations should be completed on the individual worker performing the job because each individual performs a job in a slightly different manner. Ideally, the evaluation should prioritize which risks pose the greatest risk to an individual, then interventions should be planned accordingly.

Ergonomic evaluations for work task related (also called biomechanical) risks may take the form of observations, direct measurement, or standardized tests in addition to self-reported surveys and simple checklists. Surveys and checklists provide a quick means of identifying which jobs may be hazardous should be analyzed further. Direct observation and measurement can provide more specific information which may be necessary (NIOSH, 1997; Sanders, 2004). OSHA and NIOSH provide multiple resources for public use including ergonomic checklists, and The NIOSH Lifting Equation. The NIOSH Lifting Equation is widely used in manual material handling jobs when workers are lifting, handling, and carrying equipment or product on a regular basis (NIOSH, 1994).

A job analysis must be performed prior to analyzing risk factors. A job analysis identifies the *activity demands* and includes the specific tasks, motions, equipment specifications and durations involved in lifting, carrying, and manipulating objects (for a complete discussion see Ellexson, 2004).

Ergonomic Interventions

ANTHROPOMETRIC PRINCIPLES

Anthropometrics is the study of human dimensions such as height and limb length. Anthropometrics also includes physical capacities such as lifting, carrying, and grasping (Pheasant, 2001). When designing a workspace for a group, knowledge of anthropometrics is a starting point for ergonomic interventions. Clients' sizes and capacities need to be identified relative to their jobs in order to create an efficient work environment.

Ideally, each type of equipment is designed to fit the specifications of each worker. Realistically, however, managers in industry purchase equipment and plan workstations to accommodate most workers, including the largest man (95th percentile) and the smallest woman (5th percentile) in order to keep costs reasonable. Anthropometric charts provide reference data on the sizes of typical worker populations. However, some of this information may not be accurate for today's increasingly diverse workforce of women, older adults, workers with disabilities, and workers from different ethnic backgrounds. Therapists must identify workforce characteristics and take direct measurements when feasible.

The process of planning a work area for workers (or users) takes anthropometric data and equipment criteria into account. For example, if a factory decides to buy chairs for all shop workers including lab technicians, assembly persons, and clerical workers, the procurement specialist must identify *who* will be using the chairs and the distinct needs or criteria for each work group. The lab technicians may need a chair with height adjustment that will accommodate a high lab bench; the assembly workers may need a sit/stand chair to allow alternate positions, and the clerical workers need lumbar and thoracic support for comfort in a seated position all day. All workers' chairs need to accommodate their particular body sizes.

Four main categories of anthropometric criteria are used in designing ergonomic workstations:

- *Clearance* refers to planning enough space for headroom, legroom, and elbowroom.

- *Reach* refers to the locating controls, materials, and equipment within close proximity to a worker.

- *Posture* refers to organizing the job so that a worker can assume a neutral posture to the work surface and controls.

- *Strength* refers to the muscle strength and grip strength related to lifting or carrying weighted loads.

In order to accommodate the largest range of users, clearances should be designed for the largest user (95th percentile), whereas reaches should be designed for the smallest user (5th percentile) (Pheasant, 2001).

Categories of Interventions

Ergonomic interventions modify, adapt, and in some cases compensate for hazardous job tasks that present excessive physical stresses to the body. Ergonomic interventions are categorized in terms of whether the intervention changes the design of the job, changes the way the job is performed, and/or offers a means to protect a worker while performing the job. Most often, recommendations will include suggestions from all categories of interventions in order to thoroughly manage the problem. Ergonomic interventions, called controls by OSHA, are categorized as *engineering controls, administrative controls,* and *work practice controls* (OSHA, nd). Each of these will be discussed below.

ENGINEERING CONTROLS

The ideal ergonomic solutions are those that will improve the design of the workstation or job task for all those performing the job. *Engineering controls* are recommendations in the design of the equipment, workstation layout, work processes, transport of materials, design of the tools, and mechanical assists that will minimize inherent risks in the job. Engineering controls are considered to be the preferred way to solve or mitigate problems (NIOSH, 1997).

Standing Workstations

The design of both sitting workstations and standing workstations is based on anthropometry and principles of body mechanics during dynamic tasks. Optimal heights of *standing workstations* depend not only on the height of the individual performing the task but also on the type of work performed. Kroemer and Grandjean (2001) suggest that workers who perform precision work while standing should work at surfaces whose heights are 2 inches to 4 inches above the elbow with the elbow flexed to about 90 degrees. This height allows for proximal stability while performing detailed work. For light assembly, workstation surfaces are typically 2 inches to 4 inches below elbow height; heavy work surfaces are 4 inches to 5 inches below the elbow to allow for additional force or effort from the shoulders and trunk to assist in the work.

Other intervention considerations for standing workstations are the flooring and prolonged standing position. Workstations should provide supportive or cushioned flooring in order to minimize stress to the low back and prevent leg and foot fatigue. Anti-fatigue mats can cover hard flooring at individual workstations where necessary. Rails or stools elevate 1 foot allowing workers to alleviate strain from the lower back. Sit-stand chairs allow workers to the options to change postures (Kroemer & Grandjean, 2001).

When standing stations are used for lifting and packaging, mechanical assists can compensate for a worker's muscle strength and thus minimize worker fatigue and injury. Conveyor systems and carts or containers with wheels can decrease the need to carrying items. Mechanical assists such as pallet jacks, cranes, and other mechanical hoists can lift a product to an optimal position to be handled or bring products to desired destination.

Sitting Workstations

Workers in seated workstations strive for a neutral sitting posture with options for variability and movement. The neck should be upright or slightly flexed, shoulders at one's side, hips flexed greater than 90 degrees, elbows flexed from 90 degrees to 100 degrees, wrists in neutral without deviation, lumbar curve supported, and feet flat on floor.

The comfort of sitting workstations is highly dependent upon the design, fit, and adjustability of a chair. Many variations in chair designs exist; however, all ergonomic chairs should have the following adjustable features:

- *Adjustable chair height*: Individuals who share workstations will need to adjust their chairs at the start of a shift. Workers may also change chair heights during the day according to the work surface height and task. Generally, the chair height should be adjusted so that the elbows are level with the work surface or slightly higher.

- *Seat angle:* An individual should be fully seated on the chair with the hips in greater than 90 degrees of hip flexion. This position will minimize pressure on the discs of the spine yet still allow for use of the hands.

- *Seat pan:* The seat pan should be wide enough and deep enough to support the thighs without touching the posterior aspect of the knees. The edges of the seat pan should be rounded with padding to distribute the pressure of the ischial tuberosities.

- *Back rest:* The backrest should support both the lumbar curve and thoracic region. This support is especially important for office workers who spend the majority of time at their desks.

- *Footrests:* Feet need to be resting on the floor or on footrests in order to relieve pressure on the thigh and low back. Inexpensive footrests can be purchased or made from wooden platforms. Phone books can also provide temporary fixes.

- *Armrests:* Armrests may support the arms when they are held in the same position for much of the task. However, armrests may interfere with getting close to the desk and keyboard for office workers.

- *Base:* The chair base should have five points or casters for the greatest stability.

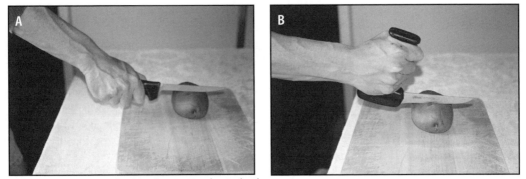

Figure 6a-3. (A) Standard knife. (B) Pistol-grip knife.

Computer Workstations

The criteria for ergonomic computer workstations encompass those discussed for sitting workstations, in addition to further guidelines for interfaces with the keyboard and monitor. The worker should be directly facing the monitor and viewing the screen with a downward gaze of about 15 degrees. The monitor should be positioned about an arm's length away from the worker. Those with bifocals and progressive lenses may find sitting in a more reclined posture (110 degrees of hip flexion) with the monitor tilted slightly backwards will enable them to view the monitor without straining their necks (Hedge, 2004).

Workers should use their wrists in a neutral (straight) position for keying in order to avoid compression to the median nerve. Keyboards are commonly positioned in a "negative tilt" in order to accommodate this position. Document holders should be used when inputting data or text from a paper. Use of a document holder minimizes eye and neck movements required to shift between the documents and the computer screen. The document holder should be placed as close to the monitor as comfortably possible. The mouse should be positioned close to the keyboard within easy reach of the user (for further information on computer workstation ergonomics, refer to Hedge, 2004; Noack, 2005; Sanders, 2004).

Tool Design

Ergonomic tools must be designed to fit the anatomical structures of the hand while fulfilling the functions of the task. Many traditional tools place pressure on the soft tissue structures of the hand, which may contribute to injury over a period of time. Traditional pliers, for example, are designed with a short handle that places pressure on the thenar eminence near the thenar branch of the median nerve. Over a period of time, such pressure may injure the soft tissue structures. Many other tools, such as traditional scissors and can openers, also place pressure on delicate hand structures. Use of traditional tools, such as hammers, saws, wrenches, and screwdrivers, causes the worker to assume an ulnarly deviated position of the wrist during use. This position places further stresses on the forearm musculature.

Many tools are now being designed to distribute pressure across a larger area of the hand and improve the position of the hand and wrist. Ergonomic pliers, for example, extend the handle through the palm and provide coated rubber padding to the handles. Saws, knives, and other tools are being designed with a "pistol grip," which includes a vertical handle design that places the wrist in neutral relative to the working area of the tool (Figure 6a-3). Table 6a-2 provides a list of design principles that should be incorporated into ergonomic tools.

Table 6a-2

DESIGN PRINCIPLES THAT SHOULD BE INCORPORATED INTO ERGONOMIC TOOLS

- Handles with round edges and rubber coating.
- Tool handles that extend through palm.
- Loop handle designs with spring openings.
- Pistol grip for vertical surface.
- Inline grip for horizontal surface.
- Balanced tools to avoid excess torque during use.
- A trigger strip rather than a trigger button.
- Tools designed for either hand (R or L).

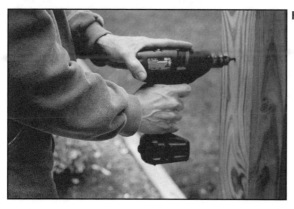

Figure 6a-4. Power drill with pistol grip.

Table 6a-3

COMMON MEANS TO REDUCE FORCE

- Use mechanical assists such as conveyor systems, pallet jacks, and overhead cranes to transport items.
- Use handles or hand slots to improve ability to carry containers or packages.
- Use a counterbalance sling support to hold a tool in place while using the tool.
- Keep the center of gravity of tools closest to worker.
- Break down a heavy load into smaller loads if possible (although this practice may increase the repetitions).
- Reduce handle slipperiness by increasing the coefficient of friction on the handle.
- Clean and maintain controls in order to minimize resistance during operation.

Principles to Reduce Force

The quip "power with motors rather than muscles" holds true for ergonomic design. Efforts to reduce the force in a task focus on decreasing the resistance a worker must overcome in order to complete a task. This may involve decreasing the weight of loads, decreasing the resistance to operate a machine, or decreasing the weight of a tool during use. Figure 6a-4 shows a power drill with a pistol grip. Table 6a-3 identifies common means to reduce force.

Table 6a-4
COMMON MEANS TO REDUCE REPETITION
• Enlarge job tasks to include more variety of movements and components. • Mechanize using power tools. • Automate the job. • Enlist other workers to assist in the job.

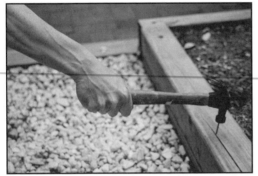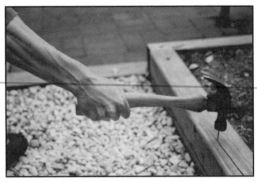

Figure 6a-5. (A) Poor and (B) good hammer design.

Principles to Reduce Repetition

Repetition is difficult to minimize without the use of automation. However, efforts can be made to decrease repetitive exposures to each individual by enlarging the job tasks so an individual is not performing a repetitive cycle or job all day. Some examples of means to reduce repetition in a job are provided in Table 6a-4.

Principles to Reduce Awkward Postures

Work in awkward positions places excess stress on musculature and may entrap muscles and tendons against boney structures or soft tissue structures. Awkward postures are most apparent when workers perform tasks requiring forward bending and twisting of the back, use of the hands above the shoulders, or lifting with a load away from the body. The adage, "bend the handle instead of the wrist" implies good handle or workstation design should be encouraged (Figure 6a-5). Many jobs can be modified so the product or process is positioned at elbow or waist height. Typical recommendations are provided in Table 6a-5.

ADMINISTRATIVE CONTROLS

Situations exist in which the work equipment or work environment cannot be changed. In such cases, administrative controls may become the primary source of interventions. Administrative controls are management policies that determine how the job can be organized or "administered" to reduce individual worker risks. These controls may include providing proper training for the workers, making sure the equipment and work area is maintained properly and scheduling worker according to job task needs (NIOSH, 1997).

Administrative controls should be used in conjunction with engineering and work practice controls in order to effectively manage a safe work environment. While administrative controls address how the job is organized and workers trained, the overall *culture* of the workplace also impacts the degree to which supervisors, managers, and workers will support safety and ergo-

Table 6a-5

TYPICAL WORKPLACE RECOMMENDATIONS

- Use fixtures to tilt parts such as vice grips.
- Adjust the work height to avoid forward bending at the waist.
- Use turntables to hold the work.
- Rotate the part so that the wrist is straight.
- Position work close to elbow height.

nomic interventions. A culture of workplace safety will prioritize safe worker practices over extremely high work productivity standards, recognizing healthy workers are key to a viable business (Krause, 1997; Melnik, 2004). The following recommendations help to minimize hazardous workplace exposures and situations for individual workers.

- Train workers properly for the job.
- Allow the worker to control the pace of the job.
- Enlarge the job to include a variety of workers' skills.
- Rotate workers through hazardous jobs if workers' skills are comparable.
- Maintain the equipment regularly.
- Schedule breaks to allow for rest and recovery.
- Provide a new employee conditioning period.
- Educate workers on risk factors and symptoms of overuse.
- Monitor workers' symptoms regularly.
- Offer modified duty programs for injured workers.

WORK PRACTICE CONTROLS

Work practice controls are those measures a worker can take to protect him- or herself on the job. Such controls include not only using PPE, but also utilizing the correct body mechanics, sitting posture, and proper technique that was provided through training. Work practice controls are important in industries that have fewer options for changing the task design.

Work practice controls focus on means by which individual workers can take responsibility for protecting themselves. Whereas a company can provide optimum equipment and tools, breaks, and job variety, the individual worker must be committed to using and adjusting the equipment properly and following body mechanics programs. Most workers have good intentions of working injury free and following company guidelines when first beginning a job. However, over time, some workers tend to take short cuts or rearrange a workstation in order to hasten job completion. These changes often increase the risk of injury. Workers benefit from ongoing "reminders" and training sessions to emphasize the importance of adherence to safe practices (Melnik, 2004). The following work practice controls are important for workers to follow:

- Use PPE: gloves, safety glasses, helmets, knee pads.
- Follow correct body mechanics.
- Stretch throughout the day.
- Use proper work technique.
- Adjust workstations as needed.

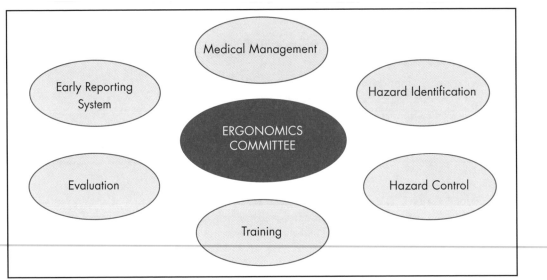

Figure 6a-6. Ergonomics committee (adapted from Warren, N. [2004]. The expanded definition of ergonomics. In M. Sanders (Ed.), *Ergonomics and the management of musculoskeletal disorders*. St. Louis: Butterworth-Heinemann).

Other Interventions

OTs are well aware of individual worker differences that can impact a job. For example, those who work with greater speed and intensity at work tend to be at higher risk for MSDs (Feurerstein, 1996). Accordingly, workers who continually seek perfection in a job may also place undo stresses on their emotional and physical status (Feurerstein, 1996). Since MSDs result from the accumulation of strains throughout the day and over time, a worker's hobbies, home responsibilities, and level of stress may contribute to the development of MSDs (Sanders, 2004).

The OT's understanding of a worker's injury and lifestyle can contribute greatly to success in return-to-work programs. OTs may educate and train workers in using the least amount of force to accomplish a job (such as computing for video display terminal workers or scaling for dental hygienists). OTs can help workers identify sources of stress and offer stress reduction programs to enhance work and home coping. Finally, OTs can also encourage a healthy lifestyle including good physical and mental health in an overall workplace wellness approach.

A Comprehensive Ergonomics Program

The overturned ergonomics standard provided recommendations about comprehensive management of MSDs through ergonomic intervention. An ergonomics program should include identification of worker hazards or risk factors, means to control the risks, and training on proper work procedures, use of body mechanics, and safety precautions. Additionally, early reporting of MSD symptoms, medical intervention, and a return-to-work program are effective means of limiting the severity of injury and keeping the worker engaged in the worker role even during rehabilitation. These program components are presented in Figure 6a-6 surrounding an ergonomics committee that provides input to all facets of the program (Warren, 2004).

Melnik (2004) provides strategies for keeping an ongoing ergonomics program viable, active, and visible to all employees. Such strategies include management commitment and employee involvement in program planning and execution. OTs need to understand the culture of the company and develop ergonomic programs that are flexible and creative in order to maintain ongoing support of its employees.

Ergonomics for Older Workers

The participation of older adults in the workforce (aged 55 and older) has steadily increased from 55.1% in 1982 to 56.2% in 1992 and 61.9 % in 2002. By the year 2012, the labor force participation rate of older adult workers is expected to be 65% (Toosi, 2004). While the rates of labor participation are increasing, many employers have not recognized the physical needs of older workers, their unique motives for working, and the experience that they can offer to a younger workforce. In fact, a recent study of 2001 retirees conducted by the American Association of Retired Persons (AARP) (2003) found the major reasons retirees work or seek employment are to remain productive (73%), stay mentally (68%) and physically (61%) active, earn money (51%), do something enjoyable (49%), be around people (47%), help people (44%), and learn new things (20%). Additionally, at least 70% of the retirees seek a work environment where they can engage in new work experiences and interact with other people. Hence, older adults are motivated to work by social and health reasons rather than income alone.

This section will outline some changes associated with aging that may impact the workplace. It will offer interventions that can modify and compensate for physical losses associated with aging.

IMPACT OF AGING ON WORK CAPACITIES

Age-related losses in physical and functional capacities vary greatly among older adults. The extent to which changes in capacities affect work performance depends to a great extent on the work being performed. In general, older adults may experience age-related changes in sensory, cognitive, and neuromuscular status.

Visual changes may include decreased near vision, difficulty focusing, blurred vision, problems with color discrimination, difficulty recognizing moving objects, and difficulty seeing at low levels of illumination (Bonder & Wagner, 2001). These changes may impact work environments that have glare due to direct lighting or shiny surfaces, low levels of illumination or work tasks that require careful scanning or discriminating features of a task. Visual impairments such as cataracts and macular degeneration make such changes more pronounced.

Hearing ability may become diminished for higher frequencies and for speech recognition, particularly under stress (Bonder & Wagner, 2001). In work situations with high background noise and high demands for rapid communication, deficits in hearing may impact work performance.

Musculoskeletal changes may occur in muscle and tendon tensile strength, ligament flexibility, joint mobility, and posture. Muscle strength in older adults declines due to a decreased number and size of skeletal muscle fibers. However, older adults who remain physically active show only moderate declines in strength. In the workplace, changes in muscle strength may reduce the maximum loads that can be lifted, slow walking speed, and decrease endurance for large muscle, aerobic tasks (Leveau, 1992).

Although past research has documented the gradual decline of cognitive abilities with increasing age, current research is finding that cognition for older adults is not a single construct that maintains or declines as a whole. Research studies suggest that older adults are able to solve simple everyday problems and arithmetic problems with the same accuracy as younger adults. However, they tend to be slower at solving more complex tasks than younger adults. Older adults seem to have difficulty holding many items in working memory and retaining knowledge of word processing commands. They benefit from being challenged in a cognitive task and improve performance over time in order to match job demands. Most researchers suggest, however, that these deficits seem to be at the high range of intellectual capabilities and may not be a detriment in everyday work-related tasks (Chueng & Strough, 2004; Oberauer, Wendland, & Kliefl, 2003; Schooler, Mulatu, & Oates, 1999).

ERGONOMIC INTERVENTIONS FOR OLDER WORKERS

With these physical changes in mind, the following interventions focus on specific adaptations for older adults, acknowledging that these design changes universally increase the ease of work performance for all workers.

Engineering Controls

Older workers should make use of mechanical assists to assist with lifting and seek to minimize lifting manual loads when possible. Work environments should be well-lit, following the higher illumination ranges suggested for older workers in various tasks (Kroemer & Grandjean, 2001). Ergonomic tools should be routinely introduced in order to reduce the hand forces needed. Other ergonomic aids such as ergonomic box cutters, glare filters, and an ergonomic mouse should be individually adapted to the worker.

Workers with visual changes should identify the low vision adaptations that may be relevant to the workplace such as clocks, watches, and signage with large numbers or typeface (Bonder & Wagner, 2001). Employers should design offices with appropriate contrast in colors, hand-rail support, and non-slip flooring to enhance the safety and work performance of workers.

Since most older workers will be using the computer for some aspect of work, software design should be older-worker friendly in order to minimize eye fatigue and improve the speed and retention of computer skills. Fisk, Charness, Rogers, Czaja, Sharit & Sharit (2004) recommend a software screen set-up that enlarges critical information and minimizes distractions. Software should place minimal demands on working memory by keeping directions simple and visually available, providing drop-down menus, minimize switching from one screen to another, and limiting visual searches.

Administrative Controls

The AARP (2003) specifically addressed the preferred work environment for an older worker. An *elder-friendly* work culture is one in which the experiences and opinions of older adult workers are respected and valued. Such workplaces should provide flexible or part-time scheduling so older adults can take off time to care for relatives as needed.

Fisk et al. (2004) suggests that training for older adults should be thorough yet self-paced with ample time to learn tasks and practice tasks prior to performing them on the job. Training programs should build on previous experiences of older workers to enable them to make cognitive associations for new job tasks. Cuing, ongoing visual instructions, and developing new work habits may assist in compensating for any cognitive deficits in speed or working memory. The process of progressing an older worker from simple to complex tasks in a training program may facilitate the older worker's adaptation to new work environments.

The job should be organized so that older workers work alongside other colleagues in order to provide support, socialization, and the opportunity for intergenerational contact. As for any worker, the job should allow for creativity and challenge. Companies may consider creatively scheduling breaks throughout the day in order to avoid fatigue in the older worker.

Work Practice Controls

Older adult workers need to take the same precautions as younger workers to protect themselves. However, they need to be even more vigilant in executing proper body mechanics and considering further joint protection techniques. Such techniques may include using more adaptive devices to open, cut, or handle boxes as described. They may consider purchasing prescription eye safety wear.

Ergonomics can improve the experience of workers so work is not a means to the end, but a productive and self-fulfilling experience that goes beyond implications for material income. Honor the unique individual qualities of each worker.

Industrial Rehabilitation

History of Industrial Rehabilitation and Occupational Therapy

Dr. Leonard Matheson is considered to be one of the founding fathers of industrial rehabilitation. Dr. Matheson renewed our interest in work interventions during the 1970s by incorporating clinical expertise related to specific diagnoses with task analysis and work environments (www. ot.wustl.edu) He transformed the clinic into a shop or factory, allowing for more effective reproduction of critical job duties and therapeutic intervention to facilitate recovery of lost work skills, abilities and tolerances. Injured workers would present themselves daily for up to 12 weeks and engage in functional work tasks designed and graded to advance the ability and tolerance of the given injured worker. In time, this gave way to many forms of industrial rehabilitation that have grown and changed to meet the needs of today's injured worker (www.ot.wustl.edu).

Components of an Industrial Rehabilitation Program

Industrial rehabilitation refers to work programs whose goals are to remediate a client's injury in order to return to the workforce. Industrial rehabilitation may be appropriate for workers who have psychiatric and/or physical disabilities. Although the focus of this chapter is physical disabilities, psychosocial issues have been addressed throughout as appropriate. Rehabilitation may include means to increase clients' overall strength, endurance, and job-specific skills as well as prevocational skills such as punctuality and following directions. Programs may include compensation for deficits in skills such as teaching clients to use lifting aids to compensate for limited strength.

Safety Restrictions and Concerns

Prior to engaging a worker in the work hardening process, the worker should be cleared medically. Concerns that should be considered are tachycardia, resting heart rate above 110, blood pressure significantly above 140 systolic and 90 diastolic, and other unstable medical conditions, such as recent development of kidney stones (Demers, 1992).

Implications for the Americans with Disabilities Act

The worker's ability to meet the critical job demands determines the individual's ability to return to performing the job. The Americans with Disabilities Act (ADA) suggests a worker protected under the ADA can perform the essential job functions (29 C.F.R. § 1630.2(m)), or those functions that cannot be completed by another employee, with reasonable accommodation. According to the ADA, reasonable accommodations may include environmental modifications, job modifications, or the use of specific equipment that will allow the employee to perform the essential job functions (ADA, 1990, 42 U.S.C. § 12111[9]). These accommodations must be requested by the employee and must not cause undue hardship for the employer (42 U.S.C. § 12111[10]). The determination of undue hardship is a relative term based on the size of a given company. Reasonable accommodation to a small company could mean provision of a small inexpensive cart that could be pushed so loads did not need to be carried. Reasonable accommodations for a larger company could mean installing a hoist and crane system to automatically transport an object so the product is not manually handled. The OT serves as an expert at assisting employers in adapting actual vocational demands and means of accommodation.

Acute Rehabilitation

Therapy delivered by OTs at the acute stage of industrial rehabilitation focuses on the recovery of body structures such as soft tissue injuries, joint trauma, ligamentous sprains, and muscle strains. Injuries are typically treated the day of injury or as soon as medically appropriate. The acute phase of care can last up to 3 months. Early, but appropriately controlled movement allows for effective control of symptoms and avoidance of chronic conditions (Prosser & Conolly, 2003).

As explained in Chapter 2, various modalities including ice, heat, iontophoresis, and electrical stimulation are utilized by the therapist to control inflammation, pain, and swelling. Manual therapies, muscle energy, myofascial and craniosacral therapy may also be used to address painful symptoms (Bracciano, 2000). It should be noted that some interventions stated above require continuing education beyond entry-level skills. Special care should be taken to assure the normal joint and tissue integrity above and below the site of treatment is maintained. Functional activity is graded to offer enough stress to facilitate proper healing, not exacerbate the injury. The focus of intervention is expedited care to allow the worker to resume performance skills and normal work routines.

Therapists should make an effort to understand the worker's personal belief mechanisms about injury and recovery and educate him/her as to the most effective process for recovery. Addressing the emotional content of the injury is equally as important as treating the worker's actual physical complaints. The worker may have competing advice from medical, legal, and work arenas, all of which impact recovery. Concerns outside of the worker's actual injury may include pressure from decreased financial resources as well as chronic pain. New roles (homemaker or child care provider) may become a barrier to returning to work or exploring alternate means of employment.

Often, the worker cannot readily resume full duty and may need a modified duty job for a short time. OTs assist physicians in determining the extent of limitations. Simple functional evaluations or more formal Functional Capacity Evaluations (see next section) provide objective data for this process (Isernhagen, 1995). It is crucial that the therapist encourage the worker to take responsibility for his/her own well-being. Health club membership or other effective means of fitness training, weight loss, tobacco cessation, and ergonomic equipment should all be encouraged as a normal part of healthy living.

On-Site Programs

The birth of on-site programs was stimulated from the need to offer more effective means of intervention to larger corporations. The concept is to offer effective intervention with the least amount of lost time (Yassi, 2005; Jacobs, 1991; Key, 1995; Niemeyer & Jacobs, 1989). Depending on the company size and injury, on-site care can range from the provision of an occupational health nurse and a 3-day-a-week therapist to larger offerings including x-ray equipment and daily rehabilitation. The on-site facility offers the injured worker immediate care, follow-up intervention, and rehabilitation without having to visit an emergency room or off site clinic (Isernhagen, 1995).

A benefit of on-site therapy is that the therapist is able to directly assess the worker's ability to engage in given work tasks, understand the factors that contribute to injury, and effectively plan intervention toward returning to previous work capacity. All care providers at on-site facilities are keenly aware of the work environment and work nature. This is especially important when decisions are being made about work readiness, modified duty, and ergonomic modifications. On-site programs typically offer more direct communication between medical provider, employer, therapist, and worker. The venue creates more effective understanding and limits information delay.

Subacute Rehabilitation

Subacute intervention begins typically after resolution and healing of an injury, somewhere between 3 and 6 months after injury. The injury itself is stable, although it may have become a persistent or chronic condition. At this stage, the elapsed time since injury may present with ramifications that are as significant as the original injury. For example, workers may have become deconditioned and may present with guarding of the involved extremity due to prolonged painful conditions.

Occupational therapy intervention scenarios focus on addressing long-term complaints, specific work activities that result in exacerbations, and new manifestations that are born from long-standing conditions. Therapists may continue to utilize modalities appropriate for subacute conditions (continuous ultrasound, moist heat, transcutaneous electrical stimulation). Updating of home exercise programs should also be considered to facilitate recovery. More likely, the therapist will need to focus on regaining time limited ROM, joint excursion quality, and pain management (Isernhagen, 1995).

Return to Work Fitness

Following subacute therapy, a worker may need to be placed in a brief program intended to build tolerance, stamina, and strength. A return-to-work fitness program offers the worker a supervised fitness program that targets specific needs and weaknesses in order to transition back to work. Partial engagement of actual duties in the form of modified duty may be beneficial and be included in the work fitness program. The program prescribes fitness activities graded to the worker's level of physical capacity and offers recommendations for a program that can be followed independently at a local fitness facility, community center, home gym, or home exercise program. The worker should understand the balance between sustaining adequate fitness to insure tolerance to work and overtraining, which further stresses musculature.

Work Hardening and Work Conditioning

Work hardening incorporates work fitness but focuses further on improving the functional limitations that have developed from a given injury. Work hardening typically consists of injury intervention, specific fitness training, specific work act simulation, conditioning, body mechanics training, and safe work practice training. The objective is to reestablish a sense of normal work momentum by fabricating an environment that simulates the eventual full work demands that will be expected of the worker. Workers simulate tasks to build up a tolerance to the stresses associated with work performance. With time, the worker can readily tolerate the stresses without setback or exacerbation of injury (Demers, 1992).

The client in a work hardening program is expected to resume normal ADL and prework rituals prior to participation in the program. Specifically, the worker is expected to rise, shower, dress, and eat breakfast as would be expected prior to going to work. The worker is then expected to arrive to work hardening on time and ready to invest in the program. A typical work hardening program can be 5 days a week and 8 hours long.

Work hardening is generally provided in a group setting by a multidisciplinary team of providers. The team typically consists of OTs, physical therapists, medical providers, rehabilitation nurses, case managers, and may also include psychology and sociology professionals. The team works collaboratively to provide consistent intervention in all facets of the program (Demers, 1992). Work hardening is effective in returning an injured worker to the most optimal level of functional ability where employment opportunity readily exists. Outcome studies on the return to work status of clients in work hardening programs suggest 50% to 88% of all workers return to work and remain at work at least 6 months after discharge from a program (Scully-Palmer, 2000).

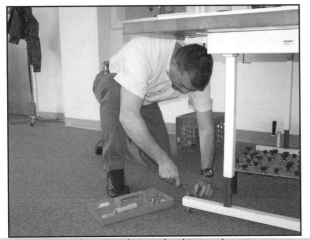

Figure 6a-7. Client simulating plumbing task.

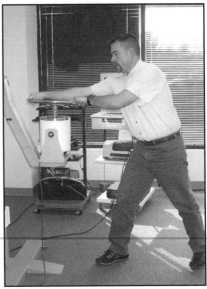

Figure 6a-8. Client simulating plumbing task.

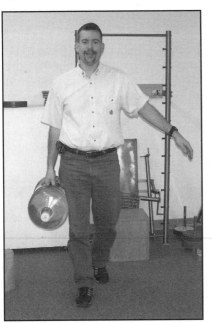

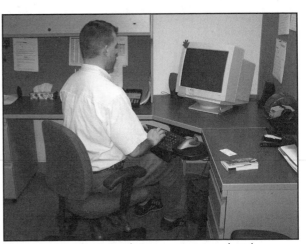

Figure 6a-9. Client simulating common work task.

Figure 6a-10. Client simulating common work task.

Work hardening equipment typically incorporates actual work samples from industry as well as equipment that simulate job motions. Work samples may include actual kegs of beer, saws, hammers, plumbing, or electrical tools that allow workers to practice their trade in a clinical environment. Job simulation equipment simulates specific tasks using computerized equipment that provides numerous attachments and adjustments to enable practice in similar positions and resistance levels as the actual job. Low tech work samples, ramps, lift boxes, work frames, and assembly kits are also seen across the country. Figure 6a-7 identifies a client simulating a plumbing task that are similar to the motions and equipment that he would need to perform on the job. Figures 6a-8 through 6a-10 provide additional examples and descriptions.

> ## Table 6a-6
> ## BASIC COMPONENTS OF A FUNCTIONAL CAPACITY EVALUATION
>
> - Health interview and physical exam.
> - Grip/pinch/dexterity tests.
> - Posture and activity tests.
> - Manual material handling/weighted negotiation (Lifting).
> - Job simulation.
> - Cardiovascular tests were relevant.
> - Behavior profile.
> - Reliability of effort determination.

The work hardening program assesses the worker's injury and current functional status using a baseline evaluation called a Functional Capacity Evaluation (FCE). The goal of the FCE is to identify the functional attributes of an injured worker, compare these skills with the known job demands, and determine whether the worker can perform the essential job functions fully, with restrictions, or not at all. *Essential functions*, as stated earlier, are those tasks that must be completed in order for the worker to be wholly competent in terms of performing his/her job. Essential functions are comprised of *critical demands* that constitute the physical nature and quantities of work associated with the essential functions. Work is also often comprised of nonessential functions and demands that are typically associated with a given duty but are not criteria for competence.

The results of the FCE are compared to the demands of the job in order to develop an intervention plan that will increase the client's functional status to the level necessary to resume normal work participation (Chaffin & Andersson, 1984). The FCE specifically defines an individual's ability to perform work-related performance skills and performance patterns (Isernhagen, 1995). Various FCEs evaluate cognition, vision, and mentality; however, most FCEs directly relate to the Workers' Compensation focus on a worker's physical ability. For example, a carpenter who recently underwent a rotator cuff repair would need to strengthen his shoulder in order to hammer overhead, ascend a ladder, and operate a circular reciprocating saw. The carpenter, given the time away from work, would likely also need to recover his aerobic capacity and general work tolerance. The OT would offer the carpenter functional and exercise-based activities to address these issues so that the worker could resume his past job. Table 6a-6 identifies the basic components of a FCE. The most simplistic subtests of an FCE are typically universal, but variations in procedure, methodology, and test components exist. The FCE components will be specific to evaluator philosophy, job demands, and intervention approach. Figure 6a-11 shows a client performing a weighted lifting component from the floor to mid-thigh height.

Aspects of the FCE can also be used as part of normal occupational therapy evaluation and intervention, especially in the Industrial Rehabilitation arena, where a progressive understanding of the worker's functional abilities is needed to know how to adjust, update, or advance therapy. Specific FCE subtests (bending, squatting, reaching, lifting, etc.) can be used to provide meaningful information to medical providers relative to establishing "recuperative posts" or "temporary alternate work" opportunities.

Overall, the work hardening program should instill a sense of growing independence so that the OT offers more encouragement than direction by the end of the program. The worker is ready and able to return to the rigors of employment with the needed fitness, conditioning, and mindset to address the dynamics of full-time work participation and the physical dynamics of the actual work itself.

Figure 6a-11. Client performing a weighted lifting component from the floor to mid-thigh height.

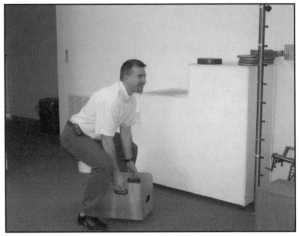

Work Conditioning

Work conditioning differs from work hardening in that typically no team is present to collaboratively treat the worker. According to Jacobs & Jacobs, work conditioning is defined as, "An intensive work-related, goal-oriented conditioning program designed specifically to restore systemic neuromuscular functions (e.g., strength endurance, movement, flexibility, motor control) and cardiopulmonary functions. The objective of a work conditioning program is to restore physical capacity and function to enable the patient/client to return to work" (2004, p. 250). Workers engaged in work conditioning generally present to the therapy setting and engage in a combination of physical exercise, stretching, fitness, aerobic conditioning, body mechanics training, and some limited involvement in work-related functional tasks. Work conditioning can occur either as an individual program or a group setting with several workers completing the program together. The workers may not share similar work demands but are encouraged to offer each other positive reinforcement and an effective level of competition or peer pressure. Work conditioning often lasts 2 to 4 hours a day and may occur several days per week (Niemeyer and Jacobs, 1989).

Work conditioning does not require an extensive clinical environment in terms of exercise equipment to be successful: a treadmill, some weights, and a floor mat are typical of many programs. Similar to work hardening, the work conditioning program instills within the worker the importance of continuing the daily fitness and exercise routines that have been established. However, less work simulation is performed prior to returning to the job.

Body Mechanics Training

Both work hardening and conditioning share as part of their intervention strategies health promotion activities such as education and training specific to body mechanics and safe work practice. Body mechanics focuses on teaching workers to use their bodies effectively and safely. Training focuses on teaching workers how heavy loads affect their bodies, possible consequences of cumulative stress, as well as anatomy and kinesiology of the back and shoulders (Melnik, 2004).

Many approaches to body mechanics exist. Three common lifting techniques for lifting objects from the ground include squatting, semi-squatting, and stooping (Straker, 2003; Melnik, 2004). Although positions vary, most approaches maintain that lumbar lordosis, or "locking in the spine," is the safest position for the back. Principles include keeping the load close to the body, keeping the back straight, and avoiding twisting the back. Since twisting places significant torque on the back, workers are trained to move *with* the load taking small steps, pivoting their feet, or stance shifting instead of fixing their feet and twisting from their low back. Workers must anticipate the weight of the load and expect load shifting for unsecured objects (Greene & Roberts, 2002). Workers in health care such as certified nursing assistants (CNAs) must learn how to apply lifting principles to transferring clients in health care facilities.

Although most body mechanics programs focus on proper use of the low back, shoulders also present with lifting concerns. Overuse of the shoulder may cause tendonitis, which may lead eventually to a rotator cuff tear. In order to prevent this sequela, workers are trained to keep loads close to the body and avoid reaching with loads. Positions that place excessive torque on the shoulders are lifting above chest level or greater than 90 degrees of shoulder flexion/abduction. The worker's hand coupling (relationship of hand to object to be lifted/moved) may be modified to identify the most effective means to handle loads in a given lift.

Safe Work Practice

Safe work practice advances body mechanics training to the entire behaviors associated with meaningful work. The worker is taught to consider every aspect of the given job in terms of physical stress and the opportunity to physically respond to the stress by ideal work practice and/or adaptation of the demand. Advanced problem solving is encouraged to allow a level of preparedness for the possible outcomes of a given demand. Workers are trained to remain in full attention to their physical acts. Therapy can set the stage for safe work practice by providing dynamic activity that does not follow a routine or level of repeatability. A simple training tool is having the worker respond to weighted medicine balls that are caught in various scenarios off rebounding equipment. Workers must anticipate the trajectory and decelerate the ball, all the while maintaining proper spinal and shoulder posture. Safe work practice inherently includes body mechanics training but goes further to instill a sense of general safety for all vocational participation.

Pain Management

Another extension of work hardening and work conditioning is the arena of pain management. This intervention is focused on workers whose pain issues supersede the actual functional implications of their given injury or injuries. Two intervention approaches exist to address this issue: behavioral and functional.

Behavioral Intervention

Behavioral intervention is typically a team-oriented intervention composed of the same professionals as a formal work hardening program. Intervention consists of work hardening and work conditioning, except the worker's identified pain behaviors are literally "disacknowledged" by the team. The worker with pain is rewarded only for functional gains and assertive dialogue about any symptoms. The worker is medically weaned off of all pain medications, as it has been determined the worker's pain is present despite pain medication; therefore, it is determined the medication is only an extension of pain behavior and no longer therapeutic. Additionally, intervention extends beyond the worker to the worker's family or support network, such that family and significant others are trained to not enable the worker's current pain paradigm. This program is very demanding and can be quite stressful to both the worker and the therapist. The worker elects to adopt wellness behaviors or fails the program by not adopting healthful beliefs. The therapist needs to fully understand the end goal in order to encourage functional and therapeutic activity despite the worker's pain (Guzman, Esmail, Karjalainen, Malmivaara, Irvin & Bombardier, 2001).

Functional Restoration

The goal of *functional* restoration is to offer a safe environment for the worker to resume normal movement, activity, and vocational/avocational involvement. Strategies are provided to offer effective pain management such as ice, pacing, and conditioning. The worker's medical provider may offer strategic medications to maximize the worker's tolerance and pain modulation to facilitate success in the program. Ideally, the worker will graduate from the program with a renewed sense of self and ability. Pain modulation should be a personal concern and no longer a public one with effective pain therapy being made available to the worker.

As in work conditioning, functional restoration focuses on maximizing physical ability through exercise, aerobics, weighted activity, and activities that promote normal movement patterns. The worker's pain issues are not denied but rather intellectualized so that workers can understand how to use their bodies despite the pain. Permission is given to work through pain or to accept pain. Many of these workers are overtly fearful that their pain somehow represents some level of fragility or structural instability within their bodies. This creates a tendency to minimize activity in order to avoid pain. This strategy may be effective during the acute phase of injury but remains counterproductive in the chronic phase because the decreased movement and activity results in range limitations that continue a cycle of pain (Schonstein, Kenny, Keating, & Koes, 2003).

As with all forms of intervention, it is paramount that the OT be able to instill a sense of importance in the worker about maintenance of skills and ongoing fitness and health. Many clinics offer some form of "after care" where the worker can return informally and use the clinic as a health club and check in with the care team. This service offers a good bridge upon completion of a formal program, but should be time limited so that workers ultimately take full responsibility for themselves.

Outcomes of Work Hardening Programs

Work hardening programs strive to prepare a worker to return to the job. However, if the worker does not achieve the physical capacities necessary for the workplace, the employer may further use discharge assessments or FCEs to understand how to modify the relevant work area or job process in order to allow the worker to be competent. The worker may also be referred to vocational retraining, which attempts to retrain the worker for potential vocations at the physical demand levels identified by the completed FCE. A final scenario is that the worker may never return to employment and use the FCE to gauge a financial award to the worker to compensate him/her for any suffered injury or condition.

In summary, the overall goal is that the worker experiences a satisfying job or career that promotes personal satisfaction and competency in a healthful work environment. Ergonomic and industrial rehabilitation services can offer prevention, modification, and remediation services to promote worker health. Dr. Matheson eloquently captures this sentiment with his quote, "After you save a person's life, the only thing that is more profound is to re-establish competency at work" (personal communication, 2005).

SUMMARY QUESTIONS

1. Define ergonomics and its relation to occupation.
2. Discuss the difference between work hardening and work conditioning.
3. Discuss compensation/adaptation strategies for individuals who are retired.
4. How might a perceptual deficit impact the safety of a worker? Choose a specific example of a profession in the discussion.

REFERENCES

Alexander, C. K. (2004). Work programs practice: Aiming for successful context management. *OT Practice*, 9(7), CE-1-CE-6.

American Association of Retired Persons (2003). *Staying ahead of the curve: The AARP working in retirement study*. AARP Knowledge Management: Washington, DC.

American Occupational Therapy Association (2002). Occupational therapy practice: Domain and process. *American Journal of Occupational Therapy, 56*, 609-639.

Americans with Disabilities Act, 34 C.F.R. §1630 (1999).

Americans with Disabilities Act. 42 U.S.C. §12111 (1990).

Atwood, M. J. (1992). Adolescent learning in two environments. *Work, 2*(2), 61-81.

Baker, N. & Sanders, M. (2004). The individual worker perspective. In M. Sanders (Ed.), *Ergonomics and the management of musculoskeletal disorders*. St. Louis, MO: Butterworth-Heinemann.

Bing, R. K. (1989). Work is a four-letter word! A historical perspective. In S. Hertfelder, & C. Gwin (Eds.), *Work in progress: Occupational therapy in work programs*. Rockville, MD: AOTA.

Bonder, B. R., & Wagner, M. B. (2001). *Functional performance in older adults* (2nd ed.). Philadelphia: F.A. Davis.

Bracciano, A. G. (2000). *Physical agent modalities*. Thorofare, NJ: SLACK Incorporated.

Brady, S., Mayer, T. G., & Gatchel, R. J. (1994). Physical progress and residual impairment quantification after functional restoration, Part II. Isokinetic trunk strength. *Spine, 19*, 395-400.

Chaffin, D. B., & Andersson, G. (1984). *Occupational biomechanics*. New York: Wiley.

Chueng, S., & Strough, J. (2004). A comparison of collaborative and individual everyday problem-solving in younger and older adults. *International Journal of Aging and Human Development, 58*(3), 167-195.

Cole, M. B. (1998). *Group dynamics in occupational therapy* (2nd ed.). Thorofare, NJ: SLACK Incorporated.

Demers, L. (1992). *Work hardening: A practical guide*. Boston: Andover Medical Publishers.

Ellexson, M. (2004). Job analysis and worksite assessment. In M. Sanders (Ed.), *Ergonomics and the management of musculoskeletal disorders* (pp. 283-298). St. Louis: Butterworth-Heinemann.

Erikson, E. (1997). *The life cycle completed: Extended version*. New York: W.W. Norton & Company.

Feuerstein, M. (1996). Workstyle: Definition, empirical support, and implications for prevention, evaluation, and rehabilitation of occupational upper-extremity disorders. In S. D. Moon, & S. L. Sauter (Ed.), *Beyond biomechanics: Psychosocial aspects of musculoskeletal disorders in office work*. Bristol, PA: Taylor and Francis.

Fisk, A. D., Charness, N., Rogers, W. A., Czaja, S. J., & Sharit, J. (2004). *Designing for older adults*. New York: CRC Press.

Green, D. P., & Roberts, S. L. (1999). *Kinesiology: Movement in the context of activity*. St. Louis: Mosby.

Guzman, J., Esmail, R., Karjalainen, K., Malmivaara, A., Irvin, E., & Bombardier, C. (2001). Multidisciplinary rehabilitation for chronic low back pain: systematic review. *BMJ, 322*, 1511-1516.

Harvey-Krefting, L. (1985). The concept of work in occupational therapy: A historical review. *American Journal of Occupational Therapy, 39*, 301-307.

Hedge, A. (2004). *Ergonomic guidelines for arranging a computer workstation: 10 steps for users*. Retrieved on Nov. 1, 2004 at: http://ergo.human.cornell.edu/ergoguide.html

Isernhagen, S. J. (1995). *Work injury management*. Gaithersburg, MD: Aspen Publishers.

Jacobs, K. (1991). *Occupational therapy: Work-related programs and assessments* (2nd ed.). Boston: Little, Brown and Company.

Jacobs, K., & Jacobs, L. (2004) *Quick reference dictionary for occupational therapy* (4th ed.). Thorofare, NJ: SLACK Incorporated.

Karasek, R., & Theorell, T. (1990). *Healthy work: Stress, productivity and the reconstruction of working life*. New York: Basic Books.

Key, G. L. (Ed.). (1995). *Industrial therapy*. Philadelphia: Elsevier/Mosby.

Kirsh, B., & McKee, P. (2003). The needs an experiences of injured workers: A participatory research study. *Work, 21*, 221-231.

Kjellen, U. (2000). *Prevention of accidents through experience feedback*. New York: Taylor & Francis.

Krause, T. R. (1997). *The behavior-based safety process* (2nd ed.). New York: John Wiley.

Kroemer, K. H. E., & Grandjean, E. (2001). *Fitting the task to the human* (5th ed.). Philadelphia: Taylor & Francis.

Leveau, B. F. (1992). *Williams's and Lissner's biomechanics of human motion* (3rd ed.). Philadelphia: WB Saunders.

Matheson, L. (1988). How do you know that he tried his best? The reliability crisis in Industrial Rehabilitation. *Industrial Rehabilitation Quarterly*, Spring.

Mayer, T., Taber, J., Bovasso, E., & Gatchel, R. J. (1994). Physical progress and residual impairment quantification after functional restoration, Part I: Lumbar mobility. *Spine, 19*, 389-394.

Melnik, M. (2004). Implementing an effective injury prevention process. In M. Sanders (Ed.), *Ergonomics and the management of musculoskeletal disorders* (pp. 242-360). St. Louis: Butterworth-Heinemann.

Murphy, K. R., & Davidshofer, C. O. (2001). *Psychological testing principles and applications* (5th ed.). New Jersey: Prentice Hall.

National Institute of Occupational Safety and Health (1994). *Applications manual for the revised NIOSH lifting equation, DHHS (NIOSH) Publication No. 94-110*. Cincinatti, OH: NIOSH Publications Dissemination.

National Institute of Occupational Safety and Health (1994). *Elements of Ergonomic programs: A primer based on workplace evaluations of musculoskeletal disorders. DHHS(NIOSH) Publication No. 97-117*. Cincinnati, OH: NIOSH Publications Dissemination.

National Institute of Occupational Safety and Health (1997). *Musculoskeletal disorders and workplace factors: A critical review of epidemiologic evidence for work-related musculoskeletal disorders of the neck, upper extremity and low back*. US Department of Health and Human Services DHHS (NIOSH) Publication No. 97-141.

National Institute of Occupational Safety and Health (1989). *Occupational exposure to hand-arm vibration* [DHHS pub no. 89-106]. Cincinnati: US Department of Health and Human Services.

National Research Council. (1998). *Work-related musculoskeletal disorders: A review of the evidence*. Washington, DC: National Academy Press.

Niemeyer, L., & Jacobs, K. (1989). *Work hardening: State of the art*. Thorofare, NJ: SLACK Incorporated.

Noack, J. (2005). Development of an employer-based injury-prevention program for office workers using ergonomic principles. *OT Practice, 10*(7), CE-1-CE-7.

Oberauer, K., Wendland, M., & Kliefl, R. (2003). Age differences in working memory: The roles of storage and selective access. *Memory & Cognition, 31*(4), 563-569.

Occupational Safety and Health Administration. (1991). Ergonomics program management guidelines for meatpacking plants. Retrieved on Feb. 16, 2005, at http://www.ergoweb.com/resources/reference/guidelines/meatpacking.cfm

Occupational Safety and Health Administration. (nd). Home page. www.osha.gov

Oxenburgh, M. (1997). Cost-benefit analysis of ergonomics programs. *American Industrial Hygiene Association Journal, 58*,150-156.

Pheasant, S. (2001). *Bodyspace*. London: Taylor-Francis.

Prosser, R., & Conolly, W. B. (2003). *Rehabilitation of the hand & upper extremity*. St. Louis: Butterworth-Heinmann.

Ramazzini, B. (1717). *De morbis artificum diatriba*. In W. Wright (Trans, 1940), *The diseases of workers*. Chicago: University of Chicago Press.

Rice, V. (Ed.). (1998). *Ergonomics in health care and rehabilitation*. Woburn, MA: Butterworth-Heinemann.

Sanders, M. (Ed.). (2004). *Ergonomics and the management of musculoskeletal disorders*. St. Louis: Butterworth-Heinemann.

Sanders, M. S., & McCormick, E. J. (1993). *Human factors in engineering and design*. New York: McGraw-Hill, Inc.

Schonstein, E., Kenny, D. T., Keating, J., & Koes, B. W. (2003). Work conditioning, work hardening and functional restoration for workers with back and neck pain. *Cochrane Database Syst Rev., 1*, CD001822.

Schooler, C., Mulatu, M. S., & Oates, G. (1999). The continuing effects of substantively complex work on the intellectual functioning of older workers. *Psychology and Aging, 4*(3), 483-506.

Scully-Palmer, C. (2000). Outcome study: An industrial rehabilitation program. *Work, 15*, 21-23.

Silverstein, B. A., Fine, L. J., & Armstrong, T. J. (1987). Occupational factors and carpal tunnel syndrome. *American Journal of Industrial Medicine, 11*, 343-358.

Smith, M. J., & Carayon, P. (1996). Work organization, stress and cumulative trauma disorders. In S. D. Moon & S. L. Sauter (Eds.), *Beyond biomechanics: Psychosocial aspects of musculoskeletal disorders in office work* (pp. 23-42). Bristol, PA: Taylor and Francis.

Snook, S. (1987). Approaches to the control of back pain in industry: job design, job placement, and education/training. *Spine: State of the Art Reviews, 2,* 45-59.

Stacey, W. (2001). The stress of progression from school to work for adolescents with disabilities... What about life progress? *Work, 17*(3), 175-182.

Stein, F., & Cutler, S. K. (1998). *Psychosocial occupational therapy.* San Diego: Singular Publishing.

Straker, L. M. (2003). A review of research on techniques for lifting low-lying objects: 2. Evidence for a correct technique. *Work, 20,* 83-96.

Tichauer, E. R., & Gage, H. (1977). Ergonomic principles basic to hand tool design. *American Industrial Hygiene Association Journal, 38,* 622-634.

Toosi, M. (2004). Labor force projections to 2012: The graying of the U.S. workforce. *Monthly Labor Review, 127*(2), 37-57.

Trombly, C., & Radomski M. (Ed.) (2002). *Occupational therapy for physical dysfunction* (5th ed.). Philadelphia: Lippincott Williams & Wilkins.

Warren, N. (2004). The expanded definition of ergonomics. In M. Sanders (Ed.), *Ergonomics and the management of musculoskeletal disorders.* St. Louis: Butterworth-Heinemann.

Washington University in St. Louis. (2005). Meet the faculty. Retrieved on June 12, 2005, from www.ot.wustl.edu

Yassi A. (2005). Health promotion in the workplace—The merging of the paradigms. *Methods Inf Med. 44*(2), 278-84.

6b Retirement/Volunteer and End of Life Issues

Marilyn B. Cole, MS, OTR/L, FAOTA

CHAPTER OBJECTIVES

By the end of this chapter, the student will be able to:

☑ Define **retirement and volunteerism** as they pertain to the *Occupational Therapy Practice Framework (Framework)*.

☑ Describe specific **models/frames of reference** as related to retirement and volunteerism.

☑ Comprehend common problems noted in the retirement process.

☑ Delineate between the roles of the **occupational therapist** (OT) and the **occupational therapy assistant** (OTA) as they pertain to the occupations of retirement and volunteerism.

☑ Comprehend and identify related **physical and psychological implications** as related to decreased independence in retirement and volunteerism.

☑ Describe the impact of **contextual factors** upon retirement and volunteerism.

☑ Identify appropriate retirement and volunteerism intervention strategies based on various **performance skills and client factors**.

☑ Identify general retirement and volunteerism **remediation** strategies.

☑ Identify compensation/adaptation intervention strategies related to retirement planning.

☑ Identify specific volunteerism **compensation/adaptation** strategies.

☑ Identify general retirement and volunteerism **maintenance** strategies.

RETIREMENT

RETIREMENT DEFINED

Retirement may be defined as withdrawal from one's position or occupation, or from active working life. Although usually associated with older adulthood (ages 60 to 65), retirement may occur at any age and for a variety of reasons. A retirement age of 65 was first proclaimed by Chancellor Bismarck of Germany in 1889. He chose this age by adding 20 years to the average life expectancy for his day, which was 45. In 1935, the United States government adopted age 65 as the age at which older adults became eligible for retirement pensions (Social Security). Individuals in 1900 spent 3% of their lives in retirement, as compared to 25% to 35% or 20 to 35 years today (Chop, 1999). This section explores both voluntary retirement and mandatory retirement due to changes in health status.

Retirement preparation and adjustment appear under the work area of occupation in the *Occupational Therapy Practice Framework* (*Framework*) (American Occupational Therapy Association [AOTA], 2002). The role of occupational therapy in this area includes "determining aptitudes, developing interests and skills, and selecting appropriate avocational pursuits" (2002, p. 620). This implies the need to replace the worker role by restructuring one's time (temporal organization) and establishing new performance patterns, routines, and roles. Logical outcomes of this process might be linked with occupational therapy's role in the areas of leisure and volunteerism.

Retirement and Health

The obvious link between retirement and health suggests that loss of the worker role can precipitate the onset of declining health. Research correlates retirement with increased risk for a broad range of health conditions, including increased stress (Perreira & Sloan, 2001; Lo & Brown, 1999; Sharpley, 1997), depressive symptoms (Szinovacz & Davey, 2004), alcohol consumption (Perreira & Sloan, 2001), declines in both physical and mental conditions (Gallo, Bradley, Siegel, & Kasl, 2000), suicide (Di Mauro, Leotta, Giuffrida, Distefano, & Grasso, 2003) and a significantly increased risk of mortality (Morris, Cook, & Shaper, 1994). Variables affecting health in retirement identified by researchers include marital status (Szinovacz & Davey, 2004), socioeconomic status (Wilson, 2001), health insurance (Baker, Sudano, Albert, Borawski, & Dor (2002), Social Security retirement incentives (Gruber & Wise, 1999), mental attitude (Reitzes & Mutran, 2004; Mayring, 2000; Fletcher & Hansson, 1991), gender (Geerts, Ponjaert-Kristoffersen, Verbandt & Verte, 1999; Quick & Moen, 1998; Hanson & Wapner, 1994), and life narratives and coping style (Jonsson, Josephsson, & Kielhofner, 2001).

Theories of Retirement and Older Adulthood

Most theories addressing the retirement transition are derived from the developmental theories of older adulthood. Jung and Erikson are most often mentioned in the interdisciplinary literature, and these will be discussed in the upcoming section on end of life issues. Theories of retirement are the subject of debate in the health-related literature. The first debate involves how one makes the transition from working life to retirement. Some theories argue that retirement signals an abrupt change at a more or less predictable age; these are called *age and stage* theories. The other side of this issue looks at all of adult life as a continuation of development into old age. The second debate revolves around the role engagement versus disengagement in life activities plays in the ongoing health and well-being of older adults.

AGE AND STAGE VERSUS CONTINUITY

According to Daniel Levinson's adult transition theory, retirement is a part of the late life transition into older adulthood. A transition begins with a re-evaluation of one's life with regard to life satisfaction and meaning, and often entails the reformulation of goals and priorities. A transition ends when the necessary changes in the structure of one's life are created to allow for continued growth and exploration of new life priorities. This transition normally occurs between the ages of 60 and 65 (Levinson, 1978). *Continuity* theory (Atchley, 1989) suggests that as adults age, they make adaptive choices that tend to preserve existing internal and external structures and strive to maintain their self-identity and existing perceptions of self and the world. One occupational therapy application of continuity theory is Velde and Fidler's Lifestyle Performance Model (2002). In looking at the intrinsic gratification component of an individual's lifestyle, notably some activities continue across the individual's lifetime. However, with advancing age, while interest in a specific activity such as baseball remained, an individual's level of participation changed. A longitudinal study of the retirement process as an occupational transition (Jonsson, Josephsson, & Kielhofner, 2001) attempts to support continuity theory in its use of narratives to link past, present, and future for a group of older workers interviewed before, during, and after retirement. However, an important result of this study, despite the anticipations of the ongoing narrative, "retirement was often full of surprises and temporary periods of turbulence" (p. 44), resonates more closely with Levinson's transitions theory.

DISENGAGEMENT VERSUS ACTIVITY THEORY

Traditionally, two opposing theories have been used to explain retirement and its consequences for occupational health and well being: *disengagement* theory, originally introduced by Cumming and Henry (1961), involves an older adult's inevitable mutual withdrawal from his/her major life roles and responsibilities, which results in decreasing interaction between the aging individual and others in the social systems to which he/she belongs. Some specific findings of these researchers are:

- Older adults become increasingly preoccupied with the self.
- Certain institutions in society promote disengagement.
- Aggressiveness decreases and passivity increases with age.
- Decreased concern for social norms is evident.
- Withdrawal is voluntary as older adults have a greater desire for solitude.
- For many older adults, disengaging means a lower level of life satisfaction.

Disengagement theory has undergone severe criticism for several decades because it reflects the biomedical model that equates aging with sickness and declined function. The notion that all elders are incompetent and on the verge of dying is politically unacceptable in today's culture. Our society makes every attempt to discourage social policy that ignores the elderly (Adams, 2004). Furthermore, the disengagement theory threatens the basic premise behind most publicly funded social programs, which assume that staying active means staying healthy.

Accordingly, occupational therapy has largely dismissed disengagement theory during the last half-century. According to Bonder (2001), a wide variety of recent studies report little change occurs (after retirement) in the number of activities or the intensity of participation. This suggests that while some roles may be lost, such as paid work, other roles, such as volunteering, quickly replace them.

Activity theory (Havighurst, 1961) has contradicted disengagement theory almost from the beginning. This theory proposes that greater continued engagement in activities leads to greater life satisfaction in the later years. OTs have embraced this theory, as have most senior social programs over the last half-century. Many research studies have confirmed the positive effect activity participation has on the health and well-being of older adults. A good deal of medically oriented research has demonstrated the continued competence of older adults, as well as their inclination and suitability for continued employment or avocational involvement. Elders themselves resist the notion of retirement, as evidenced by a recent article on the *Retirement Living* Website entitled "Aging Baby Boomers Shun the 'R' word" (retrieved 11/12/04). The well-elderly study, a well-known randomized controlled trial (Clark, Azen, Zemke, Jackson, Carlson, Mandel et al., 1997; Jackson et al, 1998) supports occupational therapy interventions that help community living older adults to stay active and involved.

THE THIRD AGE AND OTHER CONTEMPORARY THEORIES

More recent theorists have attempted to create a compromise between the disengagement and activity theories. Atchley (1975, 1976) defined retirement as a four-stage process: honeymoon, disenchantment, reorientation, and termination.

1. Honeymoon phase: New retirees actively pursue projects previously precluded by employment, such as traveling or remodeling their homes.

2. Disenchantment phase: Realization retirement hasn't worked out as they had hoped, requiring retirees to cope with the negative realities of retirement such as loss of income.

3. Reorientation phase: Re-evaluation of life leads to restructuring of one's lifestyle, including a search for meaningful occupations and establishing a new daily routine.

4. Termination: Advanced aging and the onset of disability necessitate dependence on others.

Atchley's theory, which has been validated in more recent studies (Reitzes & Mutran, 2004), paved the way for the current separation of young-old from old-old.

Peter Laslett's (1997) idea of separating young retirees from the older ones has growing credibility in light of recent research. Laslett divided life into four stages:

1. Childhood and preparation for work.

2. Employment and raising one's family.

3. Third age beginning with retirement and ending with the onset of disability.

4. Old age and dependence.

The term *Third Age* represents a change in the culture of aging based upon the reality of an extended life expectancy and a delayed onset of age-related functional decline. The Third Age concept has spawned a worldwide plan of action on aging: to provide for continued growth and education for successful aging to the "young old" and to better prepare them for the Fourth Age of dependency and physical decline (Baltes & Smith, 2001). Several thousand Universities of the Third Age (U3A) have opened across the globe, beginning with the University of Toulouse in 1973, the two major archetypes being French and British U3A models (Formosa, 2000). Most offer educational programs based on the preference of members, including instruction in crochet, dressmaking, bridge, and wine appreciation, as well as the study of a broad range of age-related topics dubbed *educational gerontology* (Withnall, 2002). Predictably, typical elderly participants (students) tend to fall within the 60 to 70 age cohort (Formosa, University of Malta, retrieved 4/22/05).

COMMON PROBLEMS IN RETIREMENT

The literature on retirement discusses a broad range of positive and negative consequences. Many older adults view retirement as a long-awaited liberation from responsibility, an increase in leisure time, and an opportunity to pursue more creative endeavors (Cohen, 1999). This may indeed be true when retirement is voluntary, accompanied by adequate financial and social pre-planning, and the retiree remains healthy and energetic. However, even the most healthy and well-prepared retirees seem destined to struggle with the transition to retirement. As Clark, et al. (1997) predicted, the process requires an active involvement in the redesign of one's lifestyle. The following is a summary of some of the predictable problems with adjusting to retirement:

- Loss of the worker role.

- Lack of time structure.

- Changes in social interactions and relationships.
- Loss of purpose or daily meaning.
- Financial factors and loss of income.
- Increased stress.
- Decline in social status.

Loss of the Worker Role

Working involves more than bringing home a paycheck. For many, working becomes very much a part of one's identity. In leaving work after many years of employment, the new retiree may also be leaving behind a vast social network that provided a major source of social and emotional support. People in Western cultures incorporate a strong work ethic that sustains them through educational programs, vocational training, and their income earning years. However, this same ethic provides little incentive for learning to relax and enjoy life, causing most to arrive at retirement largely unprepared.

Lack of Time Structure

This may be the biggest challenge of all. Work provides a daily structure for most of one's life, through a more or less routine activity (performance) pattern. The *Framework* defines performance patterns (habits) as "Automatic behavior which is integrated into more complex patterns which enable people to function on a day-to-day basis…" (AOTA, 2002, p. 623). Younger adults who manage their time effectively often spend 75% to 90% of their day in routines (Cole, 1998). In effect, the loss of these well-learned routines necessitates a large investment of energy in restructuring one's time in ways that are satisfying and meaningful. Assisting retirees in redesigning their lifestyle is an important role for OTs working with this age group.

Changes in Social Interactions and Relationships

After many years of interaction with colleagues and coworkers, retirees often find themselves suddenly disconnected from important social networks. When family relationships and friendships outside of work have not been nurtured along the way, retirement often involves the need to rebuild one's social circles. People who attempt to continue connections with former coworkers often find these relationships unfulfilling. Retirees may need the assistance of OTs in finding new occupations within which to build shared experiences with others.

Loss of Purpose or Daily Meaning

Retirees whose identity is highly invested in their worker role are more likely to experience feelings of depression after leaving work. The loss of pleasure in daily activities can lead to a loss of self-worth accompanied by feelings of helplessness and hopelessness. Part of retirement planning needs to address the exploration of leisure interests and potential volunteer roles that the client finds engaging and meaningful. The types of occupations retired individuals find meaningful vary widely. According to Warr, Butcher, & Robertson (2004), occupations in the "family and social" and "church and charity" domains most highly correlate with affective well-being and life satisfaction. The Jonsson, Josephsson, & Kielhofner (2001) study confirms the importance of *engaging occupations* in the achievement of life satisfaction in retirement. An engaging occupation is one infused with meaning, enjoyment, challenge, intensity, and a commitment or connection with others (the community). This finding gives positive guidance for occupational therapy interventions with those anticipating or transitioning into retirement.

Financial Factors and Loss of Income

Statistics tell us that many Baby Boomers reaching retirement age in the next 3 to 10 years will not be financially prepared (Hershey & Mowen, 2000). For others, retirement will be accompanied by pensions or lump sum retirement plan payouts that will need careful management in order to provide sufficient monthly income to sustain retirees for another 20 to 25 years. Major marketing efforts in the United States focus on this trend, offering investments, financial advisement, long-term care insurance, and retirement community housing options in many appealing locations. Still, a large percentage of retirees will need assistance with adjusting their lifestyle to a lower or fixed income. The *Framework* (2002) defines financial management as "using fiscal resources, including alternate methods of financial transaction and planning and using finances with long-term and short-term goals" (p. 620). Finances have a profound effect on one's lifestyle. OTs may need to assist retirees in restructuring their living arrangements, daily habits, and activity patterns to accommodate changes in economic resources.

Increased Stress

On Holmes' (1978) Social Readjustment Rating Scale, retirement ranks number 10 out of 43 stressful life events, yielding a stress score of 43 out of 100. Sharpley (1997) used a Self-Perceived Stress in Retirement Scale to study the effects of stress on retirees from 6 months to 5 years post-retirement. Three factors were found to produce stress: 1) missing work, 2) personal health, and 3) relationship issues. Parsons (2003) looked at the effects of stress on overall lifespan. He noted the longevity of "well nourished humans of the modern era" cannot be entirely explained by the propensity for stress resistance, and evolutionary theories of aging need to be considered. Krause (1986) found that older women living alone are more vulnerable to the effects of chronic life strain and stressful life events. McAndrew (2002) notes that many stressful life events can coincide with retirement, having a cumulative effect on the older adult. For example, retirement (stress score 45), may be accompanied by a personal injury or illness (53), a change in financial status (38), a change in number of marital arguments (35), a change in living conditions (25), and revision of personal habits (24), yielding an overwhelming level of stress for the retiree. OTs may be called upon to assist clients in identifying stressors, developing or supporting coping mechanisms, and establishing new routines to reduce or manage stress (see Table 6b-1).

Decline in Social Status

Work often provides a basis for social status, not only because of the income generated, but also because of one's position within the work organization. Persons having a powerful position within a corporation enjoy a feeling of control over others and their own working conditions and environment. This feeling of control may be difficult to duplicate in avocational pursuits after retirement. Because of the strong work ethic of Western cultures, gainful employment in any capacity implies a higher level of social status than that of unemployment. After retirement, it is inevitable that some older adults will be viewed differently by others in their social circles and communities. The Third Age movement has done much to counteract the negative stigma of retirement. Riley and Riley (1994) envision a *non-age differentiating society* without age expectations for school, work, or retirement. These researchers identified a *structural lag* that exists with regard to societal attitudes about work and retirement. Ageism in society still creates barriers for older adults seeking continued career growth or experiences in lifelong learning. OTs can evaluate social contexts in the immediate, community, and institutional environments and assist clients with overcoming these barriers to continued participation through engagement in meaningful occupations with others.

Table 6b-1

Holmes' Social Readjustment Rating Scale

Life Event	Mean Value
1. Death of spouse	100
2. Divorce	73
3. Marital separation from mate	65
4. Detention in jail or other institution	63
5. Death of a close family member	63
6. Major personal injury or illness	53
7. Marriage	50
8. Being fired from work	47
9. Marital reconciliation with mate	45
10. Retirement from work	45
11. Major change in the health or behavior of a family member	44
12. Pregnancy	40
13. Sexual difficulties	39
14. Gaining a new family member (through birth, adoption, elder moving in, etc.)	39
15. Major business readjustment (merger, reorganization, bankruptcy, etc.)	39
16. Major change in financial state (a lot worse or better off than usual)	38
17. Death of a close friend	37
18. Changing to a different line of work	36
19. Major change in the number of arguments with spouse (a lot more/less)	35
20. Taking on a mortgage (purchasing a home or business, etc.)	31
21. Foreclosure on a mortgage or loan	30
22. Major change in responsibilities at work (promotion, demotion, transfer)	29
23. Son or daughter leaving home (marriage, attending college, etc.)	29
24. In-law troubles	29
25. Outstanding personal achievement	28
26. Spouse beginning or ceasing work outside the home	26

continued

Table 6b-1, continued

HOLMES' SOCIAL READJUSTMENT RATING SCALE

Life Event	Mean Value
27. Beginning or ceasing formal schooling	26
28. Major change in living conditions (building a new home, remodeling, deterioration of home or neighborhood)	25
29. Revision of personal habits (dress, manners, associations, etc.)	24
30. Troubles with the boss	23
31. Major change in working hours or conditions	20
32. Change in residence	20
33. Changing to a new school	20
34. Major change in usual type or amount of recreation.	19
35. Major change in church activities (+/-)	19
36. Major change in social activities (clubs, dancing, movies, visiting, etc.)	18
37. Taking on a mortgage or loan less than $10,000 (purchasing a car, TV, freezer, etc.)	17
38. Major change in sleeping habits (a lot more/less sleep or change in part of day when asleep	16
39. Major change in number of family get-togethers (a lot more/less than usual)	15
40. Major change in eating habits (a lot more/less or very different meal hours or surroundings	15
41. Vacation	15
42. Christmas	12
43. Minor violations of the law (traffic tickets, jaywalking, disturbing the peace, etc.	11

Note: If events over past year add up to greater than 200 points, person is at risk for stress-related health conditions.

Reprinted with permission from Holmes, T. (1978) Life situations, emotions, and disease. Psychosomatic Medicine, p. 747. Copyright U. of Washington Press.

RETIREMENT INTERVENTIONS

While much has been written about OTs' role with the elderly, little attention has been given to retirement specifically. This section will review individual and group approaches to the various aspects of retirement.

Early Retirement

The incidence of early retirement in the United States has declined in recent years, partly due to an increasing scarcity of younger workers. Of those who do retire early, approximately 30% do so because of ill health. For these individuals, a decrease in financial wealth due to loss of income has a statistical relationship with a worsening of disability and an increased need for health services (Disney, Grundy, & Johnson, 1994).

PREVENTION

There is evidence that interventions that promote worker adaptation and employer accommodation following the onset of a health impairment may enable workers to keep their jobs or continue to be gainfully employed (Daly & Bound, 1996). A 6-month occupational health intervention program for workers (age 50+) at risk for early retirement demonstrated a 50% reduction in early retirement (De Boer, van Beck, Durinck, Verbach, & Van Dijk, 2004). Clients whose illness or injury has caused a leave of absence from their current jobs with the expectation of returning to work may be good candidates for such prevention programs.

Clients' use of strategies such as incorporating relaxation or exercise into their work routines or changing the movements used to accomplish work tasks are examples of worker adaptations. Using adaptive equipment, such as sound enhanced telephones or adapted computer keyboards, may be initiated by either client or employer. Examples of accommodations made by the employer include flexible working hours to accommodate rest or exercise breaks, physical changes in positioning such as ergonomic office chairs, or changes in task demand such as conference calls replacing on-site meetings. OTs may play a consulting or advisory role with clients and their employers to make mutually beneficial adjustments to the work situation in order to prevent the necessity of early retirement.

Self-assessed poor health has been found to be a strong predictor of early retirement due to mental disorders, musculoskeletal disorders, and cardiovascular diseases (Karpansalo, Manninen, Kauhanen, Lakka, & Salonen (2004). In workers with chronic low back pain, anxiety and the perception of control by others contributed significantly to the incidence of early retirement (Harkapaa, 1992). In another study, a positive link was found between cigarette smoking and early retirement due to permanent disability (Rothenbacher, Arndt, Fraisse, Aschenderlein, Fliedner, & Brenner, 1998). These findings provide evidence of the need for group preventive programs in the workplace.

ESTABLISHING, REMEDIATING, AND MAINTAINING WORK FUNCTIONS

When illness or injury causes temporary inability to work, the OT's role in rehabilitation may focus on work readiness. Specific interventions may be designed to build skills related to an identified work role, as well as building range of motion (ROM), strength, and endurance while performing simulated work tasks. These areas are explained in Chapter 6a.

COMPENSATION/ADAPTATION

When health conditions prevent a return to former employment, the OT's role is somewhat similar to working with an older retiree. Persons facing early retirement need help in making the transition to a new life structure. An assessment of skills and aptitudes may lead to recommendations for volunteer work, alternative part-time work, and/or participation in community organizations. However, there are some essential differences that OTs must consider when working with early retirees.

A younger retiree may wish to continue family or social roles that are different from those of an older adult. New areas of socialization with peers of a similar age group may be needed. When working with a younger retiree, special attention should be given to the client's life stage, and the occupations that can facilitate continued growth and development. For example, a single or divorced young adult for whom dancing and bicycling are no longer physically possible could participate in discussion groups or organizational fundraising with others in his/her age group. An individual with a specific health condition, such as a cancer survivor, might find it meaningful to volunteer to help others with a similar condition.

Middle aged retirees might find volunteer caregiving roles meaningful, or roles that utilize their special skills and talents in more creative ways. For example, in the case study at the end of the chapter, Debi worked as a nursing supervisor in a busy surgical unit prior to her stroke at age 47. Afterwards, she discovered she had a latex allergy that was exacerbated by the routine use of latex gloves and other equipment during medical procedures. In the year of rehabilitation following her stroke, Debi used her computer to establish an online information center for other latex allergy sufferers, a role that allowed her to use her medical background to help others by managing the Web site from the comfort of her home.

Retirement Planning in Older Adulthood

Most sources agree that preplanning has a positive effect on smoothing the transition into retirement (Nuttman-Shwartz, 2004), as well as life satisfaction afterwards (Reitzes & Mutran, 2004). Some of the factors associated with a successful retirement include a feeling of well-being, relatively good health, continued social interactions, and an optimistic outlook (Mayring, 2000). An older retirement age (Salokangas & Joukamaa, 1991) and a high frequency and variety of social contacts (Reeves & Darville, 1994) are correlated with greater life satisfaction in retirement.

PREVENTION

Hershey and Mowen (2000) examined financial preplanning skills through the use of hypothetical retirement scenarios requiring the participant to apply problem-solving and decision-making strategies. They concluded that both financial knowledge and personality constructors predicted the extent of preretirement planning. One of the most significant findings of this study for OTs is the need for future orientation and an ability to visualize the future. Thus, in addition to the need for education and training with regard to financial planning, occupational therapy prevention groups can be designed to focus on the ability to visualize personal future scenarios, to predict the consequences of alternative modes of behavior, and to make conscious choices regarding steps required to achieve one's goals. Furthermore, these researchers suggest that different preplanning strategies may be required for different personality types. OTs are well-prepared to develop group activities utilizing different learning styles to promote these essential skills for adequate retirement planning.

Allen's Cognitive Levels (ACLs) assessments may help OTs to identify clients who lack the ability to visualize the future. In considering the ACLs, an essential difference between levels 5 (trial and error) and 6 (planned actions) involves the lack of ability to anticipate consequences. Those clients identified as below level 6 might therefore be considered at risk, or lacking the essential skills necessary for adequate retirement planning.

Transitions at Retirement: Establishing, Restoring, or Maintaining (Remediation) the Occupational Areas, Skills, and Patterns for Health and Well-Being

Considering recent theoretical developments and research with regard to retirement, clients in the Third Age must be treated differently from those of the 80-plus age group. The preponderance

The following is a time line beginning the year you were born and continuing to 10 years from today. Please place an X along this line to record each major event of your life, including year.

- Birth
- Graduations
- Marriage
- Moving to new location
- Birth of children
- Employment changes
- Retirement
- Personal injury or illness
- Specific leisure pursuits begun
- Important volunteer positions initiated or ended
- Any other important life events

X_____X _____X
Birth   Now   Death

Figure 6b-1. Timeline evaluation at retirement with future perspective.

of evidence points toward a continuation of active involvement in occupations and interactions with others as the key to successful retirement for the 60 to 80 age group. OTs need to recognize that the transition to retirement is a process, one that many retirees handle poorly without professional help. Several adult developmental theories can guide occupational therapy interventions for this age group. Some of the tasks are reappraising the past, re-examining one's values and goals, evaluating and nurturing selected social connections, rebalancing one's time, recognizing age- and health-related adaptations, and redesigning one's lifestyle. Each of these tasks will be discussed in the following sections.

REAPPRAISING THE PAST

In individual work, the OT may facilitate this process by asking thoughtful questions, or through evaluation activities. One useful tool in looking back over one's life is to create a timeline. The client identifies significant life events along a continuum from birth to the present. Extending the timeline 10 years into the future will give the OT an indication of the client's future time perspective (Figure 6b-1).

In the case of Matt, several major changes cluster around specific years, creating a pattern of crisis and recovery, with work being the main means of coping. As this individual approaches retirement, pacing the changes and establishing alternate coping strategies is critical.

Reminiscence is another way OTs may facilitate life reappraisal (Parker, 1995). The occupational therapy perspective in planning reminiscence groups (unlike recreational groups) should focus specifically on the client's perceptions of life's accomplishments and disappointments, and on identifying client coping strategies that have failed or succeeded in the past. The outcome of this group activity may assist clients in identifying the unmet goals and meaningful occupations that will be continued into retirement.

RE-EXAMINING ONE'S VALUES AND GOALS

A natural outgrowth of the re-evaluation process may be to affirm or change one's values. The value of building wealth leads young adults to spend most of their time and energy advancing their career. In retirement, clients will need to redirect their energy toward other values, such as deep-

Figure 6b-2. Grandpa's changing roles in retirement.

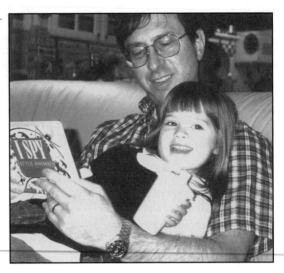

ening their relationships with others, or contributing to their communities. Identifying enduring values builds a foundation for setting occupational priorities after retirement, such as joining community organizations (socialization), volunteering for social causes (altruism), engaging in health promoting or creative activities (physical and mental health), or becoming more active grandparents (meaningful family relationships). Awareness of values increases the likelihood that clients will set occupational priorities that are meaningful and satisfying in their retirement years. OTs may examine values as a part of the evaluation process, or create individual or group interventions that focus on awareness of one's values.

EVALUATING AND NURTURING SELECTED SOCIAL CONNECTIONS

Continued socialization has been recognized by researchers as one of the most important factors for successful aging. At retirement, daily interactions with coworkers is lost, putting new retirees at risk for social isolation. Family connections, which may not have been nurtured while working, often cause stress rather than satisfaction according to some studies. Some married retirees find their newfound togetherness 24/7 to be more intrusive than satisfying (Szinovacz & Davey, 2004). An important intervention for occupational therapy may involve identifying occupations that retired couples enjoy doing together, as well as a rebalancing of home maintenance, financial management, and social planning activities.

Retirees with grandchildren may want to change their grandparenting style with retirement (Figure 6b-2). Neugarten and Weinstein (1964) identified five patterns of grandparenting:

1. Formal: Limited contact with grandchildren with no parental responsibilities.

2. Fun-seeking: Frequent informal contact focused on sharing leisure activities.

3. Surrogate: Assuming parental responsibilities in the absence of parents who may be working or otherwise unavailable (usually grandmothers).

4. Conveyer of family wisdom: Special role of transmitting family history, culture, or traditions, and of giving advice (usually grandfathers).

5. Distant figures: Contact limited to ritualistic events, such as birthdays and holidays.

Researchers have found the fun-seeking and distant styles are more common for grandparents under 65 years, and both frequency of contact and role may change with retirement. In an unpublished study of meaningful activities for older adults in the United States and Costa Rica, family relationships and interactions with adult children and grandchildren was the number one priority for both cultures (Cole, 2001).

Rebalancing One's Time

Some developmental theories identify a change in time perspective in older adulthood to *time left to live*, incorporating a recognition of the approaching end of life. Awareness of death gives a new importance to making each day count. With this in mind, OTs can take a closer look at the way clients spend their time, with the following goals:

- Eliminating occupations that have little meaning, such as watching TV.

- Identifying gaps in time that can be available for meaningful occupations such as volunteering, socializing, exercising, or creative pursuits.

- Recognizing or establishing routines for obligatory activities such as self-care, home maintenance, grocery shopping, and paying bills.

- Balancing occupational areas of avocation, leisure, self-care, and sleep to meet the older adult's changing physical and psychological needs.

A good occupational therapy evaluation for this area is the occupational Activity Configuration, which asks clients to keep track of what they are doing each hour of the day for 1 week. Filling this out with family members may assist elderly clients who have memory difficulties (Table 6b-2).

The outcome of an activity configuration is a discussion of one's temporal organization. The *Framework* defines *temporal organization* as a performance process skill that involves the "beginning, logical ordering, continuation, and completion of steps and action sequences of a task" (AOTA, 2002, p. 622). OTs need to help older adults to perform occupations more efficiently in order to pace themselves and conserve energy for their most meaningful tasks. Often this means the intentional learning and practice of routines until they become automatic, requiring less physical and mental energy. For example, forming the habit of assembling all ingredients and equipment for a specific meal before beginning the preparation saves one the time and energy of making multiple trips to the refrigerator or pantry. Using routines for taking care of basic needs enables the client to spend more time and energy on enjoyment and socialization.

Recognizing Age- and Health-Related Adaptations

As noted by Velde and Fidler (2002), while one's interest in specific activities may endure over one's lifetime, the individual's level of participation may change. OTs assist clients who have health conditions that prevent them from engaging in the occupations that create meaning for them. For example, an older client who once enjoyed mountain climbing might need to adapt hiking plans for more level terrain, wear supportive footgear, and limit the length and pace of exploratory walking.

The older adults in Figure 6b-3 are not permitted to garden outside their small apartments, even if they felt energetic and flexible enough to do so. Occupational therapy students have helped them adapt their interest in gardening by potting and learning to care for houseplants.

Another occupational therapy approach that sheds light on the role of occupation in well-being is the concept of personal projects (Christiansen, Backman, Little, & Nguyen, 1990). In their study of 120 adults, perceived progress in completing personal projects that represented meaningful occupations for individuals was highly correlated with well-being. Engaging occupations, a related concept, were identified by Jonsson et al (2001) as those that evoked a depth of passion or feeling, with a specific meaning for the retiree. The presence or absence of engaging occupations "appeared to be the main determinant of whether participants were able to achieve positive life experiences as retirees" (p. 428).

Table 6b-2

OCCUPATIONAL ACTIVITY CONFIGURATION

	Mon.	Tue.	Wed.	Thurs.	Fri.	Sat.	Sun.
1 am							
2 am							
3 am							
4 am							
5 am							
6 am							
7 am							
8 am							
9 am							
10 am							
11 am							
Noon							
1 pm							
2 pm							
3 pm							
4 pm							
5 pm							
6 pm							
7 pm							
8 pm							
9 pm							
10 pm							
11pm							
Midnight							

REDESIGNING ONE'S LIFESTYLE

The well elderly study (Clark, et al, 1997) mentioned earlier gives a good example of an occupational therapy intervention program with Third Age older adults. These researchers point out that older adults often have "neither the knowledge nor the ability to determine health-relevant consequences of their occupations" (1998, p. 329). Eight modules are identified, which guide small groups (8 to 10) of community living older adults through an "occupational self-analysis (p. 330)." Each module forms a structure for several group meetings, which includes some form of didactic presentation, peer exchange, direct experience, and personal exploration. The format allows members to learn, discuss, problem-solve, and make choices according to their own interests and needs. The module content areas are as follows:

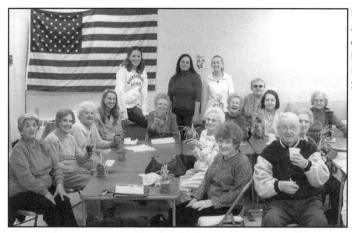

Figure 6b-3. Occupational therapy group intervention: from outdoor gardening to caring for houseplants (photo courtesy of Elm Terrace Senior Housing, Stratford, CT).

1. Introduction to the power of occupation: Discussion of how occupational choices affect well-being and create daily structure and meaning.

2. Aging, health, and occupation: Building healthy occupational habits and activities.

3. Transportation: Alternative ways to access and participate in the community.

4. Safety: In the home and neighborhood, crime prevention strategies, body mechanics.

5. Social relationships: Dealing with loss, maintaining friendships, and finding new friends.

6. Cultural awareness: Learning and sharing diverse aspects of group members and appreciating how culture shapes our daily occupations and social expectations.

7. Finances: Learning skills of budgeting, managing money, and engaging in affordable occupations.

8. Integrative summary: Lifestyle redesign journal. Reviewing the collected occupational knowledge and experience of the group using writing and photographs to construct individual roadmaps for the road ahead.

Lifestyle means many things, but for the older adult transitioning to retirement, it always means change. OTs have the skills to assist older adults in thinking about what needs changing, restructuring their time to accommodate the changes, and balancing occupations to maintain or restore health, socialization, and personal fulfillment.

END OF LIFE ISSUES

Theories of Old Age

Jung and Erikson pioneered the extension of adult development theory into later life. Jung (1933) observed the tendency for introversion in later years, focusing on more philosophical and spiritual issues. Of eight stages focusing on psychosocial development, Erik Erikson's final two stages apply to older adulthood: Generativity versus self-absorption, and ego integrity versus despair (Erikson, 1963; Schuster, 1992; Westermeyer, 2004). Although Erikson envisioned his eight stages as epigenetic, requiring resolution of conflicts in a defined hierarchy, the tasks are potentially reversible and do not necessarily follow a rigid sequence or specific timing (Vaillant, 1993). The primary focus of generativity is "the culmination of adulthood when the individual becomes a responsible guide or mentor for the next generation." More recently, two aspects of generativity have been identified by McAdams, Hart, & Maruna (1998): 1) a desire to play an active role in the next generation, and 2) empathy or compassion for others. The extension of generativity into old age was demonstrated by Shmotkin, Blumstein, & Modan (2003), who found that volunteer roles resulted in more positive psychological functioning and reduced mortality risk for the 75 to 94 age group. The primary focus of Erikson's integrity phase is the personal satisfaction with one's accomplishments and contributions, giving importance to the tasks of reminiscence and life review, the late life resolution of unfinished issues, and reconciliation of rifts with significant others in the past.

FOURTH AGE AND OTHER CONTEMPORARY THEORIES

While Laslett's theory represents a continued hierarchy of developmental stages, it acknowledges the relative health and vitality of the 60 to 80 age group as compared with octogenarians (over 80), who may exhibit the characteristics of disengagement found by Cumming and Henry so long ago. In fact, several studies over the last decade have confirmed some aspects of disengagement for this older age group. Johnson & Barer (1992) found that 50% of those over 85 years could be considered disengaged. Signs of this were: 1) a redefinition of social boundaries, 2) a change in time orientation, and 3) a decrease in emotional intensity. For the Fourth Age elders, a voluntary narrowing of one's social circle has been recognized as *Socioemotional Selectivity Theory (SST)* (Carstensen, 1992). Longtime friendships and family relationships take on a deeper meaning, while more superficial relationships are dropped. This voluntary disengagement allows older adults to conserve emotional energy, pace themselves, and reduce worry about others (Adams, 2004). Another study supporting SST suggests social supports provided by new acquaintances within retirement communities are not as meaningful, and do not replace the support of long-term friendships (Potts, 1997).

The Fourth Age adult's time orientation changes to focus on the present, while future and past diminish. Future becomes less relevant as death approaches, while the past fades away along with the loss of contemporaries who remember them when they were younger. Emotional intensity appears to diminish in elders who have come to terms with mortality, perhaps because they have nothing left to fear. Those over 85 spend more time sleeping, and feel fairly comfortable with spending time alone (Larson, Csikszentmihalyi, & Graef, 1982).

Gerotranscendence, another contemporary outgrowth of disengagement theory, focuses on the positive potential of cognitive changes that occur as the aging individual constructs a new reality, one that shifts from pragmatic and materialistic to a more cosmic and transcendent worldview. This internal, contemplative way of life, which trades in meaningless socialization for solitude, appears to be accompanied by an increase in life satisfaction (Tornstam, 1989, 1997, 2000). The cosmic dimension, which conceptually unites the past and present, may symbolize true wisdom for the older individual. In this state, the individual feels free to select only activities that are meaningful and to ignore the necessity for social reciprocation or convention.

Joan Erikson, Erik's wife and frequent collaborator, wrote at age 93 about the need for solitude as a possible Erikson's Ninth Stage, a "deliberate retreat from the usual engagements of daily activity... a paradoxical state which does seem to exhibit a transcendent quality (Erikson & Erikson, 1997, p.25)."

Adams (2004) compared the changes in investment in activities and interests between the young-old (65 to 74) and the old-old (75 to 94). Her findings support specific aspects of disengagement, socioemotional selectivity, and gerotranscendence theories, and can guide OTs in determining appropriate interventions for this population. Adams found interest in some activities diminished significantly from the Third to the Fourth Age, while other interests remained keen. In summary, this study found that after 85, interests shift away from active instrumental pursuits requiring physical or social effort, and toward more social, intellectual, and spiritual pursuits (Adams, 2004, p.103). See Table 6b-3 for a summary.

Table 6b-3

ADAMS' RESEARCH ON CHANGING INVESTMENT IN ACTIVITIES IN ELDERS' LIVES

Less Interested After 85	*More Interested After 85*
Making and creating things	Hearing from family and friends
Shopping and buying things	Spiritual life/prayer
Making plans for the future	Pleasure in small things
Keeping up with hobbies	Visit with family
Entertaining others in my home	Religious services
Social events with new people	Reading, puzzles, computer
Taking care of people and things	Getting together with old friends
Meeting new people	Keeping up with current events
Concern with others' opinions of me	Worrying about friends/family's problems
Feeling I should share opinions and advice	Being a good neighbor
Spending time with others	

Adapted from Adams, K. B. (2004). Changing investment in activities and interests in elders' lives: Theory and measurement. *International Journal of Aging and Human Development, 58,* 87-108.

OTs need to be aware of the signs of gerotranscendence, and to avoid forcing unwelcome socialization upon Fourth Age older adults. Those activities in Table 6b-3, column 2 can serve as a guide in planning meaningful activities for this age group.

Preparing for Long-Term Care

Many older adults do not plan ahead for the time when they will be dependent on others for their care, probably for the same reasons they do not plan for retirement—being unable or unwilling to visualize their future. With Baby Boomers reaching retirement age soon, many marketing efforts focus on planning for long-term care, but these efforts focus mostly on investment in retirement communities and purchasing long-term care insurance.

Moving to a Different Location

By definition, Fourth Agers have at least one disability that causes them to be dependent on others. Choices need to be made about who will provide needed services. Cultural beliefs vary widely concerning family caregiving, and it cannot be assumed that Grandma will move in with one of her adult children. Alternative choices are staying in one's home with adaptations for safety and function and daily visits by health care professionals; moving into specialized housing, such as an assisted living facility, or entering a nursing home. Crist (1999) compared the quality of life among these choices for older adults with an average age of 87. She found specialized housing offered the highest quality of life related to socialization, while nursing homes offered the lowest quality of life. In each of these choices, OTs adapt the home environment to maximize occupational performance in IADL and self-care, recognizing changes in personal routines and habits are difficult for the older age group. Elders who choose to live alone may need assistance in finding resources to take care of basic necessities. OTs need to be knowledgeable about community services including housekeeping, transportation, and socialization opportunities that are not beyond the abilities of the elder client.

Changes in residence and living conditions cause stress at any age, but may be more stressful for the older adult who simultaneously faces a decline in health status. An older adult who has well-learned routines for self-care may be able to function fairly independently in a familiar environment, but the same individual may be totally dependent in an unfamiliar one. OTs may need to work with the elder and caregivers to re-establish self-care routines in a new setting, and to bring in familiar objects, such as quilts, pictures, books, or a wall clock with a familiar look and sound. For example, one older adult who tended to get agitated found it a great comfort to sit and rock in a familiar rocking chair that was brought in by her daughter.

Scaling Down Belongings

The transition of moving to smaller living quarters involves making decisions about what to keep, and what to give away, sell, or discard. Tasks such as these require a high level of cognition. When a Fourth Age client shows signs of mild dementia, the sorting of belongings may require the help of a family member. Some tasks for the OT, family, and client in this area are determining criteria for: 1) what to keep, 2) what to discard, and 3) who will be the recipients of discarded items.

- Which clothing items will be appropriate for the anticipated environment, and which will require the least care and effort with independent dressing?
- What kitchen or bathroom items will be needed in the new location?
- What objects will be needed for meaningful leisure pursuits?
- Which items of furniture will fit safely/limit obstacles in the new location?
- Gathering personally meaningful items such as photographs, letters, souvenirs, or artwork for storage in the minimum amount of space (scrapbooks, wall shelves).
- Deciding what items of value will be given to important or significant others.
- Finding charities or other needy recipients for items in good condition that are no longer needed.

Scaling down becomes more difficult as one ages, and may become overwhelming when the elder has collected many belongings over a lifetime. Organizing objects and spaces in one's task environments is a process skill defined by the *Framework* (AOTA, 2002). For the elder client, removing clutter will increase functional performance in ADL and IADL tasks.

Safety Issues in Physical, Cognitive, and Sensory Loss

A recent conversation with older adults living in a senior housing project focused on their fear of falling. Many of these elders had health conditions that affected their mobility, including arthritis, hip or knee replacement surgery, multiple sclerosis, and low vision. Their fear of falling prevented them from performing health maintenance activities, like walking around the block, or taking public transportation to community social activities and services. This exemplifies one of the many barriers to participation that could be addressed by OTs.

Allen's Cognitive Disabilities model guides occupational therapy interventions for cognitive decline. The ACL Screening, the Routine Task Inventory, and the Allen Diagnostic Module provide the OT with an opportunity to observe a client's level of problem solving in ADLs. Guidelines of environmental adaptations, caregiver education, appropriate adaptive equipment, and assistance required for maximum functional independence within safety parameters may be found in Allen, Blue & Earhart (1995; 2001).

UNDERSTANDING COGNITIVE MODES OF PERFORMANCE

For sensory loss, many adaptations are available, such as sound enhanced telephones and large print books. However, the OT's role will often be to adapt specific activities and environments to enable desired occupational performance. For example, inserting textured tape on the numbered dial of the microwave enables the client with low vision to choose the correct number of minutes for heating up a frozen dinner independently. Discussion with older adults regarding other safety issues may include: driving safety, walking safety, meal preparation safety, use of home appliances, reaching for items in high or low cabinets, home repair activities, and yard work or gardening. Communication devices and accessibility in case of emergency is another important consideration for OTs working with elders living alone. See Chapters 3 and 4 for more information regarding adaptation of ADLs and IADLs.

Hospice Care: Occupational Therapy Roles

When the end of life is near, clients may qualify for hospice care through a doctor's certification of limited life expectancy. A broad range of health conditions may be the cause, including cancer, AIDS, Alzheimer's, Amyotrophic Lateral Sclerosis (ALS), and congestive heart failure (CHF). Hospice care may be provided at specialized facilities, or in the client's own home, guided by the following five principles:

1. Pain and symptom control—For comfort, not cure.
2. 24-hour care available in familiar and comfortable surroundings.
3. Diagnostic honesty—Full openness with client and family.
4. Quality of life for client—Respect for preferences and choices.
5. Bereavement care for the family.

According to AOTA, occupational therapy's role in hospice care is to contribute to a comprehensive plan involving the client and family in daily living activities of work, leisure, and self-care (AOTA, undated brochure). OTs work to enable occupations as follows:

- Enabling occupations that help client tie up loose ends, such as:
  - Mounting and labeling photographs.
  - Writing down experiences or family history.
  - Writing letters or e-mailing estranged relatives or friends.
  - Finishing personal projects.
- Continuing routine occupations that maintain the client's sense of well-being.
  - Independence in self-care as desired (see Chapter 3).
  - Care of pets, gardening (see Chapter 4).
  - Sharing meals with significant others.
  - Distance participation in meaningful group activities (e.g., computer, camera cell phone, conference calls) (see Chapters 7 and 8).
- Enabling occupations that deepen spiritual experience.
  - Participation in religious rituals, discussions, or reading.
  - Giving away belongings that symbolize connection with others.
  - Craft projects that have symbolic meaning, memorial quilts, jewelry making.
  - Remembering, thanking, or forgiving others through occupations, such as writing poems, stories, cards, artwork or music, or giving gifts.
  - Planning one's own funeral, with or without family input.

In the hospice setting, OTs need to advocate for conditions that help clients make the most of their time left to live. Assessing clients' roles, routines, and occupational priorities become a basis for occupational therapy client advocacy with the health care team. Sometimes lowering medication may be preferred to enable client choice, and the distraction of occupation can serve to diminish the experience of pain. Terminally ill clients often prefer to endure some pain in order to continue valued social roles or deal with end of life issues through engagement in occupations. Energy conservation becomes an important strategy for occupational therapy, so clients can engage in occupations that have the highest priority for them. For example, clients may choose to have self-care tasks done by others, so they can save their energy for communication with significant others, event planning, or creative efforts (Jacques, 2002; Marcil, 2005).

Most hospice programs do not include occupational therapy services because they are unaware of the valuable services occupational therapy can provide (Tigges & Marcil, 1988). These authors suggest that OTs approach hospice programs through volunteering, offering educational presentations, or doing pilot research projects to demonstrate occupational therapy's value for terminally ill clients.

VOLUNTEERING

VOLUNTEERING DEFINED

Volunteering refers to unpaid work. The word implies that persons participate in volunteer roles by choice, and these roles have some purpose or usefulness for others, the community, or society. According to the US Department of Labor, in 2004, 34.2% of persons age 35 to 44, 32.8% of persons 45 to 54, and 30.1% of persons 55 to 64 volunteered at least once through or for an organization. Teenagers had a 29.4% volunteer rate (the highest increase over previous years), while those 65 and over averaged 24.6%, with this number declining as age increased. Those employed full- or part-time had a higher volunteer rate than those not in the workforce (2004).

According to Wyant & Brooks (1993), the concept of volunteering is becoming broader. In addition to the traditional volunteer or charity organizations, volunteering refers to community service learning, student internships, and court-ordered programs. These areas define the more formal volunteer roles. The more informal work activities people do without pay might include caregiving for children or aging relatives, home and yard maintenance, or providing occasional help to one's neighbors and friends. The domains of concern for OTs outlined by the *Framework* are volunteer exploration and volunteer participation (AOTA, 2002).

Volunteer exploration is defined as "determining community causes, organizations, or opportunities for unpaid work in relationship to personal skills, interests, location, and time availability" (AOTA, 2002, p. 621). In this aspect of volunteering, the tasks are similar to those required for seeking paid work. The client's knowledge, skills, and interests need to be evaluated and matched to available opportunities for local volunteer positions. For some clients, OTs may need to take a closer look at the tasks, and determine the activity demands required in the volunteer "jobs" being considered. AOTA (2002) defines *task demand* as "the aspects of an activity, which include the objects, space, social demands, sequencing or timing, required actions, and required underlying body functions and body structure needed to carry out the activity" (p. 624). A part of exploration also considers time availability. The OT may need to look at a client's overall use of time to determine how much time would be optimal for the individual to devote to volunteering.

Volunteer participation is defined by AOTA (2002) as "performing unpaid work activities for the benefit of identified, selected causes, organizations, or facilities" (p. 621). OTs may assist clients in establishing needed skills, building or remediating required abilities for the tasks involved, and/or making the necessary adaptations to enable the client to participate in a volunteer experience safely.

PURPOSE OF VOLUNTEERING

Giving back to the community; working for valued causes; making new friends; learning new skills; and finding expression for one's talents, skills, and creativity are some of the many reasons why people volunteer. It cannot be assumed that the motivation for volunteering is always altruistic. Different reasons for volunteering have been associated with different age groups. For example, children and adolescents may volunteer for the purpose of increasing their understanding of, or empathy for, disadvantaged groups such as the homeless (Karafantis & Levy, 2004). Kuperminc, Holditch, & Allen (2001) suggest that adolescents who volunteer benefit from a greater sense of connection to their communities, a better work ethic, and a greater concern for the welfare of others. For adolescents, this finding may suggest youths at risk for problem behaviors might volunteer as a preventive measure.

Young adult students may seek or be required to volunteer in unpaid internships with the purpose of learning and acquiring job-related skills. Internships form a part of the standard training of certain professions, occupational therapy among them. Volunteer roles for students in many different fields, including business, communications, journalism, and the law, may lead to future employment opportunities. New graduates and those temporarily unemployed may view volunteering as a continuation of their career path, or an opportunity for finding "the key to the boardroom door" (Graff, 1993). Six motivational factors were identified by Okun, Barr, & Herzog (1998): career, enhancement, protection, social, understanding, and values.

In midlife, parents who experience a diminished caregiving role as their children grow up may fill the void with volunteer activities. Full-time workers and breadwinners have little time to devote to volunteering. However, recent efforts have been made to structure volunteer opportunities outside the 9 to 5 work day (www.wallstreetvolunteers.org). Those with chronic mental or physical illness may seek volunteer work as an alternative to competitive employment. This group is of special concern for OTs, who may need to help clients overcome both internal and external barriers to volunteer participation.

Because of the unavailability of younger volunteers, organizations have turned to retired older adults to fill the need. In 1987, 38% of persons over 65 served as volunteers in some capacity (Chambre, 1991). According to another source, 26% of older adults volunteer for organizations, 29% informally help the sick or disabled, and 33% help or care for their grandchildren (Caro & Morris, 2001). For many older adults, volunteering replaces the lost worker role, fills gaps in increased leisure time, and provides meaning or purpose in daily activities. However, Ewald (1999) points out that volunteering does not provide meaning if it is considered busy work. Good matches need to be made between an individual's talents and a real need in the community for the elder "to mentor, educate, assist, and guide the next generation" (p. 325). Here again, OTs need to develop knowledge of volunteer opportunities in order to use activity analysis and synthesis in matching volunteer roles with client abilities and priorities.

BENEFITS OF VOLUNTEERING

Benefits of volunteering differ for different age groups, and are closely tied with the reasons for volunteering. For children and adolescents, service to the community, and broadening understanding and empathy for diverse social groups is an important benefit. However, to enact this benefit, the volunteer experience must be combined with education and a facilitated discussion of the meaning of the service, a potential role for OTs working with youth.

For students and young adults, career exploration and networking for future career development might be paramount. Public education, public service, and law enforcement are examples of areas that build volunteer skills and understanding of how the system works. Occupational therapy students regularly volunteer as a prerequisite for educational program admission. Additionally, OTs themselves may find volunteering useful in paving the way for community-based employment or advocacy.

While volunteering can have mutual benefits for persons of any age, recent research tells us those who benefit the most from volunteering are older adults. This age group has been widely studied, and the results demonstrate that volunteering prevents depression (Musick & Wilson, 2003), increases physical and psychological health (Greenfield & Marks, 2004; Backes, 1993), increases well-being (Morrow-Howell, Hinterlong, Rozario, & Tang, 2003; Wheeler, Gorey, & Greenblatt, 1998), and in many cases, prolongs life (Musick, Herzog, & House, 1999). For this reason, occupational therapy interventions with this population should include volunteer exploration, placement, and ongoing problem solving in the volunteer workplace.

Volunteer Interventions: Occupational Therapist Roles

Guiding the Exploration Process

Evaluation of the client's skills and abilities, as well as limitations and barriers, is the first concern of the OT. In many ways, preparing to volunteer resembles preparing a resumé for employment, and in fact, some volunteer placement agencies require the potential volunteer to submit a resumé. Many community organizations depend on volunteers to supplement the work of paid employees. This requires a commitment of time and energy and potential volunteers need to be willing to make such a commitment.

Assessing Client Reasons for Volunteering

The next step in searching for volunteer opportunities requires a clarification of the client's reasons for volunteering. Some common reasons are:

- Substitute work role, career exploration, learn new skills.
- Altruistic, "furthering a cause I believe in."
- Socialization, make new friends.
- Structure time, get out of the house and do something useful for others.
- Egoistic, use talents, be creative, mentor others.
- Leisure focus, "do something I enjoy."

Interventions that assist clients in clarifying their volunteer desires and specific interest areas will greatly facilitate the location of appropriate opportunities.

Where to Find Volunteer Opportunities

One only needs to enter the word "volunteering" on any Internet search engine to find thousands of volunteer opportunities (Table 6b-4).

Many Internet clearinghouses identify organizations within a few miles of one's local area and classified according to specific areas of interest. However, many clients, especially those with a lower socioeconomic status, may not have Internet access or the skills necessary to use these services. The OT should be prepared to search the Internet and narrow down options that are appropriate for the client. To do the job right, the OT needs to investigate the job descriptions for

Table 6b-4

EXAMPLES OF VOLUNTEER CLEARINGHOUSE WEBSITES

Volunteer Group	Internet Address
Retired Senior Volunteer Program (RSVP)	www.seniorcorps.gov
Quintessential Careers (paid & unpaid)	www.quintcareers.com/volunteering.html
Service Corps of Retired Executives (SCORE)	www.score.org
Volunteers in Service to America (VISTA)	www.friendsofvista.org or www.recruit.cns.gov
AARP Community Service Website	www.aarp.org/about_aarp/community_service/index.html or www.aarp.org/community_service
Woman's Day volunteers	www.womansday.com/volunteer
End Childhood Hunger	www.strength.org
Volunteer Talent Bank (VTB)	www.serviceleader.org/old/advice/seniors/html
Foster Grandparents	www.seniorcorps.org/joining/fgp
Senior Companion Program	www.seniorcorps.org/joining/scp
National Retiree Volunteer Center (NRVC)	www.voa.org/tier3_cd.cfm
Volunteer Abroad	www.volunteerabroad.com
Volunteer Match	www.volunteermatch.org

volunteers and to analyze the specific tasks required. Follow-up phone calls or on-site visits may be required to assess the many task demand and contextual factors involved, especially for clients with a disability that must be accommodated.

Volunteer Roles

Once the client skills and priorities have been identified, client reasons for volunteering need to be matched with the types of volunteer jobs available. One volunteer clearinghouse (www.nottinghamcvs.co.uk) categorizes the types of volunteer roles as follows:

- Practical, immediate action: Concrete tasks like feeding the homeless.
- Helping people solve their problems: Advocacy, crisis intervention.
- Getting the organization's job done: Managing, office tasks, fundraising.
- Concern for people and relationships: Providing caregiving, social support.
- Influencing and promoting change: Political action, lobbying for social change.

Clients need to feel that the volunteer role they perform has both a personal and an organizational meaning, and this requires a good match between meeting client needs, such as socialization or an outlet for skills and creativity, and meeting the needs of recipients of service. According to Merrill (2000), for persons to view their volunteering positively and sustain their interest, there needs to be a balance between giving and taking.

Common Barriers to Volunteer Participation

Many other factors contribute to this mutual satisfaction of needs and include adequate training and coordination of volunteers, clear expectations of the volunteer role, adequate supervision and positive reinforcement, flexibility in time constraints, and willingness to accommodate to physical and social contexts. When problems arise, the OT may facilitate mutual problem solving in the volunteer workplace.

LACK OF STRUCTURE

Volunteer roles vary widely in the amount of structure they provide. Some, such as the AARP Driver Safety Program, are highly structured with specific job descriptions and a training program for each role (AARP, 2004). Others, such as friendly visitor programs, depend on the volunteers to structure their own schedule and work. Studies of burnout and dropout show that volunteers are more likely to leave a volunteer job because of too little structure and role ambiguity (Ross, Greenfield, & Bennett, 1999). The OT can work with clients and volunteer supervisors to organize and structure the volunteer role according to the needs of both.

INADEQUATE SUPERVISION

For direct service roles, such as adult literacy or soup kitchens, feedback in the form of appreciation or suggestions may come directly from the recipients. Volunteers in these types of settings report an increase in satisfaction with volunteering. However, there are many behind the scenes, fundraising, or administrative roles that do not provide much feedback or appreciation. Volunteers need guidance and feedback in order to serve more effectively and to reap the benefits of volunteering, such as daily meaning and a sense of well-being. Some organizations have performed their own studies of volunteer retention and have developed strategies for giving needed feedback, such as recognition events or awards. However, OTs can advise volunteer organizations in providing the effective supervision to meet the needs of specific clients or client groups. For example, volunteers with mental health issues need a great deal of reassurance and direction with regard to appropriate social behaviors and boundaries. Knight (2004) identifies several keys to continued volunteer participation for those with mental health conditions, including peer support networks, utilization of home health aides, individual case management, and crisis intervention programs.

THE STIGMA OF DISABILITY

Perhaps the most disturbing barrier to volunteer participation is social stigma. The social attitudes of volunteer recruiters play an important part in the successful placement of those with mental or physical disabilities. A study by Lauber, Nordt, Falcato, and Rossler (2002) found two categories of social attitudes toward volunteers in psychiatry: 1) antipathetic, including a negative view of mental illness and a desire for social distance, and 2) socially responsible, including a positive attitude and an interest in social issues. Advocacy is needed to overcome the barrier of stigma for all types of disability, and this may become the focus of occupational therapy for specific clients who wish to participate in specific community services.

Unreasonable Expectations

Some areas of volunteering involve greater levels of stress and emotional burden than others. In studying volunteer burnout with persons with AIDS, emotional overload was a common reason for dropout (Ross, et al, 1999). Caregiving roles for many special populations have a similar risk, and this needs to be considered in the occupational therapy volunteer role analysis. Some volunteers have a greater capacity for emotional involvement than others. For example, those who volunteer in bereavement or Hospice programs need a high tolerance for dealing with the intense emotions of others (Mitchell & Shuff, 1995). Physical limitations also place volunteers at risk for burnout, such as too many hours or not enough coverage for specific roles. Older adults may need to consider energy limitations and fatigue when scheduling volunteer hours.

Time Constraints

In assisting clients with volunteer roles, the OT needs to be aware of the balance of activities that make up a client's lifestyle. Linda Fried, director of the Center for Aging and Health at Johns Hopkins University, suggests 15 hours a week of volunteering is needed for older adults to reap health benefits. However, the amount of time clients can devote to volunteer roles will vary widely, and OTs need to consider each client's individual needs. Working with activity patterns, daily routines, and time management become the focus of occupational therapy in this area.

Physical and Social Contexts

Volunteers with disabilities will need a variety of physical and social adaptations to the contexts of volunteer roles. Physical adaptations will be similar to those needed for adapting work settings and work task demands. Social support has perhaps the greatest influence on volunteer satisfaction and well-being (Sadler & Marty, 1998). Positive relationships with volunteer coworkers is a powerful motivator in volunteer retention and sustained interest. Many older adults depend on volunteering to meet their needs for social contact, while others need to feel needed, useful, and appreciated. Building social environments that support volunteer participation must include opportunities for social interaction and positive reinforcement.

Enabling Client Opportunities for Community Involvement

The enduring truth that helping others also helps yourself cannot be questioned. Yet many organizations report severe shortages of volunteers, while many qualified and motivated people never consider volunteering. Community clearinghouses and listings don't go far enough in matching potential volunteers with the right placements. This would be an excellent role for future occupational therapy community efforts.

Helping Others Like Yourself

Many human interest stories in the media showcase the therapeutic value of victims and survivors helping others like themselves. Most self-help organizations have come into existence this way, including Alcoholics Anonymous, Breast Cancer Support Service, American Society of Pain Management, Compassionate Friends, and Weight Watchers. The timing of one's involvement in public sharing of one's experiences is critical, and different for each individual. In the continuum of adaptation to chronic illness, early stages of shock, denial, and anger do not lend themselves well to any interventions, peer or otherwise. OTs may create group interventions that focus on the transition from denial to acceptance of one's illness or injury and the limitations it imposes on continued participation in life. The success of occupational therapy interventions that remediate or compensate for disability may depend on client readiness to accept such help. Peer volunteers may be a valuable resource in creating such readiness for therapy. As occupational therapy becomes effective in enabling occupational performance, clients might be encouraged to join self-help groups that encourage sharing of experience and group problem-solving.

Public Service at the Community Level: Advisory Boards, Senior Centers, Consumer Groups

Occupational therapy roles with volunteers include encouragement of participation on appropriate advisory boards, community leadership groups, and advocacy groups. In the case example of Al (at the end of the chapter), advisory board participation led to continued employment opportunities after an involuntary retirement due to illness. Clients need to be empowered to participate in their communities at whatever level they are able. As OTs become more knowledgeable about public service opportunities, they will more easily find ways to involve clients who would benefit from such connections.

Advocacy for Self and Others

Several studies have reported the need for parents of children with disabilities to learn the role of advocacy for their children (Lawlor & Mattingly, 1998; Pearl, 1993). Volunteering with school systems, community service organizations, and health agencies are all good ways to learn how the system works, how to make it work for you, as well as finding helpful connections for enacting social change. Adults with acquired illness also identify "the system" of health service delivery to be a major obstacle to accessing services like occupational therapy that would enable their continued participation in important life roles (Macdonald, 1998). Advocacy groups for other causes such as Defenders of Wildlife, and American Society for the Prevention of Cruelty to Animals (ASPCA) offer a variety of volunteer opportunities that can be easily found on their websites.

Religious, Ethnic, and Political Organizations

These organizations offer volunteer opportunities across the lifespan. As people age, connections with their religious and cultural background take on deeper meaning. Volunteering may be a good way for older adults to keep in contact with others who share similar values and beliefs.

Informal Caregiving as "Volunteer" Work

As a final word, family members and friends who regularly perform caregiving need to be recognized for the very important role they play in the lives of clients. In client-centered care, family caregivers may be equal partners in choosing, planning, and carrying out therapeutic interventions. The burden of caregiving should be considered when designing meaningful occupational therapy interventions, and support for the caregiver needs to be included in the process. OTs should treat this form of volunteering with the highest respect and admiration.

CASE EXAMPLES

Case Study #1: Al

Al is a 65-year-old heart transplant recipient who has been retired for the past 10 years. He is married to his wife of 44 years, the father of three adult sons, and grandfather of three. Prior to his heart failure, Al enjoyed a successful career as an industrial engineer. Born with a heart defect, Al's leisure pursuits tended to be passive and public service oriented. They include power boating and wine making, photography and painting, church treasurer, president of Civitan, treasurer of the local Power Squadron, and board of directors at a local marina.

Table 6b-5

AL'S TYPICAL WEEK—37 HOURS VOLUNTEER, 23 HOURS LEISURE, AND 44 HOURS SOCIAL OCCUPATIONS

	Mon.	Tues.	Wed.	Thurs.	Fri.	Sat.	Sun.
1 am	Sleep	Sleep	Sleep	Sleep	Sleep	Sleep	Sleep
2 am	"	"	"	"	"	"	"
3 am	"	"	"	"	"	"	"
4 am	"	"	"	"	"	"	"
5 am	"	"	"	"	"	"	"
6 am	"	"	"	"	"	"	"
7 am	"	"	"	"	"	"	"
8 am	Coffee w/retirees	Coffee	Breakfast	Coffee w/retirees	Coffee at Bagel King	"	"
9 am	w/retirees	Volunteer newsletter prep	Volunteer budget prep	w/retirees	Coffee at Bagel King	Volunteer meeting	Coffee at Bagel King
10 am	Computer	Volunteer newsletter prep	Volunteer budget prep	Photos on computer	Shop for wine-making supplies	Volunteer meeting	Coffee at Bagel King
11 am	Pay bills	Volunteer newsletter prep	Purchase supplies for event	Photos on computer	Shop for wine-making supplies		
Noon	Volunteer	Lunch	Purchase supplies for event	Photos on computer	Shop for wine-making supplies		
1 pm	Volunteer	Volunteer	Lunch on boat	Lunch with Sikorsky retirees	Shop for wine-making supplies	Fund raising event	Boating with wife & friends
2 pm	Shopping	Banking	Lunch on boat	Lunch with Sikorsky retirees		Fund raising event	Boating with wife & friends
3 pm	Shopping	Read mail	Boat work	Lunch with Sikorsky retirees	Make wine	Fund raising event	Boating with wife & friends
4 pm	Painting	Read mail	Volunteer inventory	Update volunteer files	Make wine	Fund raising event	Boating with wife & friends
5 pm	Painting	Dinner	Volunteer inventory	Update volunteer files	Make wine	Fund raising event	Boating with wife & friends
6 pm	Dinner	Condo board meeting	Dinner out with wife	Update volunteer files	Make wine	Clean up	Boating with wife & friends
7 pm	Dishes	Condo board meeting	Dinner out with wife	Dinner	Volunteer dinner in another town	Dinner out with friends	Dinner out with family
8 pm	Board meeting	Condo board meeting	Read mail	Dishes	Volunteer dinner in another town	Dinner out with friends	Dinner out with family
9 pm	Board meeting	Condo board meeting	Computer e-mail	Read mail & paper	Volunteer dinner in another town	Dinner out with friends	Dinner out with family
10 pm	Board meeting	Wine/snack	Computer e-mail	Read mail & paper	Volunteer dinner in another town	TV	Dinner out with family
11pm	TV	TV	TV	TV	TV	TV	TV
Midnight	Sleep	Sleep	Sleep	Sleep	Sleep	Sleep	Sleep

Al's experience gives us some insights regarding the transition to retirement. Although his retirement was involuntary and unexpected, his active public service prior to his illness paved the way for volunteer and part-time employment in retirement (Table 6b-5). His appointment to the Waterfront Harbor Management Commission before his heart transplant led to his appointment afterwards as Stratford Harbormaster, a part-time, paid position. He continues his roles in former community groups, and additionally, has become a mentor to other heart transplant recipients, currently serving as Chairman of the Heart Transplant Advisory Commission.

Case Study #2: Debi

Debi led a very active lifestyle for 25 years, working as a cardiopulmonary nurse, married and raising two boys, working as ski instructor and sailing instructor during weekends and free time. For some reason, she suddenly developed a latex allergy that went undiagnosed until it almost killed her. At age 47, Debi suffered a stroke, which required her to spend several weeks in a semi-comatose state in the ICU. Hospitals are very dangerous places for someone with a latex allergy because objects containing latex are everywhere, including blood pressure cuffs, stethoscopes, disposable gloves, oral and nasal airway tubes, tourniquets, syringes, electrode pads, and IV tubing, not to mention balloons and elastic bands. The allergy complicated her recovery in many undetermined ways, which led to her postretirement vocation.

Occupational therapy issues for Debi included dressing and basic ADL strategies, neurodevelopmental treatment (NDT) for her right sided hemiparesis, and communication interventions for aphasia. Debi's top priority task was using her laptop computer to communicate. Unfortunately, occupational therapy did not help her with this task in her biomedically oriented rehabilitation program. Hopefully, that would be different today.

Debi's case demonstrates how clients can turn their own disability into a volunteer advocacy role. In the years following her stroke, Debi used her knowledge of nursing and her own experience to create and publish a latex allergy newsletter, which originated on her laptop computer and reached out to other latex allergy sufferers internationally. Debi has thoroughly researched the medical objects containing latex, alternative equipment, and procedures for filtering the toxic materials for patients, and has presented this information at conferences for nurses and other medical personnel. She has written letters and testified at public hearings to influence public policy regarding latex labeling and usage. A network of fellow sufferers now regularly contributes to the informational website she has created.

Case Study #3: Matt

Matt climbed the corporate ladder the hard way, going to college at night while driving a truck to support a wife and three children until he earned a BS in marketing at age 30. Major events in his life include some major losses, including the untimely death of his younger brother and father, a bitter divorce, and being fired from two corporate jobs. At age 53, after 20 years with the same corporation, he was "downsized," this time with a 2-year severance package. Matt reported that 90% of his personal identity is tied up in his work role. Remarried for 22 years, he had poor relationships with his three adult children, but a close one with his sister's family. The same year Matt retired, he and his wife moved from a large home to a two bedroom condo on the water. After a period of relief from stress and sleeping late, Matt's health began to decline. With no daily structure, and bereft of a highly valued work role, Matt became preoccupied with symptoms of a stomach ulcer, acid reflux, and arthritis in his knees and shoulder. Signs of depression, insomnia, and generalized anxiety soon joined the rapidly expanding list of medical complaints.

Occupational therapy assessment included the timeline in Table 6b-6. Occupational therapy interventions included leisure exploration, volunteer exploration, and daily time structuring. Re-establishing daily routines in a new location became the first priority. A dog that used to run freely outside now needed to be walked on a leash. Regular hours for rising, dressing, showering, dog walking, mealtimes, and bedtime addressed the depression and insomnia (combined with medication). Additionally, Matt took on some of the household tasks like laundry and kitchen clean-up because his wife still worked full-time. Leisure choices from the past—scuba diving and downhill

Table 6b-6

MATT'S TIMELINE

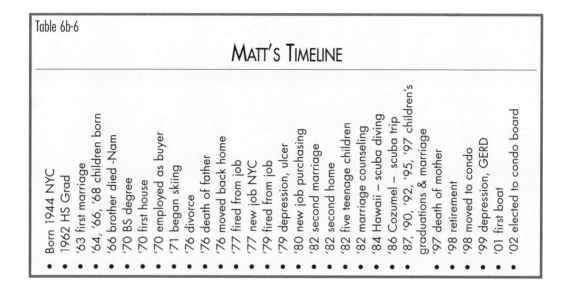

Born 1944 NYC • 1962 HS Grad • '63 first marriage • '64, '66, '68 children born • '66 brother died -Nam • '70 BS degree • '70 first house • '70 employed as buyer • '71 began skiing • '76 divorce • '76 death of father • '76 moved back home • '77 fired from job • '77 new job NYC • '79 fired from job • '79 depression, ulcer • '80 new job purchasing • '82 second marriage • '82 second home • '82 five teenage children • '82 marriage counseling • '84 Hawaii – scuba diving • '86 Cozumel – scuba trip • '87, '90, '92, '95, '97 children's graduations & marriage • '97 death of mother • '98 retirement • '98 moved to condo • '99 depression, GERD • '01 first boat • '02 elected to condo board •

skiing—required travel to distant locations. Matt, now living on the water, decided to take up swimming and boating instead. Afternoons he swam in the condo pool; he began attending boat shows and signed up for a local sailing course. Eventually, with regular walking, his arthritis symptoms subsided and he began meeting neighbors during walks with the dog. Volunteering had never interested Matt in the past. However, an opportunity presented itself when neighbors invited him to join the condo finance committee. He soon discovered his corporate purchasing experience could assist the condo in getting the best prices for needed goods and services. A year later, Matt was elected to the condo board of directors.

SUMMARY QUESTIONS

1. Discuss three common problems related to retirement.

2. Discuss potential barriers to volunteerism and how occupational therapy intervention strategies may overcome these barriers.

3. Discuss two strategies in which occupational therapy may assist in enabling client opportunities for community involvement.

4. Discuss how the stigma of disability may affect client participation in volunteer programs. How can the OT facilitate participation?

REFERENCES

Adams, K. B. (2004). Changing investment in activities and interests in elders' lives: Theory and measurement. *International Journal of Aging and Human Development, 58,* 87-108.

Allen, C., Blue, T. & Earhart, C. (2001). *Understanding cognitive performance modes.* Ormond Beach, FL: Allen Conferences.

American Association of Retired Persons. (2004). *Volunteer with the AARP driver safety program.* Retrieved November 12, 2004, from www.aarp.org/life/drive/drivervolunteer.

American Occupational Therapy Association. (2002). Occupational therapy practice framework: Domain and process. *American Journal of Occupational Therapy, 56,* 609-639.

Atchley, R. C. (1989). Continuity theory of normal aging. *Gerontologist*, *29*, 183-191.

Atchley, R. C. (1976). *The sociology of retirement*. New York: Halsted.

Atchley, R. C. (1975). Adjustment to loss of job at retirement. *International Journal of Aging and Human Development*, *6*, 17-27.

Backes, G. M. (1993). Importance of social volunteering for elderly and aged women. *Zeischrift fur Gerontolologie und Geriatrie*, *26*, 349-354.

Baker, D. W., Sudano, J. J., Albert, J. M., Borawski, E. A., & Dor, A. (2001). Lack of health insurance and decline in overall health in late middle age. *New England Journal of Medicine*, *345*, 1106-12.

Baltes, P. B., & Smith, J. (2002). *New frontiers in the future of aging: From successful aging of the young old to the dilemmas of the fourth age*. Keynote paper retrieved 4/22/05, from www.valenciaforum/Keynotes/pb.html.

Bonder, B. R. (2001). The psychosocial meaning of activity. In B. R. Bonder & M. B. Wagner (Eds.), *Functional performance in older adults* (2nd ed.). Philadelphia: F. A. Davis.

Bornstein, R. (1992) Psychosocial development of the older adult. In C. S. Schuster & S. S. Ashburn, *The process of human development: A holistic life span approach* (pp. 893-896). Philadelphia: Lippincott.

Brooks (1993).

Caro, F. G., & Morris, R. (2001). Maximizing the contributions of older people as volunteers. In S. Levekoff, Y. K. Chee, & S. Noguchi (Eds.), *Successful and productive aging*. New York: Springer.

Carstensen, L. L. (1992). Social and emotional patterns in adulthood. *Psychology and Aging*, *7*, 331-338.

Chambre, S. M. (1991). Volunteerism by elders: demographic and policy trends, past and future. In *Resourceful aging: Today and tomorrow, conference proceedings, Vol. II, volunteerism*. Washington, DC: AARP.

Chop, W. (1999). The social aspects of aging. In W. Chop & R. Robnett, *Gerontology for the health care professional*. Philadelphia: F. A. Davis.

Christiansen, C. H., Backman, C., Little, B. R., & Nguyen, A. (1998). Occupations and well-being: A study of personal projects. *American Journal of Occupational Therapy*, *53*, 91-100.

Clark, F., Azen, S., Zemke, R., Jackson, J., Carlson, M., Mandel, D., et al. (1997). Occupational therapy for independent-living older adults: A randomized controlled trial. *Journal of the American Medical Association*, *278*, 1321-1326.

Cohen, G. D. (1999). Human potential phases in the second half of life. *American Journal of Geriatric Psychiatry*, *7*, 1-7.

Cole, M. B. (1998). Time mastery in business and occupational therapy. *Work: A Journal of Prevention, Assessment, & Rehabilitation*, *10*, 119-127.

Cole, M. B. (2001). *Meaningful occupations of older adulthood across cultures*. Unpublished manuscript.

Crist, P. A. (1999). Does quality of life vary with different types of housing among older persons? A pilot study. In E. D. Taira & J. L. Carlson (Eds.), *Aging in place: Designing, adapting, and enhancing the home environment*. Binghamton, NY: Haworth Press.

Cumming, E. & Henry, W. (1961). *Growing old: The process of disengagement*. New York: Basic Books.

Daly, M. C. & Bound, J. (1996). Worker adaptation and employer accommodation following the onset of a health impairment. *Journal of Gerontology, Series B: Psychological Sciences and Social Sciences*, *51*, S53-60.

De Boer, A. G., van Beek, J. C., Durinck, J., Verbeek, J. H., & van Dijk, F. J. (2004). An occupational health intervention programme for workers at risk for early retirement: A randomized controlled trial. *Occupational & Environmental Med*, *61*, 924-929.

Di Mauro, S., Leotta, C., Giuffrida, F., Distafano, A., & Grasso, M. G. (2003). Suicides and the third age. *Archives of Gerontology and Geriatrics*, *36*, 1-6.

Disney, R., Grundy, E., & Johnson, P. (1994). *The dynamics of retirement: Analysis of the retirement surveys*. Research report N. 72. Retrieved 4/22/05, from www.dwp.gov.uk/asd/asd5/72summ.asp.

Erikson, E. H. (1963). *Childhood and society*. New York: Norton.

Erikson, E. H., & Erikson, J. M. (1997). *The life cycle completed*. New York: Norton.

Ewald, P. D. (1999). Future concerns in an aging society. In W. C. Chop & R. H. Robnett (Eds.), *Gerontology for the health care professional*. Philadelphia: F. A. Davis.

Fletcher, W. I., & Hansson, R. O. (1991). Assessing the social components of retirement anxiety. *Psychological Aging*, *6*: 76-85.

Formosa, M. (2000). Older adult education in a Maltese University of the Third Age: a critical perspective. *Education and Aging*, *15*, 315-334.

Gallo, W. T., Bradley, E. H., Siegel, M., & Kasl, S. V. (2000). Health effects of involuntary job loss among older workers: Findings from the health and retirement survey. *Journal of Gerontology, Series B: Psychological Sciences and Social Sciences, 55*, 131-140.

Geerts, C., Ponjaert-Kristoffersen, I., Verbandt, C., & Verte, D. (1999). Women and their retirement: Adaptation as a dynamic assessment process. *Tijdschrift voor genterologie en geriatrie, 30*, 6-11.

Graff, L. L. (1993). The key to the boardroom door: policies for volunteer programs. *International Journal of Volunteer Administration, 11*, 30-36.

Greenfield, E. A., & Marks, N. F. (2004). Formal volunteering as a protective factor for older adults' psychological well-being. *Journal of Gerontology, Series B: Psychological Sciences and Social Sciences, 59*, S258-264.

Gruber, J., & Wise, D. (1999). Social Security, retirement incentives, and retirement behavior: An international perspective. *EBRI Issue Brief, 209*, 1-22.

Hanson, K., & Wapner, S. (1994). Transition to retirement: Gender differences. *International Journal of Aging and Human Development, 39*, 189-208.

Harkapaa, K. (1992). Psychosocial factors as predictors for early retirement in patients with chronic low back pain. *Journal of Psychosomatic Research, 36*, 553-559.

Havighurst, R. (1961). Successful aging. *Gerontologist, 1*, 8-13.

Hershey, D. A., & Mowen, J. C. (2000). Psychological determinants of financial preparedness for retirement. *Gerontologist, 40*, 687-697.

Holmes, T. (1978). Life situations, emotions, and disease. *Psychosomatic Medicine, 9*, 747-754

Jackson J., Carlson M., Mandel D., Zemke R., & Clark, F. (1998). Occupation in lifestyle redesign: The well elderly study occupational therapy program. *American Journal of Occupational Therapy, 52*, 326-336.

Jacques, N.D. (2002). Working with the dying older patient. In C. B. Lewis (Ed.), *Aging: The health-care challenge* (4th ed.). Philadelphia: F. A. Davis.

Johnson, C. L., & Barer, B. M. (1992). Patterns of engagement and disengagement among the oldest old. *Journal of Aging Studies, 6*, 351-364.

Jonsson, H., Josephsson, S., & Kielhofner, G. (2001). Narratives and experience in an occupational transition: A longitudinal study of the retirement process. *American Journal of Occupational Therapy, 55*, 424-432.

Jung, C. G. (1933). *Modern man in search of a soul.* New York: Harcourt, Brace & World.

Karafantis, D. M. & Levy, S. R. (2004). The role of children's lay theories about the malleability of human attributes in beliefs about and volunteering for disadvantaged groups. *Child Development, 75*, 236-250.

Karpansalo, M., Manninen, P., Kauhanen, J., Lakka, T. A., & Salonen, J. T. (2004). Perceived health as a predictor of early retirement. *Scandinavian Journal of Work and Environmental Health, 30*, 287-92.

Knight, E. L. (2004). Exemplary rural mental health services delivery. *Behavioral Healthcare Tomorrow, 13*, 20-24.

Krause, N. (1986). Social support, stress, and well-being among older adults. *Journal of Gerontology, 41*, 512-519.

Kuperminc, G. P., Holditch, P. T., & Allen, J. P. (2001). Volunteering and community service in adolescence. *Adolescent Medicine, 12*, 445-457.

Larson, R., Csikszentmihalyi, M. & Graef, R. (1982). Time alone in daily experience: Loneliness or renewal? In L. A. Peplau & D. Perlman (Eds.), *Loneliness: A sourcebook of current theory, research, and therapy.* New York: Wiley-Interscience.

Laslett, P. (1997). Interpreting the demographic changes. *Philosophical Transactions of the Royal Society of London Biological Sciences, Series B, 352*(1363): 1805-1809.

Lauber, C., Nordt, C., Falcato, L., & Rossler, W. (2002). Determinants of attitude to volunteering in psychiatry: Results of a public opinion survey in Switzerland. *International Journal of Social Psychiatry, 48*, 209-219.

Lawlor, M., & Mattingly, C. (1998). The complexities embedded in family centered care. *American Journal of Occupational Therapy, 52*, 259-267.

Levinson, D. (1978). *The seasons of a man's life.* New York: Ballantine Books.

Lo, R., & Brown, R. (1999). Stress and adaptation: Preparation for successful retirement. *Australia and New Zealand Journal of Mental Health Nursing, 8*, 30-38.

Macdonald, K. C. (1998). *Adaptation to physical disability: The experiences of five women aged fifty to sixty.* New York University: Dissertation.

Marcil, W. (2005). Hope without a future. *Advance for Occupational Therapy, 21*(6), 18-19.

Marek, A. C. (2005). 48 Volunteer. In Fifty ways to fix your life (p. 84). *US News & World Report*, Dec. 27, 2004 – Jan. 3, 2005.

Mayring, P. (2000). Retirement as crisis or good fortune? Results of a quantitative-qualitative longitudinal study. *Zeischrift fur Gerontolologie und Geriatrie, 33*, 124-133.

McAdams, D. P., Hart, H. M., & Maruna, A. S. (1998). The anatomy of generativity. In D. P. McAdams & E. de St. Aubin (Eds.), *Generativity and adult development* (pp. 7-43). Washington DC: American Psychological Association.

McAndrew, J. M. (2002). Stress and aging. In. C. B. Lewis (Ed.), *Aging: The health-care challenge* (4th ed.). Philadelphia: F.A. Davis.

Merrill, J. (2000). You don't do it for nothing: women's experiences of volunteering in two community well woman clinics. *Health Soc Care Community, 8*, 31-39.

Mitchell, C. W., & Shuff, I. M. (1995). Personality characteristics of hospice volunteers as measured by Myers-Briggs Type Indicator. *Journal of Personal Assessment, 65*, 521-532.

Morris, J. K., Cook, J. G., & Shaper, A. G. (1994). Loss of employment and mortality. *British Medical Journal, 308*, 1135-1139.

Morrow-Howell, N., Hinterlong, J., Rozario, P. A., & Tang, F. (2003). Effects of volunteering on the well-being of older adults. *Journal of Gerontology, Series B: Psychological Sciences and Social Sciences, 58*, S137-145.

Musick, M. A., Herzog, A. R., & House, J. S. (1999). Volunteering and mortality among older adults: Findings from a national sample. *Journal of Gerontology, Series B: Psychological Sciences and Social Sciences, 54*, S173-180.

Musick, M. A., & Wilson, J. (2003). Volunteering and depression: The role of psychological and social resources in different age groups. *Social Science and Medicine, 56*, 259-269.

Neugarten, B. L., & Weinstein, K. (1964). The changing American grandparent. *Journal of Marriage and the Family, 26*, 199-204.

Nuttman-Schwartz, O. (2004). Like a high wave: Adjustment to retirement. *Gerontologist, 44*, 229-236.

Okun, M. A., Barr, A. & Herzog, A. R. (1998). Motivation to volunteer by older adults: A test of competing measurement models. *Psychol Aging: 13*, 608-621.

Parker, R. G. (1995). Reminiscence: A continuity theory framework. *Gerontologist, 35*, 515-525.

Parsons, P. A. (2003). From the stress theory of aging to energetic and evolutionary expectations for longevity. *Biogerontology, 4*, 63-73.

Pearl, L. (1993). Providing family centered intervention. In W. Brown, S. Thurman, & L. Pear (Eds.), *Family-centered early intervention with infants and toddlers: Innovative cross-disciplinary approaches* (pp. 81-101). Baltimore: Brookes.

Perreira, K. M., & Sloan, F. A. (2001). Life events and alcohol consumption among mature adults: A longitudinal analysis. *Journal of Studies on Alcohol, 62*, 501-508.

Potts, M. K. (1997). Social support and depression among older adults living alone: The importance of friends within and outside of a retirement community. *Social Work, 42*, 348-362.

Quick, H. E., & Moen, P. (1998). Gender, employment, and retirement quality: A life course approach to the differential experiences of men and women. *Journal of Occupational Health and Psychology, 3*, 44-64.

Reeves, J. B., & Darville, R. L. (1994). Social contact patterns and satisfaction with retirement of women in dual career/earner families. *International Journal of Aging and Human Development, 39*, 163-75.

Reitzes, D. C., & Mutran, E. J. (2004). The transition to retirement: stages and factors influence retirement adjustment. *International Journal of Aging and Human Development, 59*, 63-84.

Retirement Living Information Center (2004). Aging baby boomers shun the "R" word. Retrieved 11/12/04 from, www.retirementliving.com/RLart229.htm.

Riley, M., & Riley, J. (1994). Age integration and the lives of older people. *Gerontologist, 34*, 110-115.

Rosenkoetter, M. M., & Garris, J. M. (1998). Psychosocial changes following retirement. *Journal of Advanced Nursing, 27*, 966-976.

Ross, M. W., Greenfield, S. A., & Bennett, L. (1999). Predictors of dropout and burnout in AIDS volunteers: a longitudinal study. *AIDS Care, 11*, 723-731.

Rothenbacher, D., Arndt, V., Fraisse, E., Zschenderlein, B. Fliedner, T, & Brenner, H. (1998). Early retirement due to permanent disability in relation to smoking in workers of the construction industry. *Journal of Occupational & Environmental Medicine, 40*, 63-68.

Sadler, C. & Marty, F. (1998). Socialization of hospice volunteers: Members of the family. *Hospital Journal, 13*, 49-68.

Salokangas, R. K., & Joukamaa, M. (1991). Physical and mental health changes in retirement age. *Psychotherapy and Psychosomatics, 55*, 100-107.

Schuster, C. S. (1992). Development frameworks of selected stage theorists. In C. S. Schuster & S. S. Ashburn, *The process of human development: A holistic life span approach* (pp. 893-896). Philadelphia: Lippincott.

Sharpley, C. F. (1997). Psychometric properties of the self-perceived Stress in Retirement Scale. *Psychological Reports, 81*(1), 319-322.

Shmotkin, D., Blumstein, T., & Modan, B. (2003). Beyond keeping active: concomitants of being a volunteer in old-old age. *Psychological Aging, 18*, 602-607.

Szinovacz, M. E., & Davey, A. (2004). Honeymoons and joint lunches: effects of retirement and spouse's employment on depressive symptoms. *Journal of Gerontology, Series B: Psychological Sciences and Social Sciences,, 59*, 233-245.

Tigges, K. N., & Marcil, W. M. (1988). *Terminal and life-threatening illness: An occupational behavior perspective.* Thorofare, NJ: SLACK Incorporated.

Tornstam, L. (1989). Gerotranscendence: A reformulation of disengagement theory. *Aging, 1*, 55-63.

Tornstam, L. (1997). Gerotranscendence: The contemplative dimension of aging. *Journal of Aging Studies, 11*, 143-154.

Tornstam, L. (2000). Transcendence in later life. *Generations, 23*(4), 10-14.

U. S. Department of Labor (2004). *Volunteering in the United States, 2004.* Retrieved 4/27/05, from www.bls.gov/news.release /volun.nr0.htm.

Vaillant, G. E. (1993). *Wisdom of the ego.* Cambridge: Harvard University Press.

Velde, D., & Fidler, G. (2002). *Lifestyle performance: A model for engaging the power of occupation.* Thorofare, NJ: SLACK Incorporated.

Warr, P., Butcher, V., & Robertson, I. (2004). Activity and psychological well-being in older people. *Aging Mental Health, 8*, 172-183.

Westermeyer, J. F. (2004). Predictors and characteristics of Erikson's life cycle model among men: A 32 year longitudinal study. *International Journal of Aging and Human Development, 58*, 29-48.

Wheeler, J. A., Gorey, K. M., & Greenblatt, B. (1998). The beneficial effects of volunteering for older volunteers and the people they serve: a meta-analysis. *International Journal of Aging and Human Development, 47*, 69-79.

Wilson, S. E. (2001). Socioeconomic status and the prevalence of health problems among married couples in late life. *American Journal of Public Health, 91*, 131-135.

Withnall, A. (2002). Three decades of educational gerontology: Achievements and challenges. *Education and Aging, 17*, 87-102.

Wyant, S., & Brooks, P. (1993). The changing role of volunteerism. *Pap Ser United Hospital Fund NY*, April (23): 1-37.

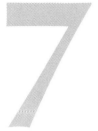

Leisure

Robert DeMatteo, OTR/L
Margo Ruth Gross, EdD, LMFT, LMT, OTR/L
Kim Mikenis, MPH, OTR/L

CHAPTER OBJECTIVES

By the end of this chapter, the student will be able to:

☑ Define **leisure** as it pertains to the *Occupational Therapy Practice Framework (Framework)*.

☑ Describe specific **models/frames of reference** as related to leisure.

☑ Comprehend **safety issues** as related to leisure.

☑ Delineate between the roles of the **occupational therapist** (OT) and the **occupational therapy assistant** (OTA) as they pertain to the occupation of leisure.

☑ Comprehend and identify related **physical and psychological implications** as related to decreased independence in leisure.

☑ Comprehend issues related to leisure in **specific settings**.

☑ Comprehend issues related to leisure when **using objects or equipment**.

☑ Describe the impact of **contextual factors** upon leisure.

☑ Identify appropriate leisure intervention strategies based on various **performance skills and client factors**.

☑ Identify specific leisure **compensation/adaptation** strategies.

☑ Identify general leisure **remediation** strategies.

☑ Identify leisure compensation/adaptation intervention strategies related to **vision, perception, and cognition**.

☑ Identify general leisure **maintenance** strategies.

INTRODUCTION

Leisure time has different meanings for individuals from different cultures, ethnic identities, gender identities, and social classes, affecting the way in which OTs utilize the concept for intervention. According to the *Random House Dictionary*, leisure is, "time free from the demands of work or duty, when one can rest, enjoy hobbies or sports, etc." (1987, p. 1100). The *Framework* further defines leisure as, "A nonobligatory activity which is intrinsically motivated and engaged in during discretionary time, that is, time not committed to obligatory occupations such as work, self-care, or sleep" (Parham & Fazio, 1997, p.250)" (AOTA, 2002, p. 621). Figure 7-1 depicts the components of leisure according to the *Framework*. Certainly, the meaning of leisure or the

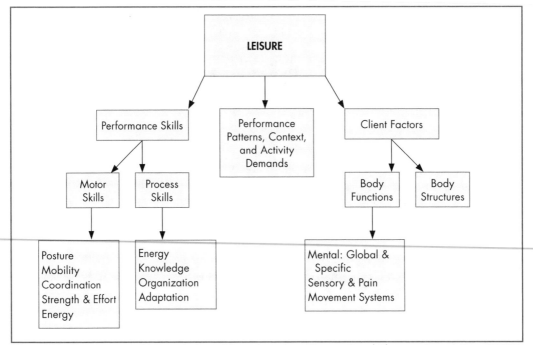

Figure 7-1. Components of leisure (adapted from American Occupational Therapy Association. [2002]. Occupational therapy practice framework. *American Journal of Occupational Therapy, 56*(6), 609-639.).

"free" time spent outside of paid work has both an objective and subjective understanding for each individual. This phenomenological point of view needs to be elucidated by engaging clients in a discussion to uncover what leisure time means to them, personally. Professionals need to be aware of their own biases, beliefs, and assumptions about leisure, as well as to be as open-minded as possible during such an interview.

In order to develop satisfactory performance skills for participation in leisure activities that are client-centered, questions involving the client's freedom of choice, level of motivation, and desired amount of relaxation or enjoyment need to be proposed. Leisure time, in balance with work and rest, is central to a person's well-being and is validated by a sense of perceived satisfaction and fulfillment in the activity. The perception of leisure or recreational activities as "leisurely" may or may not be held by a particular client; instead, free time may be seen as providing opportunities for novelty, excitement, interaction with others, or even escape from involvement with the larger community (Edginton, Jordan, DeGraaf, & Edginton, 1995). The needs met by a particular leisure activity may be simplistic, as in the case of providing relaxation, or the needs can be multifaceted, including avenues for emotional expression, creative expression, physical exercise, relationship-building, respite from interaction, cognitive stimulation, entertainment, or self-improvement.

The occupational therapy assessment process, using semistructured and open-ended questioning, ought to sufficiently uncover areas that could provide satisfaction in a variety of contexts for leisure fulfillment. Eliciting the clients' story in such a way as to encourage the development of analogies or metaphors can help explain their experiences with some cohesiveness. Assessment tools need to be chosen to match the factors that are consonant to clients' culture, age, and level of physical as well as psychological involvement. Another semistructured assessment is to use a calendar for 1 week, and ask the client to write down every activity he/she engages in, from waking up to going to bed. Asking questions informally while the client is completing the form will reveal the balance, or lack thereof, in work/productivity, leisure/recreation, and self-care/rest. A list of possible leisure time pursuits is included at the end of this chapter to serve as a guide for an interview.

Healthy communication and social skills, impulsive control, relaxation techniques, and self-esteem are just a few factors that can be enhanced through leisure pursuits. The OT, however, must be aware of the coexisting mental health functioning of the client along with the physical disability, as well as the client's leisure interests. The humanistic nature of occupational therapy addresses the "whole person," not just the simple components such as bilateral grip strength and functional mobility, and with a thorough occupational profile and analysis of occupational performance, a complete "picture" of the client can be achieved.

LEISURE EXPLORATION

Assessments and Evaluations

OTs promote and educate clients about the importance of living a balanced life composed of time for self-care, work, school, leisure, and social participation. One of the imperative tasks of OTs is to determine the interests and values of clients, a task that helps to include the clients in intervention, develop rapport between client and therapist, and assist with client motivation. The frame of reference or model used might determine the choice of evaluation and assessment tools. An excellent resource by I. E. Asher (1994) is listed in the Reference section. Each frame of reference has a different perspective on leisure exploration and it can be useful to blend approaches for a well-rounded initial assessment.

Several assessment tools exist to further explore a client's ability to engage in leisure; the most commonly used standardized assessments include the Allen Cognitive Level Test (ACL), the Kohlman Evaluation of Living Skills (KELS), and the Performance Assessment of Self-Care Skills (PASS). In addition to these tests, an abundance of information can be gathered by using informal assessments such as leisure checklists, role checklists, and ongoing assessment using worksheets such as those developed by Gross and DeMatteo (1998). These can be used individually or in groups to identify values, habits, and preferences for leisure activities. Commonly used evaluation tools utilized by OTs to assess a person's ability to engage in leisure tasks are described below, although the available resources in text or in digital form are varied and worth exploring by the OT.

THE ALLEN COGNITIVE LEVEL TEST

The ACL is a cognitive level screening tool designed by Claudia Allen. This leather-lacing task is administered to clients to provide the OT with an expedient measure of how a person learns (Allen, Earhart, & Blue, 1992). The strengths of this assessment include a relatively speedy format for administration and scoring, an excellent opportunity to observe problem-solving skills, and recommendations on how to best facilitate a client's capacity to learn. The authors' experience has identified weaknesses in this tool to include scoring discrepancies based on a client's past experience with stitching, and difficulties in administration to clients without adequate bilateral upper extremity (UE) functioning. A larger version of the task is available for clients with low vision.

THE KOHLMAN EVALUATION OF LIVING SKILLS

The KELS is a task-based, interview-style living skills evaluation developed by Linda Kohlman-Thomson and is often used by OTs to create discharge recommendations and assist the treatment team when planning for a client's transition into the community. The evaluation is divided into the following five subsections: self-care, money management, work/leisure, transportation, and telephone (Thomson, 1992). The leisure section of the KELS inquires as to whether the client engages in leisure activities alone and with others as well as when the client last engaged in leisure activities.

THE PERFORMANCE ASSESSMENT OF SELF-CARE SKILLS

The PASS is an evaluation designed by Rogers and Holm (1994). This evaluation is a testing tool developed to assess a person's ability to perform living skills. The PASS is primarily task-based with 26 testing sections. Skill performance can be tested by administering Task #22: IADL: (Leisure) Playing Bingo. The client is first instructed in the rules of the Bingo game and then asked to mark the numbers called and identify when Bingo occurs; the OT assesses whether the client marked the numbers heard correctly and whether he/she were aware when Bingo had occurred.

INFORMAL LEISURE CHECKLISTS

OTs often administer informal leisure checklists, as this type of testing can be an easy and effective way of determining a client's past, present, and future interests in leisure. An informal leisure checklist also may seem less threatening to a client than a formal evaluation. The checklist often provides numerous visual cues of varying types of leisure activities such as bowling, jogging, art, and playing a musical instrument.

Intervention Implications

If formal and informal testing yields deficiency in leisure engagement, then the OT designs an intervention plan with the client to address leisure needs. Each intervention plan will be inherently different given individual client interests and the type of clinical care setting in which the intervention will take place. Other factors to consider when designing an intervention plan to address leisure skills include issues in context and accessibility, such as cultural barriers, physical barriers, financial barriers, transportation barriers, and temporal barriers. For example, if the client said she would like to attempt international travel and she is currently in a financially disadvantaged situation, the barrier to developing this leisure interest would be financial. The OT may still assist the client in developing this interest by introducing the client to the travel section of the library and bookstore. The OT can also assist the client in locating (in newspapers, bulletin boards, and on the Internet) local lectures of persons who have engaged in foreign travel.

Additional factors to consider when designing occupational therapy intervention for leisure skills are the activity demands, such as appropriateness of activity, supplies, funds, staff time, and location of activity. For example, rather than provide adult clients with a psychiatric diagnosis (regardless of their specific diagnosis) on an inpatient unit with a box of crayons and pages to color, offer plain paper and colored pencils or markers. In order to uphold the dignity of the client, every attempt should be made by the OT to make interventions as age-appropriate as possible. A list of questions and concerns has been provided below. These should be reviewed prior to the initiation of an activity.

Additional Factors to Consider

- Will the planned leisure activity be meaningful and of interest to the client?
- Is the activity age-appropriate?
- What supplies are needed to plan for the desired leisure intervention?
- Does the facility have the budget to allow for the desired leisure intervention?
- Is there enough staff available to assist with the intervention?
- Will the desired leisure intervention fit within the timeframe of the planned session?
- Where will the intervention occur—on the facility grounds or in the community?
- If in the community, how will transportation be arranged and which staff members are able to assist?

- Will the client need a pass or doctor's order if the leisure activity is off the unit?

- Does the client need medical clearance from the doctor to engage in the leisure activity?

- Is this a leisure activity the client can pursue in the community once discharged from occupational therapy? Does the leisure intervention have carryover?

Adapting Leisure

OTs often must adapt a leisure activity to the individual needs of the client. For example, planning for a leisure intervention involving dance movements for adult clients who have had a traumatic brain injury (TBI) would be quite different from planning the same intervention for adult clients who have had a myocardial infarction (MI), or heart attack.

For the group of clients who have had a TBI, some factors to consider include:

- Are the clients able to initiate movement?

- Do any of the clients have a seizure history?

- Do perseverative movements or thoughts impede task function?

- Is sexual impulsivity a problem for any of the clients in the group?

- What is the range of motion (ROM) and grade of muscle tone of the affected limb(s) among the participants? Are the participants on any restrictions of movement?

- How do the cognitive deficits, if applicable, from the TBI impede the participants' ability to learn?

- Will the participants be seated in wheelchairs?

In comparison, some factors to consider if planning a similar intervention for a group of clients who have had a MI include:

- Are there any activity restrictions, such as lifting?

- How much endurance do the participants have? Can they tolerate a regular session or would two short sessions be more appropriate?

- Do any of the participants require closely monitored vital signs, such as blood pressure and oxygen saturation?

- Should the group include education regarding stress reduction, healthy lifestyle, risk factors, etc, as well as a physical task?

The fact that the group for individuals with TBI has a markedly higher number of considerations than the group for individuals with MI highlights the point that some group activities require much more adaptation than others depending on the make-up of the group.

Leisure Activity Adaptations

Nearly any leisure activity can be adapted with the cooperative effort of problem solving that occurs between the OT and the client. Often a creative, problem-solving approach, with a healthy dose of humor, needs to be applied to persist until an adaptation is considered satisfactory by the client. The following are just a few of the many ways in which leisure activities can be adapted. These suggestions have been grouped by client factors and processing skills.

CLIENT FACTORS: ROM, STRENGTH, AND COORDINATION

- Clients with UE deficits can join in a game of cards with the use of a plastic cardholder.

- Card sorters can be used in place of shuffling for clients with decreased coordination.

- Bowling ramps can be used with a client who may be unable to lift the ball. With this device, the bowling partner can line up the bowling ramp according to the direction of the bowler prior to the push of the ball.

- For clients with decreased UE strength or decreased coordination, throwing the bowling ball "granny-style" can be attempted. The client bends both knees and throws the ball toward the pins with both hands.

- For clients with more significant deficits in strength, be sure to use lighter weight bowling balls, or instead, attempt duckpin-bowling, which uses lighter balls.

- For clients with decreased hand strength, a table clamp can be used to hold the pages open for reading.

- For clients with decreased grip strength, use larger-handled paintbrushes, markers, and pencils. Other options are to make a universal cuff or cut cylindrical foam tubing to be placed over art utensils.

- Tape large strips of sheet paper on the wall when engaging a client in mural art while also working on increasing UE strength.

- Use tape to hold paper in place during art activities if the client only has unilateral UE functioning.

CLIENT FACTORS: SENSATION/PAIN

- For clients who have decreased grip strength due to a sensory loss, use larger handled paintbrushes, markers, and pencils.

- Making a universal cuff or cutting cylindrical foam tubing to be placed over art utensils can make gross grasp positions capable of utilizing tools more efficiently.

- Keeping all materials within the clients' visual perimeters will allow them to check on the impact of tool use and prevent injuries.

CLIENT FACTORS: ENDURANCE/ENERGY

- The amount of endurance and need for rest must be determined by the evaluation and reassessed with client feedback and input during this collaborative process.

- A pattern of gain can be documented with relation to time involvement, amount of focused concentration, and requests for break times.

PROCESSING SKILLS: COGNITION AND PERCEPTION

- Upon evaluation, the level of cognitive ability can establish parameters for single- or multi-step tasks that will guide the choices for intervention activities.

- Establishing the purpose and motivational factors will also guide the depth of intellectual challenge or lack of challenge required from the client.

- The visual motor and perceptual motor abilities can potentially limit the complexity and speed of required tasks within each recreational activity.

- For bowling, create a line down the center of the lane using brightly colored, removable electrical tape.

- Use brightly colored adhesive tape to make a border around the paper for a client with neglect or hemianopsia.

PROCESSING SKILL: VISION

- Clients with low vision can play cards by using a deck of cards with enlarged numbers and face cards.

- For bowling, create a line down the center of the lane using brightly colored, removable electrical tape.

- Use books with large print and be sure there is ample reading light. A clip-on book light would be helpful.

- Many books can be found on tape and CD for clients with significant visual impairments.

Leisure by Intervention Setting

Economic realities, physical conditions, or physical access to leisure or recreational pursuits can be potential barriers for a person dealing with a temporary or permanent disability. Community agencies offering recreational facilities may not be architecturally accessible to some populations with disabilities, and some clients' lack of ability to advocate for increasing the availability of services can serve to limit opportunities. Organizational barriers can be related to communication or language deficiencies on the part of the staff, or lack of knowledge related to adaptive devices used to assist physically challenged individuals.

There is a role for occupational therapy in creating outreach programs within community programs to reduce the lack of understanding, ignorance, or fear on the part of management or staff. Creation of new service delivery options in library settings, indoor bowling, skating arenas, gyms, or swimming clubs would help to deliver multiple avenues for leisure and recreational activities for varied populations.

When the OT creates a plan for developing a person's leisure skill intervention, he/she must consider the setting in which the intervention will occur. For example, typical settings can include hospital rooms, rehabilitation rooms, inpatient psychiatric units, community settings, or homes. If the client is in a hospital room and has a strong interest in playing basketball, it is understandable that the client will not be able to run up and down the halls of the hospital dribbling the ball. How can his/her interest in basketball be adapted? Perhaps by using a suction-cup basketball net and foam ball or by matching players' names to their respective teams, certain clients would be more successful executing the skills necessary for a successful recreational experience. Discovering what the client's leisure interests are at the time of administering formal and/or informal occupational therapy testing is essential for guiding the client and will help to foster a better rapport.

The following are examples of leisure activities that can be adapted for use in occupational therapy interventions among the more common client care settings.

HOSPITAL ROOM (FOR BED-BOUND CLIENT)

- Card decorating and card writing.
- Artwork.
- Board games and cards.
- Making tissue flowers.
- Origami.
- Exercise.
- Painting fingernails.
- Decorating flower pots.

- Making potpourri satchels.
- Collage.
- Crossword and perceptual puzzles.
- Knitting, sewing, and crochet.
- Reading the "funnies."

Rehabilitation Room or Clinic Setting (For Individual or Group Sessions)

- Foam basketball with suction cup net.
- Suction cup or safety darts.
- Video and computer games.
- Board and card games.
- Exercise.
- Word search and crossword puzzles.
- Dancing.
- Singing and karaoke.
- Cooking.
- Letter writing.
- Listening to music.
- Playing piano or keyboard.

Inpatient Psychiatric Unit (for Individual or Group Sessions)

- Artwork: painting, drawing, clay, papier-mâché, collage.
- Making jewelry.
- Card design.
- Indoor gardening.
- Decorating tee shirts.
- Painting ceramic figurines.
- Stained glass (plastic).
- Dance.
- Exercise.
- Pet therapy.
- Writing in journal.
- Writing poetry.
- Reading portions of plays aloud.
- Cooking.
- Creating weekly newsletter with articles written and illustrated by clients.
- Bingo.
- Crafts.

COMMUNITY PSYCHIATRIC SETTING

- Planning and participating in an ice cream social.

- Creating art, planning and participating in an art exhibit.

- Creating parade float and walking with float during parade.

- Baking and hosting a bake sale.

- Trips to local community leisure resources such as libraries, museums, art galleries, animal shelters, parks, and farms.

- Starting a bowling or softball team.

- Creating crafts throughout the year and having an annual craft sale.

- Involving clients in making plans to go to events such as basketball and baseball games, theater, movies, or political rallies.

- Initiating a community garden.

Leisure and Safety

With participation in leisure activities, there are varying levels of potential injury that are evident throughout the continuum of life. Examples of a temporal approach include: the 7-year-old who falls off a swing and scrapes both knees; a 16-year-old who fractures her radius while playing high school field hockey; the 40-year-old who acquires a torn meniscus while skiing down the black diamond trail; or the 70-year-old who nicks his hand during a woodworking project. Analysis of acceptable risk and those leisure activities that need to be adapted, modified, or as the last resort, restricted is part of the interrelated process of evaluation, intervention, and therapeutic outcomes. The OT is aware of safety concerns associated with body structure/function as well as activity demands (objects, social demands, space demands, and sequencing). Of course, the general therapeutic goal is for the individual to take part in leisure activities in the safest manner possible. While leisure exploration and evaluation of leisure has already been discussed in this chapter, the leisure planning activity sheet (Figure 7-2) will address safety concerns as an individual researches areas of interest.

Client Factors (Body Structure/Function) Related to Activity Demands/Medical Contraindications and Precautions

Before a client can take part in any leisure activity, body functioning as related to safety of activity demands must be determined. This information can be obtained through the medical chart and by consulting with the treating MD and nurse. A fall risk assessment is a common safety factor. Another would be cardiac precautions. Can the individual who is 75 years old and is 2 months status post-MI, take part in the team-building group parachute activity? An immediate question would be, what metabolic equivalents (METS) are required to perform the specific leisure activity? Are isometric fitness activities safe? It is also important to not assume only older adults have cardiovascular precautions. Individuals of all ages can have physical activity restrictions for a multitude of medical issues.

Understanding precautions related to the impact of medication on body functions is also vital. Many medications may be sedative in nature and cause hypostatic changes. Other medications could be activating, while others may cause sensitivity to certain foods, temperature, and/or direct sunlight. Imagine the impact this information could have on an occupational therapy community outing if a group of clients wanted to arrange a picnic in a local park on a sunny day. Medication, the effects from food, and the natural environment could be easily overlooked.

Client Leisure Planning Activity Sheet

1) Name the leisure activity that you want to enjoy:

_____

2) Identify the date of the activity:_____

3) Identify the specific location and address: _____

_____

_____

4) What will be the travel time to the location as well as the return time?

_____

5) What mode of transportation will be needed?

_____

6) Is the site accessible for your functional mobility needs (i.e., ramp, elevator)?

_____

7) How much time do you plan to devote to the activity?

_____

8) What will be the financial cost of the entire activity including transportation?

_____

9) Do you plan to go alone or will there be others with you? Describe:

_____

10) Describe safety concerns: _____

11) List three numbers you would call for assistance in case of an emergency:

_____

_____

_____

12) Describe your expectations for this community activity. What do you want to experience?

_____

_____

Figure 7-2. Sample form created by Robert DeMatteo, OTR/L.

Physiological factors must always be considered. An example would be the use of a product containing latex, such as balloons; a client could have an allergic reaction if he or she is predisposed to that type of sensitivity. Does the client have a pacemaker or any type of vitals monitor, and will a specific electronic leisure item interfere with physiological functioning?

Another consideration is being aware of the client's special dietary restrictions.

Some clients may have food allergies, such as peanuts, dairy products, certain fruits, or shellfish. Again, this information can be obtained by asking the client, checking the medical chart, and consulting with caregivers and medical staff. It is critical to know the ingredients being used for the task of food preparation, such as with cooking groups.

General health and wellness should also be promoted. Obesity, diabetes, and heart disease are common health problems in the adult population. Certain medications have side effects that can cause increased appetite and weight gain. Common occupational therapy leisure group activities have included such things as baking cakes, brownies, and sweets. It would not be appropriate to have a leisure cooking or baking activity with high sugar or high fat items with clients who have the above-mentioned concerns. Alternative healthy food choices should be presented as part of general care such as with low fat and low- or no-sugar products. For more information on wellness, see Chapter 9.

As part of any activity involving eating and drinking, body structure and body function is analyzed. The OT would inquire about issues of dysphasia and other feeding issues. Are there contraindications for certain foods due to aspiration risk? Can the client safely chew, swallow, and digest the food planned for the activity? Speech and language pathologists and dietitians can work together with OTs regarding these issues. For more information regarding eating/dysphagia, see Chapter 3.

General precautions related to body structures and functions must also be considered for fitness and sports-related leisure activities. The potential for injury increases with these types of activities. Consider what would be required if a client wanted to snowboard, kickbox, skateboard, play lacrosse, or weights. A thorough task analysis is essential. An OT can research a specific fitness activity through consulting with sports coaches, fitness trainers, local gyms, clubs, and websites. Clinicians associated with sports medicine and physical therapy may also be resources.

ACTIVITY DEMANDS

Activity demands, according to the *Framework* (AOTA, 2002), include the objects/materials used during leisure tasks, the space demands or physical environment where the task is completed, the social demands of the task, such as rules of a game, as well as the required body functions/structures discussed above. Each of these activity demands has safety concerns that need to be addressed.

Objects/Materials: General Information for All Settings

Whether it is an inpatient hospital setting, partial-hospital program, skilled nursing facility, a group home, a community clubhouse, or a home-care environment, the following precautions apply:

- The OT must be aware of the chemical contents, temperature, stress indications, and general safety precautions related to leisure materials. This is especially evident with arts and craft materials. Certain glues, inks, wood stains, and oil paints contain toxins and skin contact is contraindicated. Special ventilation may also be required to utilize some of these products. Some materials could be flammable or harmful if ingested.

- The OT must analyze if use of the materials matches the age and cognitive/behavioral skills of the client. Consider the scenario of an individual with an Allen's Cognitive Level of 4.0 who wanted to engage in oil painting as a hobby. At first, the activity appears to be a safe and healthy pastime, but with further analysis the potential for harm is discovered. The client lives in a one room, windowless apartment and plans to use turpentine in open coffee cans as a medium for the oil paint. The activity does not match the space demands or physical environmental requirements for safe participation. The client also smokes. Decreased insight into how the vapors from the solvent could be harmful as well as the risk of fire is noted. After researching painting supplies, the OT learns that acrylic paint can mix with water and there is decreased risk of harmful fumes and combustion. The acrylic is substituted for the oil paint and the activity is modified so the client can still partake in her desired leisure interest.

The OT can obtain product information by reading chemical content and caution labels. Certain inpatient settings, such as hospitals and skilled nursing facilities, have material data sheets. The OT can also consult with craft and hardware stores or even the manufacturer regarding product safety.

Other leisure products such as modes of transportation, safety gear, and electronics also have various safety precautions. For example, an OT would consider the activity demands of operating a bicycle as related to the general functioning of the rider. Imagine if the client wanted to participate in four-wheeling with a recreational quad-bike, water-ski, or use a snowmobile. Safety concerns are evident for such tasks. Similar safety concerns are also present for more common activities such as a client expressing interest in driving to see a movie. The basic safety questions for all forms of locomotion would be: Could the individual drive in an appropriate manner? Is there a need for a driving evaluation? Is the client aware of safety precautions?"

The OT should be aware of the proper way for a client to wear such items as a safety helmet, knee/elbow pads, a chest protector, a groin cup, and safety goggles. Roller skating, playing football, and welding a metal sculpture are just a few activities that utilize safety gear. It is important to remember that using protective gear does not mean the risk of injury is totally eliminated. For example, a safety helmet in batting practice can reduce the force of a ball hitting an individual's head, but the person's face and neck are still vulnerable to harm. Many safety items have force, impact, and weight limitations. The baseball helmet may be effective to a certain amount of foot-pounds of pressure per square inch before cracking. Awareness of the manufacturer's product precautions and guidelines for safety items is a critical part of proper task analysis.

Knowledge of the proper electrical plugs and outlets as related to such devices as radios, electric musical instruments, electronic games, and computers is important. A safety concern would be whether the power strip is overloaded with various plug-ins. The OT would also be aware of any signs of malfunctioning, worn, or damaged leisure materials. When possible, the client should also be encouraged to check for item defects.

Many social and leisure activities involve food. An OT may facilitate a leisure cooking group, such as a holiday lunch party or a community client picnic. Often, the clients may bring in food items from home as part of the activity. The general precautions for all food include:

- Is the food fresh?
- Is it thoroughly cooked?
- Was it refrigerated properly?
- Was it handled properly, ie, did the client wash his/her hands during preparation?
- Are the utensils clean?

Objects/Materials: Physical Disabilities With the Comorbidity of Behavioral Health Issues (Objects in Relation to Mental Functions)

Part of leisure task analysis is knowledge of the materials associated with the activity and the safety precautions. The safety precautions are closely related to the **global and specific mental functions** of the client. This is especially evident among populations with behavioral health issues in inpatient psychiatric settings, group homes, skilled nursing facilities, and TBI programs. While arts and crafts task activities are common occupational therapy modalities in these settings, proper selection and storage of the materials is critical because suicidal and self-harming behavior is a factor with some clients. Some examples of materials to be concerned with include items referred to as "sharps," such as latch-hooks, scissors, and knitting needles. Other items include yarn and ribbon, which can be doubled up to make a noose; a paintbrush or a sharpened colored pencil, which has the potential to puncture; a simple plastic bag used to carry craft materials, which can cause asphyxiation; even a common paperclip or a staple from the binding of a magazine can be bent and used to scratch or lacerate. Unfortunately, when performing a task analysis, the OT must think in terms of the protection of the client and the staff. Awareness of the client's psychiatric history and behavioral status is always the first step. Again, checking the chart and consulting with the nursing staff and the MD is critical.

An example of a safety scenario is when a client who can safely take part in a task leisure activity on the unit has materials that another client may try to take in order to cause self-harm. The OT must be vigilant regarding who is allowed to have the materials and who is not. Consider the example of clients in an inpatient neurorehabilitation unit making wooden ornaments for the holiday during an occupational therapy task/leisure group. The clients want to keep their crafts, although the OT understands the balsa wood can be snapped to make a jagged point. The clients who made the ornaments do not have aggressive or self-harming behavior, and they ask to keep their projects in their rooms on the unit. The OT needs to take the ornaments and put them in a locked storage area because of another client who was not in the group but is still in the facility, and has a history of decreased impulse control and violent outbursts. As a result, it would be highly unsafe for the ornaments to be lying around. The OT consults with the clients and assures them that they may have their ornaments back when they are discharged to go home.

The following list regarding the storage of leisure materials is valid for both inpatient and outpatient settings:

- A written inventory of all the items is highly recommended.

- A count should be made both before materials go out to be used by the clients and when they are returned (e.g., how many scissors were given to the group and how many were collected at the end).

- On the inventory list, there should also be an indication of the storage site area (e.g., locked ventilated storage cabinet, third locked drawer in occupational therapy office).

- A sign out/sign in time along with staff signatures is beneficial in tracking items (Figure 7-3).

Activity Demands/Social Demands

Many leisure activities involve such components as physical touch, socializing with peers and members of the opposite sex, competition, and the encouragement of humor and laughter. With these components, there could be related safety issues. Consider a client who sustained a TBI and now has frontal-lobe syndrome or a client who had right hemisphere CVA. Decreased impulse control, difficulties modulating frustration and anger, impairment of abstract thinking/higher-level judgment, and misinterpretation of social cues are just a few elements of the symptomology. What might happen if a client with the above-mentioned issues took part in a group hug as part of a team-building leisure activity? Decreased control related to sexual impulses and inappropriate touching could be a risk factor. Leisure pursuits that involve competition, from a simple board game to more intense activities like a tennis or basketball game, could be triggers for angry outbursts. The client may have difficulty tolerating the outcome of losing. An example of this is how the client with impulse control issues could react if spiked at the net while playing volleyball. Humor, jokes, and lighthearted teasing can also be misconstrued as insulting. Often in team sports, a coach may try to motivate a person by verbally "pushing" the individual to do better. Comments like, "Go! Go!" and "You're too slow! Pick up the pace!" may at first seem like appropriate encouragement, but again, due to impairment of higher-level cognition, the client could have an adverse emotional reaction. A literal pat on the shoulder may cause a client to retaliate with a

Date:	Item:	Quantity:	Time-Out:	Time-In:
	Scissors	10		
	Latch-hooks	7		
	Glue gun	3		
	Cans of wood stain	5		
	Spools of twine	2		
	Long-handled paint brushes	13		
Signature:				

Figure 7-3. Example of an OT Leisure Material Safety Sheet. Created by Robert DeMatteo, OTR/L.

physical outburst, injuring the first individual. Some clients with physical disabilities may have other types of coexisting cognitive or behavioral health issues such as anxiety disorders, social phobias, and histories of post-traumatic stress disorder (PTSD). Consider the example of a client with paraplegia who also has severe panic attacks, and is asked to introduce herself for the first time in an occupational therapy leisure group. While promoting socialization and the enhancement of quality of life is the therapeutic goal, the person instead may be experiencing a spike in stress and highly uncomfortable psychological and physiological responses. Another example could be a client with multiple sclerosis who has a history of physical and sexual abuse. Intimacy issues and difficulties with physical touch are noted. Holding hands in a team building exercise or interacting with other male group members may be viewed by this client as adverse.

Concerning all the above-mentioned cognitive and behavioral issues, participation in leisure pursuits is still facilitated, although with implementation of modification, adaptation, prevention, relearning, and new learning. By promoting the client to take part in a leisure role, there is the opportunity to address cognitive impairments, inappropriate social conduct, impoverished and dominating habits, as well as pathologies related to psychosocial issues.

Activity Demands, Space Demands, Sequencing

These factors will be covered when the Client Leisure Activity Planning Sheet is completed, with discussion and exploration to assess the necessary adaptations required for successful execution of the activity by the client. Certain occupational therapy settings may create limitations until the full community reinvolvement phase is underway.

GENERAL PRECAUTIONS FOR COMMUNITY LEISURE ACTIVITIES

One of the many client-centered goals of occupational therapy is for the individual to partake in and enjoy healthy leisure activities out in society. Community outings such as client picnics, visiting a bookstore, going to a restaurant, or viewing a play can be highly therapeutic experiences to promote learning, adaptation, individual satisfaction, and enhancement of general quality of life. However, along with the value of community integration activities, there are added safety concerns. For example, there is no longer the support of a controlled environment such as a hospital or a rehabilitation facility. In implementing a community-based leisure activity, objects and their properties, space demands related to physical context, social demands, sequence and timing, required actions, and client factors need to be analyzed. The basic question would be: Can the client safely tolerate the event? The following are examples of safety factors for consideration:

- The number of staff needed to facilitate and supervise the outing as related to the acuity of the client and/or number of clients in a group.

- The type of transportation needed and the accessibility to the client, such as a van with a lift versus a public bus.

- The accessibility of the site to the client (e.g., wheelchair ramps, elevators, level walkways, and bathrooms).

- Knowledge of the site as related to additional safety hazards (e.g., near a lake, near a road with traffic, or near a heavy crime area).

- Knowledge of the closest hospital in case of emergency.

- Having access to communication lines in case of an emergency (e.g., more than one cell phone, or access to a land-line if cell phone service is not responding).

- Knowledge of accurate directions to the site and an alternative route in case of traffic issues.

- Knowledge of accurate travel time and the duration of the leisure event.

- Awareness of the client's medication schedules and other time-based procedures, such as breathing interventions, colostomy, and catheter routines.

- Safety implications related to weather (e.g., can the client tolerate direct sunlight, heat, and humidity? Can the client tolerate cold?)

- Having a back-up plan for temporary shelter if there are weather or temperature changes.

- Bringing umbrellas and extra warm clothing in case of weather changes.

- Staff trained in CPR and first aid.

- OT and staff having an established, written emergency protocol for community outings.

Precautions Related to Utilization of the Internet and Computers

With the creation of computers and the Internet, there has been wide participation in leisure activities within the virtual context. Due to the massive popularity of video games, music downloading, and chat rooms for socialization and with the various types of virtual activities there are related risk factors. A common precaution involves the question regarding whether or not the video game or Web site is age-appropriate for the client. Concerning an adult client, the question would be, "Does the individual have the global mental functions to access a particular type of media with no adverse effects?" It is common for an Internet subscriber to be bombarded with junk email advertising adult Web sites, cheap prescription medication, and stock investments. There is also the real potential to unfortunately acquire dominating habits such as addiction to pornography or mail order prescriptions. The easy access of buying online could also lead to shopping addiction. In addition, there is also the widespread danger of identify theft. The Internet can be an effective leisure outlet for many individuals, but activity demands must correspond with client factors. Consider the scenario of a client with an ACL of 5.0 who has a history of cerebral palsy, and has decreased self-esteem due to difficulties with body image. The client's left UE has a manual muscle testing rating of "poor" due to neurological pathology. Muscle wasting is evident and the limb hangs inoperable by his side. The client often states he is "ugly" because of his arm. Past hospitalizations for major, recurrent, severe depression are noted. The client lives alone in an apartment building for individuals with disabilities. He reports difficulty with socialization and expresses to the OT that he is often lonely. After saving up for a computer as part of an intervention goal, he begins to utilize the Internet and is soon bombarded with emails offering various chat services for a monthly fee. The client has access to a credit card and starts to give out his personal information online, including his social security number. The client reports, "I made a bunch of new girlfriends." The potential for the client to be taken advantage of is high. The OT intervenes and provides safety education as part of leisure planning. The client agrees to utilize a SPAM-blocking feature offered by his Internet service. Money management and proper use of a credit card is addressed as well as alternative social leisure outlets.

The right of access and privacy is an additional issue concerning an adult client's use of the Internet or other types of media. If the individual can utilize Web sites, chat rooms, or purchase items online with no adverse effects, then there is no need for a therapeutic intervention. The OT must not try to restrict an adult client's right to access information, read particular material, listen to certain types of music, or communicate with another individual just because it may seem offensive. It is important to realize that the OT's moral or religious values must not impede the client-centered approach.

COMMUNITY LEISURE FOR THE ADULT WITH PHYSICAL DISABILITIES

In analyzing therapeutic outcomes, a common indicator for improvement in function and independence is to be active and involved in one's own society. This is evident with participation in leisure. With an emphasis on a client-centered approach balanced with considerations for safety, the OT should encourage the client to partake in leisure activities out in the community. This is accomplished by consideration of the following:

1. Identification of client's leisure interests and leisure goals.

2. Analysis of activity demands related to client factors.

3. Adhering to safety issues.

4. Access/transportation to community leisure sites.

5. Verifying the community leisure site is accommodating to the client.

6. The leisure intervention plan allows for modification, adaptation, learning, and relearning.

7. Quality of life is always promoted.

Additionally, for the OT to facilitate effective leisure participation, it is paramount to have a working knowledge of what the client's community has to offer (refer to the adult community leisure list later in this chapter). This is further analyzed on a continuum as to which activities have no cost, to a minimal charge, to moderately expensive, to expensive. Cost, however, is all relative to the individual's income. A specific client may be on Social Security disability and only receives $500 dollars a month to pay rent for a subsidized apartment and to buy food. Paying $9.50 for admission to a movie and $7.00 for popcorn and a soda may seem extravagant. Another client with a different financial situation may be able to hire personal aides and dine at upscale restaurants. With this point understood, a real-world generalization is that most clients tend to have some financial limitations. The OT, in collaboration with the individual, has to be creative in leisure planning while adhering to a budget.

Despite financial restrictions, another common obstacle to community leisure is transportation. A common statement made by some clients is: "I want to get out more but I have no way to get there. I can get a medical cab to my office visit but that is it. I'm stuck if I want to do anything fun." The lack of transportation is due to many factors. A few examples are: 1) the client does not drive or has stopped driving, 2) the client lives in a location were there is no bus service or other types of mass transit, and 3) the transportation available does not accommodate the client's mobility needs (the wheelchair cannot fit in the back of the family's car). The OT can assist the client in problem-solving these obstacles by being aware of what supports are available in the community. Transportation factors such as driver retraining and acquisition of modified vans and cars are separate interventions. Consider identification of the following:

- Area bus routes, time schedules, and rates related to the client's location.
- Area train and subway routes, time schedules, and rates related to the client's location.
- Taxi services and rates.
- Discount transit pass programs for clients with disabilities.
- Van services offered by community mental health clubhouse programs.
- Community senior shuttles.
- Religious/church organizations that offer rides.
- Safe transportation can be offered by family and friends.
- Knowledge of transportation options that are handicap accessible.

Interrelated with financial and transportation factors, another recommendation for effective leisure planning is for the OT to venture out physically into the client's community and see what leisure pursuits are available. Taking a drive around after work to conduct some "reconnaissance" will truly help to understand the environment, activity demands, safety issues, and the leisure sites.

Leisure Psychosocial Issues: Addiction

In the various populations in which occupational therapy is implemented, there is often the diagnosis of substance abuse or substance dependency. This includes clients with physical disabilities and not just those with coexisting mental health issues. In certain scenarios, these issues are openly identified, while at other times they can be far from evident. For example, there can be a teen with paraplegia who is starting to experiment with cannabis; a client with a history of TBI who is taking part in an outpatient partial hospital program and is addicted to cocaine; a 40-year-old male machine operator who is receiving a splint for carpal tunnel syndrome at a hand therapy clinic and reports having chronic pain issues, but is also addicted to oxycodone and exhibits medication-seeking behavior; and the 75-year-old who is status post-CVA, receiving occupational therapy on a home-care basis, has a history of alcoholism, and is now addicted to Ativan.

One of the core principles of occupational therapy is to promote quality of life through working with the client to extinguish maladaptive habits and acquire alternative healthy roles and routines. In regards to substance abuse and addiction, one of the many areas of functioning that is adversely affected is participation in healthy leisure activities. Occupational therapy can assist in a client's recovery by enhancing sober leisure pursuits. Usually, this is one of the major occupational therapy intervention goals in both inpatient and outpatient mental health settings. Clients with addiction issues often report that their leisure activities revolve around "using." Bars, dance clubs, keg and dorm parties, sporting events, and concerts are just a few examples of places where alcohol and street drugs are common. These events and activities can also be outlets for socialization. A common dilemma for clients in recovery is making decisions regarding keeping or ending friendships with individuals who also have drug and alcohol issues. Many clients in early rehabilitation often express that they feel lonely and bored with the prospect of no longer being able to "party" or to hang out with certain people. A key slogan in 12-step recovery programs is "changing people, places and things" (Anonymous, 1984). Occupational therapy can assist with this concept by facilitating involvement in new leisure activities and social outlets that are drug- and alcohol-free. A few examples that clients could consider:

- Connecting with a local gym or YMCA.
- Going out to eat with sober friends rather than to a bar.
- Seeing a movie.
- Going to coffee houses and hearing live music.
- Attending Alcoholics Anonymous (AA)/Narcotics Anonymous (NA) social events such as sober dances and picnics.

The OT should also consult with the client and analyze what sober leisure interests he/she has had in the past. A major goal of recovery is to regain previous healthy habits and roles. It is important to identify if the client has specific talents that can be fostered into sober leisure pursuits. It may be discovered in an occupational therapy session that the client has talent for such things as drawing, sculpture, playing an instrument, softball, creative writing, repairing vintage cars, singing, etc. The OT would encourage the client to restart a specific leisure interest as long as it did not trigger a relapse. The additional therapeutic benefit of fostering personal creative talents is the enhancement of self-worth and self-esteem.

Another addiction that is not always initially identified is gambling. There has been a surge of gambling addiction in the United States, as evidenced by a 13% increase in calls to the gambling addiction line in 2004 (Online Casino, 2004). This increase can be attributed to the development of new casinos, online Internet betting, state lotteries, and televised poker tournaments. Gambling addiction can be a devastating illness where an individual can literally lose everything, such as life savings, automobile, home, relationship with family, and sense of self-worth. A particular profile for the illness is the "escape gambler" (Gamblers Anonymous, 2005). This type of behavior involves gambling not for the purpose of acquiring money or for the excitement of winning but rather to distract and "numb" the individual from emotional pain. Some older adults can be prone to this condition due to psychosocial and physical stressors such as:

- Death of a spouse.
- Decreased contact with family and friends.
- Boredom.
- Decline in physical health and independence.

Additionally, weekly bingo and senior bus trips to casinos can be contraindicated for some clients. Even facilitating an occupational therapy leisure group where the activity has win/lose competitive components can be a trigger to gambling.

Alcohol, street drugs, pain medication, benzodiazepines, and gambling are common addictions, although shopping, sex, and overeating all have the potential to be addictive. These activities are often related to adult leisure. When an OT is facilitating leisure planning with a client, it is important to be vigilant about potential addiction issues. This is valid for pediatrics, teens, adults, and the geriatric population. It is also, again, valid for clients with physical disabilities. A goal of occupational therapy is to promote participation in sober, healthy leisure pursuits.

POTENTIAL LEISURE ACTIVITIES LIST

The following is a list of additional activities to assist with leisure planning and implementation. Potential safety and budget issues have been mentioned when appropriate. These options could be reviewed by OTs with clients and help the client to problem-solve as to which leisure interests are appropriate. In some cases, clients can then investigate independently and in other cases, clients may require additional assistance from the OT. Resources to locate leisure activities include:

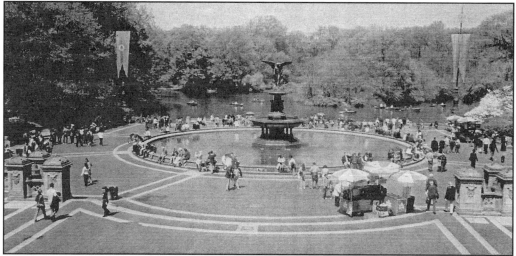

Figure 7-4. Clients should be encouraged to utilize available parks among other resources (Photo of Central Park courtesy of Robert DeMatteo).

- Leisure sections of area newspapers.
- Events offered by the public library.
- Events offered at area community colleges (some programs allow clients to audit classes for free).
- Senior center programs.
- Mental health community clubhouse programs.
- Church social programs.
- Parks and recreation programs (Figure 7-4).
- Adult continuing education programs (e.g., Learning Annex).
- Leisure events sponsored by AA/NA (e.g., picnics, sober dances).

Movies

- Multi-cinema complexes.
- Art house theaters.
- Second-run movie theaters that offer reduced admission.
- Bargain matinee specials/senior discounts.
- Film programs offered at local libraries and colleges.
- Movie theaters that offer accommodations for the hearing impaired.
- Film study classes and discussion groups at area colleges.

Places to Eat in the Community

- Listings of area restaurants (including prices).
- Obtaining discount coupons for restaurants offered in local newspapers.

- Identification of restaurants that offer early bird specials.
- Calendar of potluck dinners offered by area community organizations or church groups.
- Lunch and dinner programs offered by community mental health clubhouses.
- Identification of restaurant sites that are contraindicated for clients with obesity or special dietary needs (e.g., an all-you-can-eat buffet). Identifying sites that offer healthy cuisine would be a therapeutic goal.
- Identification of eating establishments that do not offer alcohol (for clients with substance abuse issues).

Bars, Dance Clubs, Live Music Venues, Singles Clubs, Comedy Clubs

- Area listings as well as cover charge prices.
- Identification of times and days when there is no cover charge.
- Obtaining free admission passes on establishment websites.

These types of community leisure outlets are only appropriate for adult clients who have the mental functions to safety interact within these types of environments. It is contraindicated for clients with substance abuse or addiction issues to take part in the above-mentioned sites. Sober dance parties sponsored by AA/NA are a safer alternative.

Coffee Houses

- Can be a safe, alternative adult social setting without the element of alcohol.
- Identification of coffee houses that offer nightly live music or poetry readings.
- Listings of bookstores that have an in-house café (e.g., Barnes and Noble, Border's).
- Internet cafés.
- Safety concerns regarding client's ability to tolerate caffeine is noted.

Fitness/Sports Outlets

- List of area gyms.
- YMCA (identify if local branch offers scholarships and reduced rates for clients with financial constraints).
- Martial arts clubs/schools.
- Yoga classes.
- Tai Chi Chuan classes.
- Local running tracks.
- Mall walking programs.
- Public tennis courts.
- Public and private golf courses.
- Water aerobics programs.
- Community swimming pool programs.
- Community marathon programs.

- Wheelchair basketball leagues.
- Area softball leagues (can be sponsored by various community programs, such as parks and recreation, community mental health, AA/NA).
- Skiing/snowboarding outlets.
- Hunting, shooting ranges, archery clubs.
- Fishing events.
- Bicycle clubs or events.
- Rollerskating tracks.
- Indoor rock-climbing gyms.
- Viewing community sporting events—high school, college, professional.
- Parks and recreation and adult continuing education programs offer various adult fitness and sports options.

Nature Leisure Outlets

- Listing of area parks.
- Walking and hiking trails (client should understand difficulty ratings related to specific routes).
- Hiking clubs.
- Area beaches, lakes, ponds.
- Nature walks or organized education programs.
- Bird watching groups.
- Area zoos and aquariums.

Art/Creative Expression Outlets

Fine art and craft classes are offered at area art schools, colleges, parks and recreation programs, adult continuing education programs, and senior centers (some colleges allow individuals with disabilities, especially seniors, to audit or take classes for reduced rates) (Figure 7-5).

- Involvement in area art shows, craft bazaars.
- Visiting art exibits, galleries, museums.
- Music lessons of all types.
- Joining an area chorus or choir.
- Attending concerts, musical events of all types.
- Attending plays, musicals, local theater events.
- Taking acting classes.
- Taking part in a theatrical production.
- Joining a poetry or creative writing group.
- Taking part in a book club.

Figure 7-5. Clients should be encouraged to investigate and pursue leisure interests such as art.

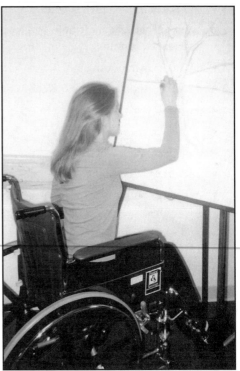

CASE STUDY #1: TOM, TRAUMATIC BRAIN INJURY

Tom is a 34-year-old white male who sustained a TBI due to a motorcycle accident. He was in a coma for 3 days. Multiple bilateral lower extremity (LE) fractures were noted. After an actual hospitalization and 2 months of inpatient rehabilitation, he was transferred to an outpatient neurorehabilitation program. Occupational therapy, physical therapy, and speech therapy were implanted as part of the intervention protocol. Tom presented with periodic lability, impulsivity, and decreased frustration tolerance due to damage to the frontal and prefrontal cortex. ACL score was 5.0. Partly through analysis of occupational performance, it was indicated that higher-level judgment was impaired as related to accessing his needs and safety. Tom expressed that he wanted to ride his motorcycle again, despite having periodic difficulties with spatial relations, visual tracking, sustained and divided attention, and topographical orientation. A labored gait was noted due to 5 centimeters (cm) of bone being removed from his left femur and the insertion of internal fix-caters and rods. Bilateral UE structure, muscle strength, and sensation were within functional limits; however, there was periodic decreased gross motor coordination.

Prior to the accident, Tom's occupational profile showed he was a successful builder and general contractor. He had an associate's degree in business from an area community college. It was accepted that the client had functioned at an ACL rating of 6.0. He was never married and had recently ended a long-term relationship with a girlfriend. No children were noted. Tom expressed his only family contact was with his elderly aunt, who was his caregiver as a child. The team social worker noted in the psychosocial report that Tom's father died when he was 5 and his mother was unable to parent due a long history of major chronic depression and substance abuse issues. No specific religious affiliation was reported. Tom stated, "I don't go to church or anything like that, but I do believe in God." His major social support was with two close male friends he described as his "riding buddies." Reportedly, the two friends were in weekly contact with the client.

The neurologist deemed it unsafe for Tom to drive any vehicle at this time due to neurovisual impairment and difficulties with attention. There was also a single episode of a seizure during his acute hospitalization. Tom became angry and tearful when he was informed of the restriction during a treatment team/client meeting. The OT informed Tom that as he progressed in his therapy there would be the possibility of partaking in a driving evaluation. The client continued with his therapy at the outpatient program while returning to his apartment to live alone. Weekly visiting nurse services were implemented to monitor the client's medication schedule. Transportation to his therapy was provided by medical livery. The client experienced feelings of periodic loneliness and boredom, especially on the weekends when his friends could not visit. Before the accident, the client spent the majority of his weekends biking with his friends and going to bike shows. Tom continued to describe himself as a "biker." He often wore his leather vest and Harley Davidson tee shirts to the intervention program. During one occupational therapy session, he stated, "You have to understand the scene, the whole culture of it all. I miss it so much." There was no history of substance abuse or problematic drinking, but he did frequent bars as another major social outlet.

Within the following weeks, his friends took him out for a "few beers" to celebrate his recovery. Tom missed his outpatient therapy on one of the Mondays. He reported feeling irritable, fatigued, and nauseated. At a meeting with the neurologist, he was told it was highly contraindicated to drink alcohol. Tom stated he only had two drinks. It was explained that alcohol lowers inhibitions and can impair higher-level judgment. As related to the head injury, a small amount of alcohol can intensify symptoms of impulsivity and decreased emotional modulation. Tom then admitted he did get "loud" that night and his friends had to calm him down. It was further explained that his brain is slowly healing and alcohol retards neuronal plasticity. Drinking was also contraindicated because it hindered the therapeutic effects of the client's schedule of antidepressants and seizure medication. Tom expressed feelings of disappointment and frustration as he was told it was best if bars were off-limits. He stated, "First you tell me I can't ride my bike anymore, and now you are saying I can't go to my favorite sports bar with my friends! This is hell! What am I going to do with my life? I'm so bored!"

The client was directed to occupational therapy. The recent intervention plan/intervention goals had involved increasing function with instrumental ADLs (i.e., organizational skills for shopping, budgeting, and accessing the community bus service). As part of the intervention review, it was evident that the client required assistance with leisure planning and social outlets. Tom was presented with a leisure checklist to formulate all current and past leisure interests. An initial occupational therapy short-term goal was for him to identify at least three sober leisure pursuits within 1 week. The proceeding goal was for him to choose one of the three activities and to partake in it. The OT was promoting a collaborative process between the practitioner and the client. Earlier, Tom stated that he sometimes felt the members of the treatment team were against him because of all of the restrictions (i.e., being told not to ride his motorcycle, no drinking). During the occupational therapy session, Tom brightened, wrote "Tae Kwon Do" on the back of the leisure checklist and said, "I want to do this again." He reported he was very active in martial arts when he was in his late teens to early twenties and he won multiple trophies in state tournaments. "I know a school in the area. I can train there."

The OT was unsure what participation in Tae Kwon Do meant. A task was given to the client to find the listing of martial arts schools in the phonebook. Tom agreed to let her call the academy to obtain information. She also researched the subject on the Internet. She discovered that Tae Kwon Do was a highly athletic activity that entailed dynamic kicking and punching. Sparring was also part of the sport, which involved kicking to the head. During the next occupational therapy session, Tom brought in his old sparring equipment, which included padded headgear, gloves, and shin protectors.

He expressed, "I use to kick butt when I was younger. I can't wait to give it another try. I'll wear this stuff and I will be okay."

Upon examining the equipment and consulting with the instructor at the martial school, the OT knew there was the potential for various injuries even with protective gear. The protective helmet in particular was of concern because its main purpose was to prevent lacerations and bruising but not protect against coup-counter-coup forces from a blow. Additional concerns were the client's cognitive and emotional status. Tom continued to present with lability and periods of angry outbursts. There was a deviant safety concern regarding his ability to have control during such an intense experience as sparring. Decreased function related to spatial relations, visual tracking, and balance during dynamic movements, and general bilateral UE and LE coordination were addition issues. There was a fall risk. The client had decreased insight into the potential for harm. It was crucial that another brain injury not be sustained. The leisure activity demands did not match with the client's body structure and body function.

The next path in clinical reasoning was the promotion of compensation, modification, and adaptation. The client was experiencing drastic changes in independence and was being told that activities and social outlets he once enjoyed were now dangerous. The client also had periodic difficulty accepting the rationales for the restrictions due to changes in higher-level judgment and reasoning. There was the fine balance of maintaining a client-centered approach to leisure while adhering to safety concerns. The OT consulted with the martial arts teacher and inquired about modifying participation in the classes and omitting sparring. The instructor expressed he would be willing to work with Tom on a one-to-one basis and have him perform basic forms and moves that he could do safely. The OT consulted with the physical therapist regarding balance, LE strength, and coordination issues. The physical therapist gave a list of exercises that were appropriate. The client did not have any cardiac restrictions. Upon presenting the information to the entire treatment team, the OT was allowed to go off-site to visit the martial arts school to perform a task analysis. The martial arts instructor showed a basic routine of conditioning such as stretching, various types of abdominal exercises, and push-ups, as well as simple stances, punches, and kicks. The instructors assured her that there would be no emphasis on fighting but rather on strengthening the body, building endurance, and improving coordination.

Another off-site visit at the martial arts school was arranged, this time with the client. Safe use of the transit/bus system was also part of the outing and intervention implementation. The OT observed while Tom took part in the workout with the instructor. Initially, the exercises were performed slowly, then gradually increased as Tom felt more comfortable. Despite a few moments when the client briefly lost his balance and had difficulty coordinating left and right moments of his arms, there were no overt signs of frustration or angry outbursts. There was instead an apparent elevation in mood and affect. Tom expressed that it was the best he felt since his accident. The instructor also introduced Tom to deep breathing techniques and had him attempt a few moments of meditation.

A leisure goal was set that involved the client taking part in a 45-minute private session at the martial arts school with the same instructor, once a week, for a month. Money management and transportation goals were also interrelated with the plan. Tom was given the task of calculating his weekly budget in order to pay for the sessions. The martial arts instructor agreed to give a substantial reduced rate to help Tom in his recovery. The bus schedule was reviewed and Tom began to attend the private classes.

As part of the intervention review, the client and his treatment team deemed the leisure plan/target outcomes successful. The physical therapist and the OT both noticed increased dynamic balance when ambulating as well as more efficient functional mobility. Improvement in visual tracking and spatial operations were also noted. The client also appeared more relaxed and had decreased signs of irritability.

Toward the end of the month, Tom stated he now wanted to take part in classes with the other martial arts students at the school. He said that while he really enjoyed the one-to-one sessions, he missed the camaraderie of training with other individuals. "When I was in classes in the past I made a lot of pals. It was more exciting. We sometimes went out to eat as a group after training. It got to be like family. We even had holiday parties together." Tom reported that he still had a lot of idle time on his hands and his "riding buddies" were not seeing him as much.

The client's request was discussed in the treatment team. Tom still presented with periodic lability despite the recent gains with a more stable mood and affect. The risk of another head injury was also an ongoing safety factor. Additionally, the martial arts instructor expressed that he had concerns about liability issues. He stated he did not want Tom to get injured or have an outburst and hurt another student. The consensus was that it was contraindicated for the client to take part in the general class. The client was again facing an intervention recommendation he would view as hindering his next step in improving his own quality of life. Rapport with his caretakers and the martial arts instructor was in jeopardy as well as general client satisfaction.

Another intervention review was implemented. The checklist of leisure pursuits was revisited with the client. Tom inquired about Tai Chi Chuan, another style of martial arts. The OT was not familiar with the particular activity but encouraged the client to research it at the local library. The martial arts instructor was also contacted to acquire more information. It was discovered that Tai Chi Chuan was a "soft" style of Kung Fu that did not emphasize sparring or fighting but rather balance and control. Slow, dynamic movements performed in a sequential pattern were part of the art as well as mediation, relaxation, and a focus on well-being. After another task analysis of the activity, it was deemed a safe alternative to Tae Kwon Do. The desire of the client wanting to be active in a class with others could now be safely promoted.

The client was educated in how to research community resources. Tom was directed to adult continuing education services and the area parks and recreation program. The local phonebook listings were another simple but effective way of acquiring information on the subject. Tom discovered Tai Chi Chuan classes offered at a local community college and at the YMCA (Figure 7-5). He also identified a Tai Chi club that met three times a week in town. Inquiring about prices for instruction and directions related to the bus route was facilitated as part of the intervention plan and implementation.

Within a month, the client was going two times a week for lessons. Tom reported that he now had something to look forward to on the weekends because there were Saturday classes. He also expressed that the people were very nice to him and he started to "feel part of the group." After another 4 weeks, Tom started spending time at the YMCA and began to take part in yoga classes at the urging of a new friend from the Tai Chi club.

At the intervention program, it was observed that there was increased ability with sustaining attention during occupational and speech therapy sessions, which lead to gains with organizational skills and efficiency with various instrumental activities of daily living. Marked improvement in visual tracking was noted. A driving evaluation was planned. The physical therapist reported increased dynamic balance and coordination. Tom expressed, "I feel good about life again."

SUMMARY QUESTIONS

1. Discuss the safety issues involved with leisure activities when working in an outpatient psychosocial setting.

2. Discuss the impact of physical limitations on at least two adult leisure pursuits.

3. Discuss possible compensation/adaptation strategies for the leisure pursuits chosen in question #2.

4. Discuss remediation techniques for the leisure pursuits in question #2.

Figure 7-6. Client participating in Tai Chi Chuan class (photo courtesy of Robert DeMatteo).

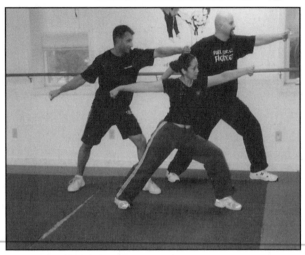

REFERENCES

Allen, C., Earhart, C. A., & Blue, T. (1992). *Occupational therapy treatment goals for the physically and cognitively disabled.* Bethesda, MD: American Occupational Therapy Association.

Allison, M. T., & Hibbler, D. K. (2004). Organizational barriers to inclusion: Perspectives from the recreation professional. *Leisure Sciences, 26,* 261-280.

American Occupational Therapy Association. (2002). Occupational therapy practice framework. *American Journal of Occupational Therapy, 56*(6), 609-639.

Anonymous. (1984).

Asher, I. E. (1994). *Occupational therapy assessment tools: An annotated index* (2nd ed.). Bethesda, MD: American Occupational Therapy Association.

Edginton, Jordan, DeGraaf, & Edginton. (1995).

Estes, C. (2000). Rethinking philosophy of leisure: A proposal for including more humanism in the curriculum. *Schole, 15,* 13-30.

Gamblers anonymous. (2005). *Profile of escape gamblers.* Retrieved June 8, 2005, from http://fargoga.org/facts/escape.htm.

Gross, M. R., & DeMatteo, R. (1998). *The healing workbook for substance dependency.* Plainview, NY: The Guidance Channel.

Law, M., Baptiste, S., Carswell, A., McColl, M. A., Polatajkop, H., & Pollack, N. (1997). *Canadian occupational performance measure* (2nd ed.). Toronto, Ontario: CAOT Publications.

Lewis, J. A., Dana, R. Q., & Blevins, G. A. (1994). *Substance abuse counseling: An individualized approach.* Pacific Grove, CA: Brooks/Cole Publishing Company.

Narcotics Anonymous. (1982). *Narcotics anonymous.* Van Nuys, CA: World Service Office.

Online Casino. (2004). *13% increase in gambling addiction help line in 2004.* Retrieved June 9, 2004, from www.onlinecasino.org/news/13-increase-in-gambling-addiction-help-line-in-2004.php.

Parr, M. G., & Lashua, B.D. (2004). What is leisure? The perceptions of recreation practitioners and others. *Leisure Sciences, 26,* 1-17.

Random House Dictionary. (2nd ed.) (1987). New York: Random House.

Rogers, J. C., & Holm, M. B. (1994). *PASS: Performance assessment of self-care skills.* Version 3.0. Pittsburgh, PA: WPIC.

Rossman, J. R., & Schlatter, B. E. (2000). *Recreational programming: Designing leisure experiences.* Champaign, IL: Sagamore.

Thomson, L. K. (1992). *The Kohlman evaluation of living skills* (3rd ed.). Bethesda, MD: AOTA.

Wilcock, A. A., Chelin, M., Hall, M., Hamley, N., Morrison, B., Scrivener, L., et al. (1997) The relationship between occupational balance and health: A pilot study. *Occupational therapy International,* 4(1), 17-30.

8 Social Participation

David M. Santoro, MBA, OTR/L
Sylvia Valerio Sobocinski, MA, OTR/L
Cristina Klippel-Tancreti, MBA, OTR/L

CHAPTER OBJECTIVES

By the end of this chapter, the student will be able to:

☑ Define **social participation** as it pertains to the *Occupational Therapy Practice Framework (Framework)*.

☑ Describe specific **models/frames of reference** as related to social participation.

☑ Delineate between the role of the **occupational therapist** (OT) and the **occupational therapy assistant** (OTA) as they pertain to the occupation of social participation.

☑ Define the role of the occupational therapist as it pertains to peer/friend interactions for adults, older adults, and adults with disabilities.

☑ Comprehend and identify related **physical implications** as related to decreased independence in social participation.

☑ Describe barriers for adults with disabilities in developing and sustaining meaningful peer/friend and intimate relationships.

☑ Describe the impact of **contextual factors** upon social participation.

☑ Identify appropriate social participation intervention strategies based on various **performance skills and client factors**.

☑ Identify specific social participation **compensation/adaptation** strategies.

☑ Identify general social participation **remediation** strategies.

☑ Identify social participation compensation/adaptation intervention strategies related to **vision, perception, and cognition**.

☑ Identify general social participation **maintenance** strategies.

INTRODUCTION

Occupational therapy practitioners direct their expertise to a broad range of human occupations and activities that make up people's lives (American Occupational Therapy Association [AOTA], 2002). Social participation activities are those associated with organized patterns of behavior that are characteristic of an individual interacting with others within a given social system (adapted from Mosey, 1996, p. 340). In an individual's life, involvement in various groups, organizations, clubs, and social systems overlap and change throughout the lifespan. Social

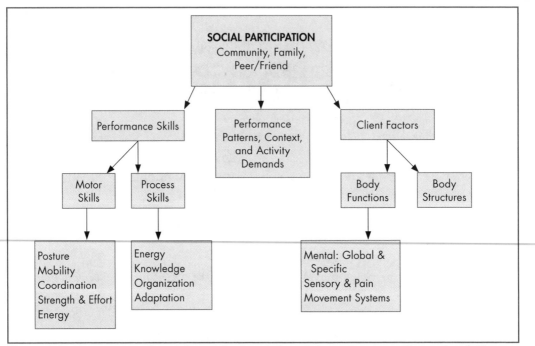

Figure 8-1. Components of social participation (adapted from American Occupational Therapy Association. [2002]. Occupational therapy practice framework: Domain and process. *American Journal of Occupational Therapy*, 56(6), 609-639).

participation activities, then, are multidimensional given the individual's physical environment and established roles and include community, family, and peer/friend interactions (AOTA, 2002).

In many ways, humans may depict portions of their own identity by their inclusion in different groups and affiliations—based upon religious or spiritual beliefs, racial identities, political parties, civic activities, interests, etc. Similarly, relationships with a spouse, sibling, grandparent, peer, boyfriend or girlfriend also influence an individual's identity and self-concept throughout the lifespan. According to the National Institutes of Health (NIH), these social and cultural factors play a central role in illness prevention, maintenance of good health and treating disease, noting that an individual's social ties, the quality of social relationships, and social resources can "mediate the effect of stress on health" (Consortium of Social Science Associations, 2000).

Faced with an onset of illness or disease, an individual's involvement in society may be altered, although his/her perception of self-identity and established habits and roles may remain the same. As a result, individuals with disabilities are five times more likely than nondisabled individuals to indicate that they are dissatisfied with their lives due to social isolation and lack of a full social life. Sixty-four percent of adults with disabilities report they are not able to get around town, attend cultural or sporting events, or socialize with friends as much as they would like (Kaye, 1997).

Thus, the OT must consider the unique significance of this performance area and what it specifically encompasses for the client throughout the service delivery process.

In this chapter, each category of social participation (community, family and peer/friend) will be explored from the adult, older adult, and adult with disability perspectives and several examples to further illustrate key points will be provided. Figure 8-1 depicts the components of social participation according to the *Framework* (AOTA, 2002).

Methods of social participation interventions, as with other performance areas, include occupation-based and purposeful activities, preparatory strategies, educational and consultative approaches, and, most significantly to this performance area, a constant therapeutic use of self by the occupational therapy practitioner. As social participation by definition consists of individuals engaging with one another, each client meeting offers the therapist a unique opportunity to model effective information exchange strategies, interpersonal boundaries, and the building of therapeutic social relations.

Specific frames of references for social participation interventions, including the Model of Human Occupation (MOHO), Cognitive Disability, and Sensory Motor approaches will also be further examined, as well as the importance of safety considerations and psychological implications of the intervention process.

As a client-centered approach, the therapist must incorporate various cultural, physical, social, personal, spiritual, temporal, and virtual conditions that influence the individual's performance in social participation (AOTA, 2002). These contexts are unique to the client, are often interrelated, and influence how the client creates his/her own personal identity. In this chapter, specific examples of social participation within these unique conditions are further examined.

Performance patterns related to daily life, including habits, roles, and routines, impact a client's ability to participate in various meaningful social relationships and activities (AOTA, 2002). This complex relationship between these patterns, a client's sense of self, and involvement in social systems are further addressed later in this chapter. Considerations on the activity demands of social activities, including the various aspects required to carry out meaningful social behaviors, will also be discussed. Finally, the role of the OTA as a contributor to the intervention process of social participation will also be examined.

METHODS OF INTERVENTIONS

The role of the occupational therapy practitioner may be multilayered when identifying and collaboratively implementing client social participation goals. According to the *Framework* document (AOTA, 2002), performance skills and patterns are impacted by the context in which the client operates, the specific demands of the activity, and individual client factors. Therefore, as a professional, not only must the OT take into account the client's age, but also the physical, mental, and social contexts of the individual as well. Since the challenge of occupational therapy is to maximize occupational (functional) performance in everyday activities, varying levels of intervention may be required to ensure that carryover of intervention approaches is consistently exhibited.

The World Health Organization (WHO) (2001) defined social participation for the lifespan as "the nature and the extent of an individual's involvement in life situations." The extent to which an individual becomes involved in daily social activities may be limited by disability. Hence, the challenge of developing meaningful interventions lies in the accurate assessment of the client's abilities and learning styles, and by choosing the best combination of interventions for the individual's successful occupational performance. A comprehensive intervention process includes three sub-steps: the development of the intervention plan, the implementation of the intervention, and intervention review. With each successful intervention, the OT establishes a meaningful approach to care with client input, includes the client in the process of intervention, and develops a plan to ensure carryover of the intervention is achieved. Although there are many forms of intervention used by an OT, the primary methods of intervention that will be addressed in the framework of this text are:

- Therapeutic use of self
- Direct service
- Education and training
- Consultation

Therapeutic Use of Self

Defined as an increased awareness of one's own values, beliefs, and attitudes (AOTA, 2002), this powerful method of intervention incorporates modeling into the intervention process. A young adult with MR who has difficulty maintaining physical boundaries in social situations may require concrete and tangible physical as well as verbal cuing by the therapist in one-to-one and small group activities. This may begin with modeling remedial behaviors such as proper eye contact and gestures, to advanced activities such as verbal pleasantries, awareness, and assessment of proprioception or position in space strategies. These latter skills may require not only verbal instruction, but also role-playing, videotaping, and other visual mechanisms for feedback. In this instance, it will be the role of the OT or OTA to determine the client's cognitive abilities and capacities for learning in order to later choose the appropriate level and type of intervention for successful performance. The true testament of successful intervention would be the exhibition of appropriate social skills not only in role-playing sessions, but also in everyday encounters. Successful intervention is measured by the quality and duration of carryover regarding learned techniques in all situations faced by the client.

Direct Service

Although direct service to clients is a small piece of what occupational therapy practitioners offer, it is the cornerstone of intervention. Comprised of multilevel approaches, direct service has as an overall goal to improve occupational performance of the individual client (Scheinholz, 2001). Direct service includes the screening process to determine the need for occupational therapy service, as well as the formal assessment and intervention plan development, discharge planning, education, and the implementation of a maintenance plan. By tailoring the intervention plan to the individual, the occupational therapy professional hopes to remediate and maximize functional performance. Social participation goals may include the establishment of an intervention plan as well as activities that allow for the client to achieve organized patterns of behavior expected of an individual in community settings and in peer/friend or family relationships (AOTA, 2002). Examples of direct service interventions using remedial, compensatory, and adaptive approaches will be explored later in this chapter.

Education and Training

The type and level of education and training that are appropriate and most beneficial for clients depend highly on cognition and the ability to process new information and adapt it to all relationships and environments (Allen, 1996). The role of the occupational therapy practitioner in the establishment of social performance goals is two-fold. It includes the ability to determine how best the client learns, and to educate and train the client using approaches that generate successful outcomes.

For example, John, a 21-year-old male with mental retardation, is seeking meaningful recreational activities that will allow him the ability to meet with people in his community. John has been followed by OTs throughout his high school years and a year-end Individualized Education Plan (IEP) goal for John is to join a community organization. From the client interview, observation, and assessment, the occupational therapy practitioner determines that for John to be successful with carryover of learned social techniques, he must be verbally cued through conversations when meeting an individual for the first time. In addition to the verbal cuing process, he also requires that the activity be modeled for him. Thus with this two-tiered approach, John is able to demonstrate successful new learning. The methodology chosen by the OT will have a direct effect on carryover of skill to multiple activities and situations. The educational process of identifying methods and tools that facilitate learning are then enhanced through repetitive and structured training sessions.

The process of identifying an individual's learning style, however, may only be gathered from an observation and interview. Additionally, the barrier of an individual's lack of insight into socially acceptable behavior must first be overcome for successful interaction in the individual's social system (Mosey, 1996). From an occupational therapy perspective, education and training build the skills necessary for lifelong adaptive learning and success.

Consultation

Often the expert skills of an OT are sought to enhance the performance of a client or organization. In this method of intervention, the OT may provide either direct or indirect service functions for the purpose of problem solving. Referring back to John, once his learning style has been identified and education and training components offered, the OT may then be required to problem-solve areas of concern that may be identified by the client or those interacting with him. For example, John continues to attend a bingo group at a local family center, but frequently interrupts the group with questions about the last number called. While direct services may be indicated in this situation, the OT may attend a bingo group session and determine that John's issue may be resolved by a change in seating location that enables him to not only hear but see the letter and number being called. An understanding of John's cognitive abilities and learning style from previous assessment led the OT to successful consultation in this instance. It is the skill and experience level of the OT that is used to enhance the individual and group function.

FRAMES OF REFERENCE/PRACTICE MODELS

This section will briefly consider the following frames of reference or practice models as they relate to the performance area of social participation: Model of Human Occupation (MOHO), Occupational Adaptation (OA), Ecology of Human Performance (EHP), Person-Environment-Occupation (PEO) model, Cognitive Disabilities model, and Sensory Motor model.

Model of Human Occupation (MOHO)

MOHO is a client-centered systems model that provides a framework for understanding a client's occupational strengths and limitations. MOHO incorporates a systems view of how an individual interacts with the environment to "create a network of conditions which influence an individual's motivation, actions, and performance" (Barrett & Kielhofner, 2003, p. 213).

When planning an intervention strategy to increase social participation from a MOHO perspective, the therapist needs to specifically address how values, roles, volition, and habituation impact social participation. What social activities are most important and meaningful to the client? Consider roles: Does this individual have roles that encourage involvement in social groups and activities? Has the individual recently lost important roles due to illness? Can the client re-establish these roles or do new roles need to be acquired (Barrett & Kielhofner, 2003)? For example, an older adult female with a cerebral vascular accident (CVA) may be struggling with the loss of ability to cook holiday meals for her extended family, a role she has held for many years and from which she derived a sense of pride.

- *Consider habituation*: What kind of habits or social routines did the individual have prior to the onset of illness, and what routines does the individual currently have? For example, a young mother with a diagnosis of multiple sclerosis may no longer be able to drive her children to the playground for the morning play group, which provided her with an opportunity to socialize with other mothers while their children enjoyed playing together.

- *Consider volition*: Does the client feel motivated to participate in activities with others or does he/she feel too exhausted, embarrassed, or stigmatized by illness or disability to socialize? For example, a male with dysphasia may no longer feel comfortable going out to participate in community activities involving food secondary to embarrassment regarding dietary restrictions and the need to thicken beverages.

- *Lastly, consider how the environment impacts social participation*: Do the client's interactions with others support positive occupational performance? Perhaps well-meaning family members are overprotective and make it difficult for the individual to regain independence, or perhaps community-based facilities are no longer physically accessible. For example, does a woman with multiple sclerosis stop attending the parent-teacher organization meetings at her son's grammar school because she can no longer drive herself, or is it because her family is worried it will be too tiring for her to go out in the evening?

Occupational Adaptation

This relatively new model, developed by Schkade and Schultz, "provides an additional dimension to the understanding of occupation and adaptation and their relationship to health" (Reitz & Scaffa, 2001, p. 65). The therapist works in collaboration with the client to focus on the process of adaptation in response to occupational challenges. An intervention plan is then developed to address occupational readiness and occupational activity. First, occupational readiness addresses deficits in performance skills, and then the client works on tasks to promote the occupational role he/she would like to master. For example, to enhance the role of hostess for a woman with rheumatoid arthritis who enjoys entertaining, occupational readiness may include the implementation of energy conservation and proper positioning techniques to allow her to meet her goal of meal preparation for a few friends.

"From an OA standpoint, occupation plays a significant role as a facilitator in social participation" (Barrett & Kielhofner, 2003, p. 222). Significantly, this model has also been used for research, including a study examining community integration following CVA, and may be relevant to consider in terms of researching various ways people adapt to restore social participation following illness.

Ecology of Human Performance

Developed at the University of Kansas, the EHP emphasizes the importance of context, which is relevant to social participation (refer to context examples previously discussed in this chapter).

The EHP model introduces five levels of therapeutic intervention approaches: establish/restore, adapt, alter, prevent, and create. Of these approaches, the *create* level is particularly suited for development of community-based wellness programs, as it does not assume a disability is present (Dunn, Brown, & McGuigan, 1994; Reitz & Scaffa, 2001, p. 65). Wellness programs often provide a secondary gain of increased community exploration and social interaction. Examples would be the creation of a walking club for seniors, or an intergenerational program involving school-aged children. Among other benefits, both programs would increase opportunities for socialization as well.

Person-Environment-Occupation

The PEO model is an interdisciplinary model that incorporates the Canadian Association of Occupational Therapists (CAOT) guidelines and theories for client-centered practice. "Occupational performance is the outcome of the transaction of the person, the environment and the occupation" (Barrett & Kielhofner, 2003, p. 229). Using this model to increase the occupation of social participation, the therapist can consider client factors affecting the individual, specifically body functions and body structure (AOTA, 2002). For example, cognitive capabilities, sensory functions such as vision and hearing, and pain issues impact an individual's ability to engage in meaningful social activities. As a result, the therapist should consider the environment and the opportunities the individual has for interacting within the environment. Is it safe, welcoming, and accessible, or are there barriers posing challenges to mobility and interaction with others?

Cognitive Disabilities

Claudia Allen uses a leather lacing activity, known as the Allen Cognitive Level test (ACL), as a screening tool to determine the client's cognitive level, which is measured on a scale of 1 to 6. Implications for social participation include the ability to predict the level of assistance the client will need for safety in the community, his/her capability for new learning, and socialization skills/communication style (Allen, Earhart, & Blue, 1992). The therapist should consider contexts, and structure the environment to provide a "just right challenge" to maximize self-esteem and client success. For example, when addressing social participation, an individual with a cognitive level score of 4 will be able to attend only to people within his/her immediate visual field, while an individual with a cognitive level 5 score will have a broader range of social abilities, but may not fully understand how his actions affect other people.

Sensory Motor

The Sensory Motor framework is particularly appropriate for persons having central nervous system (CNS) dysfunction, schizophrenia, depression, persons with developmental disabilities, and the geriatric population. This model assumes that if an individual can effectively process sensation, it will impact confidence and self-awareness, and thus set the stage for social skill building (Bruce & Borg, 2002). Intervention goals that relate to improved social participation can include increased ability to stay focused on a task, increased tolerance of touch, improved self-image, increased self-esteem, improved body language, and interpersonal skills such as the ability to initiate conversation.

Hanschu (1998) uses an alternative sensory motor approach called the Ready Approach. It provides sensory orientation to adults with severe developmental disabilities. This model, focusing on sensory processing problems, addresses sensory defensiveness and sensory modulation difficulties. Sensory defensiveness is an overreaction of one's normal protective senses. Tactile defensiveness, for example, may result in avoiding touch from others and dislike or inability to tolerate crowds, which would have a negative impact on the client's ability or motivation to socialize in his/her community.

The therapist can consider implementing a *sensory diet*, a term coined by Patricia Wilbarger (1995) to describe the provision of the appropriate combination of sensory input to keep an optimal level of arousal and performance. An intervention could include teaching the client ways to implement calming sensory input before a social interaction. Examples of calming or organizing sensory activities include soft or slow music, slow deep breathing, deep pressure touch and joint compression, and resistive activities. The therapist needs to provide the client with choices, make it enjoyable, and provide support to help establish a routine to maintain the change.

SAFETY CONSIDERATIONS

Since interventions in social participation may take place in the community setting, several key elements of client safety must be considered: mental function, personal safety, environmental/community demands, and health and wellness concerns.

In examining a client's overall safety in the community, the OT must always keep in mind the client's abilities and limitations of **specific mental functions**, including perceptual, thought, language, and higher-level cognitive functions and how these client factors may impact his/her ability to maintain safety for during social activities outside of the clinical setting. For example, an older adult with a CVA has difficulty sustaining attention when watching traffic signs while attempting to cross a street with oncoming cars. A young adult with mental retardation has difficulty maintaining physical boundaries during encounters with strangers and often tries to embrace passersby on the street. A middle-aged woman with schizophrenia has difficulty deciding if she should give all of her money for bus fare to a homeless person on the street.

Ensuring a client's personal safety in the community most often will consist of educating the client on potentially dangerous interpersonal situations, appropriate social boundaries when talking with others, including those unfamiliar to the client and methods of seeking out help in emergency situations. In some instances, clients may also be encouraged to seek out additional educational opportunities on self-defense strategies to further promote a sense of personal empowerment in the community.

Environmental and community safety considerations ensure the client's physical well-being, most often through assessment of environmental demands and barriers, and subsequently potential fall risk factors. Environmental demands and barriers in homes and public buildings are often complex and may include uneven travel surfaces, stairs or slopes, static or moving obstacles such as furniture or pedestrians, traffic crossings, weather conditions, and even poor lighting (Clemson, Cumming & Roland, 1996; Patla, 2001). The therapist and client should collaboratively determine the severity and potential safety hazards of each environmental demand and barrier based on the client's own abilities and limitations. The therapist should realize that although some environmental demands such as traffic crossings or pedestrians cannot be avoided, others, such as challenging travel paths, can be potentially modified and directions to end locations revised (Patla, 2001).

Given the intricacy of the community setting for clinical interventions, OTs must also thoroughly assess a client's community mobility (see Chapter 4), including the client's risk of falling. Falls are the leading cause of accidental death in the home and are a contributing factor in 40% of admissions to nursing homes (DiFabio & Seay, 1997). Individual factors that may cause an increased risk of falling include being female, older age, medication use, comorbidities (such as arthritis or Degenerative Joint Disease [DJD]), physical and mobility limitations, limited vision, dizziness, and cognitive impairments (Braun, 1998).

While determining potential fall risk factors and subsequently reduction strategies with a client, therapists can discuss the client's own perceptions or fears of falling, which may further impact his/her motivation level and interest to engage in community-related activities. Not surprisingly, many elderly people appear to reduce their activity levels due to these fears (Braun, 1998).

Lastly, a category of client safety that should also be addressed is the maintenance of general health and wellness. For most clients, engaging in social activities means more personal freedom and consequently opportunities to make choices regarding one's own health care. For example, the therapist can provide factual knowledge and education to clients on basic nutrition or dietary needs based on comorbidities, healthy sleep habits, disease prevention strategies, and possibly safe sex practices. As a health care practitioner, it is important to know that people 50 years and older compose the fastest growing HIV-infected group, increasing 138% since 1993 (Moore & Amburgey, 2000). Further discussion of sexuality and intimacy as a component of social participation can be found later in this chapter.

IMPLICATIONS FOR PSYCHOLOGICAL IMPACT
ON SOCIAL PARTICIPATION

A client's psychological well-being must remain a priority for the occupational therapy practitioner during social participation interventions. As previously described in this chapter, involvement in various social and family relationships, roles, and community activities encompasses a large portion of an individual's identity. As a result, a therapist must consistently pay close attention to how the client is responding to social reintegration strategies. Clients who may have isolated themselves from past social activities, or have never had meaningful social experiences due to disability or illness, may become easily frustrated or even depressed by taking on new social and interpersonal challenges. Therapists must realize that a disability can be either a cause of or a reason for social isolation (Jongbloed & Ernest-Conibear, 1995).

Upon initial evaluation, therapists need to thoroughly assess the client's experience of self functions, including body image, self-esteem, and self-concept; interaction/communication skills, energy, and drive functions; as well as motivation, impulse control, interests, and values (AOTA, 2002). Throughout the intervention process, these functions should continue to be monitored during interactions with the client, and changes should be recognized and addressed. In most cases, changes in these aspects of psychosocial functioning may not be overtly offered by the client. For example, the client will probably not say to a therapist that he is not feeling good about himself today, but instead state "I am feeling lazy," or refer negatively to himself by stating, "I'm stupid, I can't do anything right, I hate myself," etc. In addition, there may be subtle changes in body language and posture as well as decreased eye contact. As another example, an adult client with a recent left upper extremity (UE) amputation, initially appearing eager to get back into the community, may suddenly feel uncomfortable and extremely self-conscious while at a town council meeting. Later in therapy sessions, he may appear withdrawn and disconnected during interactions with the therapist, and often comments he is "a useless man with a stump."

Thus, throughout the intervention process, clients must be encouraged to verbalize their concerns about perceived inadequacies in self-concept and social barriers. Significantly, the therapist must realize that persons with disabilities face many social obstacles and stigma within communities, often described as, "community attitudes," which can play a significant role in determining the success of reintegration into society (Jongbloed & Ernest-Conibear, 1995).

Furthermore, the therapist must maintain open lines of communication and promote an honest dialogue on potentially awkward issues (dating, sexuality, intimacy, etc). In most cases, questions or concerns on intimacy or sexuality can be quite stress provoking for a client who may already have difficulty finding his/her own personal identity in an intimate relationship after disability or illness. Regardless of the subject matter, from the initial meeting the therapist sets the stage to promote effective communication between him- or herself and the client, based upon the building of trust and mutuality, or the concept that the therapist and client will influence each other, as well as the therapist's own self-awareness (Hopkins & Tiffany, 1988; Tickle-Degnen, 1995). Thus, by taking on a *helper* role to the client, it is paramount that therapists possess strong self-knowledge of their own needs, perceptual biases, and capabilities (Hopkins & Tiffany, 1988). Per Hopkins & Tiffany (1988), the therapist's own self-confidence and ability to be honest and open in this type of relationship as well as the extent to which he/she is able to communicate "unconditional positive regard" and empathy for the client will ultimately affect the client's own ability to invest trust in the relationship (p. 109).

It is also important for the therapist to take into account the client's past psychological history, if any. Does the client have a pre-existing diagnosis of depression, or symptoms of depression, but was never officially diagnosed or treated for emotional issues? Is there a past psychiatric diagnosis other than depression or a current diagnosis based on a recent injury? For example, anxiety after a stroke is a common emotional reaction that may be caused by a psychological fear of abandonment, feelings of helplessness, as well as the client's inability to externalize concerns or misinterpretations in social interactions due to cognitive impairments (Versluys, 1995). In addition, occupational therapy practitioners must realize there is a high prevalence of psychiatric disorders and distress in individuals with chronic physical illness (Wells, Golding, & Burnham, 1988a). For example, clients living with multiple sclerosis are at risk for anxiety and depression, as they cope with what is described as "riding a roller coaster in the dark; its unpredictability can cause an individual to plummet from joy to despair" (President & Fellows of Harvard College, 1997, p. 4). Since multiple sclerosis attacks different areas of the CNS, the disease may be as individualized as the individual it affects (1997). As a result, depression can often manifest when an adult with multiple sclerosis, or any chronic illness, undergoes a struggle with issues of dependency and independence. The adult needs to maintain as much autonomy and role identity as possible, while accepting an inescapable reliance on others (Cavallo, 1989).

Given the potentially fatal risks of psychological implications, therapists should not take for granted that other practitioners involved in the client's care have addressed psychological issues or the client has independently sought interventions for these types of emotional reactions. Suicide, although not always discussed overtly during client interventions, is a real risk for a depressed client with a life altering physical disability or disease. It is estimated that persons with spinal cord injuries commit suicide two to six times more frequently than the general population (Cairns & Baker, 1993).

CONTEXT OF SOCIAL PARTICIPATION

Context is particularly relevant when working with clients to increase or improve the quality of social participation, and should be addressed throughout the lifespan. Coster (1998) defined social participation as "the extent to which a child is able to orchestrate engagement or participation in an occupation in a context which is positive, personally satisfying and acceptable to the responsible adults in society" (p. 340). This is important in considering that our adult routines and preferences are influenced by childhood experiences, and also when considering the adult role of parent and caretaker.

The physical environment, attitudes of society, and policies can either facilitate or act as barriers to social participation (Law & Dunn, 1993b). As previously described, if the client perceives a stigma attached to his illness, it will negatively impact the desire and ability to socialize in the community.

In considering older adults, a majority of widowed persons use increased social participation as an active coping strategy to deal with the negative effects of widowhood (Utz, Carr, Ness, & Wortman, 2002). This may be due in part to the social context of friends and relatives rallying around and lending support (Lopata, 1996).

When setting goals and planning interventions in concert with the client, the OT needs to consider the client's cultural background, and family beliefs and traditions regarding appropriate social etiquette, and whether the client adheres to these beliefs or has chosen another path. Also consider personal aspects, such as past and previous interests, and the client's current social support system.

Physical considerations include the client's ability to access transportation and problems posed by environmental barriers. Environmental barriers that can impact social participation include crowded, excessively noisy, or inaccessible places. Social venues posing barriers may need to be replaced with environmental supports, such as wheelchair accessible buildings and transportation.

Table 8-1	
EXAMPLES OF CONTEXT IN SOCIAL PARTICIPATION	
Context	*Social Participation Example*
Cultural	A young mother with depression participating in the tradition of Sunday dinner with the extended family.
Physical	A wheelchair bound individual finding accessible restaurants where he/she can enjoy eating out with friends.
Social	Expectations of family and friends that an elderly widow with chronic obstructive pulmonary disease (COPD) should join a senior center to avoid isolation.
Personal	A single parent with the financial means to hire a babysitter and buy movie tickets or attend a concert with peers.
Spiritual	A retired social worker volunteering to run a youth group at the local church as a way to give back to the community and set a positive example.
Temporal	An individual with arthritis choosing an afternoon, rather than a morning coffee date, so she can have adequate time to prepare.
Virtual	An adolescent making plans with friends or gathering information about upcoming events by means of email, chat rooms, or via telephone.

Adapted from American Occupational Therapy Association. (2002). Occupational therapy practice framework: Domain and process. *American Journal of Occupational Therapy, 56*(6), 609-639.

Temporal considerations would include whether the time of day of the social event is compatible with the client's energy level, time management capabilities, ability to access transportation, and pain management/medication needs. In addition, consider the client's stage of life, as well as the ability to access opportunities for social participation that are appropriate and relevant to the stage. For example, a parenting group would be relevant for a young mother, while a retired individual might choose a social event sponsored by the local senior center.

Virtual considerations would include assessing whether the use of technology, such as telephones, computers, and the Internet, is a helpful link to socializing with others, or if it keeps the client isolated by acting as a substitute for face-to-face contact. According to Letts, Rigby, and Stewart (2003), electronic aids to daily living (EADLs) can allow individuals with disabilities enhanced communication and increased community access. In a case study on using a computer as an environmental facilitator to promote post-head injury social role resumption, when given computer-related activities to enhance social participation, a client was able to re-establish his roles as a brother and son and re-establish contacts with an extended family (Gutman, 2000). Table 8-1 provides specific examples of how contexts relate to social participation.

PERFORMANCE PATTERNS RELATED TO SOCIAL PARTICIPATION

Performance patterns of behavior, including social habits, routines, and roles, need to be considered when completing an intervention plan with the client. For example, is the client shy and reserved, or outgoing and comfortable in social situations? Is he/she comfortable in large settings or does he/she prefer to socialize on a one-to-one basis or in small groups?

The *Framework* divides habits into three types: useful, impoverished, and dominating (AOTA, 2002). A useful habit would support social participation, such as checking email daily and regularly conversing with friends. An impoverished habit that would need improvement would be the avoidance of eye contact when conversing with others. A dominating habit that would impact social participation would be substance abuse. Impoverished habits can result from the inability to cope with physical or mental illness and the resulting loss of roles.

Some examples of social roles in the community include PTA president, garden club member, and volunteer at the local hospital. Examples of family roles include room mother at the local grammar school, chaperone for the school field trip, coach for the Little League team, and play group organizer. Examples of peer/friend roles that involve social participation might include tennis partners, sorority sisters, or teammates at school.

ACTIVITY DEMANDS

Previously, it was noted there must be a multitiered approach to client-centered intervention. Not only must age, disability, and physical, mental, and social contexts be considered when intervention planning for social participation, but also the demand of the activity. *Activity demands*, according to the AOTA *Framework* document (2002), define the aspects of an activity to include the objects, space, social demands, sequencing or timing, required actions, and required underlying body functions and body structure needed to carry out the activity. Persons with developmental and physical disabilities are commonly faced with barriers to successful performance such as fear of injury or reinjury, presence of pain, reduced level of energy, lack of appropriate transportation, and lack of support for participation (Oman & Reed, 1998). Table 8-2 lists examples of activity demands as they relate to social participation.

The occupational therapy practitioner must be sensitive to the perceived concerns of the client and the actual limitations the client must overcome to be successful with task performance. For example, looking back at the young adult with MR, John's abilities according to the Allen Cognitive Level and their relation to differing social abilities, we are reminded, John requires verbal cuing and modeling for successful performance (Pollard, 2000). He scores a 4.8 on the ACL, which places him at an ability to follow ritualistic tasks. John has been attending a social group for about 3 weeks and he has been able to meet one new individual and use public transportation to get across town. On the fourth week John attends the group, he enters the church hall to find the group has been moved to a new location for this week's session due to air conditioning problems. The group has been relocated to the third floor of the church rectory, so John heads in the direction of the signage. He enters the rectory and encounters a sign with an arrow pointing upward toward the flight of stairs in front of him. Since John has multiple medical and orthopedic issues, he is unable to attend the group and heads for the bus stop, angry and disillusioned. Is it normal for a feeling of disappointment to manifest in this case? *Of course.* But for John, his cognitive *and* physical abilities limited him in this situation. All too often, coping strategies are an important consideration for intervention planning for clients. Therefore, the OT must not only anticipate what barriers a client attempting to be an active participant in his/her community may face, but he/she must also instruct the client in adaptive approaches to successful performance.

ROLE OF THE OCCUPATIONAL THERAPY ASSISTANT

The primary role of the certified occupational therapy assistant (COTA) is to carry out the intervention as planned and supervised by the OTR following completion of the evaluation

Table 8-2

EXAMPLES OF ACTIVITY DEMANDS IN SOCIAL PARTICIPATION

Activity Demands	Definitions (AOTA, 2002, p. 624)	Social Participation Examples
Objects and their properties	The tools, equipment and materials used in the process of carrying out an activity	• Tools: games • Materials: clothing • Equipment: tables, chairs • Inherent properties: room temperature and set up
Space demands (physical context)	The physical environmental requirements of the activity	• Large community room for a church social function
Social demands (social and cultural contexts)	The social structure and demands that may be required by the activity	• Social rules or etiquette at a function • Expectations of other persons participating in the activity
Sequence and timing	The process used to carry out the activity	• Steps: how a social function follows a schedule • Sequence: understanding process of the bingo game
Required actions	Motor, process, and communication/interaction skills required of a individual to carry out an activity	• Motor: grasping bingo chips • Process: multiple card scanning • Communication: knowing when to announce a winning card
Required body functions	Physiological functions to support the actions of an activity	• ROM of UEs for manipulation of chips • Ability to sustain attention to caller of the game
Required body structures	Anatomical parts required to perform the activity	• Number of hands • Number of eyes

Adapted from American Occupational Therapy Association. (2002). Occupational therapy practice framework: Domain and process. *American Journal of Occupational Therapy, 56*(6), 609-639.

(Scheinholz, 2001). The OTA, although routinely supervised by the OTR, must also demonstrate sound clinical judgment for efficacy in the intervention process. The level and frequency of supervision includes the experience of the practitioners, the requirements of the regulatory agencies governing practice, and the level of need of the client(s) involved (AOTA, 2004) While the role of the OTA continues to expand as the evolution of community-based occupational therapy services continues, it is imperative that modifications to intervention approaches be done collaboratively within the OTR/OTA guidelines.

Social participation goals and interventions are often associated with community, peer/friend and family relationships. Quite often, this means interventions are performed in a community setting or the interventions require the individual to be treated in "isolation" from family members and peers since they are often not present during intervention sessions. Because of this, the competency of the OTA and the amount of supervision provided by the OT are vital. The OTA in a community setting must understand the variety of resources available to the client. The OTA must also seek the appropriate supervision necessary to insure the intervention plan is achievable and, if not, adapt it for successful client performance in collaboration with the supervising OT.

COMMUNITY ASPECTS OF SOCIAL PARTICIPATION

Community participation is characterized by AOTA (2002) as activities that result in successful interaction at the community level (e.g., neighborhoods, organizations, work, or school). All human beings seek to be members of their individual communities. For some, involvement may be in work activities, a volunteer group, a social club, or a civic organization. For those with disabilities, this membership may simply be reintegration into the community, which may require alternative approaches to performing required activities. Each of these forays has its own set of challenges, but it is the ultimate challenge of the OT to assist the client in finding the just-right path, thus overcoming the barriers to independent and meaningful functioning. Uniquely, not only do cognitive, physical, and psychosocial barriers exist through this challenge, but the ways in which to participate in community activities also differs from culture to culture (Baum & Law, 1997).

The area of occupation known as *social participation* is defined as "activities associated with organized patterns of behavior which are characteristic and expected of an individual or an individual interacting with others within a given social system" (Mosey, 1996, p. 340). The act of participating in social situations includes integration into the community, with family and with peers or friends. Importantly, the role of the OT and the intervention strategies may vary depending on the client's place along the life continuum. For purposes of this text, the discussion will focus on the adult, older adult, and adults with disabilities.

Adult Community Social Participation Roles

Social participation for an adult may include a variety of activities, but successful integration will depend greatly on the individual's desired outcomes. Socioeconomic factors may impact the adult's ability to choose meaningful activities and community size and activity opportunities may be limited as well. Other factors to be considered when assisting the client with social participation goals are the client's marital status, religion, social skill levels, and communication and interaction skills. An adult will typically seek groups or organizations with matching interest levels. Men and women may also choose group activities and social settings based upon gender differences. Further, throughout the lifespan, an individual's roles change depending upon his/her occupation and peer group. Thus, the level of community participation often depends on adult development. For example, the young adult recently graduated from college may seek entirely different social participation activities than a married adult with children and an established career.

Older Adult Social Participation Roles

Older adults quite often demonstrate a dichotomous tract with respect to their level of interaction in their community. The well-elderly may consider many options and choose a multitude of opportunities in order to stay connected with friends, families, and community. The frail older adult or the individual with significant health concerns may be at great risk for social isolation and is, quite often, the most in need of services, but the least likely to seek access to them. The healthy older adult is at the point in his/her lifespan where continued personal perceptual life value is tied into the concept of being an active member of the community. In accordance with the WHO (2001) objectives of healthy aging along the life continuum, it is clearly the role of the community-based OT, then, to assist clients with accessibility options to activities based in the community to further promote their overall sense of well-being.

Adults With Disabilities Social Participation Roles

For adults with disabilities, the physical environment, the attitudes of society, and policies can either facilitate or act as barriers to social participation (Law & Dunn, 1993b). All too often, the difference between successful community reintegration for clients and impending social isolation is the active intervention of the OT who focuses on access and participation in meaningful activities. However, when an adult with a disability is challenged to participate in a community setting, quite often both the medical model and social models of intervention are equally explored. Occupational therapy interventions are based on determining whether limits in a client's social participation relate to the client's personal factors, the demands of the occupation or activity or the external factors of the environment (Rogers & Holm, 2003).

FAMILY ASPECTS OF SOCIAL PARTICIPATION

Family social participation is defined as *activities that result in successful interaction in specific required and/or desired familial roles* (Mosey, 1996, p. 340). These activities can range from in-house celebrations, holidays, and traditions to community activities that family members participate in together. Frequency may vary from weekly dinners or religious activities to occasional functions such as family weddings or reunions involving a larger network of extended family. In addition, social participation can encompass talking to relatives on the phone or communicating via email. This more informal level of social participation is helpful in keeping families connected when they have conflicting schedules, limited access to transportation, or live far away from one another.

Family Composition

The role of each family member and overall family composition is affected by culture, family finances, general economic issues, the environment, and legislation. Family roles can include, but are not limited to, the following: mother, father, grandparent, child, sibling, spouse, partner, and widow. When considering family roles, the therapist should be aware that the scope of who is considered family has evolved and expanded in recent years for a variety of reasons. "There are more extended families, single-parent families, teenage parents, grandparents as primary caretakers, joint custody situations, and foster parents" (Wooster, Gray, & Gifford, 2001, p. 240). Divorce is more accepted by society and therefore more prevalent. In addition, it is common for divorced individuals to remarry and create blended families. Same sex relationships are also more common, with recent legislation in some states allowing for same sex marriages. All of these issues will continue to have an impact on family dynamics.

Adult Family Roles

Socioeconomic trends impact adult roles and occupations. For example, more women are college educated and consequently, more women are joining the workforce and juggling household responsibilities along with work responsibilities. In addition, more adult children are moving back into their parents' home after college to save money and defray the high cost of college loans. These adult children are marrying later and having children later in life. This trend of adult children living at home causes parents to experience the "empty nest" transition later in life, described later in the peer/friend section of this chapter.

In addition to the roles designated by position in the family, there are also the occupations adults take on that are associated with their responsibilities in the family structure—occupational roles such as wage earner, homemaker, student, cook, driver, and child care provider.

Older Adult Family Roles

Life expectancy has increased, thus impacting the nature of family, with many older adults taking on increased responsibilities. For example, many adults remain active in their communities after retirement by taking on part-time jobs or by volunteering as a way to stay connected for financial reasons, and to continue to enjoy meaningful occupation. Others remain active by helping family members with child care responsibilities. According to the U.S. Census Bureau population projections, America's elderly are expected to make up more than 20% of the population by 2050. This is a projected increase of 147% for those age 65 and over, while the projected increase for the population as a whole is only 49% (U.S. Census Bureau, 2005).

It is important for the OT, then, to have an understanding of human development and roles throughout the lifespan in order to help clients and their families cope with change and to help them maintain a healthy balance of meaningful occupations including social participation.

Dealing With Disability and Social Integration

An individual dealing with the onset of illness or disability has to learn to ask for and accept help, deal with the loss of meaningful roles, and the loss of autonomy and independence. These issues can be overwhelming and often result in depression and a decrease in social participation. The *motherhood model* compares family care to a type of social control in which adults with disabilities are treated as children. While society encourages family caring and kinship, adult dependence is often disapproved (Jongbloed, Stanton, & Fousek, 1993).

Given all the changes and losses, the individual adjusting to disability often has to deal with concurrent feelings of loneliness and social isolation. These feelings can be exacerbated by societal attitudes, stereotypes, and lack of understanding. Becker discusses the term *master status*, which overrides all other statuses (Conneeley, 2002). If the client feels stigmatized by the attitudes of others, she may adopt the new identity or "status" of a disabled individual in place of previous social relationships and meaningful occupations.

Another term, *stranger status*, describes an individual who is part of a group, yet feels that he/she is outside of it (Conneeley, 2002). This perceived outsider position can also have a negative impact on social roles and self-esteem.

Impact on Family Roles and Social Participation

When changes in roles become necessary secondary to disability, they impact not only the client, but his/her entire family. For example, if a homemaker can no longer cook meals and care for her children, she has to deal with the psychological implications of the loss of the important and defining role. As a result, her husband, extended family, and even the children will have to compensate.

Disability can also have a major impact on marriage because the changes that occur provide a challenge to both partners' communication skills, and a challenge to established habits, patterns of intimacy, and beliefs. With major advances in medical technology and improved standards of living, couples are living much longer with chronic illness and disabling conditions (Rolland, 1994a). The couple must address changing boundary issues, traditional divisions of labor, the under-current of loss, and the need to redefine their relationship. The partner with the disability may consider him- or herself a burden, while the partner who is taking on more responsibilities may feel resentment. In addition, these new feelings may trigger guilt in one or both partners. Physical limitations may also pose a challenge to the relationship. For example, physical limitations secondary to stroke or spinal cord injury have an ongoing impact on intimacy and social participation, while conditions such as multiple sclerosis or rheumatoid arthritis may have exacerbations and remissions that partners need to further manage.

It is important to note, though, that some families can develop strengthened relationships following a serious illness or disability. As described in Conneeley (2002), positive relationships evolving after such events may result in spiritual growth, increased awareness of the importance of family, and the establishment of new values.

Disability of parents causes a role reversal when adult children who have depended on their parents for many years now have to take on the responsibility of caring for one or both of their parents, grandparents, or an aging relative. At times, these adult children are still caring for their own children. The growth of this dual responsibility has been coined "sandwich generation" referring to the individual being sandwiched between two very different needs at opposite ends of the developmental spectrum. They are caught between what their children need and what their parents need, and often have little or no time to engage in their own meaningful social activities outside of the family.

Women are currently assuming a primary role when a family member needs care; however, men are increasing their roles as family caregivers, with the number of men assuming the role of primary caregiver also increasing. Issues regarding family caregivers, and meeting their needs as an extension of good client care, will be addressed in more detail later in this chapter.

An individual's living environment may create a new "family"—extended family for those separated from their biological families, families of origin due to the level of care they require, or the reality in which older family members are no longer able to care for them. For adults with developmental disabilities, peers and staff members at group homes, foster homes, and halfway houses often take on the roles of extended family. This may include celebrating holidays with residents as well as accompanying them out in to the community. For these adults, social participation is most often arranged by others, and they are usually part of a structured group of peers.

With increased lifespan, more elders are coping with disability and needing assistance to carry out daily routines. OTs often evaluate elderly clients at critical life junctures such as nursing home placement or onset of illness. Adults in nursing homes, adult day programs and assisted living programs are dealing with life changes that impact their roles and necessitate an increased dependence on others. While social opportunities in the community are often decreased for these elders, activities are provided within easy access, and in a more structured as well as safe home environment.

Family Reactions to Illness/Disability

Reactions to the onset of illness or disability by family members vary, but may include shock, denial and disbelief, anger, hostility, unrealistic expectations, or disengagement from the client.

While some families pull together, support the client, and accept the illness, others may minimize or fully deny any problems or need for a change in their routines. This presents a problem for the therapist trying to gain support for the client. For example, a lack of family cooperation may hinder follow-through on interventions such as home exercise programs. It is best for the therapist to gently approach families in shock by presenting plans as options or contingencies, and then providing educational materials as well as resources, if appropriate.

When family members react with anger and hostility, the therapist needs to empathize without personalizing the feelings and without feeding into unrealistic expectations. Assess the level of family involvement the client and family are accustomed to and support it. When family members are very involved, it may be beneficial to educate them regarding the role of occupational therapy and to routinely incorporate use of counseling skills during intervention sessions. When families have unrealistic expectations, the therapist may need to share goals and set limits while maintaining a therapeutic relationship.

At times, families may disengage for a variety of reasons, which may include frustration, feeling overwhelmed, harboring guilt, feeling burnout, or concealing resentment from previous unresolved conflicts with the family member who is now ill.

Family Caregiver Issues

Many older adults living in the community require long-term care and this care is often provided by family caregivers. Caregivers face a variety of stressors on a daily basis that including fear something will happen to their loved one, difficulties juggling work and home responsibilities, social isolation, role changes, and limited income/loss of income due to time constraints.

Social isolation is a leading contributor to stress among family caregivers. This is a common problem, especially for clients with dementia and their caregivers (Szekais, 1991). Socialization becomes more difficult for the individual as the illness progresses, and he/she may often require more assistance from the family to socialize and interact with others successfully. As socialization becomes more difficult and more assistance is required in maintaining self-care and other daily routines, socialization tends to decrease for both the caregiver and the patient. Family caregivers need ongoing support and encouragement to continue to socialize in order to maintain their own mental and emotional wellness as well as energy level. Also, it is necessary to provide opportunities for the individual with dementia to socialize in order to maintain cognitive and affective functioning (Szekais, 1991).

Family caregivers also lose important roles and take on new roles secondary to dealing with chronic illness. Lost roles may include those with leisure such as gardening, dancing, and civic duties. These roles are often no longer possible due to time constraints and energy drain placed on the individual. New roles that replace them include caregiver and case manager, which often include the added responsibilities of researching options for the loved one, dealing with finances, making arrangements for transportation and equipment, and assisting with medications.

When discharging a client home to a family caregiver, the age and physical status of the caregiver must be taken into consideration. Family training should address goals and specific procedures in a format that the caregiver can understand. If multiple family members will be assisting the client, they should all be trained to make sure care is consistent. This will be addressed further in the intervention section of this chapter.

Meeting the Needs of the Family

The family will need information about the illness, intervention, and prognosis in order to know what is expected, as well as information about the role of occupational therapy. The family will need to develop skills in order to cope with the effects of illness and the changes that will occur as a result. In addition, families will need to learn how to interact effectively with health care providers.

Lastly, the family will need support. The therapist can provide support by just listening and allowing the family to vent, deal with change, and mourn the loss of what was. The therapist can assist the family and client with decision making by outlining options within the scope of occupational therapy services. For example, the therapist can let the family know that social participation is an important occupation and within our realm of practice (AOTA, 2002).

The therapist can also help the client and family locate appropriate resources or groups that will provide additional and ongoing support, and when indicated, may help the family access respite care. Respite care can be provided inside the home or at facilities in the community. Many assisted living facilities, nursing homes, and adult day care centers provide respite care services for family members to take a much-needed vacation, or attend to personal matters without worrying about the safety of their loved one (Paulson, 1991).

In addition, local hospitals usually run a variety of support groups and community-based health programs at no or low cost. Examples range from arthritis exercise groups and cardiac rehabilitation to groups providing support to caregivers and groups for families dealing with grief and loss. These venues provide support as well as an opportunity to meet and socialize with others dealing with some of the same issues.

Involving Family

When working with families, the therapist needs to demonstrate a variety of skills and coping strategies in order to establish and maintain rapport to set the stage for appropriate interventions, which include:

- Be tolerant, respectful, flexible, knowledgeable, and compassionate.
- Further consider context, habits, and patterns of the client and family (see the occupational profile in Chapter 1).
- Be respectful of family culture and dynamics
- Be flexible, as change takes time and requires the use of creativity and clinical reasoning skills.
- Be knowledgeable: teach skills at client's level of understanding to convey knowledge appropriately.
- Grade and adapt activities and home care routines as needed for success.
- Use lay terms when talking with family members, and provide written instructions for them to refer to whenever possible.
- Work with interdisciplinary team members to provide structure and continuity.

The partnership model, proposed by Crabtree (1991), joins the family with the older adult and includes family members in therapy and decision making to validate their expertise in caregiving, and incorporate their knowledge of the family member's wishes. By involving the family early on when the older adult can partner with them in decision making, they will be more informed and less overwhelmed if they need to take over and advocate on behalf of their family member. The client will need to consent if able and give durable power of attorney to a family member if this situation occurs.

The family can become an ally in partnering with the client to maximize independence and promote community integration. In addition, the family can help the client follow through on programs to get lasting benefits from therapy. The therapist must gather information from the client and family to determine role patterns of the family, the degree to which the environment has influenced roles, and how the disability has affected occupational performance (Jongbloed et al., 1993). Specifically, the therapist needs to find out what roles each member of the family fulfills, how these roles have changed, and, most importantly, if there is role flexibility when needed. Further, the therapist needs to determine how involved family members wish to be and how the support received from family influences role maintenance for the client.

Peer/Friend Aspects of Social Participation

The performance area of social participation as it relates to peer/friend interactions consists of activities at different levels of intimacy, including engaging in desired sexual activity (AOTA, 2002). Relationships with friends or cohorts can provide meaningful experiences for individuals and are interrelated to their overall sense of wellness. In addition, the individual's gender, age, and disability status can further indicate how these social interactions, or lack there of, can impact an individual's health and involvement in his/her community.

Friendships are significant human experiences for several reasons. Friends support each other emotionally, are willing to see things from the other's point of view, and provide assistance and feedback when needed (Lutfiyya, 1997). These types of relationships also involve enjoyment, acceptance, trust, respect, mutual assistance, confiding, understanding, and spontaneity (Brintnall-Peterson, 2004). In a crisis situation or personal tragedy, an individual's close friends, outside of his/her own family of origin, can even serve as a protective factor when faced with life changing experiences and psychosocial stressors (Simmons Longitudinal Study, 2004).

Peer Versus Friend

Peer relationships are not the same as friendships. Although friendships and peer groups occur in the social context of an individual's environment, the latter may be based solely on existing common characteristics that are influential in establishing norms, role expectations and social routines (AOTA, 2002; Kindermann & Sage, 1999). Generally, peers are individuals that a person identifies or compares themselves with, who are usually, but not always, of the same age group. Acceptance by the peer group is often desirable and based on recognition of similarity (Bourne, 1998; Cook & Semmel, 1999). In addition, peer groups influence an individual's belief structure and system of rules, values, and goals based on commonality of its group members (Bourne, 1998).

Through the lifespan, an individual's peer group changes based upon the individual's roles and occupations. In adulthood, a career woman's peers may be her female coworkers. In older adulthood, a retired man's peers may be members of his fishing club. For an adult male with a recent spinal cord injury (SCI), his peer group may consist of other SCI survivors from a local sports group Often, these common peer bonds can be the basis of friendship development.

Adult Friendships

The term *social convoy* describes the network of close relationships we maintain throughout life. In general, an individual's social convoy consists of two to five close friendships and does not necessarily change during adulthood, although the actual members may change (Brintnall-Peterson, 2004). During emerging adulthood, between the ages of 18 to 30, individuals often begin to establish themselves outside of their families of origin and create a social support network of friends, colleagues, and intimate partnerships, which becomes extremely important in defining a sense of self (Simmons Longitudinal Study, 2004). Some close friendships in adulthood may actually be those first established during childhood or adolescence. Through middle adulthood, from the ages of 40 to 65, friendships and social circles are further seen as support systems that help in the adjustment of midlife transitions. During these so-called *mid-life crises*, individuals may view themselves in terms of how many years they have to live versus how many years they have lived (Rathus, 1988, p. 379).

Older Adult Friendships

Late or older adulthood begins at age 65. As we age, friendships change because of declining individual physical and mental capacities and life cycle transitions including retirement and death of spouse. Per Rathus (1988), the basic challenge for individuals in older adulthood is to maintain the belief that life is meaningful and worthwhile in the face of the inevitability of death (p. 383). Within this psychosocial development theory, an individual's support network aids in the adjustment of these life changes.

Social Isolation With Older Adults

It is important to note that older individuals are more likely to lose family members and friends due to illness and death and are more vulnerable to loneliness and social isolation (Yeh & Lo, 2004). Studies suggest that feelings of loneliness for older adults contribute to increasing functional disability, especially greater ADL dependency (2004). As a result, social relations are often still regarded as an important criterion of quality of life in old age and a key environmental factor enhancing health, participation and psychosocial security (Bukov, Maas, & Lampert, 2002; Yeh & Lo, 2004).

Gender Differences in Friendships

According to Bell (1981), there is no social factor more important than gender in leading to friendship variations. Interestingly, women tend to define friendship in terms of closeness and emotional attachment, whereas men often have less intense, more action-oriented friends. This concept is further described by Block (1980), as "convenience or activity friends," which are segmented or centered around particular activities (Traustadottir, 1993). In addition, researchers have argued that males tend to have significantly fewer close or *best* friends than females throughout the lifespan. Specifically, throughout the adult years, women seem to have larger social convoys than men and also maintain these relationships longer (Brintnall-Peterson, 2004). Although male friendships may be less intimate and fewer than their female counterparts, these relationships still serve to buffer stress and reduce depression in the same way women's friendships do (Traustadottir, 1993).

In older adulthood, similar gender trends in friendship continue. Interestingly, as females tend to have larger groups of friends, they are more susceptible to emotional stress when negative experiences happen to their cohorts. In addition, women are generally faced with a more significant psychological life adjustment after the death of a spouse, as they tend to live longer than men (Brintnall-Peterson, 2004).

Dating and Partnerships

According to Levinson, the ages of 33 to 40 are characterized by an individual's desire to settle down. Often during this transitional period, men seek independence and autonomy in their interpersonal relationships and women may have a newfound interest in childbearing and are more likely to undergo a transformation from being cared for to caring for others (Rathus, 1988). In a survey of college men and women, it was determined that several psychological traits including fidelity, warmth, sensitivity, and honesty were relatively more important in long-term relationships than physical attractiveness (1988, p. 620). Additionally, for mate selection, women often place greater emphasis on characteristics such as dependability, kindness, professional status, and fondness for children than men do and men place relatively greater importance on physical attractiveness than women (Rathus, 1988). Commonly, individuals are likely to meet their partners in work environments, social situations, and leisure time (Brown, 1996).

There are potentially several advantages of partnerships and marriage. Such companionship offers each individual various opportunities to share a wide range of experiences and promote social learning and adaptation, which further promotes motivation and emotional development (Brown, 1996). It is also well known that partnership and marriage lead to greater longevity, thus married individuals enjoy better health than those of other marital statuses (Brown, 1996; Christiansen, 1990). Specifically, in a comparison study between married and unmarried men and women, it was concluded that divorced, single, and separated individuals suffered much higher rates of disease, morbidity, disability, mental neuroses, and mortality than their married counterparts (Christiansen, 1990).

Intimacy and Sexuality

The complexity of human sexuality includes body image, self-concept, gender identity, beliefs and feelings about sex, capacities for love and friendship, social behavior, as well as overt physical expression of love or sexual desire (Gourley, 2002). Humans are considered sexual beings; therefore, sexual identity and fulfillment of sexual roles and expression are intrinsic components of the overall human experience.

An individual's ethical, religious and spiritual beliefs, cultural traditions, and moral concerns further influence patterns of sexual behavior, as well as levels of intimacy with others (Gourley, 2002; Rathus, 1988). Intimacy can be described as feelings of closeness and affection between interacting partners, the state of having revealed one's innermost thoughts and feelings to another individual, relatively intense forms of nonverbal engagement (notably touch, eye contact, and close physical proximity), particular types of relationships (especially marriage), and sexual activity (Mackey, Diemer, & O'Brien, 2000). Additionally, intimacy from a psychosocial perspective can be considered a sense that one can be open and honest in talking with a partner about personal thoughts and feelings not usually expressed in any other relationship (Mackey et al., 2000).

In general, humans crave intimacy, to love, and to be loved (Barbor, 2001). In a study of same- and opposite-gender couples, participants described intimacy as the verbal sharing of inner thoughts and feelings between partners along with mutual acceptance of those thoughts and feelings (Mackey et al., 2000). Sexuality, as a form of intimacy, is also associated with happiness, overall well-being, and also longevity; studies have shown that frequency and enjoyment of sexual intercourse are significant predictors of longevity (Nusbaum & Hamilton, 2002).

Notably, sexual function and intimacy with others should be considered relevant throughout the lifespan, as an elderly widow may be as concerned about her sexuality as a young adult (Nusbaum & Hamilton, 2002). Society views older adults as asexual beings, incapable of healthy sexual relationships. This stereotype is also predominantly significant for postmenopausal women (Gourley, 2002). In contrast, Moore & Amburgey (2000) discuss recent studies that show older adults are interested in sexual intercourse and enjoy sexual activities.

As previously mentioned in this chapter, it is significant to note that individuals 50 years of age and older are the fastest growing HIV-infected group, increasing 138% since 1993, and they comprise 11% of people in the United States diagnosed with AIDS (Moore & Amburgey, 2000). Health care workers often lack awareness of this prevalence, probably due to societal stereotypes of this age group and limited educational focus. In addition, older adults in general often lack knowledge of risk-taking behaviors and are often hesitant to discuss their sexual activities with others (Moore & Amburgey, 2000).

Adults With Disabilities and Friendships

The development of any friendship depends on the opportunity to interact with others, appropriate social and interpersonal skills, and the ability to initiate and sustain a relationship; some or all of these components are often challenging for the adult with a disability (Gordon, Tantillo, Feldman, & Perrone, 2004). Problematically, people with cognitive or mental limitations don't always understand how to interpret what others are thinking and expressing nonverbally, further impacting their ability to develop and maintain social relations (Greenfield, 2005).

As previously described in this section, many friendships maintained in young adulthood are formed during childhood and adolescence. As a result, students with disabilities who are offered mainstream educational opportunities generally have an advantage in participating more fully in society than children or adolescents who are segregated into special schools or classes (Kaye, 1997).

Most disabled young adults have extremely limited out-of-school contacts, negligible participation with organized social activities, and a predisposition towards sedentary activities (Ng, Dinesh, Tay, & Lee, 2003). Even for previously mainstreamed students with disabilities, this cycle of social alienation unfortunately worsens when young adults leave the structure of a school setting. For example, young adults with cerebral palsy tend to become less socially active and more isolated after leaving school (Ng et al., 2003).

Additionally, adults with disabilities that remain after school age years have fewer opportunities to form meaningful relationships unless social bonds were developed prior to the onset of the disability. Also, many disabled individuals primarily interact with family members, caregivers, or health care providers and others in the programs in which they participate. Notably, outside of family relations, individuals with disabilities may have no freely given and chosen relationships, thus becoming further alienated from the community and isolated from others (Lutfiyya, 1997).

Social Isolation and Disability

Social isolation is a major reason disabled adults are dissatisfied with their lives, with 51% surveyed by Harris in 1994 stating that a lack of a full social life is a problem (Kaye, 1997). Studies also indicate that high levels of loneliness negatively affect mental and physical health, as depression, anxiety, and low self-esteem appear to be related to loneliness (Hoppe, Popin, Aroonoau, Freschette, & Begin, 2001).

Although social integration for disabled persons is a significant component of the Americans with Disabilities Act (ADA), comparable surveys from the Harris group in 1986 and 1994, respectively, indicate little evidence of progress (Kaye, 1997). Researchers further argue that social isolation can also be a result of living alone, as people with disabilities are more than twice as likely to live alone as those without disabilities, according to data from the 1990 National Health Interview Survey (1997). Significantly, as the disabled population ages, this problem also increases. It is estimated that over one-third (33.9%) of those over the age of 65 with disabilities live by themselves (1997).

Barriers to Social Relationships

Friendships and interpersonal connections are obviously significant experiences for all people's lives, including those faced with a disability (Chen, Brodwin, Cardoso, & Chan, 2002; Gordon et al., 2004). As previously described, adults with disabilities may have fewer opportunities to create these bonds due to several factors, including longstanding negative social attitudes and stigma, often described as *invisible community barriers* (Gordon et al., 2004). Researchers have found that societal attitudes toward fully integrated disabled individuals in the community have become more positive in the vocational and educational arenas, but not within personal and social relations (Chen et al., 2002). In the United States, attitudes toward disability vary dramatically according to social contexts, with more positive attitudes held toward people with disabilities in work situations than in dating and marriage (Chen et al., 2002). This social rejection is evident in other cultures and is somewhat hierarchical in nature, depending on the type of disability. In a study of students in Hong Kong and Taiwan, for example, individuals with physical disabilities were viewed more positively than individuals with developmental delays and mental disorders, questionably due in part to Chinese culture, in which persons with severe mental retardation and mental illness are often viewed as a source of shame by their parents and kept at home out of public attention (Chen et al., 2002). Historically, mental illness and mental retardation have been noted to be the least socially accepted. Mental retardation specifically has also been described as "the most socially invisible of all people with disabilities" (Gordon et al., 2004).

In additional research studies, adults with disabilities have been viewed by their nondisabled counterparts as *unequals* and in most cases not perceived as potential friends. Nondisabled individuals also tend to view those with disabilities as different across several social dimensions. For example, individuals who are more socially anxious, uneasy about dating, and less likely to date, may experience an "interaction strain" between the two parties (Gordon et al., 2004).

Women in particular may have more of a challenge in social settings than their male counterparts. In a recent survey, women with physical disabilities reported significantly lower levels of self-esteem and perceptions of how others see them compared to women without disabilities. Hence, they face serious social isolation and dissatisfaction with their relationships, which also puts them at a distinct disadvantage for quality of life experiences compared to women in general (Nosek & Hughes, 2001). Per Matheson (2003), "...to be a disabled woman is to be, in the eyes of many, somehow less of a woman, less of an individual than the nondisabled people around you..." (p. 44).

Dating and Partnerships for Adults With Disabilities

Adults with disabilities are often deprived of ordinary social stimulation and the possibility of developing friendships and intimate, long-term partnerships, which are essential tools for adulthood (Brown, 1996). For many disabled persons, the concept of dating and potentially developing an intimate bond with someone else is a common desire.

Recent research notes people who acquire their disabilities early in life are more likely to delay marriage or remain single. Specifically, 40.7% of 25- to 44-year-olds with disabilities lack a live-in spouse or partner, compared to only 29.7% of the nondisabled population in the age group (Kaye, 1997). Small qualitative studies also suggest that disability limits the ability of women especially to find romantic partners and thus to form families (1997). In addition, emerging disabilities may also dissolve predisability relationships. In one study, half of the women who had relationships prior to their SCI endured the break-up of those relationships following the injury (1997).

Developmentally disabled individuals, similar to their nondisabled counterparts, also have the desire to maximize their self-fulfillment and to participate fully in mainstream life by forming intimate connections (Lerner, 2005). An adult with Down's syndrome is more likely to partner with someone else with a disability, since the majority of people with Down's syndrome mostly meet other people with disabilities (Brown, 1996). These relationships, including marriage, can increase the quality of life and self-esteem for both spouses (Lerner, 2005). However, there are multiple challenges that developmentally disabled individuals face with such relations due to their social, emotional, and adaptive limitations; difficulties accessing necessary community resources; and inappropriate involvement by significant others. Ultimately, the success of marriage and intimate partnerships depends greatly on the type of support the couple receives and how they respond overall to these challenges (Lerner, 2005).

Intimacy and Sexuality for Adults With Disabilities

Sexuality and intimacy are essential parts of an individual's self-identity and self-esteem, whether an individual is sexually active or not, married or unmarried, heterosexual or homosexual, disabled or not disabled (adapted from Versluys, 1995a, p.231). Significantly, acute or chronic disability or illness may disrupt sexual activity because it interferes with cognition, motor skills, coordination, sensory skills and the individual's sense of self, thus impacting the individual's ability to fulfill his/her identified sexual roles and habits (Dahl, 1988; Gourley, 2002). In addition, disfiguring conditions such as amputation or mastectomy or conditions such as incontinence can raise anxiety about attractiveness and may undermine an individual's self-image, inducing concern about a loss of desirability and lowered self-worth (Glass & Soni, 1999; Rolland, 1994). As described in Hendley (1996), "...a disability shatters our image of ourselves. Changes in how the body looks, loss of independence, diminishment of a traditional role—all of these can impact on our image of ourselves as sexual beings..." (p. 17).

Notably, the onset of impairments early in life often produces low social and sexual confidence, whereas individuals who become disabled in adulthood are much more aware of what has actually been lost. While the degree of adjustment to either form of disability may be no different, the process of adjustment varies. How people view their disability and who they see as responsible for managing the effects of the condition strongly influence their ability to cope (Glass & Soni, 1999). Defining sexuality as more than just a physical function is particularly important for people with disabilities (1999).

Although an individual's disability may vary, society has placed an added challenge to the already disabled individual by denying him/her a realistic and positive identity as a sexual being and the opportunity for sexual expression and fulfilling sexual relationships (Bidgood, Boyle, & Ballan, 2004). Societal attitudes, then, offer the implication persons with disabilities are not fully human, meaning that he/she does not have sexual desires, but an individual who is not able to use part of his/her body still has an equal right to full sexual expression and cognitive or mental limitations do not preclude an individual's participation in sexual activity (Glass & Soni, 1999; Gourley, 2002). The National Women's Health Information Center reports many medical professionals are often misinformed about the sexual potential of women of any age with disabilities, and as a result do not encourage them to resume normal sexual activities. In addition, older women also reported they often do not receive adequate education on sexual function related to disability (Gourley, 2002).

The sexuality of individuals with developmental disabilities has also been historically misunderstood in society. For example, allegations of individuals with developmental delays being asexual, oversexed, sexually uncontrollable, sexually animalistic, subhuman, dependent and childlike, as well as breeders of disability, have been discussed in the literature (Bidgood et al., 2004; Gourley, 2002).

In general, individuals with developmental disabilities do not always receive adequate or accurate education on sexuality or sexual relationships (Greenfield, 2005). For even severely disabled adults, the greatest factor against appropriate sexual relationships is the attitudes and knowledge base of staff with whom they are involved, as well as parents who have been responsible for their upbringing (Brown, 1996). As a result, these individuals may have difficulty conceptualizing appropriate physical interactions with others and understanding sexual feelings. The Association for Retarded Citizens (ARC) states that persons with mental retardation have the fundamental right to learn about sexual functions and relationships and should be able to make informed decisions regarding their own sexuality (Gourley, 2002).

Various intervention strategies addressing issues on sexuality, intimacy, and peer/friend interactions will be discussed later in this chapter.

Remediation/Compensation/Adaptation Intervention Strategies for Social Participation

OTs use the holistic intervention model to assist clients with social participation. Taking into account such factors as age, disability, and social skills, the therapist can assist with the transition to community activities. Across the lifespan, the challenge to be a purposeful being is at the core of an individual's identity. As always, occupational therapy intervention takes place in a three-tiered approach: 1) remediation, 2) compensation/adaptation of the task, and 3) maintenance of successful performance through caregiver education and environmental modifications. The overall approach to intervention will depend primarily on the client's abilities in performance areas and disabilities requiring intervention at the performance skill level.

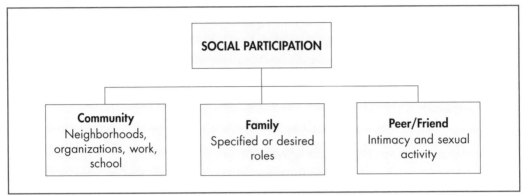

Figure 8-2. Components of social participation activities (adapted from American Occupational Therapy Association. [2002]. Occupational therapy practice framework: Domain and process. *American Journal of Occupational Therapy*, 56(6), 609-639).

OTs and OTAs work collaboratively with clients to promote desired participation in activities at home, school, the workplace, and other community life situations (Figure 8-2). This also includes successful role performance in each of these areas (AOTA, 2002). Since disease and disability may negatively impact successful role performance, the practice of occupational therapy is vital to engagement in occupation and social participation. While it is important to discuss each person's individual diagnosis and prognosis when generating a intervention plan, this section will generalize interventions with respect to social participation.

Remediation

Remediation is the act of treating a "condition" and allowing an individual to regain lost skills and function. In simplest terms, a client enters intervention with goals aimed at restoration of a prior level of functional capacity. This may be best expressed using a case study example

CASE STUDY #1: MARY, CEREBRAL VASCULAR ACCIDENT

Mary is a 70-year-old widow who lives with her daughter, son-in-law and two granddaughters in a two-level home. She drives, is completely independent with her ADLs and IADLs and is an active social participant in her church's ladies' auxiliary and religious education program, in which she serves as an instructor. Medically, she also has a history of diabetes and hypertension. While driving to church on a Sunday, Mary begins to feel dizzy and has a sudden onset of blurred vision. She loses control of her car and hits a barrier wall on the side of the road. Upon the arrival of an emergency crew and with first aid administered, she is rushed to a local hospital's emergency department. A battery of tests reveals that Mary has had a left-sided CVA with resulting visual/perceptual deficits, mild aphasia, and right-sided flaccidity of her UEs and LEs. After a brief acute hospital stay, Mary is admitted to a rehabilitation facility for continued therapy intervention.

- An OT evaluating Mary will need to take many factors into account when determining functional outcome levels.

- Goals aimed at remediation would be set to include Mary's ability to return to her daughter's home with residual motor, perceptual, process, and interaction skills restored to functionally independent levels.

- Included in this comprehensive intervention plan and identified as most important to Mary is her desire to return to teaching religious education and remaining an active member of the church auxiliary.

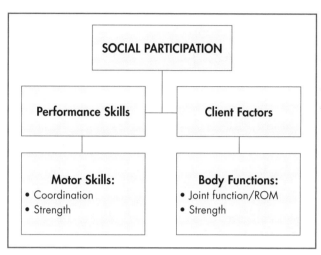

Figure 8-3. Relationship of ROM, strength, and coordination to social participation (adapted from American Occupational Therapy Association. [2002]. Occupational therapy practice framework: Domain and process. *American Journal of Occupational Therapy*, 56(6), 609-639).

- The barriers to successful occupational performance here are numerous, but since Mary is motivated to participate, an evaluation of the environment in which Mary teaches may be incorporated into the intervention plan.

- Since Mary's social participation goals are quite meaningful to her, her ability to successfully reintegrate into her church community may be predicated on her ability to regain her verbal abilities.

Compensation/Adaptation Interventions for Clients With Decreased Performance Skills/Client Factor

RANGE OF MOTION, STRENGTH, AND COORDINATION DEFICITS (FIGURE 8-3)

The compensatory approach to intervention allows for functional task independence with variations of the components of task performance. This intervention approach assumes the client will not immediately be able to restore task abilities and provides an opportunity for independent performance with an alternative approach or with the use of adaptive equipment. The OT has the ability to assist the client in achieving independence through *changing the task* or *changing the tools* for the client to achieve independence. Compensatory interventions to increase social participation for clients with motor skill deficits are included in Table 8-3, using Mary as the example.

With the social participation goal in mind, the compensatory intervention approach may shift to the community environment that Mary is seeking to re-enter. Mary's goal is to be able to socially participate in the annual holiday dinner sponsored by the ladies' auxiliary. For the past 15 years, Mary has served as the chief menu planner and hostess for the gala event. In order for her to achieve this goal, she must be able to communicate her thoughts and ideas. With her handwriting ability limited by her CVA, a compensatory approach to intervention in this example may include Mary using a tape recorder to dictate the menu to a friend or purchasing an assistive computer technology package that recognizes voice input and converts it to script. Both the tools used to perform the task, and the task itself, have been modified for successful independent performance. The OT or OTA would provide the intervention opportunities for Mary to become proficient with the tools provided.

Table 8-3

EXAMPLES OF COMPENSATION/ADAPTATION STRATEGIES FOR ROM, STRENGTH, AND COORDINATION DEFICITS

Performance Skill Deficit	Examples of Compensatory/Adaptation Intervention
ROM	• The client is instructed in hemi-dressing techniques until she can perform the tasks independently with or without adaptive equipment. • Social participation goals would include Mary's ability to self-toilet while at all functions. • Incorporating the family into intervention for caregiver education on an active assistive range of motion (AAROM) program may be vital to Mary's future success.
Strength	• The client is instructed to perform techniques in sitting and supine or gravity-eliminated planes to compensate for UE strength deficits. • Mary would then be able to meet the goal of active participation in her church group functions either at standing or seated (compensatory) levels.
Coordination	• The client is provided with elastic shoelaces and a button-hook secondary to impaired fine motor coordination of the digits. • Socially, Mary would be able to gain independence of her abilities to perform clothing management and manage barriers to access in her physical environment.

SENSATION & PAIN (FIGURE 8-4)

Like many clients with a CVA, Mary may not only have pain in the affected extremities, but also hyper- or hyposensitivity, putting her at risk for injury. In order to reach desired social participation goals and subsequent community re-entry, the client is often faced with overcoming physical barriers. In this instance, changing the task may be required to allow Mary the opportunity for meaningful performance in her social setting. The example of an alternative to a handshake or hand grasp for greeting guests at the dinner may be necessary to decrease Mary's exposure to external physical stimuli, which may cause her excessive pain or discomfort (Table 8-4).

ENDURANCE AND ENERGY (FIGURE 8-5)

Quite often, the most challenging of tasks for community re-entry to meet social participation goals is the realization that endurance, or lack of it, has an impact on ability. In order to preserve their role in social settings, many clients with physical disabilities succumb to social stigma and shun the help of an assistive device or aid that they may require. The role of the OT in these instances is to provide the client and the caregiver with education regarding energy conservation techniques and its importance for the client. In addition, it is quite common for persons with neurological impairment to have markedly reduced physical activity levels and require an assistive device or compensatory approach to activity performance to preserve energy stores and reduce the chance for falls (Table 8-5).

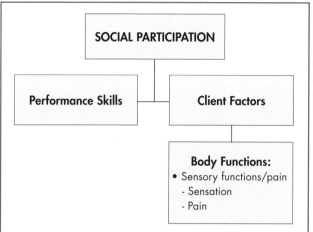

Figure 8-4. Relationship of sensation/ pain to social participation (adapted from American Occupational Therapy Association. [2002]. Occupational therapy practice framework: Domain and process. *American Journal of Occupational Therapy*, 56(6), 609-639).

Table 8-4

EXAMPLES OF COMPENSATION/ADAPTATION STRATEGIES FOR SENSATION AND PAIN DEFICITS

Performance Skill Deficit	Examples of Compensatory/Adaptive Interventions
Hypersensitivity	• The client is instructed to perform alternative methods to social greetings in lieu of a handshake due to extreme pain or hypersensitivity. • Family and friends may also be provided with education in order to insure Mary's inability to hand grasp may not be deemed a social faux pas.
Hyposensitivity	• The client is instructed to visually examine the community environment for objects that may cause physical injury until remediation techniques are deemed successful.

COGNITIVE, PERCEPTUAL, AND VISUAL LIMITATIONS (FIGURE 8-6)

Arguably, the most challenging of barriers to overcome for successful community social participation re-entry are those related to cognitive, perceptual, and/or visual limitations. A client with cognitive deficits may demonstrate differing social abilities and, despite a need for assistance, may make it difficult for caregivers and peers to advise and assist the client (Pollard, 2000). Social skills necessary for advanced participation goals may be impaired, leaving an individual and his/ her caregiver socially isolated.

Cognitive Limitations (Figure 8-7)

These process skills (Table 8-6) are vital to successful performance in the social environment. Memory impairment, specifically as it relates to the ability for new learning, may prohibit independent functioning of clients in a social setting. The establishment of routine and structure is imperative in these cases, yet the client is often faced with challenges that require external assistance. Compensatory approaches for community reintegration may focus on the client's ability to seek assistance effectively when challenged with a situation that causes anxiety (Allen, 1996).

Figure 8-5. Relationship of energy/endurance to social participation (adapted from American Occupational Therapy Association. [2002]. Occupational therapy practice framework: Domain and process. *American Journal of Occupational Therapy*, 56(6), 609-639).

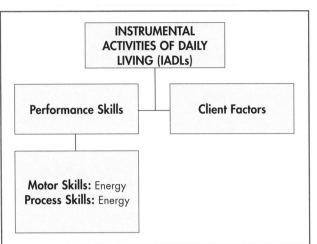

Table 8-5

EXAMPLES OF COMPENSATION/ADAPTATION STRATEGIES FOR ENERGY/ENDURANCE DEFICITS

Performance Skill Deficit	Examples of Compensatory/Adaptive Interventions
Endurance/activity tolerance	• The client is instructed in signs/symptoms of decreased endurance and its impact on physical functioning and safe performance. • Family members may also be trained to assist as needed with tasks and to recognize signs and symptoms of fatigue for Mary to minimize the potential for falls and other accidents.
Energy	• The client is instructed to perform tasks required in the social environment while sitting to conserve and/or maintain energy levels.

In addition to the process skills noted in Table 8-6, the AOTA *Framework* (2002) identifies Body Function Categories that are cognitive and perceptual in nature. These functions may be further divided into two specific categories: global mental functions and specific mental functions (AOTA, 2002).

- **Global mental functions** include arousal and orientation. The quality of social participation is, indeed, highly connected to the individual's ability to maintain a level of arousal throughout the activity, as well as to be able to participate in the "here and now" with others in the setting. Social isolation of the client and caregiver is common in situations where the client may exhibit negative behaviors and lack the ability to identify meaningful social cues.

- **Specific mental functions** include attention, memory, perception, higher-order thought processes and mental functioning (process skills, e.g., motor planning). While clients may be instructed in adaptive techniques for successful performance in a social setting, quite often deficits in higher-order/executive functioning lead to diminished participation in familiar settings due to social embarrassment. The OT or OTA in this instance may seek to find the

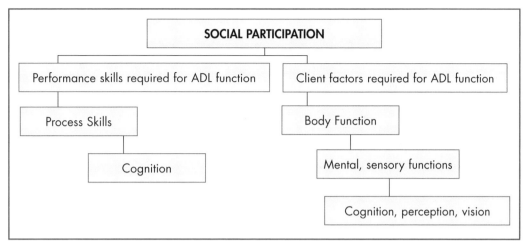

Figure 8-6. Components of performance skills/client factors related to social participation (adapted from American Occupational Therapy Association. [2002]. Occupational therapy practice framework: Domain and process. *American Journal of Occupational Therapy,* 56(6), 609-639).

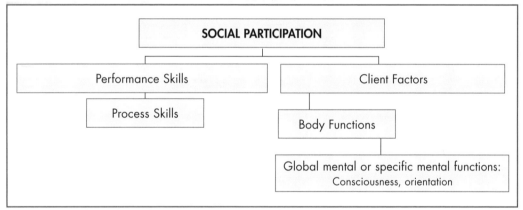

Figure 8-7. Relationship of cognition to IADLs (adapted from American Occupational Therapy Association. [2002]. Occupational therapy practice framework: Domain and process. *American Journal of Occupational Therapy,* 56(6), 609-639).

environment or social setting that matches the client's mental functioning so as to make certain success is achieved. If Mary were to have executive function deficits as a result of her CVA, instead of her taking on the role of finance chair of the dinner event as she had done in the past, she may take on the role of menu planner and preparation supervisor with assistance provided from a peer as necessary. In this sense, her goal of social participation in her community is met, while the task for which she is responsible for is adapted to meet her cognitive needs.

Perceptual Limitations (Figure 8-8)

The client may be required to have the task adapted (e.g., providing a written script for Mary of the chronological events of the dinner so she is able to be oriented to the program at all times). She may also enlist the use of a date book for visual cues and sequencing for any task she may need to perform. A walk-through of the environment with a friend prior to community entry may familiarize the client with environmental barriers to overcome and allow for routine and structured performance (Table 8-7).

Table 8-6

Examples of Compensation/Adaptation Strategies for Cognition Deficits

Performance Skill Deficit (Process Skills)	Examples of Compensatory/Adaptive Interventions
Knowledge/memory	• The client is instructed in the use of a daily planner for social activities.
Temporal organization	• The client is instructed in the use of "to do" lists in order to initiate tasks.
Organizing space and objects	• The client is visually cued through the use of lists or verbally cued for the set-up of a room for social activities. This may include the assistance of family members or peers to guide and assist the client as necessary.
Adaptation	• The client is instructed in various techniques aimed at providing alternative approaches for successful independent functioning in the social environment.

Figure 8-8. Relationship of perception to social participation (adapted from American Occupational Therapy Association. [2002]. Occupational therapy practice framework: Domain and process. *American Journal of Occupational Therapy*, 56(6), 609-639).

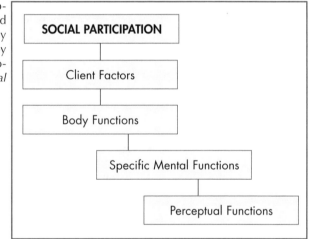

Visual Limitations (Figure 8-9)

When referring to vision in this context, the physical aspect of sight is explored. Nearly 80% of our social cuing is derived from visual feedback (Warren, 1995). If an individual has a visual impairment, intervention is especially warranted to provide opportunities for successful community reintegration. Vision, in this text, will be explored as a result of a change or loss of a visual field and also, as a broad term: *low vision* (see Chapter 5 for a definition of low vision).

The loss of vision as it relates to aging is most pronounced in the loss of visual acuity. However, neurological disease processes such as CVA, brain injury, and multiple sclerosis may also lead to visual changes, which may include the loss of a partial field of vision, also called a *field cut*. Other diseases such as glaucoma and macular degeneration lead to a syndrome known as low vision. Since lighting varies tremendously in all community environments, an individual with low

Table 8-7

EXAMPLES OF COMPENSATION/ADAPTATION STRATEGIES
FOR PERCEPTION DEFICITS

Performance Skill Deficit	*Examples of Compensatory/Adaptive Interventions*
Motor planning/apraxia	• Instruct the client using the best learning method for him/her and provide external cuing as needed for successful task performance. • The ability to succeed in social activities may depend on the ability to motor plan; therefore, family or peer training for safety may be necessary.
Visual fixation/scanning	• Instruct the client in the ability to scan all environments, objects, and people in the same methodology.
Visual inattention/neglect	• Instruct the client in head-turning strategies when meeting new people or navigating the environment so as not to miss environmental and social cues.
Body scheme	• Instruct the client to use a mirror or seek the counsel of a family member or friend prior to attending a community event to ensure that dressing, grooming, and hygiene tasks are successfully performed.
Visual discrimination	• Instruct the client in various compensatory visual techniques aimed at providing visual feedback to the client until (if) visual or perceptual issues resolve.

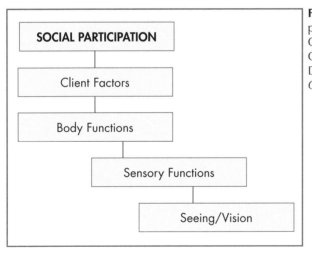

Figure 8-9. Relationship of vision to social participation (adapted from American Occupational Therapy Association. [2002]. Occupational therapy practice framework: Domain and process. *American Journal of Occupational Therapy,* 56(6), 609-639).

vision may find social participation may be limited by these barriers. For example, an individual with low vision who might have enjoyed going to lunch with friends at a restaurant may be less inclined to participate socially as the disease, and its resulting loss of quality functional vision, progresses. The OT in this role may provide compensatory strategies for the client. These strategies may include instruction in the use of magnifiers and providing contrasting color backgrounds to minimize the loss of visual discrimination. Since there is no cure for low vision, all interventions aimed at this disease will be adaptive in nature (Table 8-8).

Table 8-8	
EXAMPLES OF COMPENSATION/ADAPTATION STRATEGIES FOR VISION DEFICITS	
Performance Skill Deficit	*Examples of Compensatory/Adaptive Interventions*
Visual field loss/cut	• Instruct the client in head-turning and scanning techniques. • Arrange a neuro-opthalmology consult to assess for prism glasses.
Low vision	• Instruct the client in the use of visual assistive technology aids and lighting changes so that he/she has successfully navigated the community environment.

PERFORMANCE SKILL LIMITATIONS IMPACTING SOCIAL PARTICIPATION

Strategies to Enhance Communication/Interaction Skills

Limitations within the performance skill known as communication/interaction skills are a primary focus for occupational therapy practitioners working on social participation intervention strategies given the underlying interpersonal experiences that encompass this performance area. According to the *Framework*, communication/interaction skills refer to conveying intentions and needs and coordinating social behavior to act together with other people (AOTA, 2002, p. 622).

This performance skill includes three distinct components: physicality, information exchange, and relations, all of which are ultimately vital elements to an individual's ability to engage in meaningful social participation activities in his/her community.

Fundamentally, as previously described in this chapter, a therapist's therapeutic use of self, in which the practitioner uses his/her personality, insights, perceptions, and judgments as part of the therapeutic process, is the foundation of all intervention strategies addressing interpersonal relations (AOTA, 2002). Given the ongoing interactions between the therapist and the client in intervention sessions, the therapeutic role of the OT is of an *interpersonal coach*, in which the therapist can utilize various social intervention strategies during individual or group experiences.

Modeling

Modeling, described as the "silent influence," actually occurs every time a therapist is with a client, not just when the therapist is consciously attempting to model specific behaviors or actions (Denton, 1987). Individuals, thus, can learn by observing the behaviors and actions of a role model and then by imitating and practicing the behavior (Versluys, 1995a). Specifically, modeling activities not only provide verbal experiences through information exchange, but also nonverbal, social cues on elements of physicality. For example, the way the therapist maintains eye contact and gestures with his/her hands provides training for the client on socially acceptable nonverbal communication strategies.

As therapists offer frequent individual interaction experiences for clients, each therapy session provides a unique opportunity to further promote and practice appropriate interpersonal relations, which can then be integrated into the client's social participation endeavors in his/her community. In a group setting, models include not only the therapist, but other clients as well, which can then provide another dimension of social reinforcement to the individual (Versluys, 1995). Additionally, when out in the community, family members and peers can serve as role models to encourage carryover of appropriate communication strategies identified during therapy sessions. For example, they can model appropriate information exchange by introducing friends to the client and asking questions to initiate and stimulate ongoing conversations.

Role-Play

For communication/interaction performance skills, role-playing can also be a particularly helpful purposeful activity to practice or test new verbal and nonverbal skills and enhance the individual's awareness of feelings, attitudes, and behaviors of others to take back into effective social participation performance in the community (Denton, 1987). This type of intervention method offers an opportunity for the client to act out new interpersonal scenarios that he/she may potentially encounter in the community within a safe, nonthreatening environment, either individually with the therapist or in a group setting. Role-playing activities are often organized around a simulated situation such as being appropriately assertive or demonstrating personal boundaries in a social activity. As a result of this type of interpersonal exercise, the client may be able to further identify problems he/she he may be anticipating once out in the community (Versluys, 1995).

To further illustrate these intervention techniques in greater detail, let's use the ongoing chapter example of John, the client with mental retardation. Perhaps John is able to verbalize that he is apprehensive about going to the movies with a new friend. He is clearly nervous and somewhat pressured to have his new friend "like him." He wonders what they will talk about. How will he start off a conversation? Although the role-playing exercise cannot solely predict how the actual interaction will go, it can prepare John ahead of time and provide awareness of potential *interpersonal roadblocks*, including personal topics to avoid in conversation, inappropriate language, etc. Additionally, role-playing can offer an opportunity for individuals to practice nonverbal communication techniques including body language and positioning, as well as actual physical boundaries. For example, during a therapy session in which the therapist and client are role-playing the movie scenario, John may ask whether he should sit next to the friend or a seat away, and whether he should face the friend while talking to him before the movie begins. Again in this example, the therapist and client can collaboratively problem-solve the social outing, giving John better self-confidence in a new interpersonal event.

Videotaping

Audiovisual tools, including videotaped intervention encounters, provide a real-time feedback mechanism for educating a client on communication/interaction skills. This visual learning mechanism then provides the individual an opportunity to incorporate new or practiced behaviors that may need to be changed or altered in someway when out in the community during social participation (Denton, 1987). Obviously, the therapist should keep in mind, a drawback to this technique is that the client's overall presentation may change if he/she is acknowledging he/she is being recorded. Acting out for the camera is an example; therefore, it is suggested that videotaping be used in addition to other types of interventions.

Community Outings

Fieldtrips are occupation-based intervention activities that offer an additional opportunity for the individual to integrate communication/interaction skills outside of the clinic and into the "real world" (Denton, 1987). Initially, therapists may role model specific behaviors required for the task and gradually decrease the amount of structure and assistance offered to the client to further promote successful performance later when the client is alone, or with family and friends in the community. Community-based interventions also provide a unique way to incorporate context. In community settings, family members are often present during intervention sessions. Family can provide insight into communication issues, and support client successes. In addition, family members can also serve as effective role models to others in the community regarding how best to approach and communicate with their loved one by making necessary adaptations. For example, the sister of a client with visual impairments can model how to approach the individual so he/she can best see, and thus maximize meaningful interactions with others

PERFORMANCE AREA LIMITATIONS IMPACTING SOCIAL PARTICIPATION

Personal Hygiene and Grooming Intervention Strategies

ADLs, including personal hygiene and grooming, are activities that are oriented toward taking care of one's own body (previously described in Chapter 3). These activities are also essential components to effective social participation as they impact how others will perceive and respond to an individual during communal interactions. These social perceptions, then, are ways in which we form and modify impressions of others (Rathus, 1988). Fundamentally, these preconceived notions are considered to be basic human nature and can be formulated solely by an individual's outward physical appearance, including his/her hygiene and grooming practices.

Adults with various disabilities may have several challenges to face in completing their activities of daily living (ADLs). Often, the occupational therapy practitioner will introduce various strategies to optimize an individual's occupational performance in this area, including the use of assistive devices and/or adaptive equipment. It is expected that these techniques are then carried over by the client to utilize in his/her own environment. If the client lives with family, it is helpful for the therapist to schedule a family training session to familiarize family members with the adaptive equipment and provide ways that they can support strategies to maintain independence gained during therapy sessions, and if applicable, reinforce safety issues. See Chapter 3 for more information on ADLs.

Within the focus of self-care, the OT needs to also educate the client about social norms relating to hygiene and grooming practices in society, based upon the client's own abilities and limitations, as well as financial status. As previously described in this chapter, adults with disabilities are often faced with significant social stigma and invisible barriers that impact their ability to fully integrate into all aspects of the community. Limited knowledge and understanding of social norms of appearance may be an additional hindrance for clients while trying to reintegrate into their community.

Occupational therapy practitioners may find discussions on personal hygiene and grooming practices can initially be difficult for the client to engage in. Often there is an element of embarrassment or modesty for the client, as if they know they need to improve some aspect of their self-care, but are not quite sure how to go about it. Sometimes, the topic may be too personal for the client and he/she may not feel comfortable talking about these issues with a therapist of another gender. There may be other times when the client may be relieved that he/she is given the opportunity to talk about topics that are usually avoided in most intervention settings. It is important for the therapist to acknowledge and validate these feelings and respond to the client in a caring, yet matter-of-fact way. Verbal feedback to the client should be basic and nonjudgmental and never a *critique* of the individual's appearance. Therapists should also not take for granted that clients have had such discussions about these issues with anyone else in the past.

When beginning such conversations, the therapist may ask the client how he/she feels about his/her physical appearance. Does the client have specific concerns or questions about how he/she seem to others? The therapist should also inquire about what the client's typical self-care routine currently consists of as part of the evaluation process. While providing education on social aspects of self-care performance, various topics to address may include, but are not limited to, self-care/hygiene frequency, coordination of dress, coiffing, halitosis, use of deodorant/antiperspirant, body sprays, and colognes. Verbal and/or written information is helpful, and therapists need to provide adequate explanation on why socially these issues are important; for example, a client with a developmental delay has now joined the neighborhood social club, which he will be attending three times per week. During therapy, the occupational therapy practitioner has asked the client how often he takes a shower and changes his clothes. The client, John, explains that he showers once a week on Sundays and does his laundry on the same day. Although he demonstrates an understanding that if his clothes are stained or soiled he needs to change them before embarking out into the community, he continues to wear the same undergarments each day, is malodorous, and has unruly hair during most therapy sessions. The therapist also notes during a community outing to practice money management skills, several passersby stared and pointed at him. Additionally, the client had a difficult time getting the bank teller's attention in line, as it appeared he was being avoided. Unfortunately given John's mental limitations, the therapist realizes he is unable to pick up on subtle social cues that impact how he is perceived by others in public. Further, the OT anticipates that given his current appearance, he will not be able to optimally perform and get his social needs met in the community.

Given this scenario, the practitioner decides to approach the subject tactfully with basic concrete information to the client. She explains in simplistic terms about good hygiene practices and body functions, educating the client on how glands produce secretions causing smells and how these smells can be modified by various hygiene products. The therapist further describes the need for clean undergarments and appropriate seasonal fabrics that can act as protective agents during inclement weather or allow the body to breathe. The concept of halitosis and appropriate oral hygiene is explored. Adequate hair management and basic coiffing techniques are discussed.

The therapist notes that John appears interested in the discussion and poses several questions to her: What is the difference between deodorant and the other thing? It seems like my mouth is dry usually after I take my medications, can that make my breath smell bad to others? I have tried to comb my hair every time I leave the house but sometimes it is itchy and I scratch it, which messes it up all the time... As the therapist continues with such topics of focus during weekly intervention sessions, she notices not only improvements in the client's grooming, but in his overall presence. His posture has improved, as has his eye contact, and his affect appears brighter.

Given a client's interest and motivation to further enhance his/her appearance, the therapist can determine how much further to explore self-care issues with the client. Significantly, though, if the client continually dismisses feedback on his/her hygiene and grooming practices and is frequently not engaged in therapist-initiated conversations on such topics, the therapist probably needs to limit his/her focus on the issue. Ultimately, the client must be motivated to participate in such aspects of therapy and be willing to pursue behavioral changes in order to further impact social participation performance.

Strategies to Enhance Sexuality

An individual's sexuality, like any other meaningful occupation in an individual's life, is certainly a relevant issue considered by the OT throughout the intervention process (Gourley, 2002). As stated by the Sexuality Information and Education Council of the United States (SIECUS), individuals with disabilities have the same right to education on sexuality, sexual health care, and opportunities for sexual expression as their nondisabled counterparts (Gourley, 2002).

Unfortunately, in general, sexual expression is an important but often overlooked ADL (Estes, 2002).

It is common for clients, as well as therapists, to be potentially embarrassed or unsure how to initiate discussions about sexual activity, but clearly if such occupation is meaningful to the individual, this topic should be addressed by the therapist. Prior to discussing aspects of sexuality with a client, the therapist should have a sense of his/her own self-awareness, including bias, attitudes, and feelings, realizing clients may want to talk about aspects of this subject that the therapist may or may not feel comfortable discussing (Gourley, 2002).

In providing quality health care, sexual health should be integrated with all aspects of a client, holding equal status with physical, spiritual, social, and emotional care (Nusbaum & Hamilton, 2002). Although several health care specialties, as well as clients, are in agreement that addressing sexual health should be an integral component of intervention, there are several complex factors that interfere with addressing rehabilitation clients' sexual expression needs (Estes, 2002). Research indicates there is limited knowledge, training, and experience in the area of sexuality by OTs (Estes, 2002). In some cases, therapists may generally assume that the client has discussed such topics with other members of the health care team or if the client has not brought up the subject, that it may not necessarily be a priority for him or her at the present time. A client may legitimately feel uncomfortable talking about such topics due to his/her generational or cultural background, gender (or the gender of the therapist), or lack of self-confidence following the onset of an injury or disability (Estes, 2002). Additionally, if the practitioner avoids the topic, the client may assume the subject is inappropriate to discuss (Gourley, 2002). Subsequently, if therapists do initiate conversations on sexuality, some may also fear the client will misinterpret their intentions, which could result in accusations of sexual harassment (Estes, 2002). Ultimately, if therapists do not feel comfortable discussing or providing education on sexuality to the client, it is their professional responsibility to adequately refer the client to additional health care specialists.

While providing education on sexuality, OTs need to provide concrete, simplistic information in a nonjudgmental manner that is consistent with the client's level of mental functioning (Gourley, 2002; Nusbaum & Hamilton, 2002). Practitioners can initially approach the subject with a closed-ended question, possibly asking the client if he/she has any questions about sexuality. Although the client may refuse or not acknowledge the question during this intervention session, the therapist has at least addressed the subject and the client may then feel more comfortable in the future bringing it up. The therapist should also utilize professional judgment on determining how far to guide the conversation with the client, as to prevent or minimize anxiety or embarrassment. Frequently, practitioners can help ease the potentially uncomfortable client by acknowledging and validating his/her concerns and apprehensions.

When working with clients with developmental disabilities, it is important to keep in mind that their exposure to education on this topic is probably limited. As previously mentioned, education provided to the client with a developmental delay should flow from his/her needs and mental functions, realizing information is better processed in small doses with much repetition (Greenfield, 2005). Often, these clients may be confused or unsure as to what constitutes "normal" sexual behaviors, aspects of attractiveness to others, and levels of sexual desire. It is often advantageous for occupational therapy practitioners to reassure individuals that "normal" covers a wide range of degrees of interest in sexual relationships and behaviors (Gourley, 2002). Hence, a vital component of occupational therapy interventions in regards to sexuality, then, is to eliminate myths and misinformation (Versluys, 1995).

Therapists can offer education and information on sexuality in a variety of ways. Again, the client's needs, comfort level, abilities and limitations will guide the appropriate manner of teaching. In some instances, individual counseling sessions and or group discussions may be appropriate. Techniques often include both verbal and written education and may or may not include the partner of the client, based on the client's request. Role-play scenarios can also offer the occupational therapy practitioner a starting point when working with clients with limited mental functioning to find out what they know about intimate relationships in a nonthreatening way (Greenfield, 2005). For educating and teaching individuals who have a developmental delay, other creative intervention methods may include dolls, pictures, videos, games, and slides on topics of sexuality (Greenfield, 2005).

As sexuality is a lifelong element of an individual's identity, the occupational therapy practitioner must also initiate educational opportunities with older adult clients, based upon multiple physiological and psychological changes that can impact an individual's sexual roles and habits during this life stage. Information on the impact of aging on sexuality, including medication side effects, can be presented (Gourley, 2002). In addition, as previously described in this chapter, the number of older people infected with HIV is growing, thus therapists must consider these clients as an at-risk population for infection. Therefore, the therapist can offer open-ended opportunities to engage older adult clients to participate in a frank discussion of sexuality either individually or in a group setting, while providing basic verbal and written information based upon the clients' needs and abilities.

GENERAL MAINTENANCE INTERVENTION STRATEGIES

Once remedial and adaptive techniques addressing various client factors and performance skills have been successfully introduced and deemed to be effective, maintenance level programming provided to insure carryover of social participation not only occurs in the immediate days following intervention, but for the lifespan as well. The role of the client and caregiver education is monumental in this process. In addition to education models, clients may also be provided with lists of community resources including support groups for peer and social interaction. In the ever-changing world of health care and the shrinking resources available, occupational therapy practitioners find themselves in the role of educator from the onset to the termination of the intervention session. Even with the best intentions to remediate the problems identified, the OT is often forced to quickly move to adaptive and maintenance intervention strategies secondary to reimbursement demands and time restrictions. A client facing the challenge of social participation in a community setting must not only have the motivation to succeed, but also the willingness to explore alternative options to insure a smooth path along the road to success.

SUMMARY QUESTIONS

1. Define and discuss examples of three aspects of social participation.

2. Discuss unique issues that family/caregivers face in relation to a client's social participation.

3. Discuss strategies for the OT to involve family members in the intervention process related to social participation.

4. Explain the significance of peer/friend and intimate relationships in various stages of life as related to social participation.

REFERENCES

Allen, C. K., Earhart, C. A., & Blue, T. (1992). *Occupational therapy treatment goals for the physically and cognitively disabled*. Rockville, MD: American Occupational Therapy Association.

Allen, C. K. (1996). Allen cognitive level test manual. Colchester, CT: S&S Worldwide.

American Occupational Therapy Association. (2002). Occupational therapy practice framework: Domain and process. *American Journal of Occupational Therapy, 56*(6), 609-639.

American Occupational Therapy Association. (2004). *The reference manual of the official documents of the American occupational therapy association* (10th ed.). Bethesda: MD: AOTA.

Barbor, C. (2001, January/February). Finding real love—intimacy and alienation. *Psychology Today, 34*, 42-49.

Barrett, L., & Kielhofner, G. (2003). Theories derived from occupational behavior perspectives. In E. B. Crepeau, E. S. Cohn, & B. A. B. Schell (Eds.), *Willard and Spackman's occupational therapy* (10th ed., pp. 209-233). Philadelphia: Lippincott, Williams & Wilkins.

Baum, C. M., & Law, M. (1997). Occupational therapy practice: Focusing on occupational performance. *American Journal of Occupational Therapy, 51*(4), 277-288.

Bell, R. R. (1981). *Worlds of friendships*. Beverly Hills, CA: Sage Publications.

Bidgood, F. E., Boyle, P. S., & Ballan, M. (2004). Forty years of knowledge-SIECUS on sexuality and disability. *Sex Information and Education Council of the United States Report, 32*(2), 28.

Block, J. D. (1980). *Friendship: How to give it, how to get it*. New York: Collier Books.

Bourne, H. (1998). Peer pressure. In J. Kagan (Ed.), *Gale encyclopedia of childhood and adolescence* (pp. 493-495). Detroit, MI: Gale Research.

Bradford, E. L. (2001). *The importance of friendship*. Retrieved May 14, 2005, from the Mental Health Association in Orange County, NC Web site: http://www.mhaoc.com/lack.html

Braun, B. J. (1998). Knowledge and perception of fall-related risk factors and fall-reduction techniques among community-dwelling elderly individuals. *Physical Therapy, 78*, 1262-1276.

Brintnall-Peterson, M. (2004, March-May). Friendships are important across the years. *Happenings: Dane County Association for Home and Community Education Cooperative Extension-University of Wisconsin*, 9-10.

Brown, R. I. (1996). Partnerships and marriage in Down syndrome. *Down Syndrome Research and Practice, 4*(3), 96-99.

Bruce, M. A., & Borg, B. (2002). *Psychosocial frames of reference: Core for occupation-based practice* (3rd ed.). Thorofare, NJ: SLACK Incorporated.

Bukov, A., Maas, I., & Lampert, T. (2002). Social participation in very old age: Cross-sectional and longitudinal findings from BASE. *Journals of Gerontology Series B: Psychological Sciences and Social Sciences, 57*, 510-517.

Cairns, D., & Baker, J. (1993, October-December). Adjustment to spinal cord injury: A review of coping styles contributing to the process. *Journal of Rehabilitation, 59*, 30-33.

Cavallo, P. (1989). Teens, guilt and MS: Some guidelines to coping—multiple sclerosis. *Inside MS, 7*(3), 19.

Chen, R. K., Brodwin, M. G., Cardoso, E., & Chan, F. (2002). Attitudes toward people with disabilities in the social context of dating and marriage: A comparison of American, Taiwanese, and Singaporean college students' attitudes toward disability. *Journal of Rehabilitation, 68*, 5-11.

Christiansen, B. J. (1990). The costly retreat from marriage—married individuals deemed healthier. *Saturday Evening Post, 262*, 32-35.

Clemson, L., Cumming, R. G., & Roland, M. (1996). Case-control study of hazards in the home and risk of falls and hip fractures. *Age and Ageing, 25*, 97-101.

Conneeley, A. C. (2002). Social integration following traumatic brain injury and rehabilitation. *British Journal of Occupational Therapy, 65*(8), 356-362.

Consortium of Social Science Associations. (2000). *National institutes of health conference highlights importance of social and behavioral influences on health*. Retrieved May 14, 2005, from http://www.cossa.org/july102k.html

Cook, B. G. & Semmel, M. I. (1999). Peer acceptance of included students with disabilities as a function of severity of disability and classroom composition. *Journal of Special Education, 33*, 50-61.

Coster, W. (1998). Occupation-centered assessment of children. *American Journal of Occupational Therapy, 52*(5), 337-344.

Crabtree, J. L. (1991). Ethical dilemmas and the older adult. In J. M. Kiernat (Ed.), *Occupational therapy and the older adult: A clinical manual* (pp. 338-350). Gaithersburg, MD: Aspen.

Dahl, M. R. (1988). Human sexuality. In H. L. Hopkins & H. D. Smith (Eds.), *Willard and Spackmans's occupational therapy* (7th ed., pp. 354-358). Philadelphia: J.B. Lippincott.

Denton, P. L. (1987). *Psychiatric occupational therapy: A workbook of practical skills.* Boston: Little, Brown & Company.

DiFabio, R. P., & Seay, R. (1997). Use of the "fast evaluation of mobility, balance and fear" in elderly community dwellers: Validity and reliability. *Physical Therapy, 77,* 904-917.

Dunn, W., Brown, C., & McGuigan, A. (1994). The ecology of human performance: A framework for considering the effect of context. *American Journal of Occupational Therapy, 48,* 595-607.

Estes, J.P. (2002). Beyond basic ADLs- Sexual expression is an important but often overlooked activity of daily living. Retrieved April 23, 2005, from the Rehab Management Web site: http://www.rehabpub.com/features/42002/7.asp

Glass, C. & Soni, B. (1999). ABC of sexual health: Sexual problems of disabled patients. *British Medical Journal, 318,* 518-21.

Gordon, P. A, Tantillo, J. C., Feldman, D., & Perrone, K. (2004). Attitudes regarding interpersonal relationships with persons with mental illness and mental retardation. *Journal of Rehabilitation, 70*(1), 50-56.

Gourley, M. M. (2002). Sexuality and disability. In K. Krapp (Ed.), *Gale encyclopedia of nursing and allied health.* Vol. 4. (pp. 2203-2206). Farmington Hills, MI: Thomson Gale Group.

Greenfield, M. (2005). Talking about sexuality with individuals with intellectual disabilities: Notes from the field. *Planned Parenthood Federation of America, Inc. Educator's Update, 9*(5), 1-6.

Gutman, S. S. (2000). Using a computer as an environmental facilitator to promote post head injury role resumption: A case report. *Occupational Therapy in Mental Health, 15,* 71-90.

Hanschu, B. (1998). Using a sensory approach to serve adults who have developmental disabilities. In M. Ross & S. Bachner (Eds.), *Adults with developmental disabilities: Current approaches in occupational therapy.* Rockville, MD: AOTA.

Hendley, J. (1996). Sexual problems your doctor may not have mentioned to you—intimacy and multiple sclerosis. *Inside MS, 14*(1), 14-17.

Hopkins, H. L., & Tiffany, E. G. (1988). Occupational therapy—A problem solving process. In H. L. Hopkins & H. D. Smith (Eds.), *Willard and Spackmans's occupational therapy* (7th ed., pp. 102-111). Philadelphia: J.B. Lippincott.

Hopps, S. L., Pepin, M, Arseneau, I., Frechette, M., & Begin, G. (2001). Disability related variables associated with loneliness among people with disabilities. *Journal of Rehabilitation, 67,* 42-49.

Jongbloed, L., Stanton, S., & Fousek, B. (1993). Family adaptation to altered roles following a stroke. *Canadian Journal of Occupational Therapy, 60*(2), 70-77.

Jongbloed, L. & Ernest-Conibear, M. (1995). Regaining participation in leisure-time activities. In C.A. Trombly (Ed.), *Occupational therapy for physical dysfunction* (4th ed., pp.351-375). Boston: Williams & Wilkins.

Kaye, H.S. (1997). *Disability watch: The status of people with disabilities in the United States.* Volcano, CA: Volcano Press.

Kindermann, T. A., & Sage, N. A. (1999). Peer networks, behavior contingencies, and children's engagement in the classroom. *Merrill-Palmer-Quarterly, 45,* 143-171.

Law, M., & Dunn, W. (1993a). Challenges and strategies in applying an occupational performance measurement approach. *American Journal of Occupational Therapy, 47*(5), 431-436.

Law, M., & Dunn, W. (1993b). Perspectives for understanding and changing the environment for children with disabilities. *Physical and Occupational Therapy in Pediatrics, 13,* 1-17.

Lerner, P. (2005). Marriage for the developmentally disabled. *Spirit Magazine, 1*(1), 70-74.

Letts, L., Rigby, P., & Stewart, D. (2003). *Using environments to enable occupational performance.* Thorofare, NJ: SLACK Incorporated.

Lopata, H.Z. (1996). *Current widowhood: Myths and realities.* Thousand Oaks, CA: Sage Publications.

Lutfiyya, Z. M. (1997). The importance of friendships between people with and without mental retardation. In M. L. Hardman, *Persons with severe disabilities: educational and social issues* (pp. 101-129). New York: Allyn and Bacon.

Mackey, R. A., Diemer, M. A., & O'Brien, B. A. (2000). Psychological intimacy in the lasting relationships of heterosexual and same-gender couples. *Sex Roles: A Journal of Research, 43*(3/4), 201-227.

Matheson, L. (2003). Defined by disability. *Off Our Backs, 3*(1/2), 44-45.

Moore, L. W., & Amburgey, L. B. (2000). Older adults and HIV. *Association of Perioperative Registered Nurses Journal, 71*(Elderly Care), 873.

Mosey, A. C. (1996). *Applied scientific inquiry in the health professions: A epistemological orientation* (2nd ed.). Bethesda, MD: AOTA.

Ng, S. Y., Dinesh, S. K., Tay, S. H., & Lee, E. H. (2003). Decreased access to health care and social isolation among young adults with cerebral palsy after leaving school. *Journal of Orthopaedic Surgery, 11*(1), 80-89.

Nosek, M. A., & Hughes, R. B. (2001). Psychosocial aspects of sense of self in women with physical disabilities. *Journal of Rehabilitation, 67*(1), 20-25.

Nusbaum, M. R., & Hamilton, C. D. (2002). The proactive sexual health history. *American Family Physician, 66*, 1705-1712.

Oman, D., & Reed, D. (1998). Religion and mortality among the community dwelling elderly. *American Journal of Public Health, 88*(10), 1469-1475.

Patla, A. E. (2001). Mobility in complex environments: Implications for clinical assessment and rehabilitation. *Journal of Neurologic Physical Therapy, 25*(30), 82.

Paulson, C. P. (1991). Home care programs. In J. M. Kiernat (Ed.), *Occupational therapy and the older adult: A clinical manual* (pp. 220-239). Gaithersburg, MD: Aspen.

Pollard, N. (2000). *Allen cognitive levels: Differing social abilities.* Bethesda, MD: AOTA.

President & Fellows of Harvard College. (1997). Living well with multiple sclerosis. *Harvard Health Letter, 22*(10), 4-6.

Rathus, S. A. (1988). *Psychology* (4th ed.). Chicago: Holt, Rinehart, and Winston.

Reitz, S. M., & Scaffa, M. E. (2001). Theoretical frameworks for community-based practice. In M. E. Scaffa, (Ed.), *Occupational therapy in community-based practice settings* (pp. 51-84). Philadelphia: F.A. Davis.

Rogers, J. C., & Holm, M. B. (2003). Evaluation of areas of occupation activities and daily living and instrumental activities of daily living. In E. B. Crepeau, E. S. Cohn, & B. A. B. Schell (Eds.), *Willard and Spackman's occupational therapy* (10th ed., pp. 789-795). Philadelphia: Lippincott, Williams & Wilkins.

Rolland, J. S. (1994a). *Families, illness and disability: An integrative treatment model.* New York: Basic Books.

Rolland, J. S. (1994b). In sickness and in health: The impact of illness on couples' relationships. *Journal of Marital and Family Therapy, 20*(4), 327-347.

Scheinholz, M. K. (2001). Community-based mental health services. In M. E. Scaffa (Ed.), *Occupational therapy in community-based practice settings* (pp. 291-317). Philadelphia: F.A. Davis.

Simmons Longitudinal Study (2004). *Parental Newsletter,* 1-6.

Szekais, B. (1991). Treatment approaches for patients with dementing illness. In J. M. Kiernat (Ed.), *Occupational therapy and the older adult: A clinical manual* (pp. 192-219). Gaithersburg, MD: Aspen.

Traustadottir, R. (1993). The gendered context of friendships. In A. N. Amado (Ed.), *Friendships and community connections between people with and without developmental disabilities* (pp. 109-127). Baltimore, MD: Paul H. Brookes Publishing.

Tickle-Degnen, L. (1995). Therapeutic rapport. In C.A. Trombly (Ed.), *Occupational therapy for physical dysfunction* (4th ed., pp. 277-285). Boston: Williams & Wilkins.

United States Census Bureau. (2005). *Facts for features: Older Americans month celebrated in May.* Retrieved May 24, 2005, from http://www.census.gov/press-release/www/releases/archives/facts for features special editions/004210.html

Utz, R.L., Carr, D., Ness, R., & Wortman, C.B. (2002). The effect of widowhood on older adult social participation: An evaluation of activity, disengagement and continuity theories. *Gerontologist, 12*(4), 522-533.

Versluys, H. P. (1995a). Evaluation of emotional adjustment to disabilities. In C. A. Trombly (Ed.), *Occupational therapy for physical dysfunction* (4th ed., pp. 225-233). Boston: Williams & Wilkins.

Versluys, H. P. (1995b). Facilitation psychosocial adjustment to disability. In C. A. Trombly (Ed.), *Occupational therapy for physical dysfunction* (4th ed., pp. 377-389). Boston: Williams & Wilkins.

Warren, M. (1995). Providing low vision rehabilitation services with occupational therapy and ophthalmology: A program description. *American Journal of Occupational Therapy, 49*(9), 877-883.

Wells, K., Golding, J., & Burnham, M. (1988). Psychiatric disorder in a sample of the general population with and without chronic medical conditions. *American Journal of Psychiatry, 145*, 976-981.

Wilbarger, P. (1995). The sensory diet: Activity programs based on sensory processing theory. *American Journal of Occupational Therapy, Sensory Integration Special Interest Section Quarterly, 18*, 1-4.

Wooster, D. A., Gray, L., & Gifford, K. E. (2001). Specialized practice in home health. In M. E. Scaffa (Ed.), *Occupational therapy in community-based practice settings* (pp. 223-252). Philadelphia: F.A. Davis.

World Health Organization. (2001). Mental health: New understanding, new hope. *World Health Report, XVIII*, 178.

Yeh, S. J., & Lo, S. K. (2004). Living alone, social support and feeling lonely among the elderly. *Social Behavior and Personality, 32*(2), 129-138.

Wellness

Karen Sladyk, PhD, OTR/L, FAOTA

CHAPTER OBJECTIVES

By the end of this chapter, the student will be able to:

- ☑ Define **wellness** as it pertains to the *Occupational Therapy Practice Framework (Framework)*.
- ☑ Comprehend the **create and promote** approach to occupational therapy intervention and the relationship to wellness.
- ☑ Describe specific **models/frames of reference** as related to wellness.
- ☑ Identify related **teaching/learning principles** related to wellness.
- ☑ Delineate between the role of the **occupational therapist** (OT) and the **occupational therapy assistant** (OTA) as they pertain to wellness.
- ☑ Comprehend and identify related **physical and psychological implications** as related to wellness issues.
- ☑ Identify how an OT may be involved in wellness education.
- ☑ Identify issues related to **program planning** in wellness.
- ☑ Describe the impact of **contextual factors** upon wellness.
- ☑ Identify appropriate wellness intervention strategies based on various **performance skills and client factors**.
- ☑ Comprehend basic research questions and principles regarding wellness programs.

PRACTICE FRAMEWORK AND WELLNESS

The *Framework* (American Occupational Therapy Association [AOTA], 2002) is a document rich in detail and guidance for occupational therapy practice with individuals who have disabilities; however, the same document can guide practice in wellness and prevention. In the ideal world, disabilities would not exist and prevention techniques would keep all individuals well. Ours will never be an ideal world, so the work of the OT and OTA must assist our clients in developing wellness patterns to promote maximum health.

Areas of Occupation

Performance in the areas of occupation outlined in the *Framework* include activities of daily living (ADL), instrumental activities of daily living (IADL), education, work, play, leisure, and social participation (AOTA, 2002). All of these occupations have a wellness component to participation. Of course, each area of occupation is individualized, although various general themes can be seen. For example, a well adult is typically independent in ADLs at a level that does not call attention to him- or herself. IADL levels may vary due to the individual's context, although generally, well adults manage independently. Education and/or work depend on the adult's developmental stage, although typically, a well adult has managed these occupations at least most of his/her life. Lastly, play, leisure, and social participation are also important aspects of a well adult.

Performance Skills and Performance Patterns

If performance skills and patterns are maximized, then wellness in the areas of occupation is likely strong. Being well does not require all skills and patterns to be "normal," but the individual has developed adaptations that support health. Motor skills, process skills, and communication/interaction skills have been addressed in great detail in earlier chapters. An OT or OTA's responsibilities in traditional occupational therapy intervention is usually remediation and adaptation of problems with skills. In wellness, the practitioner is concerned with using the individual's skills to promote healthy living. For example, regular, moderate exercise (motor skills) for individuals with multiple sclerosis has been shown to have a positive impact on the quality of life (Petajan, Gappmaier, White, et al., 1996). In addition, strength exercises (motor skills) for these individuals have been shown to decrease fatigue and improve general fitness (Romberg, Virtanen, Ruutianen, et al., 2004). Less fatigue may mean the client will be able to attend his/her child's band concert and see him- or herself as a "well parent."

Performance patterns include habits, routines, and roles. These areas are not as concise and measurable as performance skills, yet they have great influence on a client's wellness. In addition, performance patterns often come with subjective bias from society and individuals. For example, most individuals agree that the habit of smoking, the routine of driving fast, and the role of drug dealer are not healthy, but others are not clear. When does shopping as a stress reducer become unhealthy? How about attending a formal church that requires time and financial commitments? Just as occupations are individualized, performance patterns are highly individualized.

Context, Activity Demands, and Client Factors

Wellness is influenced by context, activity demands, and client factors, especially context. All three are once again highly individualized, although activity demands and client factors are typically evaluated in a scientific model by the OT. Context is complicated by the different boundaries of the individual or society. For example, what is spiritual to one individual may be unacceptable to another. What is fashionable dress in one culture is not acceptable in another. What is communication face-to-face may be insulting virtually. Context is not only individual but also time sensitive. Wellness of any given individual cannot be considered until all areas of context are assessed.

Occupational Therapy Theory as a Guide to Health Planning and Wellness Programs

Frames of reference or theory to guide occupational therapy practice are extensive and rich in detail beyond what can be addressed in this chapter alone. Occupational therapy leaders all agree that a practitioner who does not use theory to guide practice is nothing more than a technical worker. Theories or frames of reference provide the professional with a guide to predict behavior and outcomes of intervention. Although the profession of occupational therapy debates the differences between theories and frames of reference and further debates the usefulness of theories inside and outside of occupational therapy, all agree that a professional uses models to guide effective practice.

Theories Developed in Occupational Therapy

Several theories have been put forward by scholars in occupational therapy, including:

- Occupational Behavior (Reilly, 1974).
- Model of Human Occupation (Kielhofner & Burke, 1980).
- Person Environment Occupational Performance (Christiansen & Baum, 1991).
- Occupational Adaptation (Schkade & Schultz, 1992).
- Occupational Science (Zemke & Clark, 1996).
- Canadian Model of Occupational Performance (CAOT, 1997).

Although uniquely different, each of these models has common themes that can be effectively used in wellness practice with occupational therapy clients. First, all of these models are client focused, respecting, and understanding of the person as a unique individual. Second, these models acknowledge that individuals do not stand alone, but are part of an environment that places demands on the individual. Third, each model acknowledges that roles and occupations are meaningful to individuals, and essential to helping the client find meaning in life. All three of these themes support wellness programming.

Theories Developed in Other Disciplines

OTs also use theories developed from other disciplines as a core for occupation-based practice. Psychodynamic, behavioral, sensory motor, and cognitive approaches help predict and explain behavior (Giroux-Bruce & Borg, 2002).

Historical figures in theory development helped shape current practice in occupational therapy. For example, the early work of Freud and Jung set the foundation for psychodynamic theory refined by Fidler's Task Oriented Group (1969). Fidler believed that clients project the same problems they have in the world when they participate in a task group. The OT can address these issues in the group, and then the individual will have better interactions in his/her world. Skinner (1971) presented theory on reinforcement and conditioning, which has lead to OTs incorporating learning contracts and behavioral techniques such as chaining, modeling, and motivation into occupational therapy practice. Sensory motor theory reinforced the brain's connection to explaining movement and behavior. Lastly, cognitive approaches underscore the importance of teaching and learning in understanding human behavior (Giroux-Bruce & Borg, 2002).

Just as the occupational therapy models presented above share a common theme, models outside of the discipline also share a common theme: the individual himself cannot be understood alone. The unconscious self, the behavioral self, the sensory motor self, and the cognitive self all contribute to understanding the whole person. The OT with an understanding of theories, in and out of occupational therapy, is best positioned to assist a client in wellness planning.

So What Are Health and Healthy Behaviors?

Health is a continuum from wellness to death. Healthy behaviors are any action humans take to maintain or promote well-being (Curtis, 1998). These are two simple definitions, yet wellness is incredibly difficult to achieve for most individuals. The topic of health is of concern to many disciplines and has been the focus of theory development and research, particularly in the last 50 years. Several models of understanding health and wellness are shared by health care professionals across many disciplines and are briefly described here.

Biopsychosocial Model

This model presents a psychological and medical model of understanding wellness. The body's physical systems, such as nervous, endocrine, digestive, cardiovascular, and immune, work in harmony to maintain wellness. Stresses from external forces impact the balance of these systems and cause sickness. Stress can be from numerous sources. Biological stress might be pollution. Psychological stress might be work performance. Interpersonal stress might include relationship issues. Physiological stress includes addictions. Any combination of stresses may cause sickness depending on the human's ability to cope (Sarafino, 2002; Taylor, 1999).

Health Behavior Theories

Bandura's work (1977) on self-efficacy and Becker's (1974) examination of locus of control help explain how individuals stay well. Locus of control shows that individuals approach healthy behaviors whether or not they believe there is control over the situation. Individuals with an internal locus of control believe their actions contribute to their health. Individuals with an external locus of control believe health is caused by fate or things outside of their control. Health care providers must assess the individual's locus of control before providing advice. Pender (1982) adds demographic, biological, social, and environmental factors to locus of control to explain how individuals receive cues from outside factors to influence their locus of control.

Health Belief Model

The health belief model examines why individuals fail to be healthy. Key to this model is the perception of the risk of unhealthy behaviors. Susceptibility, severity, benefits of behaviors, and costs/barriers are weighed by each individual before making changes in unhealthy behaviors (Rotter, 1966). An individual may make nonscientific assessments of the risks, such as, "my grandmother ate a high fat diet and never had a stroke." An individual's behavior has little to do with the message being sent by the health care worker.

Transtheoretical Model

This model examines healthy behaviors as a progression through stages (Prochaska & DiClemente, 1982). Precontemplation, contemplation, preparation, action, and maintenance map the changes in health behaviors. This model states that individuals do not necessarily go through these stages in order and often repeat stages or fail to move out of a stage towards health. Health care practitioners should consider the individual's current stage when providing advice.

IF EFFECTIVE HEALTH MODELS EXIST, WHY ARE INDIVIDUALS UNHEALTHY?

Just as no occupational therapy theory can guide all occupational therapy practice, no health theory can answer all health and wellness concerns. Theory does, however, guide our practice, providing direction when the occupational therapy practitioner needs a focus. Theory must be combined with evidence from peer-reviewed research to make the most effective intervention approach specific to each client.

What Does the Evidence Say?

Those who reimburse and consumers are demanding services be evidence-based, yet few OTs examine the literature before developing wellness programs. In addition, consumers want choices in health care, including alternative intervention methods shown to be effective. The OT must be well read in the literature and able to translate meaningful options to the consumer.

MIND-BODY CONNECTION TO VARIOUS DISEASES

A great variety of opinion regarding the effect of the mind on the body's wellness will depend upon on the type of health practitioner chosen. Some have reported as high as 90% of all diseases have an emotional root (Hafen, Karren, Frandsen, & Smith, 1996). These emotions are not imaginary diseases, but triggers to physical illness such as heart disease, digestion problems, and accidents. The immune system in human beings is known to have chemical relationships with emotions. Physiological changes at the individual's cellular level may trigger long-term effects causing disease or disability. Much research has shown emotional ties to illness, yet little is understood about the science of this process (Hafen et al., 1996). Examples of how emotions are tied to illness are presented in Table 9-1.

IMPACT OF EMOTIONAL ISSUES ON WELLNESS

As the reader can see above, emotional issues such as stress, anger, and personality may play important roles in triggering an illness or accident. What emotional issues provide triggers to wellness? Social supports, spirituality, resilience, and humor are thought to impact health in a positive manner, as described below.

SOCIAL SUPPORTS

Long-term research has shown that good health and long life are tied to the amount of social support an individual enjoys (Hafen, Karren, Frandsen, & Smith, 1996). The theory presented to explain this phenomenon is that social support: 1) enhances positive feelings and self-esteem, 2) encourages stability and mastery of the environment, and 3) acts as a buffer against stress, therefore protecting the individual from stress-induced disease and accidents (Sheldon, Cohen, & Syme, 1985). This social support provides appraisal support, helping the individual assess stressful events, tangible support such as financial resources, informational support such as advice, and emotional support including reassurance (Taylor, 1999). A social support system does not mean only a traditional family system but includes any individual supportive in a family, friend, and service circle. Coping skills in individuals within social support systems appear stronger.

SPIRITUALITY AND HEALTH

Spirituality is often confused with religion, although it should be seen as separate (Seigel, 1993; Smith, 1993). For many individuals, religion supports their spirituality, but for many others

Table 9-1

EMOTIONS AND THEIR RELATION TO ILLNESS

Accidents	Inattention due to emotional distractions makes us prone to accidents. An individual worried about falls is likely to become inactive and therefore at a great risk for falls.
Allergies and asthma	Stress causes allergy antibodies to increase and therefore trigger greater immune responses to the allergen. A child worried about his skill on the baseball team may internalize the stress and increase the chance to develop an asthma attack.
Arthritis	Several research studies have found a tie between emotional stress and the development of rheumatoid arthritis. Timing of emotional events such as divorce may indicate a relationship to the outbreak of the disease.
Back pain	Heavy lifting may not be the major factor in back pain. Back muscles may tense to emotional issues and therefore be at risk for injury.
Cancer	Cancer cells are thought to be in all individuals but our immune system effectively controls them. Stressors such as emotions or other causes may reduce the effectiveness of the immune system to fight the cancer cells leading to the need for medical assistance.
Diabetes	Individuals with depression seem to be more at risk of developing diabetes than those without; however, other issues may be trigger the depression such as environmental situations.
Heart disease and hypertension	Hypertension is a known factor in heart disease. Adrenaline released during anger speeds the heart and constricts the blood vessels, resulting in hypertension. Chronic anger may further the progress of heart disease.
Insomnia	Every individual has experienced a sleepless night due to rehashing of emotional thoughts at bedtime. Chronic insomnia interferes with the body's ability to retool.
Irritable bowel and stomach issues	An overreaction to environmental cues may trigger digestion problems for those who are hyper alert.

Adapted from Hafen, B. Q., Karren, K. J. Frandsen, K.J., & Smith, N. L. (1996). *Mind/body health: The effects of attitudes, emotions, and relationships*. Boston, MA: Allyn and Bacon.

religion is not a focus of their spirituality. It is important that the health care provider accurately assess the role of spirituality in the client's health.

Spirituality is more difficult to define than quantitative signs such as range of motion (ROM) or assessment scores. Experts in medicine and spirituality (Seigel, 1993; Smith, 1993) define spiritual health as:

- A state of well being.
- Self-forgiveness.

- Self-love and freedom.
- Peace with oneself.
- Sense of connectedness and wholeness.
- Sense of meaning, purpose, and challenge.
- Positive expectations and hope.

Spirituality is often reborn when a crisis becomes a growth experience. Often individuals report that their perspective of life changes dramatically when faced with a personal or family health crisis. Spiritual experiences are highly individualized and client-centered. Some clients report the power of prayer while others prefer relaxation exercises. Some consumers find meaning by attending formal church meetings while others enjoy volunteer work. Connectedness may be with animals, children, friends, family, or the deeper self. Spirituality is a personal faith or hope that may or may not be connected to a formal religion. Myths, shrines, customs, and healers all represent the connectedness of spirituality.

RESILIENCE

A major research focus of behavioral scientists in the new millennium has been how some children raised in horrible settings grow up to function well in society, while others in better settings have dysfunctional lives. The concept, known as resilience, applies to wellness in general. How do some individuals form a disease-resistant personality and manage stress so effectively? What makes an individual resilient? Kobasa (1984) believes social support, a sense of control, fitness, a sense of humor, self-esteem, optimism, coping skills, and hardiness of personality make an individual resilient and able to form a stress buffer zone. Hope and perseverance are major factors of resilience. Hafen, Karren, Frandsen, & Smith (1996) suggest the following skills be taught to clients to improve resilience:

- Develop creativity.
- Use personal insight to face a challenge.
- Break stressful tasks into smaller chunks.
- Turn negative perceptions into positive perspectives.
- Develop a network of social supports.
- Develop a sense of humor.
- Use compassion and empathy.

HUMOR

Just about everyone has heard "laughter is the best medicine," yet humor has just recently received attention in the scientific community. History, including the Bible (Proverbs 17:22), has documented the use of humor. More recently, Norman Cousins was credited for writing about the use of humor to reduce chronic pain. Hospitals have begun to develop humor rooms, humor television shows, or bedside humor entertainment for clients to take a laugh break because hospitalization can be a highly stressful event.

Laughing provides physiological, physical, and psychological benefits (Hafen et al., 1996). Physiologically, the brain releases endorphins while laughing. This natural response is more effective than medical pain relievers. Further, endorphins reduce inflammation and jump-start an immune response. Physically, muscles relax during laughing. Oxygen and circulation improve, benefiting the cardiovascular system. Psychologically, laughing reduces stress, provides a positive outlook for the future, and provides an outlet for emotions. Twenty minutes of humor has been shown to be equally as effective as exercise in lifting mood and decreasing anxiety (Szabo, 2003). Hafen et al. (1996) suggest the following skills be taught to clients to improve laughter:

- Watch funny movies.
- Read and collect humor.
- Share funny things with others (e-mail "laugh out loud" items).
- Do silly things at least once a week.
- Add more fun to the day and help others add fun as well.
- Remember how much fun it is to be a child.

Adult Learning Models That Support Healthy Living

Numerous books have been written about educational theories (Sladyk, 2005). This section will look at theories specific to adults, commonly called *andragogy*. *Pedagogy* is the educational foundation of schooling through high school, based on pediatric theories (Jacobs & Jacobs, 2004).

Adults like to learn differently from children. Sometimes, teachers or health care practitioners who use pedagogy techniques on adults actually insult the adult learner. Adults learn differently. Some may like to learn the way they did in primary or secondary school, and others want different approaches. The key to teaching adults is flexibility and continual assessment of meeting their learning needs (Sheckley, 1984).

Adult learners are a widely diverse group who encompass many different styles, goals, and experiences (Cross, 1988). Understanding some of the major characteristics of this group can lead to more effective application of knowledge and transfer of learning to life situations. When interpreting major characteristics of adult learning, caution should be used to avoid labeling a diverse group with limited characteristics.

We live in a complex society where continual learning is no longer a luxury, but a necessity (Cross, 1988; Wlodkowski, 1990). Adults are independent thinkers with a variety of thoughts and experiences that accompany them when embarking upon new learning. Addressing this diversity of experience and needs will help the educator or therapist succeed.

Adults come to each learning experience with an integration of all prior learning experience (Kolb, 1984). For example, if a teenager had negative experiences in high school gym class, he is likely to come to a wellness program as an adult with negative feelings. If a client has had positive experiences all during her rehabilitation program, she is likely to be open to new experiences in an outpatient clinic. The role of an adult's life experience in forming new learning cannot be minimized. Formal and informal experiences (Bandura, 1978) are included in this integration of experiences; therefore, academic success in the past may predict the openness to wellness ideas in the future. As the adult gets older, work experiences are added to this integration.

Brookfield (1990) points out that adults learn best in situations of mutual respect. Fostering the growth of the learner along a path to an ideal wellness goal is the job of the OT. Brookfield advocates that teachers help students: 1) identify and challenge assumptions and context, 2) imagine and explore alternatives, and 3) view knowledge with reflective skepticism. Simply providing the learner with information does not foster the transfer of knowledge (1990).

Chaffee (1998) states that the key to successful adult thinking is in 8 steps: 1) think critically, 2) live creatively, 3) choose freely, 4) solve problems effectively, 5) communicate effectively, 6) analyze complex issues, 7) develop enlightened values, and 8) think through relationships. He encourages adults to transform themselves though thinking and to create a life philosophy to follow. This requires a strong commitment to self-analysis, which many adults cannot call upon because of other factors. Wellness or lack of wellness is illustrated in this model when other factors interfere with the adult's ability to live freely.

Adult behavior is an interaction of person and environment (Bandura, 1978). Although most individuals believe the learner's responsibility is to learn, learners will act on their learning within the structure of their environment. In some cultures, women are not expected to be learners. Teaching an individual from this environment may be difficult but effective if the wellness educator considers the restrictive environment to be the learning environment. For example, wellness education for new mothers can be effective if it includes the elderly women of the community as part of the "teachers."

In general, when addressing the unique learning needs of adults, several themes emerge. Adults bring with them an educational history that may or may not be positive. Adults learn through their experiences (experiential learning). Motivation can support new learning; however, adults typically learn within their own environments. Mutual respect plays an important role in adult learning. All of these factors can influence the transfer of training to life situations. All of these factors, if negative, can cause a negative loop that is recursive and self-fulfilling. The goal of the wellness educator is to manage these factors in a way that is positive to the adult learner (Sladyk, 2005).

EFFECTIVE WELLNESS EDUCATION

Before effective wellness planning can begin, some general issues known in health care apply to wellness. First, individuals cannot be "scared healthy," and second, basic teaching and learning skills used in any rehabilitation setting apply to wellness.

Scare Techniques Do Not Work

There have been some very moving advertising campaigns in the media, including "this is your brain on drugs," cars falling off schools, and famous actors with cigarettes in their noses. Many individuals may remember a DARE officer in school or seeing a plastic, moveable model of lungs addicted to cigarettes try to take a breath. All of these show the negative effect of unhealthy behaviors, yet drugs, cigarettes, and fast driving remain problems. Scare campaigns are not effective teaching methods but can open a discussion if the audience is concerned about the topic. Too often, a scare campaign can lead to denial and turn some individuals away from the topic (Kerr, 1999). Scare techniques might affect rapport building with clients and resistance might follow. A wellness practitioner must understand where the client is currently functioning in order to plan an effective wellness intervention plan. Scare techniques must be well thought out before being added as a teaching tool to a wellness program.

Teaching and Learning Principles

Teaching and learning methods have been a part of occupational therapy from the early years of practice, although Mosey's (1986) book on psychosocial occupational therapy was one of the first to link educational theory and psychological theory with occupational therapy intervention (Sladyk, 2005). Mosey detailed 16 principles to guide therapist-client interaction in learning. Learning principles do not provide firm rules but provide a base to begin to facilitate learning. One principle may carry more importance with one individual than another. The therapist's judgment is the key to success. The following guidelines are adapted from Mosey's (1986) work.

When teaching in wellness, the practitioner will:

1. *Use good communication skills*: Collaboration is a valued aspect of the therapeutic relationship beginning with the practitioner using good communication skills. The therapist should sit squarely towards the client without crossing arms or legs. Good, comfortable eye contact and a relaxed approach will make the client comfortable. Use open-ended questions to

probe for details about a client's wellness. For example, "What type of activities make you feel happy, Seth?" Use closed ended questions carefully and only when a specific answer is needed. For example, "Show me where you have pain during exercise, Nicole."

2. *Accept the clients for who they are*: All human beings have the right to good health and wellness. The practitioner should keep biases in check and be reflective of any behavior which appears judgmental. Understand wellness is a personal judgment of the client, not the occupational therapy practitioner.

3. *Begin the intervention at the client's current level*: This allows the individual initial success before moving on to the next level. When the individual is ready for the next level, provide what Allen, Earhart, and Blue (1992) called the "just right challenge." Remember, everyone learns at different rates.

4. *Acknowledge the client's current culture and environment*: This can include heritage, country of origin, age, gender, and memberships. The individual's assets and limitations are important to address in light of his/her culture and environment. All of these factors can have a positive and/or negative influence on returning to health. For example, membership in a street gang or social club can hinder an individual in remaining alcohol-free, but membership in a church or fitness club can help.

5. *Communicate effectively in volume and pace*: Consider how something is being said as well as what is said. Clients with hearing problems usually hear better with their eyeglasses on because they pick up on the visual cues of speech. Confused clients perform better with simple, clear cues such as "Open the paint."

6. *Encourage the client to be an active learner*: Empower the client to be the leader of his/her wellness plan. Encourage learning with all the sensorimotor components to reinforce the task.

7. *Control the consequences of learning*: Pleasurable experiences in wellness reinforce the client to want to learn again. Always process the experience, whether in a group or individually, after the learning experience. Provide opportunities to make errors and then discuss how things could go better next time. If need be, stop an experience if safety is an issue because safety is always addressed first in intervention.

8. *Provide an opportunity for trial and error*: This is empowering for the individual when consequences are controlled. Use first and last experiences to demonstrate how much the individual has improved. Stay open-minded to ways the individual wants to "try something out." The client may know better than the practitioner.

9. *Provide opportunity for practice and repetition*: No one likes to learn something by rote memory, but opportunities to practice skills provide mastery. Similar to trial and error, use the first and last experiences to show the client his/her progress. Many wellness clients like to chart or journal their progress.

10. *Encourage the client to set his/her own goals*: Wellness plans allow the client to drive the intervention rather than the practitioner writing intervention goals in the client's record. A practitioner should never solely develop goals for an individual even when goals may be influenced by insurance reviewers. Motivation and responsibility are powerful components to wellness plans.

11. *Practice skills in different situations*: Learning is often specific to an experience but practice in different situations allows the client to generalize the skill or transfer the training. For example, saying "no" to an offer of an alcoholic drink is very different in a group of non-drinking friends versus in a crowded bar.

12. *The client should understand what is being learned*: Too often the client does not understand what is being learned. This is especially true for clients with a head injury and/or confusion who also need wellness programs. Check for understanding during the processing stage of intervention. Educate staff, family, and friends at every available opportunity.

13. *Learning moves from simple to complex*: All theory in adult education, occupational therapy, and health promotion supports starting at a level at which the client can be successful. The idea of learning from simple to complex is nicely illustrated by the rating system for ski slopes—bunny trail to black diamond. An individual just learning to ski as a stress reducer would not start on a black diamond slope.

14. *Encourage creative problem solving*: Often, traditional approaches to a problem may not be the right answer for clients with nontraditional issues. The practitioner should role model and encourage his/her client to "think outside of the box." For example, fitness walking in an unsafe neighborhood might move to the inside of a local place of worship following adult religious study.

15. *Acknowledge that everyone handles stress and anxiety differently*: Learning is frustrating, stressful, and anxiety producing. Learners deal with this stress in different ways. Some shut down and become very quiet. Some get loud and angry. Some get the giggles and laugh at everything. The practitioner needs to watch for signs of stress or anxiety and process this information with the client (Sladyk, 2005).

PROGRAM PLANNING IN WELLNESS

Ideally, every wellness program has a developed protocol to outline the program from development to evaluation of effectiveness. This protocol provides written guidance to any practitioner who leads the program even if the practitioner is not the original developer. The protocol should include the following:

Frames of Reference

Any frame of reference or theory presented in this chapter can guide a wellness program. Choosing the appropriate theory requires judgment from the OT and should consider the audience, facility, and problem.

Audience

Who is the target of the wellness program? Will he/she be seen individually or in groups? Will the audience be part of an adult education program? An outpatient facility? Are the members volunteers or not? The audience of a wellness program is as varied as the general population. What works in an adult education program in a large city may not work in the suburbs.

Problem

What health problem will this program address? Can several problems be effectively addressed together or should the program focus on just one? How does the audience view this problem? The problems addressed in this area are as varied as the problems facing most communities: overeating, smoking, ADA issues, safety, and fitness.

Readiness

Is the potential audience ready to address this health concern? A program planned too early, even a well-developed program, will fail if the timing is not correct. OTs can avoid problems in this area by completing a detailed needs assessment before developing a program. This needs assessment should include a review of the literature and evidence, focus groups of potential audience members, key informants from the community, and survey of referral sources.

Actions

What actions are needed by both the leader and the participants to succeed? These are often written as program goals and client goals. Both program (administrative) and client (individual) goals should be written in measurable terms to facilitate evaluation. To facilitate action by the participant, present the most important information first. Be brief, using common language. Concepts that are difficult to understand or need to be linked to other concepts should be presented by clustering. Instructions need to be clear and presented so that the participant understands.

Materials

What financial and material supplies are needed to effectively run this program? Are administrative needs such as staff or facilities shared with other programs?

Evaluation

How will the program's goals be measured and documented?

SAMPLE WELLNESS PROGRAMS IN OCCUPATIONAL THERAPY

There are so many potential wellness programs that could be lead by occupational therapy practitioners, the limits are only fixed to the energy of the staff. Potential wellness programs and the available evidence are presented in Table 9-2. Typically, a wellness program is developed out of an urgent need or a new understanding of a need not recognized before.

Case Study #1: Julie

Julie is a mental health OT employed by the mental health services department of a community hospital. Her department services clients in both inpatient and outpatient programs with referrals to a variety of community support systems. Her department allows great flexibility in choosing frames of reference for her clients and the hospital respects the services provided by occupational therapy.

After the birth of Julie's first child, she became aware that the mental health department did little to support new mothers. Julie believed occupational therapy could provide assistance with skill building for new moms, especially those dealing with postpartum depression. Julie began discussing the topic with peers and investigating needs. She connected with the maternal health department of the hospital and found they were eager to network with the staff in mental health. Julie explained occupational therapy services to the staff in maternal health and was encouraged to develop a program for new mothers with a focus on mental health. Julie developed a program that would see new mothers individually and help them network with friends and family for support as they adjusted to a new occupation. Potential wellness programs and the available evidence are presented in Table 9-2.

Table 9-2

EVIDENCE FOR WELLNESS PROGRAMS

Wellness Program	Learning Activities	Evidence
Depression	Moderate exercise and mood	Turnbull & Wolfson, 2002; Netz & Lidor, 2003; Lovejoy & Lane, 2000; Lawlor & Hopker, 2001; Dimeo et al., 2001; Russell et al., 2003
	Social support	Oman & Oman, 2003
	Cognitive reframing	Odone, 1996; McHugh & Wierzbicki, 1998; Totterdell, 1999; Hewston et al., 2005; McKay & Fanning, 2000
Eating healthy	Mood and food	Heatherton et al., 1992; Guinn, 1991; Cools et al., 1992; Ward & Mann, 2000
	Societal issues	Schotte et al., 1990
	Stress	Greeno & Wing, 1994; Cartwright et al., 2003; Denisoff & Endler, 2000; Ng & Jeffery, 2003
Fitness	Attitude	Mack & Shaddox, 2004; Dixon, Mauzey, & Hall, 2003; Blamey & Mutrie, 2004; Chatzisarantis et al., 2005;
	Health	McKay et al., 2003; Larson & Zaichowsky, 1995; Thomas, Baker, & Davies, 2003
	Social support	Phillips, 2005; Mathias et al., 1997
	Cognitive reframing	Prestwich, Lawton, & Conner, 2003
Pain reduction	Back pain prevention	Wortman, 2003; Wilson, 1998; American Academy of Pediatrics et al., 2004
	Mind body connection	McCaffrey, Frock, & Garguilo, 2003; Atli & Loeser, 2004
	Massage or physical activity	Shealy, 2005; Teitelbaum, 2005
Sleep preparation	Sleep hygiene	Brown, Buboltz, & Soper, 2002; Sadeh, Keinan, & Daon, 2004;
	Restorative benefits	Ward, 2004; Blissitt, 2001; Bower, 2004; Trockel, Barnes, & Egget, 2000; Heuer & Klien, 2003

continued

Table 9-2, continued

EVIDENCE FOR WELLNESS PROGRAM

Wellness Program	Learning Activities	Evidence
Smoking cessation	Relaxation exercises	Kassel & Shiffman, 1997
	Stress	Kassel, 2000; Juliano & Brandon, 2002; Britt et al., 2001; Piasecki & Baker, 2000; Parrott, 2000; Shiffman & Waters, 2004; Todd, 2004
	Cognitive reframing	Ong & Walsh, 2001; Chassin et al., 2002
	Weight gain	Ludman et al., 2002
Stress reduction	Physical health	Fontana & McLaughlin, 1998; Edwards et al., 2001; Leitner & Resch, 2005
	Mental health	Dantz et al., 2003; Lumley & Provenzano, 2003; Fletcher & Fletcher, 2005
	Mind body connection	Deckro et al., 2002
	Hardiness and motivation	Judkins, 2004; Peterson & Wilson, 2004; LePine, LePine, & Jackson, 2004
	Leisure	Misra & McKean, 2000
	Social support	Misra, Crist, & Burant, 2003

Case Study #2

Applying the evidence from Table 9-2 provides challenges. A small group of Level II fieldwork students were completing their mental health fieldwork in a community clubhouse model for individuals with chronic and persistent mental health disorders. The students, under the supervision of an OT, were to develop a wellness program of their choice based on a needs assessment completed with clubhouse members and staff. The staff were very concerned with the smoking of members. Members were required to smoke outside and often were so busy smoking that they missed meetings or group activities. The students remembered from pathology class that individuals with schizophrenia had the highest smoking rate of all disabilities. The members of the clubhouse thought smoking was an issue. The students developed a smoking cessation group that met daily. The frames of reference selected were cognitive-behavioral with a health promotion influence. Activities included journaling, using the Internet for support information, psychoeducational tips for quitting, and peer support when the smoking urge came for members. On the first day, several members attended. They made a list of coping strategies based on experience and information from the American Cancer Society, including delaying a cigarette for as long as possible, making a plan, finding support, remembering the benefits of quitting, and performing relaxation exercises. Despite having the students as personal coaches, none of the members were able to reduce their smoking. The students met with the members and OT to evaluate the program. The OT reminded the students about the timing in Prochaska & DiClemente's health model (1982). Precontemplation, contemplation, preparation, action, and maintenance map the changes in health behaviors, although the staff and students jumped right to action and the members were not ready for change.

OTHER WELLNESS AND HEALTH PROMOTION IDEAS

As occupational therapy is changing in the new millennium, students and staff have wonderful opportunities to effect change in the health of our citizens. Below are brief examples of known wellness programs developed by OTs or examples of potential programs that can be developed for members of the community, either as part of a formal health care system or in alternative delivery systems such as adult education.

Accident Prevention and Home Safety

An OT connected with her local fire department can offer home safety evaluations to members of the community. A local foundation can provide a small grant to staff and buy supplies for the program.

ADA Consulting

Many communities can understand ADA, but have difficulty applying the concepts for effective living. An OT can provide this service with understanding of the *Framework* and application of environmental issues in the community.

Assistive Living Support

The goal of assistive living is independence. The OT can provide group or individual consultation to members or staff.

Community Redesign

As a follow-up to ADA consulting, communities often have funding to enhance the community but little understanding of how to enhance the independence of its residents.

Community Wellness

At times, communities get together to support one another in a goal to enhance life. Examples include blood pressure screenings, reading a common book for discussion, or getting fit together. An OT on the planning committee can bring the role of participation to wellness.

Coping and Relaxation

Adult education classes dealing with strategies for the well individual to cope and relax are popular. These classes could be held at a fitness center, night school, or a community club. Stress reduction exercises, assertiveness training, relaxation exercises, and sleep readiness can all be addressed.

Diabetes Self-Management

The management of diabetes, expected to have explosive growth in the next 10 years, is a complex issue. Diet, exercise, stress reduction, cognitive changes, attitude adjustment, skin care, and medication management are just some of the issues this wellness program can address.

Fitness

Everyone understands the role of fitness in health, although not everyone participates in fitness activities such as workouts in the gym. The OT has assessment skills to address those who fail to meet their fitness requirements. Finding meaningful activities that are also fitness activities can help clients reach their goal.

Healthy Back

A healthy back can mean a life with less pain. Injury prevention is the most effective way to address this problem, yet many individuals do not know basic body mechanics. This is a great concern to health care providers, child care workers, and laborers.

Lifestyle Redesign

The concept of lifestyle redesign (Mandel, Jackson, Zemke, Nelson, & Clark, 1999) came from the wellness studies at the University of Southern California Well Elderly Program. The basic premise is keeping individuals well through participation, occupation, and meaningful activity. Needs assessment begins the process of addressing specific populations. Activity programs are designed to help clients find meaningful experience despite changes in their lives.

Pain Self-Management

Chronic pain is not understood and is very individualized. When pain becomes chronic, individuals stop participating in life and pain medications can lead to further problems, such as addiction. Pain self-management is known to be a balance of fitness and coping skills that can allow for better participation and greater life satisfaction (Atli & Loeser, 2004).

Safe Sex

When the AIDS scare began in the early 1980s, everyone talked about the need for safe sex (Sladyk, 1990). Currently, there is little discussion or understanding among all adults. Medications have changed the face of AIDS, but sexually transmitted diseases continue to be a problem.

Smoking Reduction

As illustrated by the previous case study, quitting smoking is especially hard. A multitude of materials are available to stop smoking, yet many remain challenged to stop. An effective program uses these resources and also provides an individualized approach. OTs with training in counseling, occupation, and general health care issues are skilled in helping clients to stop smoking.

Sleep Readiness

Although sleep is not an occupation, getting ready to sleep is. The effects of too little sleep on memory, driving, and general performance is known, yet few individuals know how to enhance a quality night's sleep. Table 9-3 addresses strategies to enhance sleep, which can be used in a wellness program with clients or well community members.

Spirituality and Hope

Since spirituality is not only religion, spirituality can be addressed as an IADL or social participation activity. Spirituality experiences are highly individualized and client-centered. Activities can include humor, prayer, relaxation exercises, formal church meetings, or altruistic volunteer work. Connectedness may be with animals, children, friends, family, or the deeper self.

Table 9-3

SAMPLE WELLNESS ACTIVITIES

Activities to Promote Sleep

ADLs	Limit bed to sleeping or sexual activity. Do not nap, Take a warm bath one hour before bed. Avoid any liquid drink before bed, especially liquor or caffeine.
IADLs	Set up the bedroom to reduce distractions. If awake for more than a half hour, get up and do some other quiet activity, Get some bright light during the afternoon. Make lists of things to be accomplished tomorrow well before bedtime.
Education	Learn about other medical problems affecting sleep, such as back pain. Check medications to make sure there are no interactions affecting sleep. Consult a medical doctor or dentist for medical issues effecting sleep.
Work	Keep to a regular schedule. Learn assertiveness techniques to manage office stress. When racing thoughts occupy the mind at night, quietly tell them to stop by repeating the word "stop." Replace racing thoughts with a peaceful mantra.
Play/Leisure	Exercise regularly but never in the evening. Play with fun as the goal each day, Do gentle, relaxing back stretches before bed.
Social Participation	Find quiet time before bed to clear the mind. Socialize with positive individuals who bring joy, not stress

Teen Moms: Prevention and Intervention

Teens who become mothers before establishing other adult roles often have lifetime effects on career development, long-term relationships, and lifelong learning opportunities. Young women often see the romantic side of caring for tiny babies and are ill prepared for the exhausting role of being a mother. Prevention/wellness program goals are to delay motherhood, while teen mother programs have coping as the main focus of intervention. Both address IADLs, social participation, and education.

Weight Self-Management

Everyone knows the likelihood of keeping weight off after dieting is almost nonexistent. Hundreds of weight loss programs are available, yet none have the answer for most individuals. Just as most health behaviors are complicated, weight loss is an individualized occupation that includes lifestyle redesign. Clients need more than a weight loss plan, and they must fit the plan into their ADLs, IADLs, work, and social participation.

Designing a Simple Research Study to Demonstrate Effectiveness of Wellness Programs

When the wellness program is developed and running, it is time to measure the effectiveness for outside reviewers or funding sources. Although most OTs avoid doing clinical research, wellness programs are easy to evaluate. First begin with a research question, such as:

1. In what ways and to what extent does...
   - smoking relate to weight loss?
   - self-esteem relate to teen pregnancy?
   - fitness relate to quality of sleep?

Or,

2. Is there a significant difference between admission and discharge scores of individuals who participate in...
   - accident prevention programs?
   - diabetes self-management programs?
   - weight and fitness wellness programs?

Collect the data and use a software program to analyze the outcomes statistically. The first research question asks for a relationship and is measured with a Pearson correlation coefficient. The second question asks for a difference between two scores and is measured by a t-test. Both statistical tests are easy to do and take less than a minute to run after the data is entered into the software. Results of these measures can be used in quality assurance and risk management reports in addition to funding source reports for grants.

Summary Questions

1. Discuss how an individual may maintain wellness in his/her life and how occupational therapy may facilitate this process.

2. Discuss and justify how an individual with chronic rheumatoid arthritis may participate in a wellness program.

3. Discuss additional wellness and health promotion programs in which an OT may be involved.

4. Discuss the impact of humor and resilience upon wellness and how occupational therapy may incorporate these principles into the intervention process.

References

Allen, C. K., Earhart, C. A., & Blue, T. (1992). *Occupational therapy treatment goals for the physically and cognitively disabled*. Bethesda, MD: American Occupational Therapy Association.

American Academy of Pediatrics, American Public Health Association, National Resource Center for Health and Safety in Child Care (2004). *Child care providers' health and well being: Applicable standards from caring for our children*. Elk Grove Village, IL: Author.

American Occupational Therapy Association. (2002). Occupational therapy practice framework: Domain and process. *American Journal of Occupational Therapy, 56*(6), 609-639.

Atli, A., & Loeser, J. D. (2004). Chronic nonmalignant pain: Rational management. *Consultant, 44*(13), 1693-1701.

Bandura, A. (1977). Self efficacy: Toward a unifying theory of behavioral change. *Psychological Review, 84,* 199-215.

Bandura, A. (1978). The self-system in reciprocal determinism. *American Psychologist, April,* 344-357.

Becker, M. H. (1974). *The health belief model and personal health behavior.* Thorofare, NJ: SLACK Incorporated.

Blamey, A., & Mutrie, N. (2004). Changing the individual to promote health-enhancing physical activity: The difficulties of producing evidence and translating it into practice. *Journal of Sports Sciences, 22*(8), 741-755.

Blissitt, P. A. (2001). Sleep, memory, and learning. *Journal of Neuroscience Nursing, 33*(4), 208-223.

Bower, B. (2004). Slumber may fortify memory, stir insight. *Science News, 164*(4), 53-54.

Britt, D. M., Cohen, L. M., Collins, F. L., & Cohen, M. L. (2001). Cigarette smoking and chewing gum response to a laboratory induced stressor. *Health Psychology, 20*(5), 361-368.

Brookfield, S. D. (1990). *Understanding and facilitating adult learning.* San Francisco, CA: Jossey-Bass Publishers.

Brown, F. C., Buboltz, W. C., & Soper, B. (2002). Relationship between sleep hygiene awareness, sleep hygiene practices, and sleep quality in university students. *Behavioral Medicine, 28*(1), 33-39.

Canadian Association of Occupational Therapists [CAOT]. (1997). *Enabling occupation: An occupational therapy perspective.* Ottawa, ON: CAOT Publications.

Cartwright, M., Wardle, J., Steggles, N., Simon, A. E., Croker, H., & Jarvis, M. J. (2003). *Health Psychology, 22*(4), 362-369.

Chaffee, J. (1998). *The thinker's way: 8 steps to a richer life.* Boston, MA: Little, Brown and Company.

Chassin, L., Presson, C. C., Sherman, S. T., & Kim, K. (2002). Long-term psychological sequelae of smoking cessation and relapse. *Health Psychology, 21*(5), 438-443.

Chatzisarantis, N. L., Hagger, M. S., Biddle, S. J., & Smith, B. The stability of the attitude intention relationship in the context of physical activity. *Journal of Sports Sciences, 23*(1), 49-62.

Christiansen, C., & Baum, C. (1991). *Occupational therapy: Overcoming human performance deficits.* Thorofare, NJ: SLACK Incorporated.

Cohen, S., & Syme, S. L. (1985). *Social support and health.* London: Academic Press.

Cools, J., Schotte, D. E., & McNally, R. J. (1992). Emotional arousal and overeating in restrained eaters. *Journal of Abnormal Psychology, 101*(2), 348-351.

Cross, K. P. (1988). *Adults as learners.* San Francisco, CA: Jossey-Bass Publishers.

Curtis, K. A. (1998). Health behavior and effective patient education. In C. M. Davis (Ed.) *Patient practitioner interaction: An experiential manual for developing the art of health care* (3rd ed.). Thorofare, NJ: SLACK Incorporated.

Dantz, B., Ashton, A. K., D'Mello, D. A., Hefner, J., Leon, F. G., Matson, G. A., Montano, B., Pradko, J. F., Sussman, N., & Winberg, B. (2003). The scope of the problem: Physical symptoms of depression. *Journal of Family Practice, 52*(12), S6-S11.

Deckro, G. R., Ballinger, K. M., Hoyt, M., Wilcher, M., Dusek, J., Myers, P., Greenberg, B., Rosenthal, D. S., & Benson, H. (2002). *Journal of American College Health, 50*(6), 281-288.

Denisoff, E., & Endler, N. S. (2000). Life experience, coping, and weight preoccupations in young adult women. *Canadian Journal of Behavioural Science, 32*(2), 97-103.

Dimeo, F., Bauer, M., Varahram, I., Proest, G., & Halter, U. (2001). Benefits from aerobic exercise in patients with major depression: A pilot study. *British Journal of Sports Medicine, 35*(2), 114-119.

Dixon, W. A., Mauzey, E. D., & Hall, C. R. (2003). Physical activity and exercise: Implications for counselors. *Journal of Counseling and Development, 81*(4), 502-506.

Edwards, K. J., Hershberger, P. J., Russell, R. K., & Markert, R. J. (2001). Stress negative social exchange and health symptoms in university students. *Journal of American College Health, 50*(2), 75-84.

Fidler, G. (1969). The task oriented group as a context of treatment. *American Journal of Occupational Therapy, 23*(1), 43-48.

Fletcher, D., & Fletcher, J. (2005). A meta-model of stress, emotions, and performance: Conceptual foundations, theoretical framework, and research directions. *Journal of Sports Sciences, 23*(2), 157-159.

Fontana, A., & McLaughlin, M. (1998). Coping and appraisal of daily stressors predict heart rate and blood pressure in young women. *Behavioral Health, 24*(1), 11-16.

Giroux-Bruce, M. A., & Borg, B. (2002). *Psychosocial frames of reference: Core for occupation based practice.* Thorofare, NJ: SLACK Incorporated.

Greeno, C. G., & Wing, R. R. (1994). Stress-induced eating. *Psychological Bulletin, 115*(3), 444-464.

Guinn, B. (1991). Relationships of emotional motivators for eating and body fatness among elderly individuals living in recreational vehicle parks. *Journal of American Dietetic Association, 91*(8), 978-980.

Hafen, B. Q., Karren, K. J. Frandsen, K.J., & Smith, N. L. (1996). Mind/body health: The effects of attitudes, emotions, and relationships. Boston, MA: Allyn and Bacon.

Heatherton, T. F., Herman, C. P., & Polivy, J. (1992). Effects of distress on eating: The importance of ego-involvement. *Journal of Personality and Social Psychology, 62*(5), 801-803.

Heuer, H., & Klein, W. (2003). One night of total sleep deprivation impairs implicit learning in the serial reaction task, but not the behavioral expression of knowledge. *Neuropsychology, 17*(3), 507-516.

Hewston, R. M., Lane, A. M., Karageroghis, C. I., & Nevill, A. M. (2005). The relationship between mood-regulation and coping style among student athletes. *Journal of Sports Sciences, 23*(2), 175-176.

Jacobs, K., & Jacobs, L. (2004). Quick reference dictionary for occupational therapy. Thorofare, NJ: SLACK Incorporated.

Judkins, S. K. (2004). Stress among nurse managers: Can anything help? *Nurse Researcher, 12*(2), 58-71.

Juliano, L. M., & Brandon, T. H. (2002). Effects of nicotine dose, instructional set, and outcome expectancies on the subjective effects of smoking in the presence of a stressor. *Journal of Abnormal Psychology, 111*(1), 88-97.

Kassel, J. D. (2000). Smoking and stress: Correlation, causation, and context. *American Psychologist, 55*(10), 1155-1156.

Kassel, J. D., & Shiffman, S. (1997). Attentional mediation of cigarette smoking's effect on anxiety. *Health Psychology, 16*(4), 359-368.

Kerr, T. (1999, April 5). Scared healthy: How health scare tactics work and don't work. *Advance for Occupational Therapy Practitioners, 45.*

Kielhofner, G., & Burke, J. (1980). A model of human occupation. Part 1. Conceptual framework and content. *American Journal of Occupational Therapy, 34*(9), 572-581.

Kobasa, S. O. (1984). How much stress can you survive? *American Health, 67.*

Kolb, D. A. (1984). *Experiential learning.* Englewood Cliffs, NJ: Prentice-Hall.

Larson, G. A. & Zaichkowsky, L. D. (1995). Physical, motor, and fitness development in children and adolescents. *Journal of Education, 177*(2), 55-79.

Lawlor, D. A., & Hopker, S. W. (2001). The effectiveness of exercise as an intervention in the management of depression: Systematic review and meta-regression analysis of randomized controlled trials. *British Medical Journal, 322*(7289), 763-773.

Leitner, K., & Resch, M. G. (2005). Do the effects of job stressors on health persist over time? A longitudinal study with observational stressors measures. *Journal of Occupational Health Psychology, 10*(1), 18-30.

LePine, J. A., LePine, M. A., & Jackson, C. L. (2004). Challenges and hindrance stress: Relationships with exhaustion, motivation to learn, and learning performance. *Journal of Applied Psychology, 89*(5), 883-891.

Lovejoy, D., & Lane, A. (2000). The effects of exercise on mood changes. *Journal of Sports Sciences, 18*(1), 53-54.

Ludman, E. J., Curry, S. J., Grothaus, L. C., Graham, E., Stout, J., & Lozano, P. (2002). *Psychology of Addictive Behaviors, 16*(1), 68-71.

Lumley, M. A., & Provenzano, K. M. (2003). Stress management through written emotional disclosure improves academic performance among college students with physical symptoms. *Journal of Educational Psychology, 95*(3), 641-649.

Mack, M. G., & Shaddox, L. A. (2004). Changes in short-term attitudes toward physical activity and exercise of university personal wellness students. *College Student Journal, 38*(4), 587-564.

Mandel, D. R., Jackson, J. M., Zemke, R., Nelson, L., Clark, F. A. (1999). *Lifestyle redesign: Implementing the well elderly program.* Bethesda, MD: AOTA.

Mathias, K. E., Brynteson, P. A., Thomas, M., & Caldwell, A. (1997). An investigation of the relationships between family activity habits and children's fitness levels. *Physical Educator, 54*(3), 128-135.

McCaffrey, R., Frock, T., & Garguilo, H. (2003). Understanding chronic pain and the mind-body connection. *Holistic Nursing Practice, 17*(6), 281-290.

McHugh, K., & Wierzbicki, M. (1998). Prediction of responses to cognitive and behavioral mood inductions. *Journal of Psychology, 132*(1), 33-42.

McKay, M., & Fanning, P. (2000). *Self-esteem: A proven program of cognitive techniques for assessing, improving, and maintaining your self-esteem*. New York, NY: MJK Books.

McKay, H. A., Macdonald, H., Reed, K. E., & Khan, K. M. (2003). Exercise interventions for health: Time to focus on dimensions, delivery, and dollars; The importance of physical activity is proven, and methods of implementing exercise programmes should be urgently researched. *British Journal of Sports Medicine*, *37*(2), 98-100.

Misra, R., Crist, M., & Burant, C. J. (2003). Relationships among life stress, social support, and reactions to stressors of international students in the United States. *International Journal of Stress Management*, *10*(2), 137-157.

Misra, R., & McKean, M. (2000). College students' academic stress and its relation to their anxiety, time management, and leisure satisfaction. *American Journal of Health Studies*, *16*(1), 41-55.

Mosey, A. C. (1986). *Psychosocial components of occupational therapy*. New York: Raven Press.

Netz, Y., & Lidor, R. (2003). Mood alterations in mindful versus aerobic exercise modes. *Journal of Psychology*, *137*(5), 405-420.

Ng, D. M., & Jeffery, R. W. (2003). Relationships between perceived stress and health behaviors in a sample of working adults. *Health Psychology, 22*(6), 638-642.

Odone, C. (1996). Counsellors have taught us to avoid sadness at all costs. But sometimes it's right to feel unhappy. *New Statesman, 128*(4436), 24-25.

Oman, R. F., & Oman, K. K. (2003). A case-control study of psychosocial and aerobic exercise factors in women with symptoms of depression. *Journal of Psychology, 137*(4), 338-351.

Ong, A. D., & Walsh, D. A. (2001). Nicotine dependence, depression, and the moderating role of goal cognitions. *Psychology of Addictive Behaviors, 15*(3), 252-254.

Parrott, A. C. (2000). Cigarette smoking does cause stress. *American Psychologist, 55*(10), 1159-1160.

Pender, N. J. (1982). *Promotion in nursing practice*. East Norwalk, CT: Appleton and Lange.

Petajan, J.H., Gappmaier, E., White, A.T., et al. (1996). Impact of aerobic training on fitness and quality of life in multiple sclerosis. *Annals of Neurology, 39*(4), 432-431.

Peterson, M., & Wilson, J. F. (2004). Work stress in America. *International Journal of Stress Management, 11*(2), 91-113.

Piasecki, T. M., & Baker, T. B. (2000). Does smoking amortize negative affect? *American Psychologist, 55*(10), 1156-1157.

Phillips, B. J. (2005). Working out: Consumers and the culture of exercise. *Journal of Popular Culture, 38*(3), 525-552.

Prestwich, A., Lawton, R., & Conner, M. (2003). The use of implementation intentions and the decision balance in promoting exercise behaviour. *Psychology and Health, 18*(6), 707-721.

Prochaska, J. O., & DiClemente, C. C. (1982). Transtheoretical therapy: Towards a more integrative model of change. *Psychotherapy Theory Resource Practice, 19*, 276-288.

Reilly, M. (1974). *Play as exploratory learning*. Beverly Hills, CA: Sage Publications.

Romberg, A., Virtanen, A., Ruutianen, J., et al. (2004). Effects of a 6-month exercise program on patients with multiple sclerosis. *Neurology, 63*, 2034-2038.

Rotter, J. B. (1966). Generalized expectations for internal versus external control of reinforcement. *Psychology Monographs, 80*, 1-28.

Russell, W., Pritschet, B., Frost, B., Emmett, J., Pelley, T. J., Black, J., & Owen, J. (2003). A comparison of post-exercise mood enhancement across common distraction activities. *Journal of Sport Behavior, 26*(4), 368-374.

Sadeh, A., Keinan, G., & Daon, K. (2004). Effects of stress on sleep, the moderating role of coping style. *Health Psychology, 23*(5), 542-545.

Sarafino, E. P. (2002). *Health psychology: Biopsychosocial interactions*. New York, NY: John Wiley & Sons.

Schkade, J. K., & Schultz, S. (1992). Occupational adaptation: Towards a holistic approach to contemporary practice, part 1. *American Journal of Occupational Therapy, 46*, 829-837.

Schotte, D. E., Cools, J., McNally, R. J. (1990). Film-induced negative affect triggers overeating in restrained eaters. *Journal of Abnormal Psychology, 99*(3), 317-320.

Seigel, B. (1993). *How to live between office visits*. New York, NY: HarperCollins.

Shealy, C. N. (2005). Chronic pain management. *Townsend Letter for Doctors and Patients, 258*, 22-24.

Sheckley, B. G. (1984). The adult as learner: A case for making higher education more responsive to the individual learner. Two part series, *CAEL News, 7*(8) & *8*(1).

Shiffman, S., & Walters, A. J. (2004). Negative affect and smoking lapses: A prospective analysis. *Journal of Consulting and Clinical Psychology*, 72(2), 192-201.

Skinner, B. F. (1971). *Beyond freedom and dignity*. New York, NY: Knopf.

Sladyk, K. (2005). Teaching and learning. *Ryan's occupational therapy assistant: Principles, practices, and techniques*. Thorofare, NJ: SLACK Incorporated.

Sladyk, K. (1998). Teaching safe sex to psychiatric patients. *American Journal of Occupational Therapy*, 44(3), 284-286.

Smith, N. L. (1993, November 13). Good health: More than absence of disease. *Church News*, 7.

Szabo, A. (2003). The acute effects of humor and exercise on mood and anxiety. *Journal of Leisure Research*, 35(2), 152-163.

Taylor, S. E. (1999). *Health psychology*. Boston, MA: McGraw-Hill.

Teitelbaum, J. (2005). Pain free 1-2-3, A proven program to get patients pain free. *Townsend Letter for Doctors and Patients*, 258, 123-127.

Thomas, N. E., Baker, J. S., & Davies, B. (2003). Established and recently identified coronary heart disease risk factors in young people. *Sports Medicine*, 33(9), 633-650.

Todd, M. (2004). Daily processes in stress and smoking: Effects of negative events, nicotine dependence, and gender. *Psychology of Addictive Behaviors*, 18(1), 31-39.

Totterdell, P. (1999). Mood scores: Mood and performance in professional cricketers. *British Journal of Psychology*, 90(3), 317.

Trockel, M. T., Barnes, M. D., & Egget, D. L. (2000). Health-related variables and academic performance among first-year college students: Implications for sleep and other behaviors. *Journal of American College Health*, 49(3), 125.

Turnbull, M., & Wolfson, S. (2002). Effects of exercise and outcome feedback on mood: Evidence for misattribution. *Journal of Sport Behavior*, 25(4), 394-406.

Ward, E. M. (2004). Good night, sleep tight. Weight, immunity, and memory will benefit. *Environmental Nutrition*, 27(9), 1-2.

Ward, A. & Mann, T. (2000). Don't mind if I do: Disinhibited eating under cognitive load. *Journal of Personality and Social Psychology*, 78(4), 753-763.

Wilson, K. (1998). The manual handling of children: A 24-hour exposure. *Safety Science*, 2(2), article 7, 1-13.

Wlodkowski, R. J. (1990). *Enhancing adult motivation to learn*. San Francisco, CA: Jossey-Bass Publishers.

Wortman, A. M. (2003). Preventing work-related musculoskeletal injuries. *Head Start Bulletin*, 75. Retrieved June 13, 2007, from http://headstartinfo.org/publications/hsbulletin75/hsb75_05.htm.

Zemke, R., & Clark, F. (1996). *Occupational science: The evolving discipline*. Philadelphia, PA: F. A. Davis.

Aspects of the adult learning and teaching and learning sections were adapted from:

Sladyk, K. (2005). *Teaching and learning. Ryan's occupational therapy assistant: Principles, practices, and techniques*. Thorofare, NJ: SLACK Incorporated.

Appendix: Resources

Resources have been supplied in chapters throughout the text. While there is some overlap, this is appropriate as some suppliers provide equipment for various areas of intervention. This list is a general resource and is not intended to be "all inclusive." This appendix is intended to be an introductory tool to expose the reader to resources that may potentially be used in seeking additional information.

AQUATIC REHABILITATION

- **Aquatic Resources Network**
  302 160th Street, Suite 200
  Amery, WI 54001
  Phone: 715-248-7258
  Fax: 715-248-3065
  Worldwide web address: http://www.aquaticnet.com
  - ➢ Web site provides valuable and comprehensive resources including training opportunities, educational products, membership, and a provider\facility directory

- Text book recommendations as general resources to supplement continuing education in the area of aquatics:
  - ➢ *Aquatic Rehabilitation* (1997) by A. Cole, D. Morris, & R. Ruoti (Published by Lippincott-Raven Publishers)
  - ➢ *The Teacher's Manual of Advanced Aquatic Therapy* (1998) by A. Poteat Salzman (Available from Concepts in Physical Therapy, 1092 West Outer Drive, Oak Ridge, TN 37830)

ASSISTIVE TECHNOLOGY AND EDUCATION-RELATED RESOURCES

- **About Learning** contains products and supports related to education of those with disabilities: 441 West Bonner Road; Wauconda, IL 60084; 800-822-4628; www.aboutlearning.com

- **ABLEDATA** is a project that maintains a database of information about more than 27,000 products for people with disabilities: 8630 Fenton Street, Suite 930; Silver Spring, MD 20910; 800-227-0216; www.abledata.com

- **Alliance for Technology Access** is a national organization dedicated to providing access to technology for people with disabilities: www.ataccess.org

- **Assistive Technology Access Partnership (ATAP)** is the Rhode Island website with a list of statewide organizations and agencies, each with a targeted assistive technology focus, who work together to provide information and improve access to assistive technology for individuals with disabilities: www.atap.ri.gov

- **Association for Higher Education and Disability (AHEAD)** contains links regarding assistive technology as well as many other adult student options: www.ahead.org

- **ATIA,** The Assistive Technology Industry Association is a not-for-profit membership organization for manufacturers, sellers or providers of technology-based assistive devices and/or services: www.atia.org/em

- **CAST Universal Design for Learning** is an organization committed to the research and development of innovative, technology-based educational resources and strategies: www.cast.org

- **Equal Access to Software and Information** is a project of the Teaching, Learning, and Technology (TLT) Group, EASI serves as a resource to the education community by providing information and guidance on access-to information technologies for individuals with disabilities. EASI disseminates information on developments and advancements within the adaptive computer technology field to colleges, universities, K–12 schools, libraries, and the workplace: TLT Group; P.O. Box 18928; Rochester, NY 14618; (Fax) 716-244-9065; www.rit.edu/~easi

- **Job Accommodation Network** is an international information network and consulting resource which provides information about employment issues, the Americans with Disabilities Act (ADA), and possible employment-related accommodations to employers, rehabilitation professionals, and persons with disabilities. Callers should be prepared to explain their specific problem and job circumstances. Sponsored by the President's Committee on Employment of People with Disabilities, the Network is operated by West Virginia University's Rehabilitation Research and Training Center. Brochures and printed materials are available at no cost: West Virginia University; 918 Chestnut Ridge Road, P.O. Box 6080; Morgantown, WV 26506-6080; (Voice/TTY) 800-232-9675; www.jan.wvu.edu

- **The George Washington University HEATH Resource Center** is a national clearinghouse on postsecondary education for those with disabilities: 2121 K Street NW, Suite 220; Washington, DC 20037; 800-544-3284; www.heath.gwu.edu

- **The National Center for the Study of Postsecondary Educational Supports** focuses upon the use of individualized supports and technology to meet student's needs and promote a successful transition to chosen career: 808-956-9199; (Fax) 808-956-5713; www.rrtc.hawaii.edu

- **Independent Living Aids, Inc.** is a supplier of a variety of different AT options: P.O. Box 9022; Hicksville, NY 11802-9022; 800-537-2118; www.independentliving.com

- **MaxiAids** is a supplier of a variety of different AT options: 42 Executive Blvd; Farmingdale, NY 11735; 800-522-6294; www.maxiAids.com

- **EnableMart** is a catalog of a variety of different AT options: 400 Columbus Street, Suite 100; Vancouver, WA 98669-3413; 800-640-1999; www.EnableMart.com

- **Optelec U.S.** offers a variety of solutions for those who are blind or visually impaired: 6 Lyberty Way; Westford, MA 01886; 800-828-1956; www.optelec.com

- **RehabTool.com** offers leading-edge assistive technology products and services for children and adults with disabilities. They can help you choose the right equipment for your needs with their popular Product Search & Referral service. http://www.rehabtool.com

- **Sammons-Preston Rolyan** is a supplier of various items for those with disabilities, contains accessibility and assistive technology options: www.sammonspreston.com

- **Solutions for Humans, Inc.** is a source of solutions, consulting, training, evaluation and implementation of solutions for individuals and organizations addressing sight loss, physical impairment, ergonomic issues, communication and hearing disorders: 365A Tesconi Circle; Santa Rosa, CA 95401; 800-953-9262; www.sforh.com

- **Apple Computer Accessibility Center** is committed to helping people with disabilities attain an unparalleled level of independence through a personal computer. Apple's commitment to accessibility is evident throughout the Mac OS X operating system which is by design, easy to use, but also includes a wide variety of features and technologies specifically designed to provide accessibility to users with disabilities. Apple refers to these features collectively as Universal Access and has integrated them right into the operating system so they can be used in conjunction with a variety of applications from Apple and other developers: www.apple.com/accessibility

- **The Boulevard** is a Disability Resource Directory of Products and Services for the Physically Challenged, Elderly, Caregivers and Healthcare Professionals: www.blvd.com

- **EITAC Solutions Group** is dedicated to providing solutions that help people with disabilities live, learn, and work with greater degrees of accessibility and success through our innovative products and services. EITAC Solutions Group is an EnableMart Strategic Partner and maintains a full-service demonstration center on behalf of EnableMart: 765-775-2121; www.eitacsg.com

- **gh Braille** offers a full range of accessible media formats and software applications, including Digital Talking Books, an Accessible Testing System, Braille, and Tactile Graphics, that enable people with visual disabilities to improve their educational experience, become more competitive in the workplace, and lead more enjoyable lives: www.ghbraille.com

- **IBM Accessibility Center** responds to requests for information on how IBM products can help people with a wide range of disabilities use personal computers. While the center is unable to diagnose or prescribe an assistive device or software, free information is provided on what is available and where users can go for more details: 11400 Burnet Road; Mailstop 9150; Alston, TX 78758; 800-426-4832; www.IBM.com/able

- **Microsoft** is committed to their mission of helping customers scale new heights and achieve goals they never thought possible. Delivering on this mission means Microsoft strives to build products that are accessible to everyone—including people with disabilities and impairments: http://www.microsoft.com/enable

- **PACER Center, Parent Advocacy Coalition for Educational Rights**, is an organization whose mission is to expand opportunities and enhance the quality of life of children and young adults with disabilities and their families, based on the concept of parents helping parents. The links and resources section has information related to accessibility and assistive technology as well as other resource centers for students with disabilities: www.pacer.org/links/index.htm

- **PEPNet, the Postsecondary Education Programs Network**, is the national collaboration of the four Regional Postsecondary Education Centers for Individuals who are deaf: www.pepnet.org/Hard of Hearing

- **Recoding for the Blind and Dyslexic,** National Headquarters; 20 Roszel Road; Princeton, NJ 08540; 866-732-3585; www.rfbd.org

- **The Technical Braille Center** produces books in Braille, large print and special electronic forms for scientists, engineers and mathematicians who are blind, dyslexic or paralyzed. It also provides books for students preparing for careers in the technical professions: www.execpc.com/~chpi/techbrl.htm

- **University of Washington – DO-IT: Disabilities, Opportunities, Internetworking, and Technology** is a resource for students with disabilities. Links for AT, universal design and other items pertinent to adults with disabilities in postsecondary education are provided: www.washington.edu/doit

- **Rehabilitation Engineering and Assistive Technology Society of North America** is an interdisciplinary association of people whose purpose is to improve the potential of individuals with disabilities through the use of technology. RESNA serves as an information center to address research, development, dissemination, integration, and utilization of knowledge in rehabilitation and assistive technology settings: http://www.resna.org

- **Worldwide Disability Solutions Group** works with key education, rehabilitation, and advocacy organizations nationwide to identify the computer-related needs of individuals with disabilities and to assist in the development of responsive programs. WDSG is involved with Apple's research and development to ensure that its computers have built-in accessibility features. By working closely with third-party vendors who develop products for people with disabilities, WDSG is further able to provide information about Apple's personal computers and the technology of independence: 800-MY-APPLE (692-7753); www.apple.com/disability

- **Other useful information about products that can assist individual with mobility impairments can be found at the following websites:**
  - Don Johnston, Inc: www.donjohnston.com
  - Infogrip: www.infogrip.com
  - IntelliTools: www.intellitools.com
  - Interlink Electronics: www.interlinkelec.com
  - Origin Instruments: www.orin.com
  - Penny & Giles: www.pgcontrols.com
  - Prentke Romich: www.prentrom.com
  - Kensington: www.kensington.com
  - TASH: www.tashinc.com
  - TechAble: www.techable.org

CRANIOSACRAL THERAPY

- **The International Association of Healthcare Practitioners**
  11211 Prosperity Farms Road, Suite D-325
  Palm Beach Gardens, FL 33410-3487
  Phone: 561-622-4334
  Toll free: 800-311-9204
  Fax: 561-622-4771
  Worldwide web address: www.iahp.com
  - Web site offers certification courses, provider directory, educational products, and membership opportunities.

- **Milne Institute, Inc.**
  P.O. Box 220
  Big Sur, CA 93920
  Phone: 831-667-2323
  Fax: 831-667-2525
  Worldwide web address: www.milneinstitute.com
  - ➤ Web site lists certification and continuing education courses available as well as educational products including texts, tapes, and DVDs

Driver Rehabilitation

- **Occupational Therapists and Driving**
  Worldwide web address: www.AOTA.org/olderdriver
- **The Association for Driver Rehabilitation Specialists (ADED)**
  711 S. Vienna Street
  Ruston, LA 71270
  Toll-free: 800-290-2344 (US Only)
  Phone: 318-257-5055
  Fax: 318-255-4175
  Worldwide web address: www.driver-ed.org
- **Adaptive Mobility**
  100 Delaney Avenue
  Orlando, FL 32806-1228
  Phone: 407-426-8020

Educational Opportunities

- **The Hand: An Interactive Study for Therapists With CD-ROM** (Self-Paced Clinical Course) by Judy C. Colditz, OTR/L, CHT, FAOTA
- **AOTA Self-Paced Clinical Courses:** Continuing educational opportunities are listed by the AOTA at http://www.aota.org under the link entitled "continuing education"
  - ➤ Links are provided for current online courses, workshops, self-paced clinical courses, as well as downloadable continuing education articles
  - ➤ In addition, the AOTA CE WebFind option allows searches nationwide of opportunities available through not only the AOTA, but also AOTA-approved continuing education providers
  - ➤ *Work: Principles and Practice* by Barbara L. Kornblau, JD, OT/L, FAOTA, DAAPM, ABDA, CCM, CDMS, and Karen Jacobs, EdD, OTR/L, CPE, FAOTA, Editors
  - ➤ *Dysphagia Care for Adults* by Wendy Avery-Smith, MS, OTR/L, Cynthia McKinnon DuBose, MA, CCC-SLP, Evelyn Ince, MEd, OTR/L, Sharon Kurfuerst, MEd, OTR/L, Donna Latella, MA, OTR/L, and Catherine Meriano, JD, MHS, OTR/L
  - ➤ *Low Vision: Occupational Therapy Intervention with the Older Adult* by Mary Warren, MS, OTR/L, Editor
  - ➤ *STROKE: Strategies, Treatment, Rehabilitation, Outcomes, Knowledge, and Evaluation* by Charlotte Brasic Royeen, PhD, OTR, FAOTA, Editor

- **AOTA online courses**:
  - ➤ *Low Vision in Older Adults: Foundations for Rehabilitation* by R. G. Cole, R. Rovins, & A. Schonfeld

ERGONOMICS/WORK HARDENING

- **Human Factors and Ergonomics Society**
  P.O. Box 1369
  Santa Monica, CA 90406-1369
  Worldwide web address: www.hfes.org
- **Websites for ergonomic information, resources, and equipment:**
  - ➤ http://ergo.human.cornell.edu/ergoguide.html
  - ➤ www.ergoweb.com
  - ➤ www.osha.gov
  - ➤ www.aota.org
  - ➤ www.alimed.com
  - ➤ www.roymatheson.com

LEISURE

- **Gamblers Anonymous**
  P.O. Box 17173
  Los Angeles, CA 90017
  Phone: 213-386-8789
  Worldwide web address: www.gamblersanonymous.org
- **YMCA**
  Worldwide web address: www.YMCA.net

LOW VISION RESOURCES

- **The Internet Low Vision Society**
  Worldwide web address: www.lowvision.org
- **Smart Solution Partners**
  Phone: 845-735-1417
  Worldwide web address: www.sspdirect.com/catalog.htm
- **ABLEDATA**
  8630 Fenton Street, Suite 930
  Silver Spring, MD 20910.
  Phone: 800-227-0216, TTY: 301-608-8912
  Worldwide web address: www.abledata.com
- American Federation for the Blind (AFB)
  Phone: 800-232-5463
  Worldwide web address: www.afb.org

- **Other low vision links:**
  - ➤ www.allaboutvision.com/lowvision
  - ➤ www.magnifyingaids.com
  - ➤ www.lowvisioninfo.org
  - ➤ www.lighthouse.org

LYMPHEDEMA

- **National Lymphedema Network**
  Latham Square, 1611 Telegraph Avenue, Suite 1111
  Oakland, CA 94612-2138
  Toll-free: 800-541-3259
  Phone: 510-208-3200
  Fax: 510-208-3110
  Worldwide web address: www.lymphnet.org
  - ➤ Offers an array of resources available to clinicians including membership opportunities and educational materials
- **Academy of Lymphatic Studies**
  11632 High Street Suite A
  Sebastian, FL 32958
  Phone: 800-863-5935 (United States & Canada)
  Fax: 772-589-0306
  Worldwide web address: www.acols.com
  - ➤ Web site lists current certification and training courses available

MANUFACTURER CONTACTS FOR LOW-LOAD, PROLONGED STRETCH DEVICES OR DYNAMIC SPLINTING DEVICES

- **Dynasplint™ Systems, Inc**
  Corporate Headquarters
  River Reach, W21
  770 Ritchie Highway
  Severna Park, MD 21146
  Phone: 800-638-6771
  Worldwide web address: www.dynasplint.com
- **Empi™**
  599 Cardigan Road
  St. Paul, MN 55126-4099
  Phone: 800-328-2536
  Worldwide web address: www.empi.com
- **Saebo**
  Worldwide web address: www.saebo.com

Mental Health

- **Alcoholics Anonymous World Services, Inc**
  General Service Office
  P.O. Box 459
  Grand Central Station, New York, NY 10163
  Phone: 212-870-3400
  Worldwide web address: www.alcoholics-anonymous.org

- **N.A.M.I. (National Alliance for the Mentally Ill)**
  200 North Glebe Road, #1015
  Arlington, VA 22203-3754
  Phone: 800-950-6264
  Worldwide web address: www.nami.org
  - ➤ Founded in 1979 as the National Alliance for the Mentally Ill, it is a well-known nonprofit, self help, support and advocacy organization and a good resource for families, consumers and friends.

- **Brain Injury Association, Inc**
  1776 Massachusetts Ave., #100
  Washington, DC 20036
  Phone: 800-444-NHIF
  Worldwide web address: www.biausa.org

- **National Family Caregiver Support Program**
  Worldwide web address: www.aoa.gov/prof/aoaprog/caregiver/caregiver.asp
  - ➤ National Family Caregiver Support Program, developed by the US Administration on Aging, part of the Department of Health and Human Services.

Myofascial Release

- **Myofascial Release Treatment Centers and Seminars**
  222 West Lancaster Avenue, Suite 100
  Paoli, PA 19301
  Phone: 610-644-0136
  Toll-free: 800-FASCIAL (800-327-2425)
  Fax: 610-644-1662
  Worldwide web address: www.myofascialrelease.com
  - ➤ Web site lists certification and continuing education opportunities, articles and reviews, educational resources, and a provider directory

Physical Agent Modalities (PAMs)

- **The American Occupational Therapy Association's Position Paper** on the use of Physical agent modalities can be purchased at www.aota.org or by phone at 877-404-AOTA (2682) or by fax 301-206-9789
  - ➤ American Occupational Therapy Association. (2002). *The reference manual of the official documents of the AOTA, Inc.* (9th ed.). Bethesda, MD: AOTA. (ISBN: 1-56900-179-0, 544 pp)

- Continuing Educational opportunities are listed by the AOTA at http://www.aota.org under the link entitled "continuing education"
  - ➢ The AOTA CE WebFind option allows searches nationwide of opportunities available through not only the AOTA, but also AOTA-approved continuing education providers
- Text book recommendations as general resources to supplement continuing education in the area of PAMs:
  - ➢ Bracciano, A. G. (2000). *Physical agent modalities: Theory and application for the occupational therapist.* Thorofare, NJ: SLACK Incorporated
  - ➢ Cameron, M. H. (2003). *Physical agents in rehabilitation.* St. Louis: Saunders

REHABILITATIVE EQUIPMENT DISTRIBUTORS/SUPPLIERS

- **Sammons Preston Rolyan**
  An AbilityOne Company
  Corporate Headquarters
  270 Remington Blvd., Suite C
  Bolingbrook, IL 60440-3593
  Phone: 630-226-1300
  Fax: 630-226-1389
  Worldwide web address: http://www.sammonspreston.com
  - ➢ Web site allows for review of products, place a purchase order, listing of training opportunities\workshops, or to request a product catalog
- **North Coast Medical, Inc.**
  18305 Sutter Boulevard
  Morgan Hill, CA 95037-2845
  Phone: 800-821-9319
  Fax: 877-213-9300
  Worldwide web address: www.ncmedical.com
  - ➢ Web site allows for review of products, place a purchase order, and to request a product catalog
- **AliMed, Inc**
  297 High Street
  Dedham, MA 02026
  Phone: 800-225-2610
  Fax: 800-437-2966
  Worldwide web address: www.alimed.com
  - ➢ Web site allows for browsing of products, placing a product order, submitting and product idea, and requesting a product catalog
- **Pro-Med Products**
  6445 Powers Ferry Road, #199
  Atlanta, GA 30339
  Phone: 800-542-9297
  Fax: 770-951-2786
  Worldwide web address: www.promedproducts.com

- **Invacare Corporation**
  One Invacare Way
  Elyria, OH 44035
  Phone: 800-333-6900
  Fax: 440-329-6568
  Email: info@invacare.com
  Worldwide web address: www.invacare.com

STRAIN COUNTERSTRAIN TECHNIQUES

- **Jones Institute (originators of the Strain Counterstrain Technique)**
  7937 Corte Domingo
  Carlsbad, CA 92009
  Phone: (760)942-0647
  Fax: (760)942-0645
  Worldwide web address: http://jiscs.com
  - Web site includes listing of certification course from the originators of the strain Counterstrain technique as well as case studies, additional course offerings, and educational products

WORK SIMULATORS

- **The Baltimore Therapeutic Equipment (BTE) Work Simulator**
  Designed by the Baltimore Therapeutic Equipment Company who recently (2004) merged with Hanoun Medical Systems to form BTE Technologies, Inc. They can be contacted at:
  - BTE Technologies, Inc
    Corporate & Products Group
    7455-L New Ridge Road
    Hanover, MD 21076
    Phone: 800-331-8845
    Fax: 410-850-5244
    Worldwide web address: www.btetech.com
  - Web site offers an array of information including an overview of products available and outline of 2-day training workshops on the use of their equipment
- **The ERGOS™ Work Simulator**
  - Designed by Simwork Systems(SM) who can be contacted at:
    Simwork Systems
    4500 East Speedway Boulevard, Suite 113
    Tucson, AZ 85712
    Phone: 520-795-2222
    Fax: 520-795-4358
    Worldwide web address: www.simwork.com

- **Valpar International Corp**
  3801 East 34th Street
  Tucson, AZ 85713
  Worldwide web address: www.valparint.com

B Appendix: Assessment Grid

Amy P. Burns, MOT, OTR/L

While the primary focus of this text is adult intervention, evaluation is addressed briefly in multiple chapters. The function of the grid that appears in the following pages is to provide information regarding adult evaluations mentioned in these chapters, as well as other appropriate evaluations. Due to the large number of evaluations available, this grid is intended as a sampling, not a complete list of evaluations on each topic. The last column of the grid provides a location where the reader may look for further information. Again, this is not the only location as some evaluations are available through multiple vendors. This list is for general educational and reference purposes only and is not intended to promote sale of any products. The information provided was accurate as of publication; however, some Web sites may change after the production of this text and may no longer be available.

Assessment Grid

Posture/Balance/Mobility

Name	Standardization	Validity/Reliability	Setting Used	Areas Assessed	Information/Purchase
Berg Scale Berg et al., 1992. *Measures 14 balance items. Includes sitting and standing unsupported, sit-to-stand, transfers, picking up objects from floor, and turning.*	No	Valid & reliable.	Home or clinic setting.	Transfers, sitting, standing, balance.	Berg, K., Wood-Dauphinee, S., Williams, J.I., & Maki, B. (1992). Measuring balance in the elderly: Validation of an instrument. *Canadian Journal of Public Health*, 7-11.
Functional Reach Test Duncan, Weiner, Chandler, & Studenski, 1990. *Simple way to measure standing balance. Measures the difference between arm's length and maximal forward reach.*	Yes	Valid & reliable.	Wall and tape measure needed.	Reaching and balance.	Duncan, P. W., Weiner, D. K., Chandler, J., & Studenski, S. (1992). Functional reach: A new clinical measure of balance. *J Gerontol, 45*(6): M192-7. Duncan, P. W., et al. (1990). Functional reach: Predictive validity in a sample of elderly male veterans. *J Gerontol, 47*(3), M93-8.
Modified Gait Abnormality Rating Scale (GARS) Wolfson, Whipple, Amerman, & Tobin (1990) *Seven item assessment of gait, stepping and arm movements, staggering foot contact, hip ROM, shoulder extension, etc.*	No		Room to walk.	Hip ROM, foot contact, staggering, arm/leg symmetry, guarding.	Wolfson, I., Whipple, R., Amerman, P., & Tobin, J. N. (1990). Gait assessment in the elderly: A gait abnormality rating scale and its relation to falls. *J Gerontol, 45*(1):M12-9.

continued

ASSESSMENT GRID (CON'T)

Name	Standardization	Validity/Reliability	Setting Used	Areas Assessed	Information/Purchase
Timed Get Up and Go (TGUG) Podsiadlo & Richardson, 1991 *Measures the overall time to complete a series of functionally important tasks. Helps to identify clients with balance deficits.*	No	Valid & reliable.	Room to walk 10 feet; chair.	Balance, posture, mobility.	Podsiadlo, D., & Richardson, S. (1991). The timed "up & go": A test of basic functional mobility for frail elderly persons. *J Am Geriatr Soc, 39*(2), 142-148.
Tinetti Tinetti, 1986 *Measures a client's gait and balance.*	No	Inter-rater reliability.	Room to walk 10 feet; chair.	Balance and gait.	Tinetti, M. E. (1986). Performance-oriented assessment of mobility problems in elderly patients. JAGS, 34,119-126.
Cognition					
Autobiographical Memory Interview (AMI) Kopelman, Wilson, & Baddeley, 1990 *Interview recalling events from the clients' past including school, wedding, children, etc.*	Yes	Valid & reliable.	Quiet environment with minimal distractions.	Memory, retrograde amnesia.	www.nss-nrs.com

continued

ASSESSMENT GRID (CON'T)

Name	Standardization	Validity/Reliability	Setting Used	Areas Assessed	Information/Purchase
Bay Area Functional Performance Evaluation (BaFPE) Bloomer and Lang, 1987 *Assesses how a client might function in task-oriented settings and settings with social interaction. Uses sea shells, design blocks, and associated items.*	Yes	Valid & reliable..	Seated at table.	Memory, organization, attention span.	www.sammonspreston.com/
Behavioral Inattention Test Wilson, Cockburn, & Halligan, 1987 *Assesses unilateral visual neglect. Includes card sorting, article reading, figure/shape copying, etc.*	Yes	Valid & reliable..	Quiet environment with minimal distractions.	Unilateral visual neglect, picture recalling, line crossing, article reading, phone dialing.	www.nss-nrs.com or http://harcourtassessment.com
Cognitive Assessment of Minnesota (CAM) Rustad et al., 1993 *Assesses the cognitive abilities of adults with neurological impairments.*	Yes	Valid & reliable..	Quiet room.	Attention, memory, visual neglect.	http://harcourtassessment.com/
Contextual Memory Test Toglia, 1993 *Assesses awareness of memory capacity, strategy use, and recall in adults with memory dysfunction.*	Yes	Valid & reliable..	Quiet room with minimal distraction.	Memory, awareness of memory capacity, recall of line drawings.	http://buros.unl.edu/

continued

ASSESSMENT GRID (CON'T)

Name	Standardization	Validity/ Reliability	Setting Used	Areas Assessed	Information/Purchase
Glasgow Coma Scale *Measures response of eyes, verbal response, and motor response in numerical levels.*	No	Reliable	In hospital.	Alertness, awareness, verbal response, motor response.	*The American Heritage Stedman's Medical Dictionary* (2nd ed); Houghton Mifflin Company
Lowenstein Occupational Therapy Cognitive Assessment (LOTCA) (also LOTCA-Geriatric) Itzkovich, Averbuch, Elazar, Katz, 2000 *Assesses clients with neurological deficits and mental health issues. Tests orientation, visual/ spatial perception, praxis, visuomotor. Includes cards, blocks, pegboard.*	Yes	Valid & reliable.	Quiet environment with minimal distractions.	Orientation, perception, praxis, visuomotor, organization, thinking operations.	http://store.grovergear.com/lotcabattery.html
Luria-Nebraska Neuropsychological Battery Golden, 1991 *Reading numbers, writing words, differentiate hard/soft touch, sounds. Provides a pattern analysis of strength and weakness across areas of brain function.*	Yes	Valid & reliable.	Quiet environment with minimal distractions.	Numbers, reading, writing, touching.	WPS, Western Psychological Services

continued

Assessment Grid (con't)

Name	Standardization	Validity/Reliability	Setting Used	Areas Assessed	Information/Purchase
Mini-Mental Status Evaluation (MMSE) Folstein, Folstein, & McHugh, 1975 *Used to assess cognitive function.*	Yes	Valid & reliable...	Seated at table.	Brain injury, writing, reading, drawing.	www.minimental.com
Ranchos Los Amigos *Developed at the Rancho Los Amigos Hospital in California by the Head Injury Treatment Team Medical scale, assesses the level of recovery of a client with a brain injury and those recovering from a coma.*	No	Reliable	In hospital.	Alertness, awareness.	Original Scale coauthored by Chris Hagen, PhD, Danese-Malkmus, MA, & Patricia Durham, MA. Communication Disorders Service, Ranchos Los Amigos Hospital, 1972. Revised 11/15/74 by Danese Malkmus, MA and Kathryn Stenderup, OTR
Rivermead Behavioral Memory Test (RBMT-II) Wilson, Cockburn & Baddeley, 1995 *Assessment of gross memory impairments encountered by clients in their everyday lives. Identifies everyday memory problems and monitors change over time.*	Yes	Valid & reliable...	Quiet environment with minimal distractions.	Memory: immediate and recall.	http://harcourtassessment.com

continued

ASSESSMENT GRID (CON'T)

Name	Standardization	Validity/Reliability	Setting Used	Areas Assessed	Information/Purchase
Severe Impairment Battery Saxton, McGonigle, Swihart, & Boller, 1993 *Evaluates cognitive abilities at the lower end of the range (severely impaired dementia client). Allows for nonverbal and partially correct responses.*	Yes	Valid & reliable.	Quiet room.	Memory, completing simple actions.	http//harcourtassessment.com
Test of Everyday Attention Robertson, Ward, Ridgeway, Nimmo-Smith, 1994 *Measures selective attention, sustained attention and attentional switching. Includes map search, telephone search, elevator counting, etc.*	Yes	Valid & reliable.	Quiet room; table and chairs.	Everyday materials (map searching, phone skills, etc).	www.harcourt-uk.com/product. aspx?n=1315&s=2037&cat=2064&s key=2886
Dexterity					
Disabilities of the Arm Shoulder and Hand (2nd ed) Solway, Beaton, McConnell, & Bombardier *Quantifies upper extremity limitations*	No	Valid & reliable.	Questionnaire.	Upper extremity disability.	Institute for Work & Health: www.dash.iwh.on.ca

continued

ASSESSMENT GRID (CON'T)

Name	Standardization	Validity/Reliability	Setting Used	Areas Assessed	Information/Purchase
Jebsen-Taylor Hand Function Test Jebsen, Taylor, et al., 1969 *Assesses a broad range of hand functions used in daily activities. A 7-part test that uses common items such as paper clips, cans, pencils, etc.*	Yes	Reliable	Seated, requires adequate lighting.	Writing, page turning, lifting small/large objects, simulated feeding.	www.sammonspreston.com/
Manipulative Aptitude Test Roeder *Measures hand/arm/finger dexterity and speed through sorting and assembling.*	Yes	Valid & reliable..	Seated at a table or desk.	Dexterity, manipulative aptitude, dominant hand.	www.wisdomking.com/product140188c220087.html
Minnesota Rate of Manipulation University of Minnesota Employment Stabilization Research Institute, 1969 *Assesses unilateral and bilateral manual dexterity along with eye-hand coordination. Provides information on standing tolerance, sustained neck flexion, weight bearing, and repetitive reach.*	Yes	Valid & reliable..	Table and chair.	Manual dexterity, turning, displacing.	www.roymatheson.com/equip_dexterity.html

continued

Assessment Grid (con't)

Name	Standardization	Validity/Reliability	Setting Used	Areas Assessed	Information/Purchase
Nine Hole Peg Mathiowetz, Weber, Kashman, & Volland, 1985 *Client places 9 dowels in 9 holes while being timed.*	Yes	Valid & reliable.	Table and chair.	Finger dexterity.	Mathiowetz, V., Volland, G., Kashman, N., & Weber, K. (1992). Nine-hole peg test. In: Wade, D. T., *Measurement in neurological rehabilitation.* New York: Oxford University Press, 171. www.sammonspreston.com
O'Connor Finger Dexterity Test O'Connor *Requires hand placement of 3 pins per hole.*	Yes		Table and chair.	Predictor of rapid manipulation.	www.rehaboutlet.com
O'Connor Tweezer Dexterity Test O'Connor *Measures the speed with which a client can puck up pins with a tweezer, one at a time, and place the pin into a small hole.*	Yes		Table and chair.	Finger dexterity, fine motor coordination, speed, eye hand coordination.	www.rehaboutlet.com
Purdue Pegboard Tiffin, 1948 *Assesses gross movement of hands/fingers/arms, as well as fingertip dexterity.*	Yes	Valid & reliable.	Table and chair.	Gross movement of hands, fingers, and arms; fingertip dexterity.	North Coast Medical or Devine Medical.

continued

ASSESSMENT GRID (CON'T)

Name	Standardization	Validity/ Reliability	Setting Used	Areas Assessed	Information/Purchase
Range of Motion *The measurement of the achievable distance between the flexed position and the extended position of a particular joint or muscle group.*	Yes	Valid, not 100% reliable	Comfortable for client, chair/ mat.	Biomechanical.	Multiple sources including: Latella, D., & Meriano, C. (2003). *Occupational Therapy Manual for the Evaluation of Range of Motion and Muscle Strength.* Clifton Park, NY: Thomson Delmar Learning.
Strength Testing *The strength of each muscle group is measured on a scale of 0/5 to 5/5.*	Yes	Valid, not 100% reliable	Comfortable for client, chair/ mat.	Biomechanical.	Multiple sources including: Latella, D., & Meriano, C. (2003). *Occupational Therapy Manual for the Evaluation of Range of Motion and Muscle Strength.* Clifton Park, NY: Thomson Delmar Learning.
Sensation/Edema/Tone					
Ashworth Scale Ashworth, B. *Scale to define tone.*	No	Not tested	Any	Tone	Ashworth, B. (1964) Preliminary trial of carisoprodol in multiple sclerosis. *Practitioner, 192,* 540.
Semmes-Weinstein or Touch Test	No	Not tested	Any	Sensation hand and foot.	www.rehaboutlet.com
Volumeter *Fill container with water, measure the displaced water of both hands.*	No	Not tested	Countertop or table; need access to water faucet.	Edema, swelling of UE.	www.rehabmart.com

continued

ASSESSMENT GRID (CON'T)

Name	Standardization	Validity/ Reliability	Setting Used	Areas Assessed	Information/Purchase
Vision/Visual Perception					
Benton Visual Form Discrimination Hamsher, Varney, & Spreen, 1983 *Assesses the ability to discriminate between complex visual configurations. Book of line drawings.*	No	Valid	Seated at table, test at midline.	Neglect, neurological and psychological.	www3.parinc.com/products/product. aspx?productid=visualform
Hooper Visual Organization Test (VOT) Hooper, 1983 *Ability to visually integrate information into whole perceptions through the use of line drawings arranged in puzzles.*	Yes	Valid & reliable..	Quiet environment with minimal distractions.	Organization of visual stimuli.	http://portal.wpspublish.com/portal/page?_pageid=53,69277&_dad=portal&_schema=PORTAL
Motor Free Visual Perception Test (MVPT-3) Colarusso & Hammill, 2003 *Assesses overall visual perceptual ability.*	Yes	Valid & reliable..	Seated at table. Adequate light and free from distraction.	Visual perceptual.	www.theraproducts.com

continued

Assessment Grid (Con't)

Name	Standardization	Validity/Reliability	Setting Used	Areas Assessed	Information/Purchase
Vision/Visual Perception					
STROOP Color and Word Test Golden & Freshwater, 2002 *Reading aloud colored words. The words themselves are names of colors, but the actual color is different than the name.*	Yes	Valid & reliable..	Quiet environment with minimal distractions.	Brain function and planning.	Western Psychological Services (WPS)
Test of Visual Motor Skills (UPPER) Gardner, 1992 *Measures visual motor functioning using 16 geometric figures.*	Yes	Valid & reliable..	Seated at table. Adequate light and free from distraction.	Visual motor.	Devine Medical
Warren's Brain Injury Visual Assessment Battery for Adults (biVABA) Warren, 1998 *Assessment of visual processing ability after a brain injury.*	Yes	Valid & reliable..	Comfortable for client.	Visual perceptual processing, oculomotor function, how function is affected.	www.visabilities.com/bivaba.html
ADLs/IADLs					
Allen Cognitive Level Test (ACL) Allen, 1996 Leather lacing test.	Yes	Valid & reliable.	Environment with minimal distractions and good lighting.	Problem solving, sequencing.	www.allen-cognitive-network.org/

continued

ASSESSMENT GRID (CON'T)

Name	Standardization	Validity/Reliability	Setting Used	Areas Assessed	Information/Purchase
Arnadottir Occupational Therapy Neurobehavioral Evaluation (A-one) Arnadottir, 1990 *Determines the impact of neurobehavioral impairment on activities of daily living and mobility tasks using a 5-point scale.*	Yes	Valid & reliable.	Clinic or home setting.	ADLs severity of neurobehavioral impairment, occupational performance.	Requires training where forms can be purchased
Assessment of Motor and Process Skills (AMPS) Fisher, 1993 *Observational assessment, measures the quality of a person's ADLs. Rates the effort, efficiency, safety, and independence of ADL motor/process skills. (*Training required)*	Yes	Valid & reliable.	Various conditions.	IADLs, motor skills and processing skills.	www.ampsintl.com Special training required. Once trained, materials are supplied.
Assessment of Occupational Functioning (AOF) Watts, Kielhofner, & Bauer, 1996 *Assesses the functional capacity of residents in long-term treatment settings who have physical and/or psychiatric problems.*	Yes	Valid & reliable.	Comfortable for the client.	IADLs, MOHO, volition, habituation, performance.	Contact: jhwatts@hsc.vcu.edu

continued

Assessment Grid (con't)

Name	Standardization	Validity/ Reliability	Setting Used	Areas Assessed	Information/Purchase
Barthel Index Mahoney & Barthel, 1965 *Assesses self-care functions in older adults.*	No	Predictive validity	Individual or group evaluation.	Self-care.	www.massgeneral.org/stopstroke/ pdfs/barthel_reprint.pdf
Canadian Occupational Performance Measure (COPM) Law, Baptiste, Carswell, McColl, Polatajko, & Pollock, 2005 *Individualized outcome measure designed to detect changes in self-perception of occupational performance over time.*	Yes, but not norm referenced.	Valid & reliable.	Comfortable for client	Occupational performances and perception	www.caot.ca/copm/index.htm
Comprehensive Occupational Therapy Evaluation (COTE) Brayman, Kirby, Meisenheimer & Short *Developed in an acute psychiatric setting. Identifies 25 OT-related behaviors within 3 categories (general behavior, interpersonal behavior, and task behavior).*	Yes	Valid & reliable.	Where ever the task is performed.	Behavior.	Brayman, S. J., Kirby, T. F., Meisenheimer, A. M., Short, M. J. (1976). The comprehensive occupational therapy evaluation scale. *Am J Occup Ther, 30*(2),94-100.

continued

ASSESSMENT GRID (CON'T)

Name	Standardization	Validity/ Reliability	Setting Used	Areas Assessed	Information/Purchase
Direct Assessment of Functional Abilities (DAFA) Karagioxis et al., 1998 *Direct measurement of the instrumental activities of daily living. Used to determine functional deficits in clients with mild cognitive impairment.*	Yes	Valid & reliable.	Clinical setting, cafeteria, gift shop, and exam room.	IADLs.	Loewenstein, D., Amigo, E., Duara, R., et al. (1989). A new scale for the assessment of functional status in Alzheimer's disease and related disorders. *J Gerontol Psychol Sci, 44,* 114-121
Functional Independent Measure (FIM) UDSMR, 1993 *Scale (range from 1-7) that measures a client's ability to function with independence. Collected upon admission to rehabilitation unit, upon discharge, and after discharge.*	Yes	Valid & reliable.	Clinic or home setting.	ADLs self-care, communication, cognitive function.	www.udsm.org Training required.
Independent Living Scales (ILS) Loeb, 2003 *Offers assessment, daily living skills, self-advocacy training, and support with an issue that challenge the independence of a client.*	Yes	Valid & reliable.	Table and chairs; can be bedside.	IADL memory, orientation, money management, health, safety, etc.	The Psychological Corporation (Harcourt Brace & Company).

continued

ASSESSMENT GRID (CON'T)

Name	Standardization	Validity/Reliability	Setting Used	Areas Assessed	Information/Purchase
Index of Activities of Daily Living (ADL) Katz, 1963 *Assesses functional status as a measurement of the client's ability to perform activities of daily living independently. (No longer in print, may still be seen in some clinics.)*	Yes	Valid & reliable.	Inpatient observations.	ADL, biological and psychological function.	Katz, S., Ford, A.B., Moskowitz, R.W., Jackson, B.A, & Jaffe, M.W. (1963). Studies of illness in the aged: The index of ADL: A standardized measure of biological and psychosocial function. *JAMA, 185*, 94-9.
Kitchen Task Assessment (KTA) Baum & Edwards, 1993 *Measures organization, planning, and judgment skills through common kitchen tasks.*	Yes	Valid & reliable.	Kitchen/cooking environment.	IADL, initiation, organization, sequencing, judgment, safety.	Baum, C., & Edwards, D.F., (1993). Cognitive performance in senile dementia of the Alzheimer's type: the Kitchen Task Assessment. *Am J Occup Ther, 47*(5), 431-436.
Klein-Bell Activities of Daily Living Scale Klein & Bell, 1982 *Assesses age-related changes in activities of daily living ability. (No longer in print, may still be seen in some clinics.)*	Yes	Valid & reliable.	General Rehabilitation setting.	ADLs.	Klein, R.M., & Bell, B. (1982). Self-care skills: behavioral measurement with Klein-Bell ADL scale. *Arch Phys Med Rehab, 63*(7), 335-8.

continued

ASSESSMENT GRID (CON'T)

Name	Standardization	Validity/ Reliability	Setting Used	Areas Assessed	Information/Purchase
Kohlman Evaluation of Living Skills (KELS) Kohlman-Thompson, 1978 *Ability to function in 17 basic living skills. Assesses skill in 5 areas: self-care, safety and health, money management, transportation/telephone, and work/leisure.*	Yes	Valid & reliable.	Table and Chairs.	Self-care, safety and health, money mgt, transportation, telephone, work, leisure.	www.aota.org
Level of Rehabilitation Scale (LORS-II) Carey & Posavac, 1982 *Evaluates the success of inpatient rehabilitation programs.*	Yes	Valid & reliable.	Hospital reha-bilitation units.	ADLs	Carey, R.G., & Posavac, E.J. (1982). Rehabilitation program evaluation using a revised level of rehabilita-tion scale (LORS-II). *Arch Phys Med Rehabil, 63*(8), 367-370.
Milwaukee Evaluation of Daily Living Skills (MEDLS) Leonardelli, 1988 *Information from clients and families; establishes base-line behaviors necessary to devel-op treatment plans and guide intervention in regard to daily living skills.*	No	Valid & reliable.	Home environ-ment.	ADLs including communication, personal care, clothing care, etc.	http://buros.unl.edu/buros/jsp/ reviews.jsp?item=15192654

continued

Assessment Grid (Con't)

Name	Standardization	Validity/Reliability	Setting Used	Areas Assessed	Information/Purchase
Occupational Circumstances Assessment and Interview Rating Scale (OCAIRS) Version 4.0 Forsyth et al., 2005 *A 40-minute interview that analyzes the extent and nature of a client's occupational adaptation and participation.*	No	Valid & reliable.	Comfortable for the client.	MOHO, volitional, habituation, performance.	www.moho.uic.edu/assess/ocairs.html
Occupational Performance History Interview (OPHI-II) Kielhofner, et al., 2004 *Interview that gathers the appreciation of a client's life history, the direction in which they want to take their life, as well as the impact of a disability on their life.*	Yes	Valid & reliable.	comfortable for client	Occupational roles, daily routine, critical life events.	www.moho.uic.edu/assess/ophi%202.1.html
Occupational Self Assessment Baron, Kielhofner, Ienger, Goldhammer, & Wolenski, 2002 *This is a self-assessment of perceptions of strengths and weaknesses relative to occupational functioning.*	Yes	Valid & reliable.	Comfortable for the client.	MOHO, volitional, habituation, performance.	http://www.moho.uic.edu/assess/osa.html

continued

Assessment Grid (cont't)

Name	Standardization	Validity/ Reliability	Setting Used	Areas Assessed	Information/Purchase
Performance Assessment of Self-care Skills (PASS) Holm & Rogers, 1999 *Performance based observation tool covering functional mobility, personal care, and ADLs. Measures short term functional change in elderly after hospitalization. (Requires 2-day training workshop.)*	Criterion referenced.	Valid & reliable.	Clinic and home version.	IADL.	Special training required. Once trained, materials are supplied.
Role-Checklist Oakley *Assesses the values that clients place on their occupational roles.*	Yes	Valid & reliable.	Comfortable for client	MOHO, habituation sub-system.	To request the role checklist, e-mail Fran Oakley at foakley@rih.gov
Routine Task Inventory (RTI-II) Allen et al., 1992 *Measures the level of performance in activities of daily living through observation and questioning.*	No	Valid & reliable.	Clinic or home setting.	ADL, effect of cognitive impairmen on task performance.	www.allen-cognitive-network.org/ index.htm

continued

Assessment Grid (con't)

Name	Standardization	Validity/ Reliability	Setting Used	Areas Assessed	Information/Purchase
Environmental Evaluations					
Enabler Iwarsson & Slaug, 2001 *Norm-based environment assessment, developed to assess the accessibility of housing and its close surroundings.*	Yes	Valid & reliable.	Home environment and close surroundings.	IADLs, neurological, musculoskeletal, psychological, movement, cognition, physical.	Iwarsson, S., & Isacsson, A. (1996). Development of a novel instrument for occupational therapy assessment of the physical environment in the home methodological study on the Enabler. *Occup Ther J Res, 16(4),* 227-244. www.enabler.nu/index.html
HOME FAST Mackenzie, Byles, & Higginbotham, 2000 Screen to identify home hazards contributing to falls	No	Valid & reliable.	Home environment	Client's function within environment	Mackenzie, L., Byles, J., & Higginbotham, N. (2000). Designing the home falls and accidents screening tool (HOME FAST): Selecting the items. *Br J Occup Ther, 63,*260-269.
SAFER/SAFER-HOME Chui, Oliver, Marshall, & Letts. *Client interview/observation*	No norms, but manual available	Valid & reliable.	Home environment	Client's function within environment	COTA comprehensive Rehabilitation and Mental Health Services. Email: info@cotarehab.ca
Westmead Home Safety Assessment Clemson *Client interview/observation*	No	Minimal evidence for validity & reliability	Home environment	Client's function within environment	www.therapybookshop.com/coordinates.html Co-ordinates therapy services.

continued

ASSESSMENT GRID (CON'T)

Name	Standardization	Validity/ Reliability	Setting Used	Areas Assessed	Information/Purchase
Education					
Lifespan Access Profile	No	Not tested.	Educational.	Physical, cognitive, & emotional.	Lifespace Access (949 733-2746
Work and Retirement					
Transition to Work Inventory	No	Valid & reliable.	Work-related questionnaire.	Determine worker-job fit.	The Psychological Corporation (Harcourt Brace & Company)
Worker Environment Impact Scale (WEIS) Moore-Corner, Kielhofner, Olson, 1998 *Assesses environmental characteristics that facilitate successful employment experiences. Goal is to maximize the 'fit' of the worker and their skill to the job environment.*	No	Fair Validity and Reliability	Comfortable for the client.	Space related issues, fit of environment.	www.moho.uic.edu/assess/weis.html
Worker Role Interview (WRI) Version 10.0 Braveman, et al., 2005 *Identifies psychosocial and environmental factors that influence a client's ability to return to work.*	Yes	Valid & reliable.	Work, comfortable for client.	Physical evaluation essential job functions, psychosocial capacity to return to work.	www.moho.uic.edu/assess/wri.html

continued

Assessment Grid (con't)

Name	Standardization	Validity/ Reliability	Setting Used	Areas Assessed	Information/Purchase
Leisure					
Activity Card Sort Baum & Edwards, 2001 *Measure of activity participation*	No	Valid & reliable.	Institutional, recovering, and community versions.	IADLs and leisure.	Washington University School of Medicine, Program in Occupational Therapy www.ot.wusl.edu
Adolescent Leisure Interest Profile (ALIP) Henry, 1998 *Used to evaluate the leisure activities that clients enjoy.*	No	Reliable	Comfortable for client.	Sports, outdoor/ indoor activities, creativity.	Henry S. D. (1998). Development of a measure of adolescent leisure interests. *AJOT, 52,* 531-539.
Adolescent Role Assessment (ARA) Black, 1976 *Used to assess and identify deficiencies in the occupation choice process of adolescents.*	No	Scores lack internal consistency	Comfortable for client	Childhood play, adult work, adolescent socialization.	www.citeulike.org/user/willwade/ article/1031361
Social Participation					
Coping Inventory Zeitlin, 1985 *Profiles coping styles, as well as behaviors, that facilitate or interfere with adaptive coping. Self-administered and profiled.*	No	Self-report and observation.	Comfortable for the client.	Sensorimotor, reactive behavior, self-initiated behavior, adaptive coping.	hrrt://ststesting.com/CPOl.html

continued

Assessment Grid (con't)

Name	Standardization	Validity/ Reliability	Setting Used	Areas Assessed	Information/Purchase
Life Satisfaction Index Neugarten, Havighurst & Tobin, 1961 *Looking at 5 factors that make up total life satisfaction (pleasure, meaningfulness, feeling of success, self-image, happiness)*	Yes	Valid & reliable.	Comfortable for the client.	Activity, developmental theory, internal satisfaction.	Neugarten, B., Havinghurts, R., & Tobin S. (1961). The measurement of life satisfaction. *J Gerontol*, 16, 134-143.
Occupational Questionnaire (OQ) Kielhofner, 2002 *Self-report assessment. Client documents the main activity which he/she engages in for each half-hour throughout the morning/day/evening and identifies each activity as work, ADL, recreation, or rest. Explores the meaning of leisure from the client's perspective.*	Yes	Valid & reliable.	Clinic or home setting.	IADL, volition, activity pattern, life satisfaction, interests, values, personal causation.	www.moho.uic.edu/images/occupational%20Questionnaire.pdf
Volitional Questionnaire Version 4.0 de las Heras, Geist, Kielhofner, Li, 2003 *Observational assessment, gathers information on client's volition.*	Yes	Valid	Observations are context specific: leisure, work, ADL environments	MOHO, volition subsystem, work, leisure, intrinsic motivation, values, interests.	www.ahs.uic.edu/ahs/files/ot/student-theses/thesis%20Yanling%20li.pdf

continued

Assessment Grid (con't)

Name	Standardization	Validity/Reliability	Setting Used	Areas Assessed	Information/Purchase
Wellness					
Coping Inventory: Self-Rated Form Zeitlin *Client evaluates adaptive behavior for coping*	No	Not tested.	Any.	Habits, skills, behaviors related to coping.	www.ststesting.com
Engagement in Meaningful Activities Survey (EMAS) Goldberg & Brintnell, 2002 *Clients read statements about activities, put an 'X' in the box that best describes them (never to always).*	Yes, for research purposes only	Valid & reliable.	Comfortable for the client.	Activities.	www.haworthpress.com/store/articleabstract.asp?ID=19624
Stress Management Questionnaire (SMQ) Stein, 2003 *Identification of symptoms linked to stress and coping strategies that aid in the reduction of stress.*	Yes	Valid & reliable.	Comfortable for the client.	Coping, stressors, behavioral theory.	www.delmarlearning.com/browse_product_detail.aspx?catid=9022&isbn=0766842584&cat1ID=HCR&cat21D=OTP

Index

WAIT
...There's More!

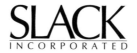